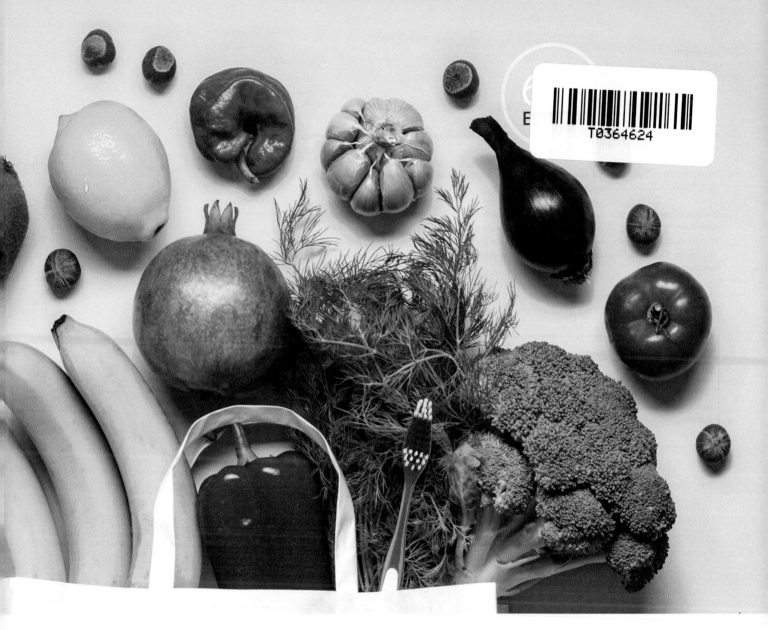

The Dental Hygienist's Guide to Nutritional Care

Lisa F. Mallonee, RDH, RD, LD, MPH
Associate Dean for Faculty Affairs
Professor, Department of Dental Hygiene
Texas A&M University College of Dentistry
Dallas, Texas

Linda D. Boyd, RDH, RD, EdD
Associate Dean of Graduate Studies
Professor, Forsyth School of Dental Hygiene
Massachusetts College of Pharmacy & Health Sciences
Boston, Massachusetts

Cynthia A. Stegeman, RDH, EdD, RDN, LD, CDE, FAND
Scientific Relations Manager in Professional Oral Health at Procter & Gamble
Cincinnati, Ohio

ELSEVIER

ELSEVIER
3251 Riverport Lane
St. Louis, Missouri 63043

THE DENTAL HYGIENIST'S GUIDE TO NUTRITIONAL CARE, SIXTH EDITION   ISBN: 978-0-323-79700-9

Copyright © 2025 by Elsevier, Inc. All rights are reserved, including those for text and data mining, AI training, and similar technologies.

Publisher's note: Elsevier takes a neutral position with respect to territorial disputes or jurisdictional claims in its published content, including in maps and institutional affiliations.

No part of this publication may be reproduced or transmitted in any form or by any means, electronic or mechanical, including photocopying, recording, or any information storage and retrieval system, without permission in writing from the publisher. Details on how to seek permission, further information about the Publisher's permissions policies and our arrangements with organizations such as the Copyright Clearance Center and the Copyright Licensing Agency, can be found at our website: http://www.elsevier.com/permissions.

This book and the individual contributions contained in it are protected under copyright by the Publisher (other than as may be noted herein).

Notice
Practitioners and researchers must always rely on their own experience and knowledge in evaluating and using any information, methods, compounds or experiments described herein. Because of rapid advances in the medical sciences, in particular, independent verification of diagnoses and drug dosages should be made. To the fullest extent of the law, no responsibility is assumed by Elsevier, authors, editors or contributors for any injury and/or damage to persons or property as a matter of products liability, negligence or otherwise, or from any use or operation of any methods, products, instructions, or ideas contained in the material herein.

Previous edition copyrighted 2019

Senior Content Strategist: Kelly Skelton
Senior Content Development Manager: Ranjana Sharma
Publishing Services Manager: Deepthi Unni
Senior Project Manager: Kamatchi Madhavan
Book Designer: Brian Salisbury

Printed in India

  Working together
to grow libraries in
developing countries

www.elsevier.com • www.bookaid.org

Last digit is the print number: 9 8 7 6 5 4 3 2 1

This sixth edition is dedicated to all dental hygiene students, faculty, and practitioners throughout the world who read and apply information from this text. Your curiosity and desire to gain evidence-based and applicable information regarding the role of nutrition in oral health continue to guide the content. We are honored to continue the intended premise of this textbook as it was originally envisioned by Cynthia A. Stegeman and Judi Ratliff Davis.

Lisa F. Mallonee and Linda D. Boyd

Gratitude to my husband Bob and children, Chris and Sabrina, who have supported me tirelessly on my academic journey, and to my grandmother, Fay Nelson, who instilled a love of learning. Special thanks to my professional mentors including, but not limited to, Dr. Carole Palmer, who recognized my potential even when I did not and pushed me out of my comfort zone on many occasions. I also want to express my thanks to Dr. Cyndee Stegeman, who first invited me to assist with the third edition of the textbook while she finished her doctoral dissertation. Cyndee was one of our "three Musketeers" because we were all registered dietitians and dental hygienists, and we embraced every opportunity to work together. We greatly miss her enthusiasm, beautiful smile, and positive energy, but we hope to make her proud by carrying her vision for the textbook forward.

Linda D. Boyd

To my husband Scott and our children, Harper and Layne, who provide me with daily inspiration, love, and support in all that I do. I am thankful for my colleagues and students who have graciously embraced my passionate desire to integrate the interrelationship of oral health and nutrition into the classroom, my conversations and my mindset as a healthcare professional. I am indebted to the mentorship provided by Dr. Cyndee Stegeman. I was first connected with Cyndee while in graduate school for my MPH with a concentration in nutrition and dietetics in the late 1990s. It was that first email that set the stage for a lasting friendship and opened the door to opportunities to collaborate as registered dietitians and dental hygienists throughout my professional career. She was and will always be one of our "three Musketeers."

Lisa F. Mallonee

Tribute

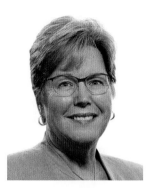

Cynthia A. Stegeman
(Permission for use of photo granted by Crest + Oral-B)

Cynthia A. Stegeman, RDH, EdD, RDN, LD, CDE, FAND was a Scientific Relations Manager in Professional Oral Health at Procter & Gamble at the time of her passing. Before moving into the corporate sector, she served as the Department Chair and a Professor in the Dental Hygiene program at University of Cincinnati. In addition to directing courses in Oral Anatomy, Histology, and Embryology, she taught Nutrition and Health Education for over 30 years. Dr. Stegeman was dually licensed as a registered dental hygienist and a registered dietitian. She was a dental hygienist for over 35 years and a long-time member of the American Dental Hygienists' Association and the Academy of Nutrition and Dietetics. She also served as the Ohio delegate to the Academy of Nutrition and Dietetics, a member of the National Board Dental Hygiene Examination test construction committee, a consultant in the evaluation process of licensure of candidates for the dental hygiene profession for the Commission on Dental Competency Assessments, an evaluator for the ADEX exam, and a Certified Diabetes Educator. She served as a speaker for numerous community and professional groups nationally and internationally and published over 80 articles on nutrition, dentistry, and diabetes. Dr. Stegeman received an Associate of Applied Science in Dental Hygiene from the University of Cincinnati, Bachelor of Science in Public Health Dentistry from Indiana University Purdue University at Indianapolis, Master of Education in Nutrition from the University of Cincinnati, dietetic internship from The Christ Hospital in Cincinnati, and Doctorate of Education in Curriculum and Instruction, Instructional Design and Technology from the University of Cincinnati.

In addition to her professional pursuits in the areas of academia and corporate education, Dr. Stegeman worked in private practice, hospitals, and the community throughout the course of her career. Her unique blend of health care experiences led to numerous publications in professional journals and invited presentations at state, national, and international conferences.

The first edition of Dr. Cynthia A. "Cyndee" Stegeman's book, *The Dental Hygienist's Guide to Nutritional Care*, was published in 1998. This inaugural textbook on nutrition specific to the dental hygienist has been adopted by dental hygiene programs throughout the country. As the author team on the sixth edition, we are honored to continue her vision. Our similar backgrounds as registered dental hygienists and registered dietitians afforded us many opportunities to collaborate on publications and initiatives. As our colleague and dear friend, we have a deep respect and commitment to all that Cyndee embodied as both a professional and as an individual. Thus she is the inspiration for our devoted efforts to continue with the sixth edition of *The Dental Hygienist's Guide to Nutritional Care*.

Lisa F. Mallonee and Linda D. Boyd

Preface

The *sixth* edition of this nutrition textbook for dental professionals!!! Why is nutrition information always changing? Concisely, nutrition is a relatively new science. It has long been recognized that certain food factors are important to health: in the early 1800s, all English ships carried lime juice, with a portion given to each sailor daily. However, isolation and discovery of the exact elements in foods and the role they play in maintaining health and preventing disease are more complicated. The B vitamins were only discovered as late as the 20th century. Scientists continue to research the nutrient content of foods, the specific physiologic uses of vitamins and minerals, and the quantity resulting in beneficial or harmful effects. Advances in technology continue to guide us in the functions and interactions of nutrients. After discovering vitamins and determining which minerals and elements are essential to health, even more food components have been discovered, such as antioxidants and polyphenols, leading to shifting recommendations and policies. Expect further changes as research delves into the effects of the microbiome and nutrigenomics in maintaining optimal health and preventing chronic diseases. The science of nutrition is further complicated by factors such as personal beliefs and food habits along with nutrient interactions. You will realize in studying this subject that nutrition is a dynamic field relevant to both you and your patients.

The study of nutrition is a rewarding topic for dental hygiene students and practitioners, not only as it relates to patient education but also for how it can affect the dental hygienist's own health. *The Dental Hygienist's Guide to Nutritional Care* is designed to show both dental hygiene students and practicing dental professionals how to apply sound nutrition principles when assessing, diagnosing, planning, implementing, and evaluating the total care of patients, as well as to help them contribute to the nutritional well-being of patients. The Academy of Nutrition and Dietetics, the American Dental Hygienists' Association, and the American Dental Association each recognize nutrition as an integral component of oral health. The dental professional should be able to assess the oral cavity in relation to the patient's nutrition, dietary habits, and overall health status. A holistic approach to dietary management of a disease by the interprofessional health care team is especially appropriate to coordinate managed health care.

Since the subject of nutrition is a hot topic in today's world, the consumer is challenged to comprehend and apply the overwhelming amount of nutritional information that can be confusing and conflicting. As the health care professional that patients may see most often, dental professionals should be able to knowledgeably and authoritatively discuss nutritional practices with their patients or provide appropriate referrals as needed.

New to This Edition

This revised edition provides the most recent developments in the field and new and improved resources for instructors, including:
- The latest federal nutrition standards, including the *2020 Dietary Guidelines for Americans* and *MyPlate*
- Content updated to support the most current evidence relevant to nutrition science and patient application.
- Information on the role of biochemistry in nutrition

Organization

Part I, Orientation to Basic Nutrition, deals with basic principles of nutrition. A basic understanding of fundamental nutrition facts enables the dental hygienist to make wise judgments about eating habits, educate patients about needed dietary changes, and evaluate the flood of new information available. Nutrient deficiencies and excesses are addressed in sections entitled *Hyper-States* and *Hypo-States*. Chapters addressing vitamins and minerals are arranged to cover the specific nutrients involved in oral calcified structures or oral soft tissues. The chapter entitled *Concepts in Biochemistry* introduces a basic understanding of biochemistry, the foundation for understanding and applying principles of nutrition. This chapter serves as a valuable resource throughout the textbook.

Part II, Applications of Nutrition Principles, addresses application of basic nutrition principles through the lifespan within ethnic groups and socioeconomically disadvantaged individuals. Because of the ever-changing, diverse population in the United States, the dental hygienist must recognize that food choices different from their own eating patterns may be nutritionally healthy. By approaching any necessary modifications with sensitivity and respect, patients are more likely to make suggested changes. Alterations in nutritional requirements and eating patterns affected by various stages of life—specifically for females, infants and children, and older adults—are discussed.

Part III, Nutritional Aspects of Oral Health, looks at factors involved in oral problems and the nutritional treatment of these problems. In these chapters, *Dental Considerations* and *Nutritional Directions* boxes provide specific information to consider during an assessment and educational dialogue by the dental professional, including (1) *physical* status and *dietary* habits; (2) *interventions*, or factors that need to be considered when caring for the patient; and (3) *evaluations* concerning the patient's ability or motivation to make changes based on what has been learned during the appointment. A nutritional assessment is a basic procedure in dental management for the nutritional well-being of all patients. This involves performing a medical and dental assessment, evaluating dietary intake/history, and educating patients about healthful changes in food choices. Many conditions or their outcome are improved by encouraging patients to eat a wide variety of foods and beverages in appropriate portion sizes or to make minor changes in food choices to improve their health.

A variety of features throughout the text help to enhance the learning experience:

- **Student Learning Outcomes:** A list of outcomes accompanies each chapter to provide a guide to the important information to acquire from the chapter.
- **Key Terms:** Definitions of unfamiliar terms for each chapter in **bold** and **blue** letters within the text; also compiled in the **Glossary** for easy reference.
- **Test Your NQ** (nutrition quotient): True-false pretests to stimulate interest in the reading assignment; answers conveniently located in the back of the book.
- **Dental Considerations:** Practical information affecting the patient's care or nutritional status.
- **Nutritional Directions:** Information to teach the patient to improve oral health and overall health status; stimulating discussions with the patient using the educational information for improvement of oral health, food choices, and/or overall health status.
- **Health Applications:** Current "hot topics" in nutrition, including the ways to obtain an adequate balance of nutrients by a vegetarian; understanding the difficulty in diagnosing persons with gluten sensitivity or intolerance, and adhering to a gluten-free diet; causes and treatment of obesity; and appropriate use of vitamin and mineral supplements.
- **Case Application:** Potential patient situations describing a clinical situation and providing the five-step care plan to help "pull it all together."
- **Student Readiness:** Questions at the end of each chapter for students to determine their comprehension of the subject.
- **Case Studies:** Practical case studies for students to test their ability to make sound judgments when faced with real-life patient scenarios.

About Evolve

The Evolve website offers a variety of additional learning tools that greatly enhance the text for both students and instructors.

For the Student

Evolve Student Resources offers the following:
- **Practice Quizzes**. Each chapter contains approximately 400 NBDHE-style questions with instant feedback answers.

- **Illustrated Case Studies**. Written scenarios with accompanying photographs, and follow-up questions present situations observed frequently. These case studies serve as an excellent review source for the NBDHE.
- **Nutrition Analysis Forms**. Printable versions of forms needed to complete the Personal Assessment Project as well as printable versions for Carbohydrate Intake Analysis and Food Diary Form.
- **MNA Mini Nutritional Assessment**. A validated nutrition screening tool that can be used to assess for malnutrition in patients 65 years and older.

For the Instructor

Evolve Instructor Resources offers the following:
- **Test Bank**. An extensive test bank makes the creation of quizzes and exams easier.
- **TEACH Instructor Resources**.
  - **Lesson Plans** organize chapter content into 50-minute class times and map to educational standards and chapter learning objectives.
  - **PowerPoints** provide lecture presentations with talking points for discussion, all mapped to chapter learning objectives.
  - **Student Handouts** are PDFs of the lecture presentations for easy posting and sharing with students.
  - **Answer Keys** provide answers to the Illustrated Case Studies in the Student Resources.
- **Image Collection**. An image collection with the illustrations from the textbook is provided for ease of incorporating a photo or drawing into a lecture or quiz.
- **Personal Assessment Project**. A classroom learning activity is provided for students to objectively assess their own personal dietary patterns, practice the process of recording and analyzing food intake for its nutritive and cariogenic value, and use nutritional and dental knowledge to contribute to better general and oral health for self and patients.

Note From the Authors

With a better understanding of the importance of food choices, the members of an interprofessional health care team can complement each other's work and provide optimal care for the patient. Even though specific amounts of nutrients are mentioned, the intent of this text is not for prescriptive use. Instead, its purpose is to provide dental hygiene students and practicing dental professionals with a relative idea of the amounts of various nutrients needed so that viable food sources can be recommended.

Lisa F. Mallonee
Linda D. Boyd

Acknowledgments

Because of the diversity of subjects presented in a general nutrition textbook, a compilation of the work of many people, whether direct or indirect, is necessary to present the current and evidence-based information that is relevant to dental professionals.

Our sincere thanks to Barbara Altshuler, formerly an Assistant Professor, Caruth School of Dental Hygiene, Baylor College of Dentistry, who "birthed" the concept of this nutrition textbook for dental hygienists and presented the idea to W.B. Saunders to develop a resource for dental hygienists to assess the nutritional status of their patients. It is an honor to continue the initial vision of Barbara Altshuler and the dedicated efforts of Cynthia A. Stegeman and Judi Ratliff Davis who brought that vision to life as authors for the previous five editions. It takes a team of experts to complete a textbook. We would like to acknowledge the hard work of Dr. Scott Tremain, Associate Professor in the Department of Chemistry at the University of Cincinnati Blue Ash, for creating a practical and usable chapter in biochemistry. Condensing complex information into one chapter is quite a feat. Another valuable contributor to the textbook is Dr. Amy Sullivan, RDH, at the University of Mississippi Medical Center who provided photos for Chapters 18–21.

We also wish to thank the many staff members at Elsevier who worked so tirelessly in the various phases of planning and producing this book. We are especially grateful to Ranjana Sharma, Content Development Manager and Kelly Skelton, Senior Content Strategist for seeing us through this project.

About the Authors

Lisa F. Mallonee, RDH, RD, LD, MPH is an Associate Dean for Faculty Affairs and a tenured Professor in the Department of Dental Hygiene at Texas A&M University College of Dentistry. Professor Mallonee's education includes a Bachelor of Science in Dental Hygiene at the University of North Carolina at Chapel Hill, a Master of Public Health with a coordinated degree in Nutrition from the University of North Carolina at Chapel Hill, and internship hours toward licensure as a Registered Dietitian at UNC Hospitals, East Carolina University Health Medical Center, Asheboro Public Health Department in North Carolina, and the Cooper Institute in Dallas Texas. She is currently pursuing her doctorate in Higher Educational Leadership. Before becoming a Registered Dietitian, she practiced full time as a Registered Dental Hygienist. Her academic career began in 2000 at Baylor College of Dentistry, which later changed its name to Texas A&M University College of Dentistry. During her first 10 years in academia, she continued to provide preventive care to patients in a community dental clinic setting. Preceding her appointment as an Associate Dean for Faculty Affairs, Professor Mallonee served as course director for the public/community health course, co-director for a nutrition seminar course provided to the undergraduate dental hygiene students, and has provided nutrition lectures in the predoctoral dental curriculum for almost 25 years. Additionally, she oversees practicum placement and thesis research as a co-director for postgraduate dental hygienists enrolled in the Master of Science in Education for Healthcare Professionals distance education program housed in the Texas A&M College of Medicine. Furthermore, she serves as a preceptor for the Baylor University Medical Center Dietetic internship program.

Professor Mallonee has actively engaged in leadership in professional organizations, including American Dental Education Association, American Academy of Dental Hygiene, and Academy of Nutrition and Dietetics. She serves as a reviewer and an expert content advisor for numerous professional publications, including *The Journal of the Academy of Nutrition and Dietetics, Journal of the American Dental Association*, and *Journal of Dental Hygiene*, and organizations, such as the National Diabetes Education Program, National Maternal & Child Oral Health Resource Center, and the American Dental Education Association. Professor Mallonee is a published author in dental textbooks and peer-reviewed journals on multiple topics pertaining to diet, nutrition, and oral health and the practical application to whole body health for dietetic and dental professionals. She is an invited speaker both nationally and internationally. As a health care professional and educator, she is committed to two interconnected goals: sharing her knowledge, expertise, and passion while promoting the value of interprofessional collaboration among dental professionals within the wider health care community for greater patient/client outcomes.

Linda D. Boyd, RDH, RD, EdD is an Associate Dean of Graduate Studies and a Professor in Forsyth School of Dental Hygiene. Dr. Boyd's education includes an Associate of Science in Dental Hygiene at Mt. Hood Community College, a Bachelor of Science in Nutrition and Food Management at Oregon State University, a combined Master of Science in Nutrition Science and Policy from Tufts University and Dietetic Internship at New England Medical Center, and a doctorate in Educational Leadership with a Specialization in Postsecondary Adult and Continuing Education at Portland State University. Before entering academia, Dr. Boyd worked in private general and periodontal practices for 20 years as a clinical dental hygienist. Her academic career began at Oregon Health and Sciences University (OHSU) School of Dentistry in Portland, Oregon as an Assistant Professor where she taught nutrition and periodontics and was involved in clinical research. Following her time at OHSU, she served as Chair of Department of Dental Hygiene at Georgia Perimeter College. After leaving Georgia, she joined Idaho State University as a Professor and Director of the online Master of Science Degree in Dental Hygiene. In this capacity she developed one of the first fully online graduate Master of Science in Dental Hygiene programs along with teaching and mentoring graduate students to be educators and leaders in dental hygiene. She then served as the Dean of the Forsyth School of Dental Hygiene for 9 years before assuming her current position as an Associate Dean of Graduate Studies where she continues to mentor graduate students in an online Master of Science degree program. Dr. Boyd has been actively involved in leadership positions in a number of professional organizations, including the American Dental Education Association, American Dental Hygienists' Association, and Academy of Nutrition and Dietetics. She has also served as a member of the National Board Dental Hygiene Examination and site visitor and Dental Hygiene Review Board Committee member for the Commission on Dental Accreditation. In addition, she is on the Editorial Review Board for the *Journal of Dental Education* and an Associate Editor for the *International Journal of Dental Hygiene* along with serving as a peer reviewer for many professional journals. Dr. Boyd has published widely on nutrition, oral health, education, and dental hygiene topics in peer-reviewed journals and textbooks.

Contents

1

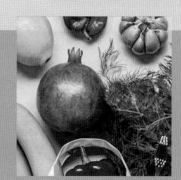

Overview of Healthy Eating Habits

STUDENT LEARNING OUTCOMES

On completion of this chapter, the student will be able to achieve the following student learning outcomes:

1. Discuss why dental hygienists and registered dietitian nutritionists (RDNs) need to be competent in assessing and providing basic nutritional education to patients.
2. List and describe the general physiologic functions of the six nutrient classifications of foods.
3. Describe factors that influence patients' food habits.
4. Explain government concerns with nutrition, as well as the purpose and objectives of *Healthy People 2030*.
5. Explain the Dietary Reference Intakes (DRIs) and its components (EAR, RDA, AI, EER, CCDR, and AMDR).
6. Describe the purpose of the *2020–2025 Dietary Guidelines for Americans*, and identify the four guidelines.

7. Discuss food components the *Dietary Guidelines* recommend to reduce in the diet.
8. Describe the purpose of *MyPlate* and the key components.
9. Identify the major food groups in *MyPlate* and recommended portions for the average adult.
10. Describe why physical activity is an important factor for an individual's overall health.
11. Practice assessment using the *MyPlate* system and demonstrate the ability to recommend improvements based on individual preferences and nutritional needs.
12. Understand and interpret the information provided on a nutritional label.

KEY TERMS

Acceptable macronutrient distribution ranges (AMDRs)
Adequate intake (AI)
Bariatric surgery
Body mass index (BMI)
Calorie (cal)
c-eq
Chronic disease risk reduction intake (CDRR)
Daily value (DV)
Dietary reference intakes (DRIs)
Energy
Enrichment
Estimated average requirement (EAR)
Estimated energy requirement (EER)
Fortification

Health claim
Healthy U.S.-Style Eating Pattern (U.S.-Pattern)
Hypertension
Kilocalorie (kcal)
Low nutrient density
Macronutrients
Micronutrients
Nutrient content claims
Nutrient-dense
Nutrients
Nutrition
Nutrition and dietetic technician, registered (DTR)
Nutrition facts label
Nutritionist

Obesity
Overweight
oz-eq
Physical activity
Physical fitness
Phytochemicals
Precursor
Qualified health claims
Recommended dietary allowances (RDAs)
Registered dietitian (RD)/registered dietitian nutritionist (RDN)
Tolerable upper intake level (UL)
Trans fatty acids
Unqualified health claims
Whole grains

TEST YOUR NQ

1. **T/F** Milk is a perfect food for everyone.
2. **T/F** According to the *Dietary Guidelines for Americans*, consumption of all sugars should be reduced.
3. **T/F** Water is the most important nutrient.
4. **T/F** Dietary Reference Intakes (DRIs) are required daily intakes essential for all patients to be healthy.
5. **T/F** Good nutrition is possible regardless of a patient's cultural beliefs.
6. **T/F** Based on *MyPlate*, two to four servings daily are needed from the fruit and vegetable group.
7. **T/F** The *Dietary Guidelines for Americans* were developed for healthy people to reduce their risk of developing chronic diseases.
8. **T/F** Sugar is the leading cause of chronic health problems.
9. **T/F** The goal of *MyPlate* is to convey the importance of variety, moderation, and proportion.
10. **T/F** The only nutrients that provide energy are carbohydrates, fats, and vitamins.

The dental hygiene profession continues to grow and rapidly move into the forefront of health care. To function as valuable members of today's interprofessional health care team, the dental hygienists must be knowledgeable in various aspects of health care. Because of the lifelong, synergistic, bidirectional relationship between oral health nutritional status, dental hygienists and registered dietitians and nutritionists need to be competent in assessing and providing basic education to patients along with collaborating and providing referrals to support comprehensive patient care.

All registered dietitians and some nutritionists are considered experts in the field of food and nutrition, but their training prepares them for slightly different specialties. A **nutritionist** may have a 4-year degree in foods and nutrition and may have been working in a public health setting assisting people in the community, such as pregnant females or older individuals, with diet-related health issues. In many states, a nutritionist is legally defined and is licensed or certified. Nutritionists work in local or state health departments and in the extension service of a land-grant university. A **registered dietitian (RD)** or **registered dietitian nutritionist (RDN)** has a minimum of bachelor's degree in foods and nutrition with training in normal and clinical nutrition, food science, food service management, research, and medical nutrition therapy. Beginning January 2024 a master's degree is required to be eligible to take the national dietetic registration examination for credentialing.[1] The credential RDN is granted by the Commission on Dietetic Registration for the Academy of Nutrition and Dietetics for those who have passed a national registration examination and who maintain updated knowledge of the field through continuing education. RDNs working in hospitals, long-term care facilities, health care providers' offices, and pharmaceutical companies may be more involved with medical nutrition therapy or specialized diets. RDNs may also work in settings dealing principally with basic nutrition, such as in schools, community and research settings, wellness and fitness centers, public health and community programs, educational institutions, and health and wellness preventive programs. The addition of the term *nutritionist* helps identify the type of work performed. Actually, all registered dietitians are nutritionists, but not all nutritionists are registered dietitians.

A **Nutrition and Dietetic Technician, Registered (NDTR)** is the one who has completed an associate degree and an accredited NDTR program with at least 450 hours of supervised practice experience or has a 4-year degree from an approved program (approved by the Accreditation Council for Education in Nutrition and Dietetics). An NDTR, like the RDN, must pass a national registration examination and receive continuing education. The DTR normally works under the supervision of an RDN in such practice areas as hospitals, clinics, and nursing homes, but they may also work independently to provide general nutrition education to healthy populations.

Dental professionals typically see patients on a more regular basis than other health care professionals; this allows observation of many physical signs, particularly oral signs, of a nutrient deficiency or medical condition that affects nutritional status before it is diagnosed. Recognition of abnormal conditions and early referral to an appropriate health care professional can lead to positive health outcomes for patients. Assessment of dietary information obtained from a patient can also uncover habits detrimental to oral health readily addressed in the dental office. Additionally, compromised oral health may affect food choices. For example, patients with missing dentition or ill-fitting dentures may avoid foods that are hard to chew and reduce the quality and variety of their diets.

Finally, dental hygienists can follow up on goals established by patients to evaluate their understanding and compliance. Overall, the dental hygienist is committed to prevention of oral disease as well as the promotion of health and wellness. All health care professionals must work together to enhance patient care. This textbook provides the dental professionals with the nutrition information needed to provide a nutrition foundation and to highlight areas pertinent to educating patients in the dental setting.

Basic Nutrition

Nutrition is the process by which living things use food to obtain nutrients for energy, growth and development, and maintenance. **Energy** is the ability or power to do work. **Nutrients** are biochemical substances that can be supplied only in adequate amounts from an outside source, normally from food. One aspect of nutrition is the integration of physiologic and biochemical reactions within the body: (1) digesting food to make nutrients available, (2) absorbing and delivering nutrients to the cells where they are used, and (3) eliminating waste products.

Nutrition is a relatively new science and still an evolving discipline. People want science to be definitive; they become confused and concerned when scientific research challenges what they assume to be factual. In nutrition, something that is considered to be true today may be disrupted by future research contradicting established beliefs. In many cases, the media exacerbate this situation by reporting new research and recommendations as soon as they are released. These findings may not necessarily be reproduced in further research. Often, it is difficult to separate a medical certainty from emerging evidence that needs further research. The pace of research has quickened; this text is based on current, well-established, and evidence-based nutrition advice. Everyone in the health care field must continue to stay abreast of ongoing research to knowledgeably respond to questions from patients.

Americans are interested in food and health issues and are concerned about their diet, their physical activity, however, many factors impact food choice and healthy eating, and physical activity. Equity and social determinants of health impact many individuals in low income communities and lead to health disparities such as higher rates of obesity and chronic disease. Overarching factors that impact healthy lifestyle behaviors include individual, social, and environmental factors.[2] At the individual level factors include personal preference (e.g., taste, texture); knowledge (nutrition literacy); skills (e.g., planning and preparing healthy meals); psychological state (e.g., emotional state, self-regulation, food craving); beliefs and attitudes (e.g., long-term benefit of healthy choices); and habits (e.g., habits learned in childhood).[2] At the social level, factors include social networks (e.g., family, peers, colleagues, and social media connections); social acceptability and expectations (e.g., cultural norms around food choice and preparation, body image expectations); marketing and media messaging.[2] Environmental factors may include food price and affordability; food availability (e.g., access to grocery stores, food insecurity); food characteristics; convenience and time; and built and natural environments (e.g., lack of transportation, geographic barriers, safe communities for walking).[2]

Physiologic Functions of Nutrients

Physiologically, foods eaten are used for energy, tissue building, maintenance and replacement, and obtaining or producing numerous regulatory substances. Nutrients obtained from foods are the following: (1) water, (2) proteins, (3) carbohydrates, (4) fats, (5) minerals, and (6) vitamins. Other naturally occurring substances in various foods, such as phytochemicals (plant chemicals) also promote health.

Of these nutrients, only proteins, carbohydrates, and fats provide energy. Alcohol also provides calories but has limited or no nutrients. The potential energy value of foods within the body is expressed in terms of kilocalorie, more frequently referred to as calorie. A kilocalorie (kcal) is a measure of heat equivalent to 1000 calories.

Nutrients work together and interact in complex metabolic reactions. Proteins, carbohydrates, and fats provide energy the body needs for metabolic processes. However, the body cannot use energy from these calorie-containing components of food without adequate amounts of vitamins and minerals. Vitamins and minerals, along with protein and water, are essential for the body to build and maintain body tissues and to regulate essential body processes.

Basic Concepts of Nutrition

Foods differ in the amount of nutrients they furnish. Any individual food can be compatible with good nutrition but should be evaluated in the context of the patient's physiologic needs, the food's nutrient content, and other food choices. The premise of personal nutrition is that, in any cultural or environmental circumstance or for any personal taste or preference, a healthy dietary pattern is possible. The total diet or overall pattern of food intake is the most important focus of making healthy choices.

Increasing the variety of healthful foods consumed reduces the probability of developing isolated nutrient deficiencies, nutrient excesses, and toxicities resulting from nonnutritive components or contaminants in any particular food. A dietary change to eliminate or increase intake of one specific food component or nutrient usually alters the intake of other nutrients. For instance, because red meats are an excellent source of iron and zinc, decreasing cholesterol intake by limiting these meats can reduce dietary iron and zinc intake.

Essential nutrients are needed throughout life on a regular basis; only the amounts of nutrients required changes. The patient's consumption of foods and beverages, stage of growth and development, sex, body size, weight, physical activity, and state of health influence nutrient requirements.

Some nutrients can be converted by the body to meet physiologic needs. Nonessential nutrients can be used by the body but either are not required or can be synthesized from dietary precursors. Precursors are substances from which an active substance is formed. An example is carotene, found in fruits and vegetables, which the liver can convert into an active form of vitamin A.

Water is the most important nutrient. After water, nutrients of highest priority are those providing energy, which must be obtained from foods or supplied from physiologic stores. The human body has adaptive mechanisms that allow toleration of modest variations in nutrient intakes. For instance, the metabolic rate usually decreases as a result of decreased calorie intake.

🦷 DENTAL CONSIDERATIONS

- Because nutrients work interdependently, a lack or excess of one can interfere with or prevent use of another. Asking the patient to record food and beverage intake for the past 24 to 72 hours allows assessment of nutrient intake.
- Evaluation of the patient's intake of food and beverages can help determine whether intake is adequate or excessive.
- Abnormalities in the oral cavity can affect systemic health and nutrition. Additionally, nutritional conditions or their treatments can affect the oral cavity or the feasibility of delivering dental care.

🦷 NUTRITIONAL DIRECTIONS

- No single food contains all the essential nutrients in amounts needed for optimal health.
- Nutritional intake can either improve or adversely affect health.

Government Nutrition Goals for Population Health

Before 1977 nutritional efforts focused on ensuring the food supply provided adequate nutrients to prevent deficiency diseases. The US government recognized health and nutritional problems related to food choices in 1977 with the *United States Dietary Goals*, which addressed excessive consumption of some nutrients.[3] In 1979, the Surgeon General issued a report confirming that 5 of the 10 leading causes of death (cardiovascular disease [CVD], certain types of cancer, stroke, diabetes mellitus, and atherosclerosis) were associated with dietary intake.[3] These reports provided comprehensive science-based objectives to improve the health of the US population and to establish national objectives for promoting health and preventing disease.

Healthy People Nutrition Objectives

Healthy People 2030: National Health Promotion and Disease Prevention Objectives, initially introduced in 1990 by the US

Department of Health and Human Services (USDHHS), established objectives and goals to measure progress in specific areas. *Healthy People* focuses on four overarching goals that include (1) increasing the quality and years of healthy life, (2) eliminating health disparities among racial and ethnic groups, (3) creating social and physical environments that promote good health for everyone, and (4) promoting quality of life and healthful development and behaviors of all age groups. In addition, the *Healthy People 2030* builds on these four goals with a focus on health equity, health literacy, well-being, and social determinants of health.[4]

Healthy People 2030 identifies emerging public health priorities and aligns them with health promotion strategies driven by the best evidence available. *Healthy People 2030* is organized into 5 topics with 359 measurable core, developmental, and research objectives to be accomplished by 2040.[5] The Healthy People 2030 has also identified 23 high priority objectives that serve as leading health indicators (LHI) to focus action on improving health and well-being.[5] For oral health professionals, the objectives of interest include: nutrition and healthy eating (27 objectives), physical activity (27 objectives), overweight/obesity (7 objectives), and 15 objectives related to oral conditions.[5]

A *Healthy People 2020* final review on these objectives found 34% targets were met or exceeded with about 21% improved.[6] However, 31% had little or no detectable change and 14% got worse.[6] For nutrition and weight status, physical activity, and oral health, 50% or more of objectives improved or met or exceeded targets.[6] Two oral health objectives met or exceeded the target and included *increased use of the oral health care system* and *reduced the portion of people who can't get the dental care they need it when they need it.*[5] Other relevant objectives are referenced throughout this text. The *Healthy People* website (https://www.healthypeople.gov/) is updated frequently, providing consumers and health care providers the opportunity to monitor progress.

Nutrient Recommendations: Dietary Reference Intakes

Recommendations for the amounts of required nutrients have undergone significant changes over the years, and the current nutrient-based reference values are collectively called the Dietary Reference Intakes (DRIs). In 1993 the Food and Nutrition Board of the Institute of Medicine (IOM, now the National Academy of Medicine which is a part of the National Academies of Sciences, Engineering, and Medicine [NASEM]) undertook this major project, which was initially completed in 2004. The DRIs, published by the National Academy of Medicine, are established by an expert group of scientists and RDNs from the United States and Canada. These groups of experts based their recommendations on the most current scientific knowledge from different types of studies involving nutrients for healthy populations. The DRIs are currently undergoing review with a joint US-Canada Dietary Reference Intakes Working Group.[7] The first DRI to be updated was energy in 2023.[7]

Previous Recommended Dietary Allowances (RDAs) focused on amounts of nutrients necessary to prevent deficiency diseases. The current DRIs also attempt to (1) estimate amounts of required nutrients to improve long-term health and well-being by reducing risk of chronic diseases affected by nutrition, for example, heart disease, diabetes, osteoporosis, and cancer; and (2) establish maximum safe levels of tolerance. The four categories of nutrient-based reference values are relevant for various stages of life. The DRIs were intended for planning and assessing diets of healthy Americans and Canadians. The DRIs are for the general population and are not meant for those with chronic disease or the malnourished. Because of emerging evidence involving potential roles of nutrients or other food substances in ameliorating chronic diseases, the National Academies appointed a committee to make recommendations for establishing DRIs for specific nutrients that could ameliorate the risk of chronic diseases. In 2017 *Guiding Principles for Developing Dietary Reference Intakes Based on Chronic Disease* ad hoc committee established guiding principles to support future DRI committees in making decisions about recommending chronic disease DRIs.[8]

DRI Values to Meet Nutritional Requirements

The Estimated Average Requirement (EAR) is the amount of a nutrient that is estimated to meet the needs of half of the healthy individuals in a specific age and gender group. This set of values is useful in assessing nutrient adequacy or planning intakes of population groups, not individuals.

The Estimated Energy Requirement (EER) is defined as dietary energy intake that is predicted to maintain energy balance in healthy, normal-weight individuals of a defined age, gender, weight, height, and physical activity level consistent with good health. The EER is similar to the EAR, and no RDA was established because consuming more calories than are needed would result in weight gain. Because energy requirement depends on activity level, four different activity levels are provided.

Recommended Dietary Allowance

The RDA is generally higher than the EAR and provides a sufficient amount of a nutrient to meet the requirements of nearly all healthy individuals (97%–98%). These recommendations provide a generous margin of safety and are intended as a goal for achieving adequate intakes. No health benefits are established for consuming intakes greater than the RDA.

Adequate Intakes

If sufficient scientific evidence was unavailable to determine an EAR or RDA, an Adequate Intake (AI) was established based on scientific judgments. An AI, which is derived from mean nutrient intakes by groups of healthy people, is the average amount of a nutrient that seems to maintain a defined nutritional state. An AI is expected to exceed average requirements of virtually all members of a life stage/gender group but is more tentative than an RDA. AI values were established for various life stages for several nutrients, including fluoride, because of uncertainties about the scientific data to determine EAR and RDA values that would reduce the risk of chronic disease.

DRI Value to Prevent Excessive Intakes

A Tolerable Upper Intake Level (UL) is the maximum daily level of nutrient intake that probably would not cause adverse health effects or toxic effects for most individuals in the general population. The potential risk of adverse effects increases as intake exceeds the UL. The term Tolerable Intake was selected to avoid implying that these higher levels would result in beneficial effects. These values are especially helpful because of increased consumption of nutrients in the form of dietary supplements or from enrichment and fortification. This recommendation pertains to habitual daily use and is based on combined intake of food, water, dietary supplements, and fortified foods, with a few exceptions: the UL for magnesium applies only to intake from nonfood sources; ULs for vitamin E, niacin, and folate apply only to fortified foods or supplement sources; and UL for vitamin A applies only to the intake of preformed retinol, regardless of the source.

DRI Values to Reduce Chronic Disease Risk

Acceptable Macronutrient Distribution Ranges (AMDRs) were established for the macronutrients, fat, carbohydrate, protein, and two polyunsaturated fatty acids, to ensure sufficient intakes of essential nutrients (carbohydrate, protein and fat), while potentially reducing risk of chronic disease. Macronutrients are energy-providing nutrients needed in larger amounts than micronutrients, for example, vitamins and minerals. The AMDR is a range of intakes for food components that provide calories; these are expressed as a percentage of total energy intake because the intake of each depends on the intake of others or of total energy requirement of the individual. Increasing or decreasing one energy source while consuming a set amount of calories affects intake of the other sources of energy. For instance, if an individual who routinely consumes 2000 cal reduces fat intake, either protein or carbohydrate intake would need to be increased to provide 2000 cal. Consuming amounts outside of the ranges increases risk of insufficient intake of essential nutrients. Recommended ranges for carbohydrates, fats, and proteins allow more flexibility in eating patterns for healthy individuals and as well as allow for individual preferences.

Chronic disease risk reduction intake (CDRR) were added to the DRI model and provide values expected to reduce the risk of developing chronic disease. The value is based on at least moderate strength evidence of both a causal and intake-response relationship between a nutrient and chronic disease risk.[9] These were first developed for the updated sodium and potassium DRIs in 2019.

Summary of Dietary Reference Intakes

Because nutrient requirements are influenced by age and sexual development, the DRIs are listed for 16 groups, separating gender groups after 10 years of age. Separate levels are established for three categories of pregnant and lactating females. Also, two age groups for the older American population are available.

These guidelines apply to average daily intakes. Meeting the recommendations for every nutrient on a daily basis is very difficult and unnecessary. These nutrient goals are intended to be met by consuming a variety of foods whenever possible.

DENTAL CONSIDERATIONS

- Use of DRIs as an assessment guide is for healthy patients only.
- An individual's exact requirement for a specific nutrient is not known for certain.
- The ULs may be used to warn patients that excessive intake of nutrients from nutritional supplements could lead to adverse effects if taken on a regular basis.
- Generally, specific foods or food groups, rather than nutrients, should be discussed with patients.
- If an individual's food consumption is below the RDA for a nutrient over several days, more food choices containing that particular nutrient should be encouraged.

NUTRITIONAL DIRECTIONS

- The DRIs are general guidelines for good health rather than specific requirements.
- Choosing a wide variety of foods will probably result in meeting established nutrient requirements.

Food Guidance System for Americans

Identification of nutrients and knowledge of their physiologic functions are significant developments. However, consumers eat and think in terms of food, not nutrients. Nutrient requirements and information must be interpreted into the "food" language that consumers understand. In 2020 the USDHHS and the US Department of Agriculture (USDA) released the *Dietary Guidelines for Americans 2020–2025* in the ninth edition of the guidelines. These *Dietary Guidelines* are based on scientific knowledge to meet nutrient requirements, promote health, support active lives through physical activity, and reduce risks of chronic disease. The *Dietary Guidelines* are the foundation for *MyPlate* (www.MyPlate.gov), released in 2011 to help consumers become healthier by making wise food choices.

Another helpful tool is the food label that helps consumers determine what kind of food and how much food to eat. Nutrition labeling, required for most packaged foods, provides information on certain nutrients. The Nutrition Facts label enumerates nutrient content of food for the serving size specified and discloses the number of servings in the package. Knowing how to interpret labels enables consumers to accurately apply *Dietary Guideline* messages that correspond to the nutrients and other information on the label.

2020–2025 Dietary Guidelines for Americans

The objective of the four key guidelines is to help consumers make healthful choices from each of the food groups that, with an awareness of calorie intake, will result in an overall healthful dietary pattern (Fig. 1.1). A dietary pattern represents all the foods and beverages consumed over time and foods and beverages act synergistically to affect health.[10] Ideally, it meets nutritional needs without exceeding limitations with regard to saturated fats, added sugars, sodium, and total calories. The long-range goal of the *Dietary Guidelines* is to prevent, or at least decrease, the rate of chronic disease and mortality. Interestingly, a recent systematic review of dietary patterns found that those with higher intake of vegetables, fruit, whole grains, legumes, nuts, unsaturated vegetable oils, fish, and lean meat or poultry were associated with a decreased risk for all-cause mortality.[11]

The *Dietary Guidelines* reference the Healthy U.S.-Style Eating Pattern (U.S.-Pattern) that indicates the number of food equivalents from each food group and subgroups for 12 calorie levels to be consumed each week for an adequate healthful diet (Fig. 1.2). Foods providing similar kinds of nutrients are grouped together and, as a rule, foods in one group cannot replace those in another (Table 1.1). This U.S.-Pattern can be adapted easily using various types and proportions of foods that Americans typically consume; however, to provide all the essential nutrients, foods need to be nutrient dense and in appropriate amounts to prevent exceeding calorie limits and other limiting dietary components. Nutrient-dense foods provide substantial amounts of vitamins

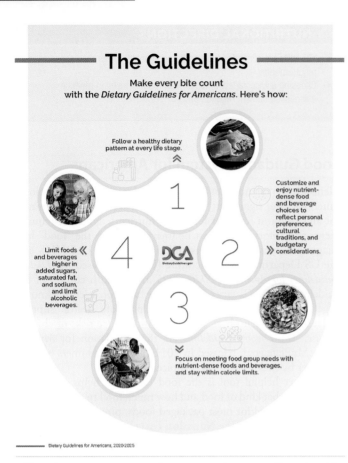

The Guidelines

Make every bite count
with the *Dietary Guidelines for Americans.* Here's how:

Follow a healthy dietary pattern at every life stage.

1

Customize and enjoy nutrient-dense food and beverage choices to reflect personal preferences, cultural traditions, and budgetary considerations.

2

DGA
DietaryGuidelines.gov

4

Limit foods and beverages higher in added sugars, saturated fat, and sodium, and limit alcoholic beverages.

3

Focus on meeting food group needs with nutrient-dense foods and beverages, and stay within calorie limits.

Dietary Guidelines for Americans, 2020-2025

• **Fig. 1.1** *2020–2025 Dietary Guidelines for Americans.* (From the U.S. Department of Agriculture and U.S. Department of Health and Human Services: *2020-2025 Dietary Guidelines for Americans.* 9th ed. U.S. Government Printing Office; 2020. DietaryGuidelines.gov.)

and minerals but relatively few calories. When many **low nutrient-density** foods or beverages (containing high fat, sugar, or alcohol) are chosen, obtaining adequate amounts of essential nutrients is difficult without excess calorie intake. The consumption of excessive calories from fats, added sugars, and refined grains reduces intake of nutrient-dense foods and beverages without exceeding calorie requirements.

Portion control is very important to stay within the desired calorie level. Portion size may be different than serving size. The amounts from each food group and subgroup change as needed among the different calorie levels to meet nutrient and *Dietary Guidelines* standards and comply with calories and overconsumed dietary components. Fig. 1.3 is a simple tool from the USDHHS that provides relationships consumers can relate to for estimating portion sizes. Within the U.S.-Pattern, serving or portion sizes are depicted as c-eq or oz-eq. Vegetables, fruits, and dairy food groups are represented with **c-eq**, which is the amount of a food or beverage considered equal to 1 cup or one portion. A serving size of many popular foods or beverages differs due to (1) concentration (e.g., raisins or tomato paste), (2) fresh produce that does not compress into a cup (e.g., salad greens), or (3) foods that are measured in a different form (e.g., meat and cheese). A serving portion of food from the grain or protein groups is equivalent to one ounce (**oz-eq**). If a food is concentrated or contains minimal amounts of water (e.g., nuts, peanut butter, jerky, cooked beans,

rice or pasta), its portion size may be less than a measured ounce (by weight). If it contains a large amount of water (e.g., tofu, cooked beans, cooked rice or pasta), it may be more than a measured ounce (weight).

The U.S.-Patterns meet the RDA for most nutrients. Vitamins D, E, iron, choline, and folate (during pregnancy) are marginal in the U.S.-Patterns for many or all age-sex groups.[12] Vitamin D has few dietary sources so fortified foods and supplements may be necessary to reach adequate intake levels.[12]

Other meal patterns endorsed in the *2020–2025 Dietary Guidelines* include the Dietary Approaches to Stop Hypertension (DASH) diet (see Chapter 12), Mediterranean-Style Eating Pattern, and Healthy Vegetarian Eating Pattern (see Chapter 5).

Key Recommendations for Healthy Eating Patterns

A healthful eating pattern includes vegetables, fruits, dairy, protein foods, and oils, as summarized in the Key Recommendations (Box 1.1).

Energy Balance

Individuals should consume a healthy eating pattern that includes all foods and beverages within an appropriate calorie level to achieve and/or maintain a healthy body weight. The basic element for healthful eating patterns is managing calorie balance, an average equilibrium between calories consumed (food and beverages) and calories expended (metabolic processes and physical activity). For a person to maintain a set weight, energy consumed from foods and beverages must equal calories expended in normal physiologic functions and physical activity. The average intake for Americans age 20 years and over from 2017 to 2020 was 2144 cal per day (1829 cal/day for females and 2483 cal/day for males).[13] Because weight loss is a challenge requiring changes in many behaviors and patterns, excess intake should be avoided. Even small decreases in calorie intake can help prevent weight gain. A reduction in daily intake of 100 calories to prevent gradual weight gain is much easier than reducing daily intake by 500 calories to lose weight. In general, the best choice for weight loss involves a change in lifestyle, both in diet and physical activity. By frequently monitoring body weight, consumers can determine whether their eating patterns are providing an appropriate amount of calories, and thus adjust food intake and/or activity level. All Americans are encouraged to achieve and/or maintain a healthy body weight to reduce the risk of chronic disease:

- Children and adolescents are encouraged to maintain calorie balance to support normal growth and development without promoting excess weight gain.
- Females are encouraged to achieve and maintain a healthy weight, and females who are pregnant are encouraged to gain weight within gestational weight gain guidelines (see Chapter 13).
- Adults who are overweight or obese should change both eating habits and physical activity to prevent additional weight gain and/or promote weight loss.
- Older adults (65 years and older) who are overweight or obese are encouraged to prevent additional weight gain. Intentional weight loss is beneficial for patients who have chronic conditions such as CVD or diabetes.

Body weight can be evaluated in relation to a person's height using **body mass index (BMI)** to determine health risks that increase at higher levels of **overweight** (BMI 25.0–29.9) and

CALORIE LEVEL OF PATTERN[a]	1000	1200	1400	1600	1800	2000	2200	2400	2600	2800	3000	3200
FOOD GROUP OR SUBGROUP[b]	Daily Amount[c] of food From Each Group (Vegetable and protein foods subgroup amounts are per week)											
Vegetables (cup eq/day)	1	1 ½	1 ½	2	2 ½	2 ½	3	3	3 ½	3 ½	4	4
	Vegetable Subgroups in Weekly Amounts											
Dark-green vegetables (cup eq/week)	½	1	1	1 ½	1 ½	1 ½	2	2	2 ½	2 ½	2 ½	2 ½
Red and orange vegetables (cup eq/week)	2 ½	3	3	4	5 ½	5 ½	6	6	7	7	7 ½	7 ½
Beans, peas, lentils (cup eq/week)	½	½	½	1	1 ½	1 ½	2	2	2 ½	2 ½	3	3
Starchy vegetables (cup eq/week)	2	3 ½	3 ½	4	5	5	6	6	7	7	8	8
Other vegetables (cup eq/week)	1 ½	2 ½	2 ½	3 ½	4	4	5	5	5 ½	5 ½	7	7
Fruits (cup eq/day)	1	1	1 ½	1 ½	1 ½	2	2	2	2	2 ½	2 ½	2 ½
Grains (oz eq/day)	3	4	5	5	6	6	7	8	9	10	10	10
Whole grains (oz eq/day)[d]	1 ½	2	2 ½	3	3	3	3 ½	4	4 ½	5	5	5
Refined grains (oz eq/day)	1 ½	2	2 ½	2	3	3	3 ½	4	4 ½	5	5	5
Dairy (cup eq/day)	2	2 ½	2 ½	3	3	3	3	3	3	3	3	3
Protein foods (oz eq/day)	2	3	4	5	5	5 ½	6	6 ½	6 ½	7	7	7
	Protein Foods Subgroups in Weekly Amounts											
Meats, poultry, eggs (oz eq/day)	10	14	19	23	23	26	28	31	31	33	33	33
Seafood (oz eq/day)[e]	2–3[f]	4	6	8	8	8	9	10	10	10	10	10
Nuts, seeds, soy products (oz eq/day)	2	2	3	4	4	5	5	5	5	6	6	6
Oils (g/day)	15	17	17	22	24	27	29	31	34	36	44	51
Limit on calories for other uses (kcal/day)[g]	130	80	90	100	140	240	250	320	350	370	440	580
Limit on calorie for other uses (%/g)	13%	7%	6%	6%	8%	12%	11%	13%	13%	13%	15%	18%

• **Fig. 1.2** Healthy U.S.-Style Dietary Pattern for Ages 2 Years and Older, With Daily or Weekly Amounts From Food Groups, Subgroups, and Components. [a]Food intake patterns at 1000, 1200, and 1400 calories are designed to meet the nutritional needs of 2- to 8-year-old children. Patterns from 1600 to 3200 calories are designed to meet the nutritional needs of children 9 years and older and adults. If a child 4 to 8 years of age needs more calories and, therefore, is following a pattern at 1600 calories or more, that child's recommended amount from the dairy group should be 2.5 cups per day. Children 9 years and older and adults should not use the 1000-, 1200-, or 1400-calorie patterns. [b]Food group amounts shown in cup-equivalents (c-eq) or ounce-equivalents (oz-eq), as appropriate for each group, based on caloric and nutrient content. [c]Amounts of whole grains in the Patterns for children are less than the minimum of 3 oz-eq in all Patterns recommended for adults. [d]All foods are assumed to be in nutrient-dense forms; lean or low-fat; and prepared without added fats, sugars, refined starches, or salt. If all food choices to meet food group recommendations are in nutrient-dense forms, a small number of calories remain within the overall calorie limit of the Pattern (i.e., limit on calories for other uses). The number of these calories depends on the overall calorie limit in the Pattern and the amounts of food from each food group required to meet nutritional goals. Calories from protein, carbohydrates, and total fats should be within the Acceptable Macronutrient Distribution Ranges (AMDRs). [e]The U.S. Food and Drug Administration (FDA) and the U.S. Environmental Protection Agency (EPA) provide joint advice regarding seafood consumption to limit methylmercury exposure for women who might become or are pregnant or breastfeeding, and children. For more information, see the FDA and EPA websites FDA.gov/fishadvice; EPA.gov/fishadvice. [f]If consuming up to 2 ounces of seafood per week, children should only be fed cooked varieties from the "Best Choices" list in the FDA/EPA joint "Advice About Eating Fish," available at FDA.gov/fishadvice and EPA.gov/fishadvice. If consuming up to 3 ounces of seafood per week, children should only be fed cooked varieties from the "Best Choices" list that contain even lower methylmercury. For a complete list please see: FDA.gov/fishadvice and EPA.gov/fishadvice. [g]Foods are assumed to be in nutrient-dense forms, lean or low-fat and prepared with minimal added saturated fat, added sugars, refined starches, or salt. If all food choices to meet food group recommendations are in nutrient-dense forms, a small number of calories remain within the overall limit of the pattern for added sugars, added refined starches, saturated fat, or alcohol. (From U.S. Department of Health and Human Services, U.S. Department of Agriculture: *2020 -2025 Dietary Guidelines for Americans*. 9th ed. Washington, DC: 2020 (Dec), USDHHS/USDA.)

TABLE 1.1	Principal Nutrient Contributions of Each Food Group				
Nutrients	Vegetable	Fruit	Meat	Milk	Grain
Protein			X	X	X
Vitamin A	X	X			
Vitamin D				X[a]	
Vitamin E	X				
Vitamin C	X	X			
Thiamin			X		X[b]
Riboflavin				X	X[b]
Niacin			X		X[b]
Vitamin B$_6$			X	X	
Folate/folic acid	X	X			X[b]
Vitamin B$_{12}$			X[c]	X[c]	
Calcium				X	
Phosphorus			X	X	X
Magnesium	X			X	X[d]
Iron			X		X[b]
Zinc			X	X	X
Fiber	X	X			X[d]

[a]If fortified.
[b]If enriched.
[c]Only animal products.
[d]Whole grains.

Serving Size Card:
Cut out and fold on the dotted line. Laminate for longtime use.

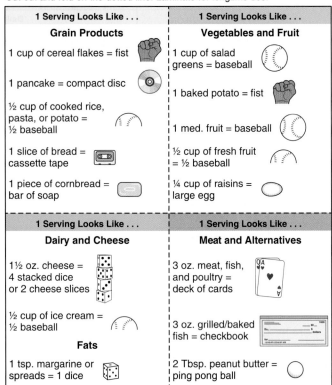

• **Fig. 1.3** Serving size card. This tool can be used when estimating appropriate serving sizes when choosing/serving foods. (From U.S. Department of Health and Human Services, National Heart, Lung and Blood Institute. *Serving Sizes and Portions: And Servings: What's the Difference?* https://www.nhlbi.nih.gov/health/educational/wecan/downloads/servingcard7.pdf.)

obesity (BMI >30.0). BMI is a reasonable indicator of body fat and can be used as a screening tool, but should not be used as a diagnostic tool.[14] BMI can be determined by using a BMI calculator (https://www.cdc.gov/healthyweight/assessing/index.html) and Table 1.2 to classify body weight category (underweight, normal weight, overweight, or obese). A BMI of less than 18.5 to 24.9 is generally considered a healthy weight; chronic disease risk increases in most people who have a BMI above 25. BMI is not appropriate for pregnant and nursing females, infants and children younger than age 2 years, or some athletes with a large percentage of muscle.

BMI reveals little about overall body composition. It is a starting point in assessing an individual's health status and risks that is noninvasive, inexpensive, and quick. Limitations of relying solely on a person's BMI include the following: (1) females tend to have more body fat; (2) BMI can underestimate body fat in an elderly person who has lost lean body mass; (3) racial/ethnic groups may have higher or lower amounts of body fat; and (4) BMI overestimates body fat in individuals who have very high levels of lean body mass (e.g., athletes).[14] On the other hand, a frail or inactive person with a normal-range BMI may have excess body fat and not appear out of shape. Additional muscle tissue aids body functions, but excessive fat interferes with normal metabolism. A healthy weight depends on the amount and location of body fat

and other health indicators, such as blood pressure, glucose, cholesterol, and triglyceride levels.

Major ethnic differences exist regarding BMI. For example, Asian Americans are at risk of health problems (e.g., diabetes) at a lower BMI than whites so a modified BMI range for normal weight is 18.5 to 22.9 kg/m², overweight range is 23 to 27.4, and obesity is defined as a BMI of 27.5 or greater.[15] Older adults tend to have a better functional capacity, fewer balance problems, lower fall risk, better muscle strength, and less malnutrition with a BMI of 27 to 28 kg/m² in females and 31 to 32 kg/m² in males.[16]

All foods and some beverages contain varying amounts of calories based on their nutrient content. Macronutrients include carbohydrates and protein that contribute 4 cal/g; fats, 9 cal/g; and alcohol, which, although not a nutrient, contributes 7 cal/g when consumed. Most foods and beverages contain combinations of macronutrients in varying amounts. There is a little evidence that any individual macronutrient has a unique impact on body weight. Calorie intake is the key factor in controlling body weight, not by manipulating the proportions of fat, carbohydrates, and protein but by balancing overall calories with energy expenditure.

A patient's calorie requirements are based on size (height and weight), age, sex, and level of physical activity. Many Americans

• BOX 1.1   *2020–2025 Dietary Guidelines for Americans:* Key Recommendations

Key Recommendations

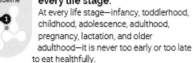

Follow a healthy dietary pattern at every life stage.
At every life stage—infancy, toddlerhood, childhood, adolescence, adulthood, pregnancy, lactation, and older adulthood—it is never too early or too late to eat healthfully.

- **For about the first 6 months of life,** exclusively feed infants human milk. Continue to feed infants human milk through at least the first year of life, and longer if desired. Feed infants iron-fortified infant formula during the first year of life when human milk is unavailable. Provide infants with supplemental vitamin D beginning soon after birth.

- **At about 6 months,** introduce infants to nutrient-dense complementary foods. Introduce infants to potentially allergenic foods along with other complementary foods. Encourage infants and toddlers to consume a variety of foods from all food groups. Include foods rich in iron and zinc, particularly for infants fed human milk.

- **From 12 months through older adulthood,** follow a healthy dietary pattern across the lifespan to meet nutrient needs, help achieve a healthy body weight, and reduce the risk of chronic disease.

Customize and enjoy nutrient-dense food and beverage choices to reflect personal preferences, cultural traditions, and budgetary considerations.
A healthy dietary pattern can benefit all individuals regardless of age, race, or ethnicity, or current health status. The *Dietary Guidelines* provides a framework intended to be customized to individual needs and preferences, as well as the foodways of the diverse cultures in the United States.

Focus on meeting food group needs with nutrient-dense foods and beverages, and stay within calorie limits.
An underlying premise of the *Dietary Guidelines* is that nutritional needs should be met primarily from foods and beverages—specifically, nutrient-dense foods and beverages. Nutrient-dense foods provide vitamins, minerals, and other health-promoting components and have no or little added sugars, saturated fat, and sodium. A healthy dietary pattern consists of nutrient-dense forms of foods and beverages across all food groups, in recommended amounts, and within calorie limits.

The core elements that make up a healthy dietary pattern include:

- Vegetables of all types—dark green; red and orange; beans, peas, and lentils; starchy; and other vegetables

- Fruits, especially whole fruit

- Grains, at least half of which are whole grain

- Dairy, including fat-free or low-fat milk, yogurt, and cheese, and/or lactose-free versions and fortified soy beverages and yogurt as alternatives

- Protein foods, including lean meats, poultry, and eggs; seafood; beans, peas, and lentils; and nuts, seeds, and soy products

- Oils, including vegetable oils and oils in food, such as seafood and nuts

Limit foods and beverages higher in added sugars, saturated fat, and sodium, and limit alcoholic beverages.
At every life stage, meeting food group recommendations—even with nutrient-dense choices—requires most of a person's daily calorie needs and sodium limits. A healthy dietary pattern doesn't have much room for extra added sugars, saturated fat, or sodium—or for alcoholic beverages. A small amount of added sugars, saturated fat, or sodium can be added to nutrient-dense foods and beverages to help meet food group recommendations, but foods and beverages high in these components should be limited. **Limits are:**

- **Added sugars**—Less than 10 percent of calories per day starting at age 2. Avoid foods and beverages with added sugars for those younger than age 2.

- **Saturated fat**—Less than 10 percent of calories per day starting at age 2.

- **Sodium**—Less than 2,300 milligrams per day—and even less for children younger than age 14.

- **Alcoholic beverages**—Adults of legal drinking age can choose not to drink or to drink in moderation by limiting intake to 2 drinks or less in a day for men and 1 drink or less in a day for women, when alcohol is consumed. Drinking less is better for health than drinking more. There are some adults who should not drink alcohol, such as women who are pregnant.

From U.S. Department of Health and Human Services, U.S. Department of Agriculture. *2020–2025 Dietary Guidelines for Americans.* 9th ed. USDHHS/USDA; 2020. https://www.dietaryguidelines.gov/

consume more calories than they need and spend large portions of their days engaged in sedentary behaviors that expend minimal calories. Consequently, many children and adults routinely consume more calories than they expend.

For weight maintenance, calorie requirements typically range from 1600 to 2400 calories daily for adult females and 2000 to 3000 calories for adult males, with variances depending on physical activity. The metabolic rate decreases with age, thus lowering calorie requirements for older adults.

Vegetables

Vegetables are primary sources of the required nutrients, dietary fiber, vitamin A (carotenoids), vitamin C, folic acid, and potassium (Table 1.3). Most vegetables are naturally low in fat and are cholesterol free. Because of their high water and fiber content, most vegetables are relatively low in calories. Dark-green vegetables provide calcium, iron, magnesium, and riboflavin. Beans are unusual because they are in both the vegetable and protein groups. Beans contain protein, fiber, calcium, folic acid, and potassium.

| TABLE 1.2 | Body Mass Index (BMI) and Corresponding Body Weight Categories for Children and Adults | |

Body Weight Category	Children and Adolescents (Aged 2–19 years; BMI-for-Age Percentile Range)	Adults (BMI)
Underweight	<5th percentile	<18.5 kg/m²
Normal weight	5th percentile to <85th percentile	18.5–24.9 kg/m²
Overweight	85th to <95th percentile	25.0–29.9 kg/m²
Obese	≥95th percentile	≥30.0 kg/m²

From Centers for Disease Control and Prevention. *Assessing Your Weight: How to Measure and Interpret Weight Status.* 2022. https://www.cdc.gov/healthyweight/assessing/index.html.

| TABLE 1.3 | Vitamin A, Vitamin C, and Fiber Contributions of Selected Fruits and Vegetables | | |

	Vitamin A	Vitamin C	Fiber
Excellent source	Bok choy Broccoli, cooked Cantaloupe Carrot Collard greens Kale Mango Papaya Romaine lettuce Spinach Sweet potato Swiss chard	Bell pepper Bok choy Broccoli, cooked Brussel spouts Cabbage Cantaloupe Cauliflower Collard greens Grapefruit Kale Kiwi Kohlrabi Mango Orange Papaya Strawberry Sweet potato Swiss chard Tomato	Avocado Prune, dried
Good source	Acorn squash Grapefruit Iceberg lettuce Tomato	Acorn squash Avocado Banana Carrot Spinach	Acorn Squash Apple with skin Banana Broccoli, cooked Brussel sprouts Cabbage Carrot Kale Kiwi Kohlrabi Pear Sweet potato

Data from U.S. Department of Agriculture, Agricultural Research Service. *FoodData Central.* 2019. fdc.nal.usda.gov.

Choosing dark-green, red, and orange vegetables; legumes (beans and peas); starchy vegetables; and other vegetables several times a week is encouraged to provide many nutrients contributed by different vegetables.

Vegetable choices include all fresh, frozen, canned, and dried options, cooked or raw, in addition to vegetable juices. Nutrient-dense vegetables are limited in the amount of salt, butter, or creamy sauces added. The U.S.-Pattern for a 2000-calorie diet includes 2½ c-eq of vegetables daily. For each vegetable subgroup, weekly amounts are recommended to ensure variety and meet nutrient needs. Despite an abundance of nutritious foods available in the United States, 90% of the US population does not meet the recommendations for vegetable intake.[10]

Fruits

All fruits or 100% fruit juices count as part of the fruit group. Fruits are naturally low in fat, sodium, and calories, and do not contain cholesterol. They are also important sources of potassium, dietary fiber, vitamin C, and folate (see Table 1.3). Fresh, frozen, canned, or dried fruits are recommended for their fiber content, but fruit juice should be minimized because it does not contain fiber and excess amounts can contribute extra calories.

Because of their high water content, fruits are more filling than juices, with fewer calories. Fruit juice can be a part of a healthy diet, but only the proportion that is 100% fruit juice counts because these products usually contain added sugars. The percentage of juice in a beverage is indicated on the package label. Fruit juices containing added sugars are classified as sugar-sweetened beverages and should be limited. The recommendation for children 6 months to 6 years old limits 100% fruit juice to 4 to 6 fluid ounces per day (infants under 6 months old should not be given any juice).[17]

At least half of the recommended amount of fruit should be from whole fruits (fresh, canned, frozen, or dried). Fruits that contain a small amount of added sugar can be chosen as long as daily calories from added sugars does not exceed 10% and total calorie intake remains within limits. With canned fruits, those containing the least amount of added sugar should be selected. The recommended amount of fruits in the U.S.-Pattern for 2000 cal is 2 c-eq daily (see Figure 1.2 for amounts for different calorie levels). Only about 80% of the population meets the fruit recommendations for the *Dietary Guidelines.*

Grains

Grains are principally carbohydrates or starchy foods and are essential for a healthful diet. The U.S.-Patterns include whole grains and refined grains, but products made with refined grains, especially those high in saturated fats, added sugars, and/or sodium, such as cookies, cakes, and some snack foods are limited. All whole-grain, refined and enriched, or fortified-grain products are included in these two groups, for example, barley, buckwheat, bulgur, corn, millet, rice, rye, oats, sorghum, wheat, and wild rice.

At the 2000-cal level, the U.S.-Pattern indicates a total of 6 oz-eq per day. Seventy-four percent of Americans are consuming more than the recommended amount of refined grains, and 98% of Americans do not meet *Dietary Guidelines* for the amounts of whole grains.[10]

Whole grains are grains and grain products made from the entire grain seed, usually called the *kernel*, which consists of bran, germ, and endosperm. If the kernel has been cracked, crushed, or flaked, it must retain all components of the original grain kernel (bran, germ, and endosperm) to be called *whole grain*. Whole wheat, oatmeal, brown rice, whole rye, and quinoa are all whole grains. When selecting whole grains, the first or second ingredient listed on the ingredient panel should contain the words *whole grain*. One oz-eq of whole grains has 16 g of whole grains; a food that contains 8 g/oz-eq or more whole grains is at least half whole grains. Product labels usually indicate the grams of whole grain to help consumers identify food choices having a substantial amount of whole grains.

The difficulty in identifying whole grains is a major barrier. Labels such as "100% wheat," "stone-ground," and "multigrain" do not guarantee that the food contains whole grain. Multiple conflicting definitions exist for identifying whole-grain products, causing confusion for consumers. Color is a poor indicator of whole grains because molasses or caramel food coloring may be added. As a result of the *Dietary Guidelines*, food manufacturers have introduced more processed foods with higher whole-grain content.

Most whole grains are a good source of dietary fiber and are needed to meet the daily fiber recommendation. Whole grains differ from a nutritional perspective, with significant variations in levels and effects of the fiber. Whole-grain products contribute more fiber, magnesium, phosphorus, and zinc than do enriched products (Table 1.4). When whole grains are refined, vitamins, minerals, and dietary fiber are lost in the process.

Most refined grains are enriched with some of the nutrients lost in the process, but dietary fiber and some vitamins and minerals are not routinely added back in the enrichment process. **Enrichment** is the process by which iron, thiamin, riboflavin, folic acid, and niacin removed during processing are restored to approximate their original levels. This process is controlled by the US Food and Drug Administration (FDA), which establishes the quantity of nutrients permitted.

Fortification is the process by which nutrients are added for one of the following reasons: (1) to prevent deficiency; (2) to restore nutrients that may be lost in storage, handling, or processing; (3) replace traditional food in the diet to avoid nutritional inadequacy; (4) and to balance nutrient content.[18] Most processed breakfast cereals are fortified to achieve nutrient levels higher than those naturally occurring in the grain. Whole grains

are a poor source of folic acid; thus rather than relying exclusively on whole grains, some cereal products fortified with folic acid should be selected. Products that are enriched with folic acid are especially important for females who are pregnant or capable of becoming pregnant. Serious birth defects may occur during early pregnancy if adequate amounts of folic acid are not consumed.[19] Despite the fact that enriched grains have a positive role in providing some vitamins and minerals, excessive amounts can result in excess calories being consumed. The recommended amount of refined grains is less than 3 oz-eq servings daily; at least one-half of an individual's grain choices should be whole grains.

Dairy and Fortified Soy Alternatives

Healthful eating patterns include fat-free and low-fat (1%) dairy products, including milk, yogurt, cheese, and/or fortified soy beverages. Soy beverages fortified with calcium and vitamins A and D are similar to milk in nutrient composition.[10] The U.S.-Pattern recommends 2 c-eq per day for children aged 2 to 3 years, 2½ c-eq for children aged 4 to 8 years, and 3 c-eq per day for adolescents and adults. Children who establish the habit of drinking milk are more likely to drink milk as adults. About 90% of the US population do not meet the dairy recommendations consistent with the *Dietary Guidelines*.[10] Most age-sex groups (except children 1–3 years old) fall below the recommended amount.

Milk products provide calcium and potassium and may be a good source of vitamin D. Fortified milk products are important sources of vitamin D. However, many milk substitutes (cheese, yogurt, and ice cream) are not fortified with vitamin D (unless made with fortified milk). Whole milk and many cheeses are high in saturated fat and can have negative health implications. Low-fat or fat-free milk products providing little or no fat should be chosen most often to avoid consuming more calories than needed. These products contain similar amounts of nutrients as the higher-fat

TABLE 1.4   Comparison of Nutrient Values of Selected Whole-Grain and Enriched Breads (1 slice)

Nutrients	Enriched White	Whole Wheat	Multigrain	Whole Grain	Rye
Protein (g)	3.0	3.98	3.47	4.0	2.72
Total dietary fiber (g)	0.6	1.9	1.9	3.0	1.9
Thiamin (mg)	0.20	0.126	0.73	0.740	0.139
Riboflavin (mg)	0.13	0.053	0.034	0.340	0.107
Niacin (mg)	1.89	1.420	1.051	1.20	1.218
Vitamin B$_6$ (mg)	0.01	0.069	0.068	0.080	0.024
Total folate (mcg)	72	13	20	Unk	48
Iron (mg)	1.10	0.79	0.65	0.72	0.91
Zinc (mg)	0.21	0.57	0.44	0.60	0.36
Sodium (mg)	120	146	99	150	193
Calcium (mg)	4.0	52.0	27.0	20.0	23.0
Phosphorus (mg)	24.0	68.0	59.0	80.0	40.0
Magnesium (mg)	6.0	24.0	20.0	32.0	13.0

Data from U.S. Department of Agriculture, Agricultural Research Service. *FoodData Central*. 2019. fdc.nal.usda.gov.

options. Fat-free milk and yogurt contain less saturated fat and sodium and more potassium and vitamins A and D than cheese; therefore decreasing the proportion of cheese-to-milk consumption improves overall nutritional intake. If a consumer does not drink milk, efforts should be made to obtain adequate amounts of calcium, potassium, magnesium, and vitamins A and D from other food sources.

The dairy group does not include high-fat products, such as butter and cream, because they are not high in calcium, riboflavin, and protein. Other milks—such as almond, rice, coconut, and hemp milks—may contain calcium but are not part of the dairy group because overall nutritional content is not similar to dairy milk and fortified soy milk.[10]

The consumption of dairy products can help children and adolescents achieve peak bone mass and reduce the risk of low bone mass and osteoporosis. In terms of oral health, evidence is emerging that higher consumption of dietary sources of vitamin D and calcium is associated with a protective effect on risk for periodontal disease in females.[20]

Protein Foods

The U.S.-Patterns include a variety of nutrient-dense forms of protein foods, including legumes (beans and peas). The U.S.-Patterns divide protein foods into subgroups, as follows, with recommended amounts of each to encourage nutritional balance and flexibility: seafood; meats, poultry, and eggs; and nuts, seeds, and soy products.[10]

These foods are important sources of protein, B vitamins (niacin, thiamin, riboflavin, and B_6), vitamin E, iron, zinc, and magnesium. A variety of foods from this group is advisable because each food has distinct nutritional advantages (Table 1.5). By varying choices and including fish, nuts, beans, and seeds, the intake of healthful fats, such as monounsaturated fatty acids and essential polyunsaturated fatty acids (eicosapentaenoic acid [EPA] and docosahexaenoic acid [DHA]), is increased.[10]

Red meats include all forms of beef, pork, lamb, veal, goat, and nonbird game (e.g., venison, bison, elk). Chicken, turkey, duck, geese, guineas, and game birds are classified as poultry. To decrease intake of saturated fats and calories, lean cuts of meat and skinless poultry should be chosen; seafood, nuts, and seeds should replace some of the meat and poultry. Fish, nuts, and seeds contain a healthy type of fat; thus they should be chosen more often than meat or poultry.

Dry beans and peas, such as kidney beans, pinto beans, lima beans, black-eyed peas, and lentils, are included in this group, as well as in the vegetable group. Dried beans and peas do not contain significant quantities of fat and are excellent sources of plant protein and dietary fiber. They also contribute other nutrients found in meats, poultry, and fish. Whether they are counted as a vegetable or a meat, several cups a week are recommended.

Seafood includes all edible marine animals from saltwater and freshwater sources, including fish (e.g., salmon, tuna, trout, tilapia) and shellfish (e.g., shrimp, crab, oysters). The adult recommendation for seafood is approximately 20% of total intake of protein foods. Moderate evidence shows that 8 oz-eq or more of seafood per week from a variety of seafood sources provides omega-3 fatty acids associated with prevention of CVD. Pregnant or breastfeeding females should avoid fish high in mercury—such as tilefish, shark, swordfish, and king mackerel—and should limit white tuna to 6 oz-eq per week.

The size portion for nuts or seeds is only ½ ounce rather than 1 ounce because of the high calorie content of these foods; thus small portions should replace other protein foods (meat or poultry). Nuts and seeds should be unsalted to control sodium intake.

Vegetarians can choose eggs, beans, nuts, nut butters, peas, and soy products to obtain adequate amounts of protein (see Chapter 5).

The U.S.-Pattern recommends 5 to 6½ oz-eq of protein foods, with the specific recommendation of at least 8 oz-eq of seafood per week. Most individuals consume adequate amounts (or more) of protein foods, but about 90% do not meet the recommendation for seafood.[10] In addition, leaner types of protein foods need to be chosen more often. Although consuming significantly higher amounts of protein may not be harmful, high-fat meats may be an undesirable source of calories, cholesterol, and/or saturated fatty acids. Protein supplements promoted to increase muscle mass may not contain nutrients important for health and should be used only after consulting a health care provider or an RDN.

Oils

Lipids (oils and fats) are not a food group, but these nutrients are important in a healthy diet as they provide essential fatty acids. Individuals should be mindful of the type and total amount of fats chosen. Oils are distinctly different from fats because oils, liquids at room temperature, contain a higher percentage of monounsaturated and polyunsaturated fats. Commonly selected oils include canola, corn, olive, peanut, safflower, soybean, and sunflower oils; these are also present in nuts, seeds, seafood, olives, and avocados. Coconut oil, palm kernel, and palm oils are called *oils* because they are derived from tropical plants, but nutritionally they are considered solid fats because they are solid at room temperature due to their high percentage of saturated fatty acids.[10]

The U.S.-Patterns contain some oils, measured in grams (g), but because they are a concentrated source of calories, amounts are limited to within calorie limits and the AMDR (20%–35% of calories) for total fat intake. Fats are classified by the type and percentage of fatty acids they contain. Polyunsaturated fatty acids, monounsaturated fatty acids, and saturated fatty acids are prevalent in American foods. Polyunsaturated and monounsaturated fats are included in the U.S.-Patterns as long as the amounts are within calorie limitations, but saturated fats are addressed in the subsequent discussion in the Nutrients to Limit section. A more detailed explanation of lipids is provided in Chapters 2 and 6.

TABLE 1.5	Excellent or Good Sources for Nutrients of Various Protein Foods	
Protein Food	**Nutrient**
Lean red meats	Iron B vitamins Zinc
Pork	Thiamin Zinc
Poultry	Potassium Niacin
Liver and egg yolks	Vitamin A Iron Zinc
Dry peas and beans, soybeans, and nuts	Magnesium Fiber Zinc

Highlights of Nutrient-Dense Foods

Nutrients of public health concern for underconsumption include calcium, fiber and vitamin D.[10]

As dental health professionals, we should focus for education on the following key ideas:

- 85% of calories per day should be focused on meeting the food group recommendations of the *Dietary Guidelines* leaving only 15% of calories for added sugars and saturated fat.[10]
- Meet recommended intakes with energy needs by adopting balanced dietary habits using the U.S.-Patterns, *MyPlate*, Mediterranean-style pattern (see Fig. 6.7), DASH Eating Plan (see Chapter 12), or Healthy Vegetarian Eating Pattern (see Table 5.5) as a guide for food choices.
- Consume a sufficient amount of fiber-rich fruits and vegetables while staying within energy needs. Per day, 2 c-eq of fruit and 2½ c-eq of vegetables are recommended for a reference 2000-cal intake, with higher or lower amounts depending on the calorie level.
- Choose a variety of fruits and vegetables each day. In particular, select from all five vegetable subgroups (dark green, orange and red, legumes, starchy vegetables, and other vegetables) several times a week.
- Adding more fruits, vegetables, whole grains, and fat-free or low-fat dairy products may have beneficial health effects and provide good sources of nutrients commonly lacking in American diets.
- Consume 3 or more oz-eq per day of whole-grain products, with the rest of the recommended grains coming from enriched products. In general, at least half the grains should come from whole grains.
- Replace most refined-grain food choices with whole-grain foods that are nutrient dense (low in added sugars and fats) to keep total calorie intake within limits.
- Because fruit juices contain little or no fiber, whole fruits (fresh, frozen, canned, or dried) are preferable choices.
- Protein-containing foods are important, but most Americans consume adequate amounts; therefore for most, including seafood as part of the protein foods is important to meet recommendations.
- Keep total fat intake between 20% and 35% of calories for adults, with most fats coming from sources of polyunsaturated and monounsaturated fatty acids, such as fish, nuts, and vegetable oils. The recommendation for total fat intake is higher for toddlers (30%–40%) and for children and adolescents (25%–35%).[10]
- When selecting and preparing meat, poultry, dry beans, and dairy products, choose lean, low-fat, or fat-free options to decrease intake of saturated fats and calories.

Nutrients to Limit

Dental providers should also focus on the following areas in regard to nutrients to limit when educating patients.

Total Calorie Intake

The U.S.-Patterns indicate food group and nutrient recommendations for calorie needs, which can only be achieved by choosing foods in a nutrient-dense form (without added sugar and lean and/or very-low-fat dairy and protein foods). To remain within a specific calorie range, a limited number of calories

• BOX 1.2   Alternative Names for Added Sugars on Food Labels

Agave	Invert sugar
Beet sugar	Malt sugar
Brown sugar	Mono- and disaccharides ending
Cane sugar/juice	in *-ose* (e.g., dextrose, glucose,
Coconut palm sugar (or coconut sugar)	fructose, lactose, maltose, sucrose)
Confectioner's sugar	Molasses
Corn syrup, high-fructose corn syrup	Palm sugar
	Raw sugar
Date sugar	Syrups (malt, corn, brown rice,
Evaporated cane juice	malt, maple, refiner's sorghum)
Fruit juice concentrate	Trehalose
Fruit sugar	Turbinado sugar
Honey	

(approximately 250–300 calories per day) are available after eating the specified amounts of all the food groups, and this is based on choosing nutrient-dense foods (see Fig. 1.2). These additional calories can be used for foods that are not nutrient dense (added sugars, additional refined starches, or fats) or to eat more than the recommended amount of nutrient-dense foods. Many foods in the American food supply provide excess calories without meeting food group recommendations to provide necessary nutrients and this excess may lead to weight gain and risk for chronic disease.

Added Sugars

Naturally occurring sugars found in fruits and milk are not added sugars. The various names for added sugars that may appear on nutrition labels are listed in Box 1.2. Consumption of foods containing added sugars makes it difficult to obtain adequate nutrients without weight gain.

Sugars, whether they are naturally present or added to the food, and grains supply physiologic energy in the form of glucose. The physiologic response of naturally occurring sugars is similar to the response from added sugars, but added sugars supply calories with few or no nutrients. Additionally, the amount, frequency, and duration of added sugar consumption are important factors in caries risk by increasing exposure to cariogenic substrates.[21]

The recommendation is to limit added sugars to less than 10% of calories per day.[10] At lower calorie levels (below 2000 calories), the amount of calories remaining after meeting food group recommendations, even using nutrient-dense foods, is less than 10% per day of the total calorie goal.[10] The limited amount of added sugars can be used to improve the palatability of nutrient-dense foods as long as calories from added sugars do not exceed 10% per day, total carbohydrate intake remains within the AMDR, and total calorie intake remains within limits.

Nonnutritive sweeteners (saccharin, aspartame, acesulfame potassium [Ace-K], and sucralose) can replace added sugars to reduce calorie intake. While much debate surrounds their use in regard to their value with weight loss, recent systematic reviews and a meta-analysis support their value as a component of weight loss to reduce added sugars in the diet.[22,23] Moderate intake of these high-intensity sugars has been deemed safe for the general population.

Saturated Fats, Trans Fats, and Cholesterol

Usually, high fat intake (more than 35% of calories) is associated with a higher intake of saturated fat, cholesterol, and excess calories. These unnecessary lipid components of food may raise undesirable blood lipids. On the other hand, if fat intake is less than 20% of calories, it may negatively impact adequate intakes of fat-soluble vitamins and essential fatty acids.[24]

Saturated fatty acids should provide less than 10% of calories and should be replaced with monounsaturated and polyunsaturated fatty acids while keeping total dietary fats within the age-appropriate AMDR. There is no dietary requirement of saturated fats for persons 2 years and older because the human body produces more than enough to meet physiologic and structural requirements. Solid fats usually contain a high percentage of saturated fatty acids. Saturated fats are consumed as food (high-fat meats and dairy products) or as ingredients in mixed dishes (e.g., burgers, pizza, hamburgers, tacos, baked goods, oils used to fry foods). These fats, abundant in the American diet, contribute significantly to excess calorie intake and exceeding the 10% per day recommendation. Only 23% of individuals meet the recommendation for less than 10% of calories from saturated fat.[10]

Trans fatty acids are no longer allowed in foods, but naturally occurring *trans* fats produced by ruminant animals are present in small quantities in dairy products and meats. They do not have the same undesirable effects as commercially produced *trans* fats.

Cholesterol is a very important component in the body for physiologic and structural functions, but adequate amounts are naturally produced; making dietary cholesterol unnecessary. Individuals should eat as little dietary cholesterol as possible while consuming a healthy diet. As a general rule, foods high in fats, such as fatty meats and high-fat dairy products, are also high in cholesterol and saturated fats. Because the U.S.-Pattern limits saturated fats, dietary cholesterol is naturally low—100 to 300 mg of cholesterol. Current intake in adults 20 years of age and older is 314 mg/day.[13] Dietary cholesterol is present only in animal foods such as egg yolk, high-fat dairy products, shellfish, meats, and poultry. Eggs and shellfish are high in dietary cholesterol but not in saturated fats.

Sodium

Sodium is an essential nutrient, but the body requires relatively small quantities available from naturally occurring sodium in foods. The natural sodium content of food only accounts for a small amount of total intake. Manufacturers and food establishments add significant amounts of sodium to prepare foods. Major sources of sodium for the US population are sandwiches including burritos and tacos (21%) followed by other prepared foods.[10] Because 71% of the sodium consumed in American diets is from processed foods,[25] the goal should be to reduce sodium added during food processing and choose more fresh and minimally processed foods.

Most Americans consume an average of 3463 mg sodium daily;[13] the recommended intake (per the *Dietary Guidelines* and CDRR [Chronic Disease Risk Reduction] level from the National Academy of Medicine) is less than 2300 mg per day for adults and children aged 14 years and older.[10] The Healthy U.S.-Style Dietary Pattern provides approximately 1,000-2,000 mg/day of sodium leaving little room for discretionary sodium intake.[10]

In general, high dietary sodium intake is associated with greater risk for cardiovascular disease and **hypertension** (high blood pressure).[26,27] Hypertension increases an individual's risk of CVD, stroke, congestive heart failure, and kidney disease. The DASH diet is recommended for people with hypertension (see Chapter 12).[28] The *Dietary Guidelines* include the DASH dietary pattern as one of the choices for a Healthy U.S.-Style Dietary Pattern.[10]

Highlights of Nutrients to Limit

- Consume a variety of nutrient-dense foods and beverages within and among the basic food groups while limiting foods containing saturated fats, cholesterol, added sugars, salt, and alcohol.
- Consume less than 2300 mg of sodium (approximately 1 tsp of salt) per day. Individuals aged 51 years and older; all African Americans; and people with hypertension, diabetes, or chronic kidney disease should further reduce intake to 1500 mg sodium per day.[29]
- Processed meats and poultry are preserved by smoking, curing, salting, and/or the addition of chemical preservatives. Processed meats, such as hot dogs and luncheon meats, contain larger amounts of sodium and saturated fats. However, these products can be part of the diet as long as sodium, saturated fats, and total calories are within limits of the U.S.-Pattern.
- To decrease intake of saturated fats, lean cuts of meat and skinless poultry should be chosen. Seafood, nuts, and seeds should replace some of the protein foods, as they are higher in monounsaturated and polyunsaturated fatty acids.
- Read nutrition labels and choose and prepare foods with less sodium.
- Choose fresh or frozen vegetables over canned versions.
- For 2000 cal per day intake, solid fats and added sugars should comprise no more than 250 to 300 cal.[10]
- Limit consumption of refined grains to three servings daily, especially those containing solid fats, added sugars, and sodium.
- Reduce the incidence of dental caries by practicing good oral hygiene and consuming sugar- and starch-containing foods and beverages less frequently.

Other Dietary Components

Alcohol

Alcohol is not a component of the U.S.-Pattern but as a substance frequently chosen by Americans, contributes to overall calorie intake. Alcoholic drink consumption was 45% in the US and 52% in Canada.[30] For adults in the US, this represented approximately 17% of total calorie intake and in Canada accounted for 11.2% of daily energy.[30,31] Females who are pregnant or anticipate a pregnancy should not consume alcohol.

Alcohol consumption can have beneficial or harmful effects depending on the amount consumed, age, and other characteristics of the person consuming the alcohol.[32] In particular, low alcohol consumption (0 to 1 drink/day) was associated with lower risk for renal cancer and dementia along with decreased mortality from colorectal cancer and hypertension.[32] Moderate alcohol intake (1–2.5 drinks/day) was associated with decreased renal cancer risk, CVD in individuals with hypertension, and all-cause mortality in those with hypertension.[32] At all levels of consumption there was a greater risk of basal cell carcinoma and at moderate and heavy levels of alcohol intake (>2.5 drinks/day) the risk for squamous cell carcinoma increased.[32]

Because alcoholic beverages supply calories with few nutrients, adequate nutrient intake without weight gain is difficult with excessive alcohol consumption.

The U.S.-Pattern categorizes adult beverages as drink-equivalents. One alcoholic beverage contains 14 g (0.6 fl oz) of pure alcohol. One alcoholic drink-equivalent (oz-eq) is defined as 12 fluid oz of regular beer (5% alcohol), 5 fluid oz of wine (12% alcohol), or 1.5 fluid oz of 80 proof distilled spirits (40% alcohol). If alcohol is consumed, it should be in moderation—up to one drink per day for females and limited to two drinks per day for males, and only for adults of legal drinking age. Moderation is not intended as an average over several days, but rather as the amount consumed on any single day.

Caffeine

Caffeine is a dietary component (not an essential nutrient) for many Americans. Caffeine functions as a stimulant in the body. Popular plant sources of naturally occurring caffeine are coffee beans, tea leaves, cocoa beans, and kola nuts, consumed as coffee, tea, and soda. Caffeine is also added to foods and beverages, such as caffeinated soft drinks, sports drinks, and energy drinks. Caffeine added to foods and beverages must be included in the ingredient list on the food label.

The amount of caffeine in frequently consumed beverages varies widely (see Box 12.1). Average intake of caffeine in the US is approximately 186 mg per day, although the Food and Drug Administration considers 400 mg per day the highest safe amount.[33,34] Females who are pregnant or capable of becoming pregnant, or breastfeeding, should follow the advice of their health care providers regarding caffeine consumption. However, low to moderate amounts (less than 300 mg/day) or about 2 to 3 cups of coffee do not adversely affect the infant.[10] Further discussion about the health effects of caffeine is provided in Chapter 12.

Highlights of Other Dietary Components

- Moderate coffee consumption (3–5 8-oz cups/day or up to 400 mg/day of caffeine)[34] can be incorporated into healthful eating patterns, but people who do not currently consume caffeine (in various forms) are not encouraged to begin.
- Adults of legal drinking age should consume alcoholic beverages in moderation—up to one drink daily for females and two drinks per day for males.
- Alcohol use is the third leading cause of death in the US. Excessive drinking is an important public health problem, not limited to college-age individuals.[35]
- Alcoholic beverages should not be consumed by some individuals, including those who cannot limit their alcohol intake; females of childbearing age who may become pregnant; pregnant and lactating females; children and adolescents; or individuals taking prescription or over-the-counter medications that can interact with alcohol, those engaging in activities requiring attention, skill, or coordination (e.g., driving or operating machinery), and those with specific medical conditions (e.g., liver disease, hypertriglyceridemia, and pancreatitis).
- Alcohol should not be mixed with caffeinated beverages or energy drinks; the stimulant effect of the caffeine may mask the depressant effect of the alcohol leading to higher consumption and possible risky behaviors such as drunk driving.[36] Alcohol mixed with energy drinks (AmED) is common in young adults and college students with a global prevalence of 37%.[36]

Physical Activity Guidelines

The principal focus of the *Dietary Guidelines* is to ensure that Americans choose foods that promote overall health and well-being.

Part of the objective to improve and/or maintain health and prevent chronic disease includes maintaining a healthy weight. Excess weight contributes to many health problems, including CVD, diabetes, and hypertension. Because of the prevalence of overweight and obesity, the *Dietary Guidelines* frequently mentions the other side of the balance—calorie expenditure, which is a significant factor in attaining and maintaining a healthy weight.

Physical Activity

Regular physical activity and physical fitness are important factors for an individual's health, sense of well-being, and maintenance of a healthy body weight. Physical activity is defined as any body movement produced by skeletal muscles resulting in energy expenditure. Physical activity is not the same as physical fitness. Physical fitness is related to the ability to perform physical activity. People with high levels of physical activity are at lower risk of developing chronic diseases, whereas a sedentary lifestyle increases the risk of weight gain and overweight, obesity, and the development of many chronic diseases.[37] Physically active individuals have longer life expectancies with better quality of life.[38] Furthermore, physical activity can help manage depression and anxiety.[39,40]

Recommendations are for 150 minutes per week of moderate-intensity aerobic activity and muscle strengthening two or more days a week.[41] Muscle strengthening includes, but is not limited to, use of resistance bands, lifting weights, using body weight for resistance, and some forms of yoga. Weight-bearing exercise like walking, jogging, dancing, pickleball, tennis, basketball, etc. increases peak bone mass during growth, maintains peak bone mass during adulthood, and reduces the rate of bone loss during aging.[42] It also may reduce the risk of osteoporosis and sarcopenia (muscle wasting).[42] Also, regular exercise can help prevent falls, common sources of injury, and disability in older adults.[42]

Physical activity may be accomplished in short bouts (10-minute periods) of moderate-intensity activity performed three to six times during the course of a day; the cumulative total is the factor in improving health status and increasing calorie expenditure. This makes it easier to plan a daily food intake pattern providing recommended nutrient requirements without exceeding calorie requirements.

In addition to physical activity, a nutrient-dense healthy diet without excess calories enhances the health of most Americans. In general, individuals should become more mindful of what they eat and their physical activity level. The *Dietary Guidelines* encourage adherence to the Physical Activity Guidelines for Americans (https://health.gov/our-work/nutrition-physical-activity) to help promote health, reduce the risk of chronic disease, and achieve and maintain a healthy body weight.

Highlights of Physical Activity Guidelines

- To prevent gradual weight gain over time, make small decreases in calories from foods and beverages and increase physical activity.
- Engage in regular physical activity and reduce sedentary activities to promote health, psychological well-being, and a healthy body weight.
- For adults to reduce the risk of chronic disease: Engage in at least 30 minutes of moderate-intensity physical activity, beyond usual activity, on most days of the week.

DENTAL CONSIDERATIONS

- The *Dietary Guidelines* do not necessarily apply to individuals with conditions that interfere with normal nutrition and require a special diet.
- Nutrient-dense foods provide substantial amounts of vitamins and minerals in relation to the calories. Suggestions for foods to recommend can be found in *MyPlate* and the *Dietary Guidelines*.
- Fats provide energy and essential fatty acids, and are important for absorption of fat-soluble vitamins A, D, E, and K, and carotenoids.
- *Trans* fats from natural sources are not considered detrimental.
- Provide the patient with a definition or example of moderation (e.g., 1 tsp salt per day or 5-oz glass of wine for a female per day).
- Many patients understand the general concepts of healthy eating, but they lack specific knowledge or motivation to help implement the recommendations. Most questions or misunderstandings are related to portion size and types of foods in each food group.
- Dental hygienists should be knowledgeable enough to provide foundational information about the food groups, whole grains, types of fats, and physical activity.
- Assess each patient's diet to determine adequacy or inadequacy related to the food groups in *MyPlate* and the *Dietary Guidelines* (For example, if a patient eliminates fruits and vegetables, vitamins A and C may be inadequate; if milk and other milk products are eliminated, calcium and vitamin D deficiencies may develop).
- Ensure that patients are aware of the number and size of servings recommended from each food group daily to obtain adequate nutrients.
- Although consumers are aware that they need to make positive dietary and lifestyle changes, putting that advice into practice is challenging and confusing (Fig. 1.4).
- The healthy eating index (HEI) scores for Americans aged 2 years and older, ranges from 51 to 63 (on a scale of 0 to 100).[10] This suggests health care providers have a key role to play in educating patients and encouraging them to choose more nutrient-dense foods.
- Remind patients that a serving size is a measured amount of food or drink (as indicated on a nutrition label) and portion is the amount actually consumed.

- Within each food group, individual foods can vary widely in the number of calories furnished; therefore knowledge about serving sizes is important.
- If nutrient-dense foods are selected from each food group in the amounts recommended, a small amount of discretionary calories can be consumed as added fats or sugars, alcohol, or other foods.
- Dairy products are poor sources of iron and vitamin C, but they are good sources of protein, Vitamins A and D, calcium, and riboflavin.
- Calorie consumption can be decreased by substituting low-fat or skim milk for whole milk. The nutrient content is the same for whole milk and low-fat milk, except for the amount of fat and calories. Skim milk (1%) or fat-free milk is recommended for all healthy Americans older than age 2 years.
- Foods in the grains group are economical as well as nutritious; they may be staple items for those in lower socioeconomic groups. However, whole-grain products may be more expensive; thus encourage patients to increase these food choices as much as possible.
- Elimination or reduction of one or more food groups will reduce the variety of food intake, thereby reducing the number or amount of nutrients consumed.
- Adults trying to lose weight should choose the lower amounts of servings from all groups and limit portion sizes.

NUTRITIONAL DIRECTIONS

- The *Dietary Guidelines* support healthy eating patterns to improve overall health and quality of life, as shown in the sample menu in Fig. 1.5.
- Choosing foods that follow the *Dietary Guidelines* will provide all the nutrients needed for growth and health.
- Make your plate look like a rainbow—consume dark-green, orange, and red vegetables; legumes; fruits; whole grains; and low-fat milk and milk products.
- Choose fewer refined grains, total fats (especially saturated fats), added sugars, and calories.
- Read food labels when choosing foods high in fiber or low in fats to determine whether the calories or grams of sugar have increased.
- Limit saturated fat intake to 20 g or less if trying to limit intake to 2000 cal daily.
- Fruits, vegetables, grains, and dairy products are important sources of many nutrients but should be chosen wisely, within the context of a calorie-controlled diet.
- By reducing frequency and duration of oral exposure to fermentable carbohydrate intake and optimizing oral hygiene practices, such as drinking fluoridated water, brushing, and flossing, dental caries can be minimized.
- A person's preference for salt is not fixed; the desire for salty foods tends to decrease after consuming foods lower in salt for a period of time.
- The recommended dietary fiber intake is 14 g per 1000 cal consumed.

- To help adults manage body weight and prevent gradual unhealthy body weight gain: Engage in approximately 60 minutes of moderate- to vigorous-intensity activity on most days of the week while not exceeding calorie intake requirements.
- For adults to sustain weight loss: Participate in at least 60 to 90 minutes of daily moderate-intensity physical activity while not exceeding calorie intake requirements (Some people may need to consult a health care provider before participating in this level of activity).
- For most adults, greater health benefits can be obtained by engaging in physical activity of more vigorous intensity or longer duration. Achieve physical fitness by including cardiovascular conditioning, stretching exercises for flexibility, and resistance exercises or calisthenics for muscle strength and endurance.

Support Healthy Eating Patterns for All

The final guideline discusses a social-ecological model for understanding individual lifestyle and motivators affecting food choices. To achieve a healthy eating pattern, food must be readily accessible and safe to eat (free from harmful diseases or bacteria). Food access is influenced by many factors, including distance to a store that stocks healthy foods, financial resources, and neighborhood-level resources (e.g., average income of the neighborhood and availability of public transportation).[43,44] An individual's perception and food preferences are also influenced by race/ethnicity, socioeconomic status, and geographic location (see Chapter 16).[45,46] The presence of a disability can limit access to healthy foods.

Healthy choices (both food choices and physical activity) should be supported by all systems (e.g., governments, education, health care, and transportation), organizations (e.g., public health, community, and advocacy), and businesses and industries (e.g., planning and development, agriculture, food and beverage, retail, entertainment, marketing, and media). All sectors have

Dietary Intakes Compared to Recommendations: Percent of the U.S. Population Ages 1 and Older Who Are Below and At or Above Each Dietary Goal

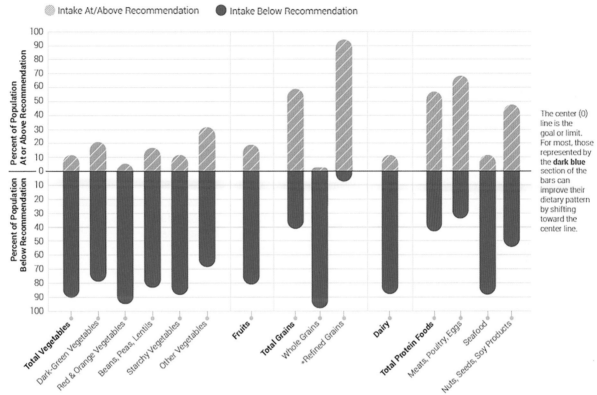

NOTE: Recommended daily intake of whole grains is to be at least half of total grain consumption, and the limit for refined grains is to be no more than half of total grain consumption.

Data Source: Analysis of What We Eat in America, NHANES 2013-2016, ages 1 and older, 2 days dietary intake data, weighted. *Recommended Intake Ranges:* Healthy U.S.-Style Dietary Patterns (see *Appendix 3*).

Dietary Guidelines for Americans, 2020-2025

• **Fig. 1.4** Dietary intakes compared to recommendations. Percent of the US population ages 1 year and older who are below and at or above each dietary goal. (From the U.S. Department of Agriculture and U.S. Department of Health and Human Services: *2020-2025 Dietary Guidelines for Americans*. 9th ed. U.S. Government Printing Office; 2020. DietaryGuidelines.gov.)

---

an important role in encouraging individuals to make healthy choices. Not only should the available food be healthy and affordable but foods must be safe (free of microbes and contaminants) to prevent foodborne illness (see Chapter 16).

MyPlate System

MyPlate is a part of a comprehensive communications initiative to promote healthy food choices. The *MyPlate* icon (Fig. 1.6), replaced the well-known *MyPyramid* symbol in 2011. The *MyPlate* food guidance system provides assistance in implementing the recommendations of the *Dietary Guidelines* and

the DRIs. About 25% of adults have heard of *MyPlate* as of 2020, and of those, about one-third had tried to follow the recommendations.[47]

The *MyPlate* icon is divided into four quadrants; each section is a different color that represents a food type. The quadrants indicate the recommended proportions on a plate for protein, grain, fruit, and vegetables at each meal, the same food groups discussed in the *Dietary Guidelines*. This icon does not indicate specific amounts to eat, however, portion sizes in relation to items consumers can relate to are shown in Fig. 1.3. The main message of *MyPlate* to consumers is: (1) fruits (red section) and vegetables (green section) should fill half the plate; (2) lean protein foods

Breakfast

1 ½ c frosted mini-wheat cereal
1 ½ c skim milk
12 oz black coffee

Mid-morning snack

12 oz water
1 oz (22) dry roasted almonds, unsalted
1 medium orange

Lunch

Sandwich with:
   1 c tuna salad with egg, low-calorie
     mayonnaise
   ¼ c thin sliced cucumber
   3 thin slices tomato
   Lettuce leaf
   2 thin slices 100% wheat bread
6 raw baby carrots
1 medium applesauce cookie
1 c grapes

Mid-afternoon snack

6 oz vanilla yogurt, low fat
12 oz herbal tea with low calorie
   sweetener

Dinner

3 oz pot roast beef, braised, lean only with
   ¼ c sauteed mushrooms
1 c white and wild rice blend,
   cooked with margarine and ¼ c
   vegetable juice
2 c garden salad with avocado, lettuce,
   tomato, carrots
   ¼ c shredded low fat Muenster
     cheese
   2 tbsp vinaigrette salad dressing
⅛ medium cantaloupe
12 oz tea with low calorie sweetener

Evening snack

3 c low fat microwave popcorn
12 oz water

Percent RDA for Female 19–30 years

Nutrient	Percent
Protein	260%
Carbohydrate	227%
Dietary fiber	128%
Added sugars	78%
Calcium	142%
Magnesium	163%
Phosphorus	300%
Iron	200%
Sodium	150%
Potassium	94%
Zinc	275%
Copper	235%
Selenium	305%
Thiamin	181%
Riboflavin	327%
Niacin	242%
Folate	228%
Vitamin B$_6$	192%
Vitamin B$_{12}$	445%
Vitamin C	197%
Vitamin A	185%
Vitamin D	73%
Vitamin E	100%
Vitamin K	282%

Percentage of calories:

Protein 22%
Carbohydrate 54%
Fat 27%

	Target	Eaten	Status
Grains	7 oz	7½ oz	OK
Vegetables	3 cups	3 cups	OK
Fruits	2 cups	2 cups	OK
Dairy	3 cups	2¾ cups	OK
Protein foods	6 oz	3½ oz	Over

• **Fig. 1.5** Making Healthy Choices: One Day at a Time. Sample menu based on the *Dietary Guidelines for Americans*. (From the U.S. Department of Agriculture and U.S. Department of Health and Human Services: *2020-2025 Dietary Guidelines for Americans*. 9th ed. U.S. Government Printing Office; 2020. DietaryGuidelines.gov.)

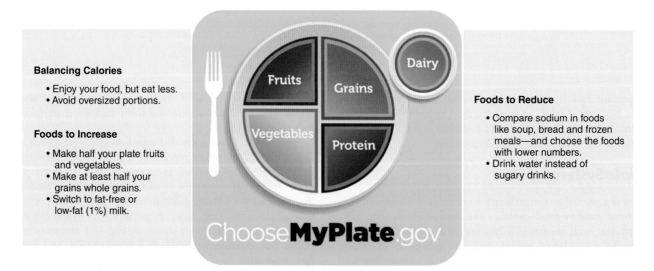

Balancing Calories

• Enjoy your food, but eat less.
• Avoid oversized portions.

Foods to Increase

• Make half your plate fruits
  and vegetables.
• Make at least half your
  grains whole grains.
• Switch to fat-free or
  low-fat (1%) milk.

Foods to Reduce

• Compare sodium in foods
  like soup, bread and frozen
  meals—and choose the foods
  with lower numbers.
• Drink water instead of
  sugary drinks.

Choose**MyPlate**.gov

• **Fig. 1.6** The *MyPlate* icon. (From United Stated Department of Agriculture. *MyPlate*. https://www. myplate.gov/.)

MyPlate, MyWins: Make it yours

Find your healthy eating style. Everything you eat and drink over time matters and can help you be healthier now and in the future.

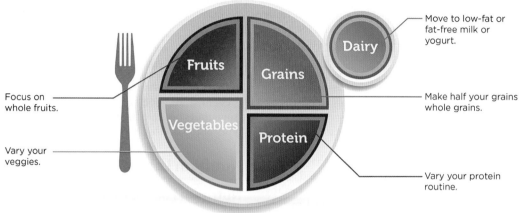

Focus on whole fruits.

Vary your veggies.

Move to low-fat or fat-free milk or yogurt.

Make half your grains whole grains.

Vary your protein routine.

ChooseMyPlate.gov

Limit the extras.
Drink and eat beverages and food with less sodium, saturated fat, and added sugars.

Create 'MyWins' that fit your healthy eating style.
Start with small changes that you can enjoy, like having an extra piece of fruit today.

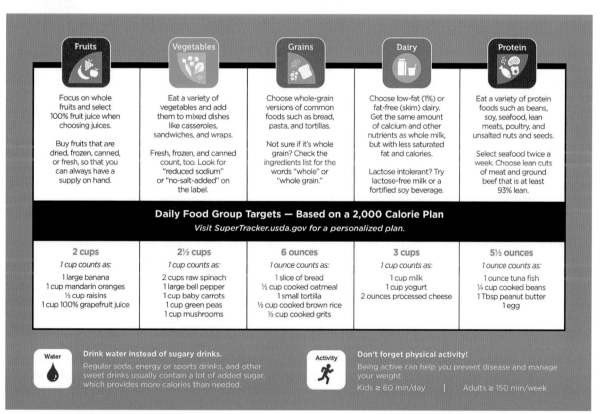

Fruits	Vegetables	Grains	Dairy	Protein
Focus on whole fruits and select 100% fruit juice when choosing juices.

Buy fruits that are dried, frozen, canned, or fresh, so that you can always have a supply on hand. | Eat a variety of vegetables and add them to mixed dishes like casseroles, sandwiches, and wraps.

Fresh, frozen, and canned count, too. Look for "reduced sodium" or "no-salt-added" on the label. | Choose whole-grain versions of common foods such as bread, pasta, and tortillas.

Not sure if it's whole grain? Check the ingredients list for the words "whole" or "whole grain." | Choose low-fat (1%) or fat-free (skim) dairy. Get the same amount of calcium and other nutrients as whole milk, but with less saturated fat and calories.

Lactose intolerant? Try lactose-free milk or a fortified soy beverage. | Eat a variety of protein foods such as beans, soy, seafood, lean meats, poultry, and unsalted nuts and seeds.

Select seafood twice a week. Choose lean cuts of meat and ground beef that is at least 93% lean. |

Daily Food Group Targets — Based on a 2,000 Calorie Plan
Visit SuperTracker.usda.gov for a personalized plan.

2 cups	2½ cups	6 ounces	3 cups	5½ ounces
1 cup counts as:	*1 cup counts as:*	*1 ounce counts as:*	*1 cup counts as:*	*1 ounce counts as:*
1 large banana
1 cup mandarin oranges
½ cup raisins
1 cup 100% grapefruit juice	2 cups raw spinach
1 large bell pepper
1 cup baby carrots
1 cup green peas
1 cup mushrooms	1 slice of bread
½ cup cooked oatmeal
1 small tortilla
½ cup cooked brown rice
½ cup cooked grits	1 cup milk
1 cup yogurt
2 ounces processed cheese	1 ounce tuna fish
¼ cup cooked beans
1 Tbsp peanut butter
1 egg

Drink water instead of sugary drinks.
Regular soda, energy or sports drinks, and other sweet drinks usually contain a lot of added sugar, which provides more calories than needed.

Don't forget physical activity!
Being active can help you prevent disease and manage your weight.
Kids ≥ 60 min/day | Adults ≥ 150 min/week

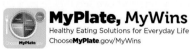

MyPlate, MyWins
Healthy Eating Solutions for Everyday Life
ChooseMyPlate.gov/MyWins

Center for Nutrition Policy and Promotion
May 2016
CNPP-29
USDA is an equal opportunity provider, employer, and lender.

• **Fig. 1.7** Start Simple with the *MyPlate* website. Used in conjunction with the *MyPlate* icon (Fig. 1.6), this concisely summarizes the food groups and portions providing 2000 calories. (From U.S. Department of Agriculture, Food and Nutrition Service. *Start Simple With MyPlate*. https://myplate-prod.azureedge.us/sites/default/files/2022-01/SSwMP%20Mini-Poster_English_Final2022_0.pdf.)

(purple section) should occupy one-fourth of the plate; (3) whole grains (brown section) should fill about one-fourth of the plate; and (4) dairy products (blue circle) should also be chosen. Fig. 1.7 is a concise synopsis of the *Dietary Guidelines*; it is available online in English and Spanish.

The key tool of this guidance system is the website, www. MyPlate.gov. The website is an interactive nutrition education tool intended to help consumers apply personalized dietary guidance to achieve a healthful lifestyle through better eating and increased physical activity. This website continues to evolve and expand to update information available.

The *MyPlate* homepage provides quick access to the food groups and their content, website organization for various age groups, social media sharing, access to online tools, and interactive quizzes to test basic nutrition knowledge. Most of the materials (brochures, tip sheets, graphics, and archived material) on the website are available in English or Spanish.

MyPlate serves as a simple, research-based icon that sends a clear message on proportionality (balance, variety, and moderation) and exemplifies what should be on a plate of healthy foods. The tools, particularly the graphics, are designed to help Americans make food choices adequate to meet nutritional needs. They also promote food choices moderate in energy level (calories) and in food components or nutrients often consumed in excess (fats, added sugars, and sodium). *MyPlate* is intended to be used as food guidance for the general public and not a therapeutic diet for any specific health condition.

The https://www.myplate.gov/ (also available in Spanish) provides numerous materials and useful information to help implement the principles of the *Dietary Guidelines* for both consumers and health professionals. Information is available for the different life stages (e.g., pregnancy, toddlers, preschoolers, teens, and adults), apps for cell phones (e.g., Shop Simple for budget friendly foods and Start Simple with *MyPlate*), *MyPlate* kitchen, activity planner, and more. The Start Simple app allows users to choose goals, see progress on goals in real-time, sync to a smartwatch, and earn badges for reaching goals.

Other Food Guides

Not all health care professionals agree that *MyPlate* is the ideal method to promote health and wellness. However, the recommendations on the *MyPlate* website are consistent with other population-based recommendations designed to control obesity, diabetes, CVD and stroke, hypertension, cancer, and osteoporosis. Although different guides were derived from different types of nutrition research and for different purposes, they share consistent messages: eat more fruits, vegetables, legumes, and whole grains; eat less added sugar and saturated fat; and emphasize plant oils.[48] Primary differences are in the types of recommended vegetables and protein sources, and the amount of recommended dairy products and total oil/fats. Overall nutrient values are also similar.

The recommendations on the *MyPlate* website are similar to the guidelines of the DASH eating plan (discussed in Chapter 12), the American Heart Association (discussed in Chapter 6), the American Diabetes Association (discussed in Chapter 7), the 2018 AHA/ACC/AACVPR/AAPA/ABC/ACPM/ADA/AGS/APhA/ASPC/NLA/PCNA Guideline on the Management of Blood Cholesterol, and the American Cancer Society. Calculated nutrient intakes associated with following any of these guidelines are generally within the ranges of nutrient recommendations of the *Dietary Guidelines*.

Canada's Food Guide

Canada has also developed a pictorial food guide to help Canadians choose food wisely (Fig. 1.8). *Canada's Food Guide* encourages consumers to find their own healthy lifestyle—a pot of gold. The website (https://food-guide.canada.ca/en/) is interactive, allowing consumers to personalize the food guide, providing recipes, tips for healthful eating and physical activity, and other educational materials.

Other Nations' Guides

Many nations eat very differently than Americans. No one food is essential for good health. People in many countries are healthy (sometimes healthier than Americans) despite eating very different types of foods. This is further discussed in Chapter 16.

Nutrition Labeling

Nutrition Facts Label

In a concerted effort by the USDA and FDA to help people make informed decisions about choosing foods to improve their health and well-being, the Nutrition Facts label graphic was designed. About 80% or 4 out of 5 adults report regularly reading the Nutrition Facts label.[49] Initially introduced approximately 20 years ago, the Nutrition Facts label was revised in 2016 to reflect new recommendations of the *Dietary Guidelines*, changes in the modern American diet, and to improve the graphics to make information clearer to consumers (Fig. 1.9).[50] The Nutrition Facts label enhances nutritional knowledge by focusing attention on information important for addressing current public health problems, such as obesity. The label indicates the nutrients in a food, enabling consumers to compare the nutrient content of various products. The labeling regulation requires that approximately 90% of all foods sold in the United States provide specific information based on the nutrient content, including imported foods.[50]

The USDA's Food Safety and Inspection Service requires packages of ground or chopped meat and poultry and the most popular whole, raw cuts of meat and poultry (such as chicken breast or steak) to have nutritional information either on the package labels or on display for consumers.[51] Currently, these products are labeled with the number of calories and grams of total fat and saturated fat in the product. For foods not packaged, the information must be displayed at the point of purchase (e.g., counter card, sign, or booklet). These nutrition labels differ from the Nutrition Facts label required by the FDA; the USDA's Food Safety and Inspection Service has proposed amending nutrition labeling for meat and poultry products to be more consistent with the FDA Nutrition Facts panel.

The updated design of the Nutrition Facts label requires calories and portion sizes to be in large bold type. Serving sizes more closely reflect the amounts of food Americans currently consume, but this amount may not be consistent with portion sizes. Packages containing between one and two servings (e.g., a 20-oz soft drink) list the calories and other nutrients as one serving because typically the full amount is consumed in one sitting. Individuals sometimes consume certain multi-serving foods in one sitting; these foods (e.g., one pint of ice cream) must indicate both "per serving" and "per package" calorie and nutrition information, displaying this information in a two-column format.

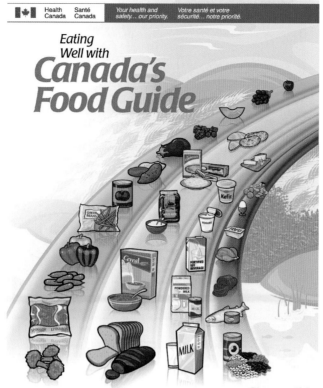

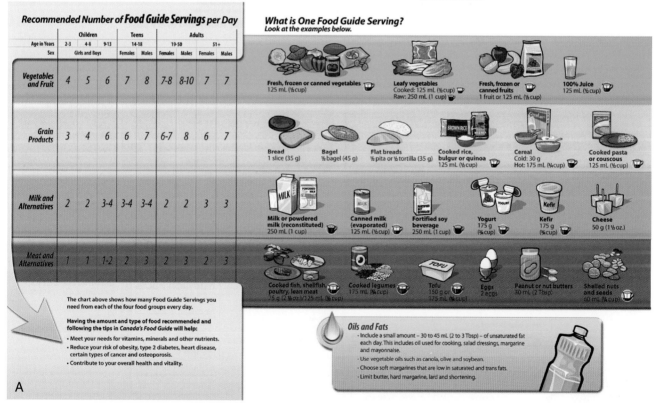

• **Fig. 1.8** Canada's food guide. (From Health Canada. *Canada's Dietary Guidelines. Canada Food Guide.* 2022. https://food-guide.canada.ca/en/guidelines/.)

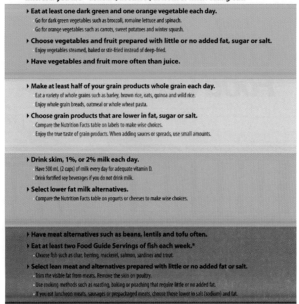

Make each Food Guide Serving count...
wherever you are – at home, at school, at work or when eating out!

▶ **Eat at least one dark green and one orange vegetable each day.**
- Go for dark green vegetables such as broccoli, romaine lettuce and spinach.
- Go for orange vegetables such as carrots, sweet potatoes and winter squash.

▶ **Choose vegetables and fruit prepared with little or no added fat, sugar or salt.**
- Enjoy vegetables steamed, baked or stir-fried instead of deep-fried.

▶ **Have vegetables and fruit more often than juice.**

▶ **Make at least half of your grain products whole grain each day.**
- Eat a variety of whole grains such as barley, brown rice, oats, quinoa and wild rice.
- Enjoy whole grain breads, oatmeal or whole wheat pasta.

▶ **Choose grain products that are lower in fat, sugar or salt.**
- Compare the Nutrition Facts table on labels to make wise choices.
- Enjoy the true taste of grain products. When adding sauces or spreads, use small amounts.

▶ **Drink skim, 1%, or 2% milk each day.**
- Have 500 mL (2 cups) of milk every day for adequate vitamin D.
- Drink fortified soy beverages if you do not drink milk.

▶ **Select lower fat milk alternatives.**
- Compare the Nutrition Facts table on yogurts or cheeses to make wise choices.

▶ **Have meat alternatives such as beans, lentils and tofu often.**

▶ **Eat at least two Food Guide Servings of fish each week.***
- Choose fish such as char, herring, mackerel, salmon, sardines and trout.

▶ **Select lean meat and alternatives prepared with little or no added fat or salt.**
- Trim the visible fat from meats. Remove the skin on poultry.
- Use cooking methods such as roasting, baking or poaching that require little or no added fat.
- If you eat luncheon meats, sausages or prepackaged meats, choose those lower in salt (sodium) and fat.

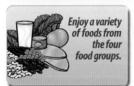

Enjoy a variety of foods from the four food groups.

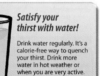

Satisfy your thirst with water!
Drink water regularly. It's a calorie-free way to quench your thirst. Drink more water in hot weather or when you are very active.

* Health Canada provides advice for limiting exposure to mercury from certain types of fish. Refer to www.healthcanada.gc.ca for the latest information.

Advice for different ages and stages...

Children

Following *Canada's Food Guide* helps children grow and thrive.

Young children have small appetites and need calories for growth and development.
- Serve small nutritious meals and snacks each day.
- Do not restrict nutritious foods because of their fat content. Offer a variety of foods from the four food groups.
- Most of all... be a good role model.

Women of childbearing age

All women who could become pregnant and those who are pregnant or breastfeeding need a multivitamin containing **folic acid** every day. Pregnant women need to ensure that their multivitamin also contains **iron**. A health care professional can help you find the multivitamin that's right for you.

Pregnant and breastfeeding women need more calories. Include an extra 2 to 3 Food Guide Servings each day.

Here are two examples:
- Have fruit and yogurt for a snack, or
- Have an extra slice of toast at breakfast and an extra glass of milk at supper.

Men and women over 50

The need for **vitamin D** increases after the age of 50.

In addition to following *Canada's Food Guide*, everyone over the age of 50 should take a daily vitamin D supplement of 10 µg (400 IU).

Eat well and be active today and every day!

The benefits of eating well and being active include:
- Better overall health.
- Lower risk of disease.
- A healthy body weight.
- Feeling and looking better.
- More energy.
- Stronger muscles and bones.

Be active

To be active every day is a step towards better health and a healthy body weight.

Canada's Physical Activity Guide recommends building 30 to 60 minutes of moderate physical activity into daily life for adults and at least 90 minutes a day for children and youth. You don't have to do it all at once. Add it up in periods of at least 10 minutes at a time for adults and five minutes at a time for children and youth.

Start slowly and build up.

Eat well

Another important step towards better health and a healthy body weight is to follow *Canada's Food Guide* by:
- Eating the recommended amount and type of food each day.
- Limiting foods and beverages high in calories, fat, sugar or salt (sodium) such as cakes and pastries, chocolate and candies, cookies and granola bars, doughnuts and muffins, ice cream and frozen desserts, french fries, potato chips, nachos and other salty snacks, alcohol, fruit flavoured drinks, soft drinks, sports and energy drinks, and sweetened hot or cold drinks.

Read the label
- Compare the Nutrition Facts table on food labels to choose products that contain less fat, saturated fat, trans fat, sugar and sodium.
- Keep in mind that the calories and nutrients listed are for the amount of food found at the top of the Nutrition Facts table.

Nutrition Facts
Per 0 mL (0 g)

Amount	% Daily Value
Calories 0	
Fat 0 g	0 %
Saturates 0 g	0 %
+ Trans 0 g	
Cholesterol 0 mg	
Sodium 0 mg	0 %
Carbohydrate 0 g	0 %
Fibre 0 g	0 %
Sugars 0 g	
Protein 0 g	

Vitamin A	0 %	Vitamin C	0 %
Calcium	0 %	Iron	0 %

Limit trans fat

When a Nutrition Facts table is not available, ask for nutrition information to choose foods lower in trans and saturated fats.

Take a step today...
- ✓ Have breakfast every day. It may help control your hunger later in the day.
- ✓ Walk wherever you can – get off the bus early, use the stairs.
- ✓ Benefit from eating vegetables and fruit at all meals and as snacks.
- ✓ Spend less time being inactive such as watching TV or playing computer games.
- ✓ Request nutrition information about menu items when eating out to help you make healthier choices.
- ✓ Enjoy eating with family and friends!
- ✓ Take time to eat and savour every bite!

For more information, interactive tools, or additional copies visit Canada's Food Guide on-line at:
www.healthcanada.gc.ca/foodguide

or contact:
Publications
Health Canada
Ottawa, Ontario K1A 0K9
E-Mail: publications@hc-sc.gc.ca
Tel.: 1-866-225-0709
Fax: (613) 941-5366
TTY: 1-800-267-1245

Également disponible en français sous le titre :
Bien manger avec le Guide alimentaire canadien

This publication can be made available on request on diskette, large print, audio-cassette and braille.

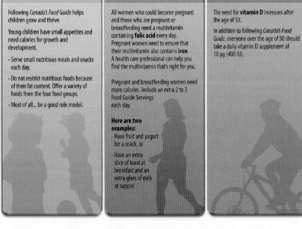

How do I count Food Guide Servings in a meal?

Here is an example:

Vegetable and beef stir-fry with rice, a glass of milk and an apple for dessert		
250 mL (1 cup) mixed broccoli, carrot and sweet red pepper	=	**2** Vegetables and Fruit Food Guide Servings
75 g (2½ oz.) lean beef	=	**1** Meat and Alternatives Food Guide Serving
250 mL (1 cup) brown rice	=	**2** Grain Products Food Guide Servings
5 mL (1 tsp) canola oil	=	part of your Oils and Fats intake for the day
250 mL (1 cup) 1% milk	=	**1** Milk and Alternatives Food Guide Serving
1 apple	=	**1** Vegetables and Fruit Food Guide Serving

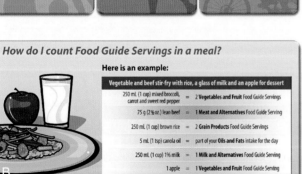

B

• **Fig. 1.8,** cont'd

Current Label

Nutrition Facts

8 servings per container
Serving size   **2/3 cup (55g)**

Amount per serving
Calories   **230**

	% Daily Value*
Total Fat 8g	**10%**
Saturated Fat 1g	**5%**
Trans Fat 0g	
Cholesterol 0mg	**0%**
Sodium 160mg	**7%**
Total Carbohydrate 37g	**13%**
Dietary Fiber 4g	**14%**
Total Sugars 12g	
Includes 10g Added Sugars	**20%**
Protein 3g	
Vitamin D 2mcg	10%
Calcium 260mg	20%
Iron 8mg	45%
Potassium 240mg	6%

* The % Daily Value (DV) tells you how much a nutrient in a serving of food contributes to a daily diet. 2,000 calories a day is used for general nutrition advice.

1. The serving size appears in large, bold font and some serving sizes were updated.
2. Calories are displayed in large, bold font.
3. Daily Values were updated.
4. Added sugars, vitamin D, and potassium are required on the label. Manufacturers must declare the amount in addition to percent Daily Value for vitamins and minerals.

• **Fig. 1.9** The Nutrition Facts Label. (From Food and Drug Administration. What's on the nutrition facts label. 9/27/2023. https://www.fda.gov/food/nutrition-facts-label/whats-nutrition-facts-label Accessed October 6, 2023.)

• BOX 1.3   **Daily Values as the Basis for Nutrition Facts Label for 2000 Calories/Day**

Total fat: 78 g
Total carbohydrate: 275 g
Dietary fiber: 28 g
Sodium: 2300 mg
Potassium: 4700 mg
Calcium: 1300 mg
Vitamin D: 20 µg

Data from FDA, Center for Food Safety and Applied Nutrition. *Daily Value on the Nutrition and Supplement Facts Labels.* FDA; 2023. https://www.fda.gov/food/nutrition-facts-label/daily-value-nutrition-and-supplement-facts-labels.

Because research indicates that the type of fat consumed is more important than the amount of fat, only total fat, and saturated fat amounts are listed. *Trans* fats appear on the label because ruminant sources, while not harmful, contribute to intake. Dietary fiber and total sugars that also indicate added sugars are all itemized under the bolded heading for Total Carbohydrate. Grams and percent daily value (%DV) for dietary fiber and added sugars must be listed. Only specific added fibers can be reflected in the carbohydrate count. Other fibers currently added to foods will be reviewed by the FDA before they can be counted. This may be confusing for consumers during the transition period. Consuming required nutrients and staying within one's calorie limit is difficult when added sugars make up more than 10% of the total calories.

Sodium, dietary fiber, and vitamin D are based on updated daily values, consistent with the National Academy of Medicine recommendations and *Dietary Guidelines* (Box 1.3). The updated footnote better clarifies the %DV and puts calories in the context

of the daily diet. Both the actual amount of nutrients and %DV are revealed for vitamin D, calcium, iron, and potassium. Survey data indicate that Americans do not consume adequate amounts of vitamin D and potassium. Vitamins A and C are no longer required because deficiencies are rare, but this information may be included voluntarily.

Daily Values (%) on the label provide a rough guide indicating whether the food contains a small or large amount of a nutrient for comparison purposes. Foods that provide 20% or more of the DV are considered high in a nutrient. The requirement to label products has resulted in reformulation of many foods to provide healthier products.

Nutrient Content and Health Claims

Two categories of claims currently can be used on foods in the United States: nutrient content claims and health claims. Nutrient content claims identify the nutrients in a product and provide information to assess its relative value.[52] Health claims describe a relationship between a food or food component and its ability to reduce risk of a disease or health-related condition.[53] These claims are based on a very high standard of scientific evidence.

Nutrient content claims describe the quantity of a nutrient in a product using words defined by the FDA, such as "free," "low," or "high." Comparative terms—such as "more" or "reduced"—can be used to indicate a difference to a similar food.[52] "Healthy," "lean," or "light" are descriptions of nutrient contents.[52] The food must meet FDA definitions to use these terms. A label cannot include an explicit or implied nutrient content claim unless it uses terms defined by the FDA. Box 1.4 defines some of the established terms and definitions used on food labels.

Health claims on foods require preapproval from the FDA; these are limited and regulated in an effort to protect consumers from false or misleading claims (Box 1.5).[53] Unqualified health claims must be supported by qualified experts agreeing that scientific evidence is available determining a relationship between a nutrient and a specific disease. Qualified health claims are supported by some evidence, but they lack significant scientific agreement; thus their claim must be accompanied by a disclaimer as specified by the FDA. Since 2002, when the FDA began allowing companies to petition for qualified health claims, fewer than 20 qualified health claims had been approved. A health claim must use the exact wording specified by the FDA.[53]

Additional Nutrition Labels

Many consumers are confused by the Nutrition Facts panel and prefer information in a quicker and easy-to-read format. Food manufacturers, supermarket chains, trade associations, and health organizations have developed comprehensive mechanisms to provide information about the nutritional quality of foods and beverages either on product packaging or shelf tags in retail setting nutrition labeling systems.

Since 1985, the American Heart Association has tried to make heart-healthy grocery shopping easier with its heart check symbol. A food has to meet certain criteria to qualify for using this symbol. The Whole Grain Council has different stamps indicating two different levels of whole grain in a serving (see Chapter 4). The Produce for Better Health Foundation's Have

• BOX 1.4 — Definitions of Commonly Used Nutrient Content Claims

Calories

- *Calorie free*: Fewer than 5 calories per RACC (reference amounts customarily consumed)
- *Low calorie*: 40 calories or less per RACC, or per 50 g of the food
- *Reduced or fewer calories*: At least 25% fewer calories per RACC than reference food

Fat

- *Fat free*: Less than 0.5 g of fat per RACC
- *Saturated fat free*: Less than 0.5 g per RACC per serving
- *Low fat*: 3 g or less per RACC, or per 50 g of the food
- *Reduced or less fat*: At least 25% less per RACC than reference food

Saturated Fat

Saturated fat free: Less than .05 g per RACC in main dishes
Low saturated fat: 1 r or less per RACC or less than 15% of calories
Less or reduced saturated fat: 25% less fat or more per RACC

Cholesterol

- *Cholesterol free*: Less than 2 mg of cholesterol and 2 g or less of saturated fat per RACC
- *Low cholesterol*: 20 mg or less or 2 g or less of saturated fat per RACC, or per 50 g of the food
- *Reduced or less cholesterol*: At least 25% less and 2 g or less of saturated fat per RACC than reference food

Sodium

- *Sodium-free*: Less than 5 mg per RACC
- *Low sodium*: 140 mg or less per RACC, or per 50 g of the food
- *Very low sodium*: 35 mg or less per RACC, or per 50 g of the food
- *Reduced or less sodium*: At least 25% less per RACC than reference food

Fiber

- *High fiber*: 5 g or more per RACC (foods with high-fiber claims must meet the definition for low fat or the level of total fat must appear next to the high-fiber claim)
- *Good source of fiber*: 2.5–4.9 g per RACC
- *More or added fiber*: At least 2.5 g more per RACC than reference food

Sugar

- *Sugar free*: Less than 0.5 g per RACC
- No added sugar, without added sugar, or no sugar added:
  - No sugars are added during processing or packaging, including ingredients that contain sugars (e.g., fruit juices, applesauce, or dried fruit).
  - Processing does not increase the sugar content to an amount higher than what is naturally present in the ingredients (a functionally insignificant increase in sugars is acceptable from processes used for purposes other than increasing sugar content).
  - The food that resembles it and for which it substitutes normally contains added sugars.
  - If it does not meet the requirements for a low- or reduced-calorie food, that product bears a statement that the food is not low calorie or reduced calorie and directs consumers' attention to the nutritional panel for additional information on sugars and calorie content.
- *Reduced sugar*: At least 25% less sugar per RACC than reference food

Healthy*

The regulatory criteria for use of the nutrient content claim "healthy" is being reevaluated, a lengthy process, but enforcement discretion may be exercised during this period. Products may use the term "healthy" in the product name or as a claim on the label or in the labeling of a food that is useful in creating a diet that is consistent with dietary recommendations. If the product is not low in fat, it should have a fat profile makeup of predominantly mono- and polyunsaturated fats (i.e., sum of monounsaturated fats and polyunsaturated fats are greater than the total saturated fat content of the food). The food must supply at least 10% of the Daily Value per reference amount customarily consumed (RACC) for at least one of six nutrients: vitamins A and C, calcium, iron, protein, or fiber, or if the food instead contains at least 10% of the DV of potassium or vitamin D. Whichever nutrient is used as the basis for eligibility should be declared in the Nutrition Facts label.

*From U.S. Department of Health and Human Services, Food and Drug Administration. *Use of the Term "Healthy" in the Labeling of Human Food Products: Guidance for Industry.* Center for Food Safety and Applied Nutrition; 2016. https://www.fda.gov/media/81606/download.

From U.S. Food and Drug Administration: *Food Labeling Guide.* https://www.fda.gov/media/81606/download

• BOX 1.5 — Health Claims Authorized by the US Food and Drug Administration

- Calcium and reduced risk of osteoporosis; calcium, vitamin D, and reduced risk of osteoporosis
- Sodium and increased risk of hypertension
- Dietary fat and increased risk of cancer
- Saturated fat and cholesterol and increased risk of heart disease
- Fiber-containing grain products, fruits, and vegetables, and reduced risk of cancer
- Fruits, vegetables, and grain products that contain fiber, particularly soluble fiber, and reduced risk of heart disease
- Fruits and vegetables and reduced risk of cancer
- Folate or folic acid and reduced risk of neural tube defects during pregnancy
- Noncariogenic carbohydrate sweeteners (D-tagatose, sugar alcohols, isomaltulose, sucralose) and reduced risk of dental caries
- Soluble fiber from certain foods (oat products, barley, and soluble fiber from psyllium husk) and reduced risk of coronary heart disease
- Soy protein and reduced risk of coronary heart disease
- Phytosterols and reduced risk of coronary heart disease

From FDA, Center for Food Safety and Applied Nutrition. *Authorized Health Claims That Meet the Significant Scientific Agreement (SSA) Standard.* FDA; 2022. https://www.fda.gov/food/food-labeling-nutrition/authorized-health-claims-meet-significant-scientific-agreement-ssa-standard

🦷 DENTAL CONSIDERATIONS

- The dental hygienist must ensure the best US-Dietary Pattern and calorie level usage based on the patient's life stage (e.g., toddler, preschooler, teen, adult).
- Review a nutrition label together with the patient and family. Ask the patient to bring in several labels of commonly used foods in the household for you to discuss.
- Encourage patients to keep portion sizes consistent with *MyPlate* and *Dietary Guidelines* along with activity level.
- On a label, point out the DVs that indicate calories (carbohydrate, fat, and protein), those indicating they should be limited (saturated fat, cholesterol, added sugars, and sodium), and how to determine whether a product contains a small or large amount of a nutrient (see Fig. 1.9).

NUTRITIONAL DIRECTIONS

- Read labels carefully. Ingredients are listed in order of quantity (by weight). Choose products that have less fat or oils or in which fats are listed last.
- Food labels are a useful tool to compare nutrient values of foods and learn valuable sources of nutrients. Fortified foods and supplements should not be purchased in an attempt to meet 100% of the RDAs because this may result in greater nutrient consumption than is needed, especially for young children. Concerns should be addressed to a health care provider or RDN.
- A product labeled "low fat" or "low sodium" may or may not be more healthy than another product. If possible, compare the Nutrition Fact labels from the modified product to the original version. In addition, the product may contain added sugar or other modified nutrients (e.g., sugar alcohols). Read the Nutrition Facts label carefully to identify the most nutrient-dense option.
- When looking at the Nutrition Facts label to compare products, consider portion sizes between products because these can vary.
- Products labeled as "dietetic," "sugar-free," or "reduced fat" may not be low in calories; this is dependent on other ingredients in the food.
- Unsweetened juices and milk contain significant amounts of natural sugars.

HEALTH APPLICATION 1

Obesity

The US population is leading the rest of the world in obesity, but this health problem has become a global issue—affecting around 14% of people worldwide.[54] Russia and the United States now have the most obese people in the world.[54] In the United States the prevalence of obesity was 41.9% in adults and 19.7% in children and adolescents according to NHANES data from 2017 to March 2020.[55] Those adults with obesity had higher medical costs than those with a healthy weight. Obesity is a threat to the world's future economy and could precipitate a catastrophic epidemic of diabetes.

As shown in Fig. 1.10, approximately 9.2% of adults were severely obese (more than 100 pounds over a healthy weight) in 2017–18, up from 4.7% in 2000.[56] Obesity is related to determinants of health and disproportionately affects racial and ethnic groups along with those with lower income and levels of education.[55] Non-Hispanic adults had the highest prevalence of obesity (49.6%) and severe obesity (13.8%).[56]

The goals of the *Healthy People 2020* (HP 2020) were to reduce the proportion of adults with obesity (NWS-03) from 38.6% at baseline (2013–16) to a target of 36%, however, with the initiation of the *Healthy People 2030* (HP 2030) cycle, the prevalence was worse at 41.8%.[5] In addition, there was an objective (NWS-04) to reduce the proportion of children and adolescents with obesity. Baseline for 2013–16 was 17.8% and the most recent data shows the prevalence increased to 19.7% so there has not been progress on meeting the objective of reducing childhood obesity to 15.5%.[5]

Other HP 2030 goals related to objectives to attain reduced obesity include (1) increase the proportion of health care visits by adults with obesity that include counseling on weight loss, nutrition, or physical activity (NWS-05); (2) six objectives related to physical activity of adults and include increasing aerobic and muscle strengthening activities (PA-10, PA-02, PA-03, PA-04, PA-05, and PA-10); (3) objectives related to increasing aerobic and muscle strengthening activities for adolescents (PA-06, PA-07, and PA-08) as well as increasing the proportion of adolescents who participate in daily school physical education (ECBP-01); and for children, there are objectives to increase aerobic activity (PA-09), engage in at least 60 minutes of physical activity/day at day care centers (PA-R01), and limiting screen time for children and adolescents (PA-13 and PA-R02).

According to the Obesity Prevalence Maps, obesity rates in three states exceed 40%, 19 states have rates between 35% and 40%, 22 states have rates between 30% and 35%, and all states have more than a 20% rate of obesity.[57] US adult obesity rates were highest in the Midwest and South and lowest in the Northeast and West.[57]

Preventing weight gain or maintaining a healthy weight is a major goal to reduce the burden of illness and its impact on reduction in quality of life and life expectancy. Obesity and overweight in adulthood go hand in hand with more than 21 diseases or conditions.[58] These include cardiovascular (hypertension, angina, heart failure, myocardial infarction, stroke), musculoskeletal (osteoarthritis, gout), endocrine (insulin resistance, type 2 diabetes), digestive (pancreatitis, liver disease), sleep apnea, respiratory (asthma), bacterial infections, skin (infections and eczema), anemia, renal failure, and certain types of cancers.[58] The conditions are interconnected and obese individuals with one condition are at 5 times higher risk for

developing a second condition and over 12 times higher risk for developing four conditions/diseases than individuals at a healthy weight.[58] Obesity along with many of these conditions is associated with risk for dental caries and periodontal disease so dental professionals are encouraged to provide education and support for healthy dietary patterns as part of the health care team.[59] These conditions impact life expectancy and quality of life.

Obesity affects many other aspects of life related to weight stigma or biases and discrimination: education, income, employability, and social position. Obesity also impacts psychological and social factors related to negative attitudes that affect interpersonal interactions.

Because overweight and obesity contribute to other health problems, their economic impact on the health care system is immense. Obesity costs more than $173 billion in health care costs in the United States and billions more in lost productivity.[60] Obesity-related medical costs in general are expected to rise significantly, especially because today's obese children are likely to become tomorrow's obese adults.[60] Reducing obesity could save billions of dollars for the health care industry.

Individuals who maintain a stable healthy weight throughout life have the lowest mortality.[61] Obesity and overweight at a young age are associated with adulthood obesity and premature death.[62] Because weight loss is so difficult, prevention of weight gain should be emphasized by health care providers.

BMI has been used as a screening tool for obesity and risk for chronic conditions. A high BMI has been considered a predictor of increased risk for mortality, but this is currently undergoing further investigation due to inconsistency in research findings.[63] Because BMI does not measure fat distribution, measures of abdominal fat may better identify risk factors for chronic disease.

Abdominal obesity increased in the United States through 2008 and waist circumference increased progressively and significantly from 37.6 inches in 1999 to 2000 to 38.8 inches in 2011 to 2012.[64] Excess fat in the abdominal area (the "apple-shaped" body) is characteristic of males, but some females also tend to accumulate more fat around the waist, especially after menopause. Accumulation of fat in the hips or thighs (the "pear-shaped" body") is typical of females. Several measures have been used to assess abdominal fat because it is associated with risk for chronic diseases such as diabetes.[65] The traditional measure has been waist circumference (WC), but other measures being explored include: a body shape index (ABSI), waist-to-height ratio (WtHR), and conicity index (CI) so health care providers need to monitor the changes that may emerge.[65]

A quick way to help determine fat intra-abdominal accumulation is waist-to-height ratio (compares the waist measurement to height). A rule of thumb to determine abdominal fat is that the waist measurement should be less than half of the person's height (Fig. 1.11). Waist-to-height ratio appears to be a more accurate predictor of cardiovascular and diabetes risk than BMI.[66]

Researchers worldwide continue to study which method of measurement is best for different genders and nationalities. Gold standard methods that determine body fat more accurately—such as magnetic resonance imaging (MRI), dual-energy x-ray absorptiometry (DEXA) scans, and bioelectrical impedance scales—are significantly more expensive and require specialized equipment.

(Continued)

◆ HEALTH APPLICATION 1

Obesity—cont'd

Obesity is a complex multifactorial disease with many contributing factors that include, but are not limited to, eating patterns and habits, physical activity, adequate sleep, genetics, certain conditions and medications, and social determinants of health (e.g., food insecurity, food deserts, access to safe environments for physical activity, socioeconomic status).[67] Ultimately consistent calorie overconsumption in excess of energy expenditure is a component of weight gain.

Genetic influence is a significant factor contributing to obesity. Body weight is affected by genes, metabolism, hormones, food choices, behavior, environment, culture, and socioeconomic status. Although genetics may increase the risk of weight gain, lifestyle changes may help to manage genetic risk.

The United States has cultivated an environment with an abundance of foods containing hidden fats and added sugars that can promote obesity. Many factors in the American culture have made food more accessible, including fast food restaurants, prepackaged food, and soft drinks. Fast foods account for 13.8% of total daily calories, averaging 309 calories/day and 36.5% of adults consume a fast food meal on a given day.[68] Non-Hispanic Black population consumes 17.4% of calories/day from fast food averaging 381 calories/day with 42.6% of adults consuming fast food on a given day.[68] However, more food purchases are made at grocery and convenience stores (63%–70% of total energy) as compared to fast food and full service restaurants (17%–26% of total energy).[69] The three food sources contributing to energy intake for children are grain-based desserts, yeast breads, and pizza; for adolescents, soda/sports drinks, pizza, yeast breads; and for adults, yeast breads, grain-based desserts, and chicken and chicken mixed dishes.[69] These foods tend to be high in added sugars, saturated fat, and sodium all of which are nutrients to be limited according to the *Dietary Guidelines*.

Weight loss of as little as 5% can have meaningful benefits for individuals with chronic disease like glycemic control in diabetes.[70] Recommendations are for 5% to 10% weight loss to provide additional benefit in risk reduction. However, weight loss is incredibly challenging so even though evidence shows a 5% weight loss has positive impact on comorbidities and health, the probability of success is low (1 in 10).[71]

Treatment of obesity has a high level of noncompliance and failure in part due to the multifactorial and complex nature of the disease. Four categories of determinants are involved in risk for weight regain and include: demographic (e.g., age, gender), behavioral (e.g., portion control, physical activity, self-monitoring of eating and weight), cognitive/psychological (e.g., mood/depression, body image, impulse control), and social and physical environmental determinants (e.g., social support, availability of healthy foods).

The incidence of obesity needs to be approached on four levels: (1) individuals need to be accountable for their food choices; (2) families must assume responsibility for foods available to their children, with parents acting as role models for healthful diet and exercise habits; (3) communities should provide opportunities for physical activity (parks, sidewalks, sports programs) and schools should provide appealing healthy food choices; and (4) more research is needed to identify optimal, effective ways of weight management.

Weight loss should be motivated by internal rather than external reasons ("I am doing this for myself," rather than "I will lose weight for my son's wedding") and requires a high level of motivation and long-term commitment for successful weight loss and maintaining a healthy weight. Weight loss involves a lifelong commitment to change one's lifestyle—regular physical activity, wise food choices, and behavior modifications.

While it is commonly believed that reducing energy intake by 3500 calories results in one pound of weight loss, this number dates back to 1958 and scientific knowledge has advanced significantly since that time. Currently mathematical equations for determining energy needs are being proposed to personalize calorie and physical activity plans for weight loss such as the Body Weight Planner (https://www.niddk.nih.gov/bwp) at the National Institute of Diabetes and Kidney Disease.[72,73]

The 3500 calorie rule significantly overestimates weight loss setting up people for disappointment. Weight loss may appear to occur fast initially due to changes in water, but in reality true fat loss is achieved slowly. A realistic goal regarding the rate and amount of weight loss must be established for each individual and using an evidence-based tool like the Body Weight Planner may be helpful. A 5% weight loss that is maintained may produce clinically relevant health improvement as previously noted.[70]

Numerous strategies have been implemented to treat overweight and obesity. No single treatment is best for everyone; each modality varies in effectiveness, risk, and cost. Review of evidence for the use of various drugs, medical devices, and surgical procedures currently being used for weight loss are beyond the scope of this text.

Popular weight loss diets are abundant. Although many different plans "guarantee" quick weight loss, no easy cure exists for weight loss. Ultimately, *diets don't work* and a healthy eating pattern like those recommended in the *Dietary Guidelines* and *MyPlate* website, regular physical activity, adequate sleep, behavior change, and stress management are the components of successful weight loss and maintenance. Setting realistic and measurable goals along with monitoring of progress are part of successful weight loss.[74] Being ready for occasional setbacks and recovering quickly support success.[74] The CDC has many resources available (https://www.niddk.nih.gov/health-information/weight-management/choosing-a-safe-successful-weight-loss-program). There are also resources for choosing a safe weight loss program (https://www.niddk.nih.gov/health-information/weight-management/choosing-a-safe-successful-weight-loss-program).

Planning is key to successful weight loss.

Indispensable to any weight-loss program is a preplanned food allotment. The *MyPlate* Plan tool (https://www.myplate.gov/myplate-plan) can be used to create a personalized plan. It provides the option of a plan to achieve a healthy weight for those who are overweight or obese. The plan can then be downloaded and it provides the number of servings for each food group. Favorite and preferred foods in each group can be selected and distributed over the day into meals and snacks to lessen feelings of deprivation, improve **satiety**, and minimize excessive food intake. Some "free" foods or beverages (foods containing less than 20 cal per serving) may be available for snacks, but regular mealtimes are important.

A weight-reduction diet should satisfy the following criteria: (1) meets all nutrient needs except energy, (2) suits tastes and habits, (3) minimizes hunger, (4) is accessible and socially acceptable, (5) encourages a change in eating pattern, and (6) favors improvement in overall health. Box 1.6 provides some questions to help determine the validity of a weight-reduction diet. Common reasons indicated for discontinuing a weight-loss regimen: (1) trouble controlling food choices, (2) difficulty motivating oneself to eat appropriately, and (3) using food as a reward.

Comprehensive lifestyle/behavioral therapy—including diet, physical activity, and behavior therapy provided by a skilled professional team of RDNs, exercise specialists, and behaviorists—have shown the highest success rate and is the cornerstone of effective treatment.[75] Behavior modification for weight control refers to getting in touch with the reality of foods being consumed and in what quantity, and when and why eating occurs (mindful eating). One of the most important components of an effective weight control program is learning new ways of dealing with old habits. Comprehensive behavior-modification programs include diet and physical activity programs individually tailored for patients. A team approach—including a health care provider, a psychologist, an RDN, and family members—is effective in helping the individual make necessary long-lasting changes in food choices and lifestyle behaviors. Self-monitoring of weight, food intake, physical activity, emotional status, and environmental factors help provide new insights to devise strategies for dealing with eating habits.[75]

Pharmacotherapy may be used in conjunction with lifestyle therapy and may be considered with health conditions that would benefit from weight loss such as diabetes.[75] Weight loss medications have come and gone over the past few decades. Some taken off the market include Redux (dexfenfluramine) and Belviq (lorcaserin). Currently the most popular drugs are used to manage diabetes such as semaglutide (Ozempic) and tirzsepatide (Mounjaro).[76]

◆ HEALTH APPLICATION 1

Obesity—cont'd

In more severe obesity (BMI ≥ 35) with one or more comorbidities, lifestyle therapy in addition to bariatric surgery (surgical procedure on the stomach or small intestine for weight reduction) may be the treatment of choice.[75] Bariatric surgery benefits have included greater weight loss, diabetes remission, reduced incidence of cardiovascular events, and hypertension.[77] Adverse side effects of bariatric surgery may include limited absorption or synthesis of many nutrients (e.g., selenium, copper, iron, B_{12}, riboflavin, folate, and vitamin K); increased risk for gastroesophageal reflux and dental erosion; and increased risk for fracture.[78–82]

The role of the oral health care professional (OHCP) in obesity is to identify health conditions that may impact oral and overall health and participate as part of an interprofessional team to refer and support the patient in making healthy choices and increasing physical activity to achieve a healthy weight.[83,84] Scoping reviews of the role of OHCPs in screening and counseling for obesity found a generally positive attitude, but the major barriers were fear of offending patients and lack of knowledge.[83,84] The approach should be non-judgmental and focus should be on the association between excess weight and link to oral health. The NIDDK has some tips for talking to patients about their weight which may be helpful.[85] A focus on the association between oral diseases (e.g., dental caries and periodontal disease)[59,86,87] and overweight and obesity along with use of national guidelines (*Dietary Guidelines* and *MyPlate*) for nutrition counseling will allow for the OHCP to be part of the team to address the obesity epidemic. OHCPs stepped up to learn to give vaccinations during the COVID-19 pandemic and this call to action is no different.

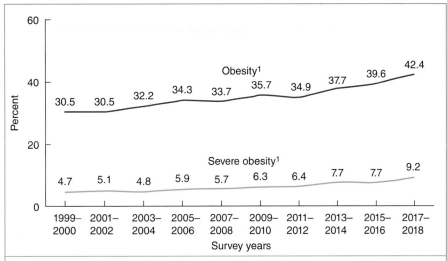

[1]Significant linear trend.
NOTES: Estimates were age adjusted by the direct method to the 2000 US. Census population using the age groups 20–39, 40–59, and 60 and over. Access data table for Figure 4 at: https://www.cdc.gov/nchs/data/databriefs/db360_tables-508.pdf#4
SOURCE: NCHS, National Health and Nutrition Examination Survey, 1999–2018.

Estimated Percentage by BMI

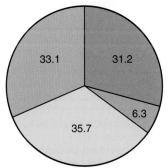

☐ Normal weight or underweight (BMI under 24.9)
☐ Overweight (BMI of 25 to 29.9)
☐ Obesity (BMI of 30+)
☐ Extreme obesity (BMI of 40+)

• **Fig. 1.10** (A) Trends in obesity and severe obesity among adults aged 20 and older, United States, 1999–2000 through 2017–18. (B) Trends in obesity and severe obesity prevalence among children and adolescents aged 2–19 years, by age: United States, 1963–65 through 2017–18. (Source: 1. Hales CM, Carroll, MD, Fryar, CD, Ogden CL. *Prevalence of Obesity and Severe Obesity among Adults: United States, 2017–2018*. National Center for Health Statistics; 2020:8. https://www.cdc.gov/nchs/data/data-briefs/db360-h.pdf.)

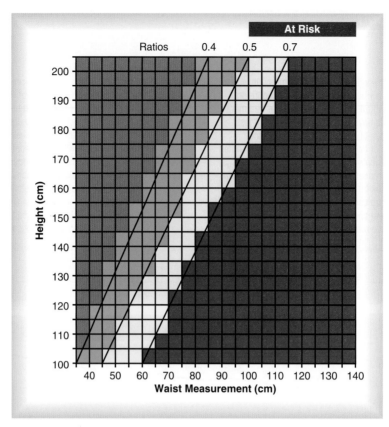

Waist-to-Height Ratio Less Than 0.5—Low Risk Level. The boundary at a ratio of 0.4 represents low risks for 'normal' body shape (green) and potentially slight risks from being underweight for height (brown).

Waist-to-Height Ratio Above 0.5—Moderate to High Risk Level. The boundary at a ratio of 0.6 represents moderate risks (yellow) and high risks (red).

• **Fig. 1.11** Waist circumference-to-height ratio chart. (Courtesy Dr. John Anderson.)

• BOX 1.6   Evaluating Weight Loss Diets or Programs

The program should evaluate the individual's body mass index and whether the weight is principally from increased fat stores or increased muscle mass and possible contributing factors.

The cost of the program should be realistic and reasonable.

The program should be adaptable for various lifestyles and something an individual can continue indefinitely.

Tips for Evaluating Safety and Effectiveness of Reduction Diets

1. Stay current with scientific research. Nutrition is a relatively new science, and new developments are still evolving to increase our knowledge base.
2. Evaluate diet trends and claims for effects on overall health.
3. Compare recommendations with known nutrition science and recommendations, such as *MyPlate* and *Dietary Guidelines for Americans.*
4. Review *MyPlate* and the *Dietary Guidelines* and compare to the diet the individual is considering to determine what food groups and nutrients would be lacking.
5. Evaluate diets using the following principles:
   • What is the weight loss recommendation?
   • What is the success rate of the program?
   • What is the basis for advertisements and endorsements?

   • Has any scientific research been done to evaluate the safety and effectiveness of the diet?
   • What is the cost of the program? Are special foods or nutrient supplements required and what do they cost? Are there other additional fees?
   • Is the program medically supervised?
   • Are any major food groups excluded?
   • Are the foods appealing to the individual? Does the program allow occasional consumption of favorite foods?
   • Is it permissible to eat in restaurants and other people's homes at least occasionally?
   • Are certain foods avoided because they cause specific problems?
   • Are certain foods used to "cure"?
   • Are dramatic statements made that contradict well-established nutrition principles or reputable scientific organizations?
   • Are exercise and behavior modification included?
   • Can an individual maintain the dietary pattern of the program for a lifetime?
   • Is there a maintenance plan?
   • Does it promote good heathy lifestyle habits?

◆ CASE APPLICATION FOR THE DENTAL HYGIENIST

A young healthy mother who has a 3-year-old son at home comes to the dental office for a 6-month recare appointment. She expresses concern about foods she should be eating and feeding her husband and son to improve and maintain their overall health for optimal growth and development of the child. She has learned a little about the food groups, the *Dietary Guidelines*, and nutrition labels from the press but does not know how to implement them.

Nutritional Assessment

- Willingness to seek nutritional information
- Desire for increased control of nutritional health habits
- Knowledge of community resources
- Cultural or religious influences
- Knowledge regarding the *Dietary Guidelines*, food nutrition fact labels, and *MyPlate* website
- Nutrition goals

Nutritional Diagnosis

Health-seeking behaviors related to lack of knowledge concerning optimal nutrition and current standards.

Nutritional Goals

The patient verbalizes correct information concerning the *Dietary Guidelines* and food labels and can name the food groups, the number of servings needed, and portion sizes from each group of *MyPlate* website.

Nutritional Implementation

Intervention: Ask the patient to write down everything she ate yesterday from the time she got up until the time she went to bed.
Rationale: This will help you tailor the information you provide to meet the patient's needs.
Intervention: Encourage variety of food intake, using *MyPlate* website. Review the number of servings needed and serving size.
Rationale: The total balance of food intake matters; the best balance incorporates variety to promote optimal nutrition. Providing the minimal number of servings prevents nutritional deficiencies in healthy individuals.
Intervention: (1) Suggest that the mother and her husband should undergo annual physical exams with blood labs if not recently done; (2) emphasize a decreased intake of saturated fats by trimming excess fat and eating smaller servings of meat (about the size of a fist or a deck of cards).
Rationale: Decreasing saturated fats helps reduce the risk of heart disease. By decreasing these saturated fats, total fat and cholesterol should be within acceptable AMDRs.
Intervention: (1) Stress the importance of eating vegetables, fruits, and grains, and (2) explain that complex carbohydrates are not fattening.
Rationale: Dietary fiber is important for healthy bowel functioning and decreases the risk of developing obesity, cancer, and diabetes.

Intervention: (1) Explain how to read labels for sugar. The names of most sugars end in "-ose." (2) Emphasize moderation of sugar intake. (3) Explain that "dietetic" and "sugar-free" do not mean that the product is low in calories. (4) Explain the relationship between sugar and tooth decay and emphasize the importance of proper oral hygiene after sugar consumption.
Rationale: Refined sugar contains calories and no other nutrients but is acceptable when used in items that contain appreciable amounts of other nutrients (e.g., a pudding would provide more nutrients than a gelatin dessert or carbonated beverage).
Intervention: (1) Stress using sodium and salt in moderation; (2) emphasize that "no salt added" does not mean that the product is low in sodium.
Rationale: Good habits that do not foster a high level of salt preference are recommended to reduce risk of high blood pressure.
Intervention: Emphasize that alcohol intake should be in moderation (one drink a day for females and two drinks a day for males).
Rationale: Alcohol is high in calories and contains few, if any, nutrients.
Intervention: (1) Review an entire label with the mother to help her understand how to interpret it. (2) Determine a serving size. (3) Explain the types of carbohydrates. (4) Determine the percentage of fat in a product by multiplying the grams of fat by 9, and compare this number with the total calories; if the amount is more than 30%, do not consume that product every day. (5) Emphasize that "no cholesterol" does not indicate that the product contains no saturated fat. (6) Point out the sodium level, and if it is greater than 400 mg, encourage its use in moderation.
Rationale: Knowledge increases compliance and allows informed choices regarding food choice.
Intervention: Refer the patient to county extension agencies or to a registered dietitian.
Rationale: These agencies and nutritional professionals provide practical guidelines through newsletters, workshops, and written materials for healthy patients wanting to improve health.

Evaluation

To determine effectiveness of care, the patient reads labels and chooses the most nutrient-dense choice. The patient states the basic guidelines for nutrition; the hygienist explains to her that serving sizes for her son are different than the standard serving size (available on the *MyPlate* website). Additionally, the patient should be able to plan a menu using recommended foods and state how to obtain and use community information/support. The patient should be able to indicate how changes in food choices would not only improve overall health, but also maintain health of the oral cavity and ensure optimal growth of her son while reducing risk of tooth decay.

---

a Plant Movement icon and Kraft's Sensible Solutions are other programs that have been developed. These food rating programs can help individuals make better food choices, as will the revised Nutrition Facts label. Furthermore, in order to make wise choices, food should be selected within the context of the whole diet.

The FDA is apprehensive about these different labeling programs, fearing they may mislead consumers about the health benefits of the food. Multiple systems may create more confusion, and other systems' criteria may not be stringent enough or consistent with the *Dietary Guidelines*. Another concern is that they may encourage consumers to choose highly processed foods and refined grains rather than fruits, vegetables, and whole grains.

The FDA has considered developing a single standardized guidance system for front-of-package labels. Whether all nutrition and health claims from the front of processed food packages will be eliminated is yet to be determined.

◆ Student Readiness

1. A patient asks you the difference between food and nutrition. What would you say?
2. Locate an advertisement on the internet or social media for a weight loss product or program and list the merits of the product or program stated in the ad. Then, list information about the product or program that might have been omitted or

should be questioned. Evaluate the product or program using information from Box 1.6.

3. Discuss popular weight loss diets and how they may have adverse effects.
4. Distinguish between nutrient recommendations and requirements.
5. Keep a record of all the foods you eat for 24 hours. Was your intake adequate as evaluated by the *Dietary Guidelines* and *MyPlate website?* In what areas did you do well? Where can you improve? Provide specific recommendations for making changes.
6. Collect nutrition labels for three similar products. Compare the nutrient values to determine which one is more nutrient dense (contains more vitamins and minerals and less saturated fat, sodium, and added sugars). Which is a better buy for the amount of nutrients it contains?
7. Discuss the pros and cons of allowing health claims on products.
8. If a food label indicates that one serving of the product has 23 g of carbohydrate and 15 g of sugar with 140 cal (total), how many teaspoons of sugar does the product contain? What percentage of carbohydrate does this product contain?

References

1. Academy of Nutrition and Dietetics. *Registered Dietitian Nutritionist Fact Sheet.* https://www.eatrightpro.org/acend/students-and-advancing-education/career-information/registered-dietitian-nutritionist-fact-sheet
2. Zorbas C, Palermo C, Chung A, et al. Factors perceived to influence healthy eating: a systematic review and meta-ethnographic synthesis of the literature. *Nutr Rev.* 2018;76(12):861–874.
3. USDA. *History of the Dietary Guidelines.* https://www.dietaryguidelines.gov/about-dietary-guidelines/history-dietary-guidelines
4. Healthy People 2030, US Department of Health and Human Services, Office of Disease Prevention and Health Promotion. *Social Determinants of Health.* https://health.gov/healthypeople/objectives-and-data/social-determinants-health
5. USDHHS, Office of Disease Prevention and Health Promotion. *Healthy People 2030.* https://health.gov/healthypeople
6. Hubbard K, Huang DT. *Healthy People 2020: An End of Decade Snapshot.* National Center for Health Statistics; 2021. https://health.gov/sites/default/files/2021-03/21%20HP2020EndofDecadeSnapshot2.pdf.
7. USDHHS, Office of Disease Prevention and Health Promotion. *Dietary Reference Intakes.* https://health.gov/our-work/nutrition-physical-activity/dietary-guidelines/dietary-reference-intakes
8. National Academies of Sciences, Engineering, and Medicine. *Guiding Principles for Developing Dietary Reference Intakes Based on Chronic Disease.* National Academies Press; 2017.
9. National Academies of Sciences, Engineering, and Medicine. *Expansion of the Dietary Intake Reference Model: Learning From Sodium and Potassium.* https://nap.nationalacademies.org/resource/25353/interactive/
10. U.S. Department of Agriculture, U.S. Department of Health and Human Services. *Dietary Guidelines for Americans.* 9th ed. 2020. dietaryguidelines.gov
11. English LK, Ard JD, Bailey RL, et al. Evaluation of dietary patterns and all-cause mortality: a systematic review. *JAMA Netw Open.* 2021;4(8):e2122277.
12. Dietary Guidelines Advisory Committee. *Scientific Report of the 2020 Dietary Guidelines Advisory Committee: Advisory Report to the Secretary of Agriculture and Secretary of Health and Human Services.* U.S. Department of Agriculture, Agricultural Research Service; 2020. https://www.dietaryguidelines.gov/2020-advisory-committee-report.
13. Agricultural Research Service, USDA. *What We Eat in America, NHANES 2017-2020.* Food Surveys Research Group; 2022. https://www.ars.usda.gov/ARSUserFiles/80400530/pdf/1720/Table_1_NIN_GEN_1720.pdf
14. Centers for Disease Control and Prevention. *All About Adult BMI.* Centers for Disease Control and Prevention; 2022. https://www.cdc.gov/healthyweight/assessing/bmi/adult_bmi/index.html
15. Shah NS, Luncheon C, Kandula NR, et al. Heterogeneity in obesity prevalence among Asian American adults. *Ann Intern Med.* 2022;175(11):1493–1500.
16. Kıskaç M, Soysal P, Smith L, Capar E, Zorlu M. What is the optimal body mass index range for older adults? *Ann Geriatr Med Res.* 2022;26(1):49–57.
17. Heyman MB, Abrams SA, Section on Gastroenterology, Hepatology, and Nutrition, et al. Fruit juice in infants, children, and adolescents: current recommendations. *Pediatrics.* 2017;139(6):e20170967.
18. Institute of Medicine (US) Committee on Use of Dietary Reference Intakes in Nutrition, Committee on Use of Dietary Reference Intakes in Nutrition on Labeling. *Overview of food fortification in the United States and Canada. Dietary Reference Intakes: Guiding Principles for Nutrition Labeling and Fortification.* National Academies Press (US); 2003. https://www.ncbi.nlm.nih.gov/books/NBK208880/.
19. Viswanathan M, Urrutia RP, Hudson KN, Middleton JC, Kahwati LC. Folic acid supplementation to prevent neural tube defects: updated evidence report and systematic review for the US Preventive Services Task Force. *JAMA.* 2023;330(5):460–466.
20. Nascimento GG, Leite FRM, Gonzalez-Chica DA, Peres KG, Peres MA. Dietary vitamin D and calcium and periodontitis: a population-based study. *Front Nutr.* 2022;9:1016763.
21. Alosaimi N, Bernabé E. Amount and frequency of added sugars intake and their associations with dental caries in United States adults. *Int J Environ Res Public Health.* 2022;19(8):4511.
22. Laviada-Molina H, Molina-Segui F, Pérez-Gaxiola G, et al. Effects of nonnutritive sweeteners on body weight and BMI in diverse clinical contexts: systematic review and *meta*-analysis. *Obes Rev.* 2020;21(7):e13020.
23. Rogers PJ, Appleton KM. The effects of low-calorie sweeteners on energy intake and body weight: a systematic review and meta-analyses of sustained intervention studies. *Int J Obes.* 2021;45(3):464–478.
24. Liu AG, Ford NA, Hu FB, Zelman KM, Mozaffarian D, Kris-Etherton PM. A healthy approach to dietary fats: understanding the science and taking action to reduce consumer confusion. *Nutr J.* 2017;16:53.
25. Harnack LJ, Cogswell ME, Shikany JM, et al. Sources of sodium in US adults from 3 geographic regions. *Circulation.* 2017;135(19):1775–1783.
26. Wang YJ, Yeh TL, Shih MC, Tu YK, Chien KL. Dietary sodium intake and risk of cardiovascular disease: a systematic review and dose-response *meta*-analysis. *Nutrients.* 2020;12(10):2934.
27. Filippini T, Malavolti M, Whelton PK, Vinceti M. Sodium intake and risk of hypertension: a systematic review and dose-response *meta*-analysis of observational cohort studies. *Curr Hypertens Rep.* 2022;24(5):133–144.
28. Filippou CD, Tsioufis CP, Thomopoulos CG, et al. Dietary Approaches to Stop Hypertension (DASH) diet and blood pressure reduction in adults with and without hypertension: a systematic review and *meta*-analysis of randomized controlled trials. *Adv Nutr.* 2020;11(5):1150–1160.
29. Whelton PK, Appel LJ, Sacco RL, et al. Sodium, blood pressure, and cardiovascular disease: further evidence supporting the American Heart Association sodium reduction recommendations. *Circulation.* 2012;126(24):2880–2889.
30. Vanderlee L, White CM, Kirkpatrick SI, et al. Nonalcoholic and alcoholic beverage intakes by adults across 5 upper-middle- and high-income countries. *J Nutr.* 2021;151(1):140–151.
31. Butler L, Poti JM, Popkin BM. Trends in energy intake from alcoholic beverages among US adults by sociodemographic characteristics, 1989-2012. *J Acad Nutr Diet.* 2016;116(7):1087–1100.e6.

32. Zhong L, Chen W, Wang T, et al. Alcohol and health outcomes: an umbrella review of *meta*-analyses base on prospective cohort studies. *Front Public Health*. 2022;10:859947.

33. Verster JC, Koenig J. Caffeine intake and its sources: a review of national representative studies. *Crit Rev Food Sci Nutr*. 2018;58(8):1250–1259.

34. Food and Drug Administration. *Spilling The Beans: How Much Caffeine Is too Much?* FDA; 2023. https://www.fda.gov/consumers/consumer-updates/spilling-beans-how-much-caffeine-too-much

35. American Public Health Association. *Addressing Alcohol-Related Harms: A Population Level Response*. APHA; 2019. https://www.apha.org/policies-and-advocacy/public-health-policy-statements/policy-database/2020/01/14/addressing-alcohol-related-harms-a-population-level-response

36. De Giorgi A, Valeriani F, Gallè F, et al. Alcohol mixed with energy drinks (AMED) use among university students: a systematic review and *meta*-analysis. *Nutrients*. 2022;14(23):4985.

37. Anderson E, Durstine JL. Physical activity, exercise, and chronic diseases: a brief review. *Sports Med Health Sci*. 2019;1(1):3–10.

38. Lee DH, Rezende LFM, Joh HK, et al. Long-term leisure-time physical activity intensity and all-cause and cause-specific mortality: a prospective cohort of US adults. *Circulation*. 2022;146(7):523–534.

39. Pearce M, Garcia L, Abbas A, et al. Association between physical activity and risk of depression: a systematic review and *meta*-analysis. *JAMA Psychiatry*. 2022;79(6):550–559.

40. Wanjau MN, Möller H, Haigh F, et al. Physical activity and depression and anxiety disorders: a systematic review of reviews and assessment of causality. *AJPM Focus*. 2023;2(2):100074. 4.

41. U.S. Department of Health and Human Services. *Physical Activity Guidelines for Americans*. 2nd ed.; 2018:118. https://health.gov/our-work/nutrition-physical-activity/physical-activity-guidelines/current-guidelines

42. American Association of Orthopedic Surgeons. *OrthoInfo: Exercise and Bone Health*; 2020. https://www.orthoinfo.org/en/staying-healthy/exercise-and-bone-health/

43. Drisdelle C, Kestens Y, Hamelin AM, Mercille G. Disparities in access to healthy diets: how food security and food shopping behaviors relate to fruit and vegetable intake. *J Acad Nutr Diet*. 2020;120(11):1847–1858.

44. Herforth A, Bai Y, Venkat A, Mahrt K, Ebel A, Masters WA Cost and Affordability of Healthy Diets Across and Within Countries. Background paper for The State of Food Security and Nutrition in the World 2020. Rome: FAO; 2020. FAO Agricultural Development Economics Technical Study No. 9.

45. McCullough ML, Chantaprasopsuk S, Islami F, et al. Association of socioeconomic and geographic factors with diet quality in US adults. *JAMA Network Open*. 2022;5(6):e2216406.

46. Wright KE, Lucero JE, Ferguson JK, et al. The impact that cultural food security has on identity and well-being in the second-generation U.S. American minority college students. *Food Sec*. 2021;13(3):701–715.

47. Wambogo E, Ansai N, Wang CY, et al. *Awareness of the MyPlate Plan: United States, 2017–March 2020*. USDHHS; 2022:14.

48. Rong S, Liao Y, Zhou J, Yang W, Yang Y. Comparison of dietary guidelines among 96 countries worldwide. *Trends in Food Science & Technology*. 2021;109:219–229.

49. USDA Economic Research Service. *Flexible Consumer Behavior Survey: Use of the Nutrition Facts Panel on Packaged Food Labels*. 2023. https://www.ers.usda.gov/topics/food-choices-health/food-consumption-demand/flexible-consumer-behavior-survey/#panel

50. US Food and Drug Administration, Center for Food Safety and Applied Nutrition. *The New Nutrition Facts Label*. FDA; 2022. https://www.fda.gov/food/nutrition-education-resources-materials/new-nutrition-facts-label

51. USDA Food Safety and Inspection Service. Nutrition Labeling: FSIS Regulated Foods. 2006. http://www.fsis.usda.gov/guidelines/2006-0006

52. FDA, Center for Food Safety and Applied. *Nutrient Content Claims*. FDA; 2022. https://www.fda.gov/food/food-labeling-nutrition/nutrient-content-claims

53. FDA, Center for Food Safety and Applied Nutrition. *Authorized Health Claims That Meet the Significant Scientific Agreement (SSA) Standard*. FDA; 2022. https://www.fda.gov/food/food-labeling-nutrition/authorized-health-claims-meet-significant-scientific-agreement-ssa-standard

54. Boutari C, Mantzoros CS. A 2022 update on the epidemiology of obesity and a call to action: as its twin COVID-19 pandemic appears to be receding, the obesity and dysmetabolism pandemic continues to rage on. *Metabolism*. 2022;133:155217.

55. Bryan S, Afful J, Carroll M, et al. *National Health and Nutrition Examination Survey 2017–March 2020 Pre-Pandemic*. National Center for Health Statistics; 2021:21. https://stacks.cdc.gov/view/cdc/106273.

56. Hales CM, Carroll MD, Fryar CD, Ogden CL. *Prevalence of Obesity and Severe Obesity among Adults: United States, 2017–2018*. National Center for Health Statistics; 2020:8. https://www.cdc.gov/nchs/data/databriefs/db360-h.pdf.

57. CDC. *Adult Obesity Maps*. Centers for Disease Control and Prevention; 2023.

58. Kivimäki M, Strandberg T, Pentti J, et al. Body-mass index and risk of obesity-related complex multimorbidity: an observational multicohort study. *Lancet Diabetes Endocrinol*. 2022;10(4):253–263.

59. Chapple ILC, Bouchard P, Cagetti MG, et al. Interaction of lifestyle, behaviour or systemic diseases with dental caries and periodontal diseases: consensus report of group 2 of the joint EFP/ORCA workshop on the boundaries between caries and periodontal diseases. *J Clin Periodontol*. 2017;44(Suppl 18):S39–S51.

60. CDC. *Overweight & Obesity: Why It Matters*. Centers for Disease Control and Prevention; 2022. https://www.cdc.gov/obesity/about-obesity/why-it-matters.html

61. Yu E, Ley SH, Manson JE, et al. Weight history and all-cause and cause-specific mortality in three prospective cohort studies. *Ann Intern Med*. 2017;166(9):613–620.

62. Lindberg L, Danielsson P, Persson M, Marcus C, Hagman E. Association of childhood obesity with risk of early all-cause and cause-specific mortality: a Swedish prospective cohort study. *PLoS Med*. 2020;17(3):e1003078.

63. Wiebe N, Lloyd A, Crumley ET, Tonelli M. Associations between body mass index and all-cause mortality: a systematic review and *meta*-analysis. *Obesity Reviews*. 2023;24(10):e13588.

64. Ford ES, Maynard LM, Li C. Trends in mean waist circumference and abdominal obesity among US adults, 1999-2012. *JAMA*. 2014;312(11):1151–1153.

65. Liu XC, Liu YS, Guan HX, Feng YQ, Kuang J. Comparison of six anthropometric measures in discriminating diabetes: a cross-sectional study from the National Health and Nutrition Examination Survey. *J Diabetes*. 2022;14(7):465–475.

66. Zhang Y, Gu Y, Wang N, et al. Association between anthropometric indicators of obesity and cardiovascular risk factors among adults in Shanghai, China. *BMC Public Health*. 2019;19(1):1035.

67. Safaei M, Sundararajan EA, Driss M, Boulila W, Shapi'i A. A systematic literature review on obesity: Understanding the causes & consequences of obesity and reviewing various machine learning approaches used to predict obesity. *Comput Biol Med*. 2021;136:104754.

68. Dunn CG, Gao KJ, Soto MJ, Bleich SN. Disparities in adult fast-food consumption in the U.S. by race and ethnicity, National Health and Nutrition Examination Survey 2017–2018. *Am J Prev Med*. 2021;61(4):e197–e201.

69. Drewnowski A, Rehm CD. Energy intakes of US children and adults by food purchase location and by specific food source. *Nutr J*. 2013;12:59.

70. Ryan DH, Yockey SR. Weight loss and improvement in comorbidity: differences at 5%, 10%, 15%, and over. *Curr Obes Rep*. 2017;6(2):187–194.

71. Kompaniyets L, Freedman DS, Belay B, et al. Probability of 5% or greater weight loss or BMI reduction to healthy weight among adults with overweight or obesity. *JAMA Netw Open.* 2023;6(8):e2327358.

72. National Institute of Diabetes and Digestive and Kidney Diseases. *Research Behind the Body Weight Planner – Integrative Physiology Section.* National Institute of Diabetes and Digestive and Kidney Diseases. https://www.niddk.nih.gov/research-funding/at-niddk/labs-branches/laboratory-biological-modeling/integrative-physiology-section/research/body-weight-planner

73. Hall KD, Sacks G, Chandramohan D, et al. Quantification of the effect of energy imbalance on bodyweight. *Lancet.* 2011;378(9793):826–837.

74. CDC. *Healthy Weight Loss.* Centers for Disease Control and Prevention; 2023. https://www.cdc.gov/healthyweight/losing_weight/index.html

75. Garvey WT, Mechanick JI, Brett EM, et al. American Association of Clinical Endocrinologists and American College of Endocrinology comprehensive clinical practice guidelines for medical care of patients with obesity. *Endocrine Practice.* 2016;22(7):842–884.

76. Lazzaroni E, Ben Nasr M, Loretelli C, et al. Anti-diabetic drugs and weight loss in patients with type 2 diabetes. *Pharmacol Res.* 2021;171:105782.

77. van Veldhuisen SL, Gorter TM, van Woerden G, et al. Bariatric surgery and cardiovascular disease: a systematic review and meta-analysis. *Eur Heart J.* 2022;43(20):1955–1969.

78. Ciobârcă D, Cătoi AF, Copăescu C, Miere D, Crişan G. Bariatric surgery in obesity: effects on gut microbiota and micronutrient status. *Nutrients.* 2020;12(1):235.

79. Liao J, Yin Y, Zhong J, et al. Bariatric surgery and health outcomes: an umbrella analysis. *Front Endocrinol.* 2022;13:1016613.

80. Lewis CA, de Jersey S, Seymour M, Hopkins G, Hickman I, Osland E. Iron, vitamin B12, folate and copper deficiency after bariatric surgery and the impact on anaemia: a systematic review. *Obes Surg.* 2020;30(11):4542–4591.

81. Saad RK, Ghezzawi M, Habli D, Alami RS, Chakhtoura M. Fracture risk following bariatric surgery: a systematic review and *meta*-analysis. *Osteoporos Int.* 2022;33(3):511–526.

82. Castilho AVSS, Foratori-Junior GA, Sales-Peres SHde C. Bariatric surgery impact on gastroesophageal reflux and dental wear: a systematic review. *Arq Bras Cir Dig.* 2019;32(4):e1466.

83. Greenberg BL, Glick M, Tavares M. Addressing obesity in the dental setting: what can be learned from oral health care professionals' efforts to screen for medical conditions. *J Public Health Dent.* 2017;77(Suppl 1):S67–S78.

84. Mallonee LF, Boyd LD, Stegeman C. A scoping review of skills and tools oral health professionals need to engage children and parents in dietary changes to prevent childhood obesity and consumption of sugar-sweetened beverages. *J Public Health Dent.* 2017;77(Suppl 1):S128–S135.

85. National Institute of Diabetes and Digestive and Kidney Diseases. *Talking With Patients About Weight Loss: Tips for Primary Care Providers.* National Institute of Diabetes and Digestive and Kidney Diseases. https://www.niddk.nih.gov/health-information/professionals/clinical-tools-patient-management/weight-management/talking-adult-patients-tips-primary-care-clinicians

86. Marro F, De Smedt S, Rajasekharan S, Martens L, Bottenberg P, Jacquet W. Associations between obesity, dental caries, erosive tooth wear and periodontal disease in adolescents: a case-control study. *Eur Arch Paediatr Dent.* 2021;22(1):99–108.

87. Abu-Shawish G, Betsy J, Anil S. Is obesity a risk factor for periodontal disease in adults? A systematic review. *Int J Environ Res Public Health.* 2022;19(19):12684.

▶ **Evolve Resources**

Please visit http://evolve.elsevier.com/Mallonee/nutritional for additional practice and study support tools.

2

Concepts in Biochemistry

SCOTT M. TREMAIN, PHD

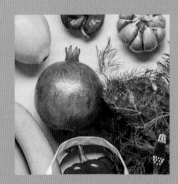

STUDENT LEARNING OUTCOMES

On completion of this chapter, the student will be able to achieve the following outcomes:

1. Explain the role of biochemistry in nutrition.
2. Discuss the fundamentals of biochemistry, including assigning biomolecules according to functional groups.
3. Discuss concepts related to principle biomolecules in nutrition:
   - Compare and contrast the structure, function, and properties of the four major classes of biomolecules (carbohydrates, proteins, nucleic acids, and lipids).
   - Outline the structure, function, and properties of monosaccharides, disaccharides, and polysaccharides.

- Outline the structure, function, and properties of amino acids and proteins.
- Compare and contrast the roles of enzymes, coenzymes, and vitamins in nutrition.
- Outline the structure, function, and property of nucleotides and nucleic acids.
- Outline the structure, function, and property of fatty acids, triglycerides, and steroids.

4. Summarize metabolism, as well as differentiate catabolism from anabolism. In addition, explain connections between metabolic pathways in carbohydrate, protein, and lipid metabolism.

KEY TERMS

Active site
Adenosine 5′-triphosphate (ATP)
Adipose tissue
Aerobic
Amino acids
Amphiphilic
Amylase
Anabolism
Anhydrous
Antioxidants
Bioactive
Bioinformation
Biomolecule
Carbohydrates
Catabolism
Chemical bonds
Cholesterol
cis isomer
Coenzymes
Condensation reaction
Covalent bond
Disaccharide
Disease
Enzymes
Epigenetics
Epinephrine
Essential amino acids (EAAs) or
    indispensable amino acids
Fatty acids (FAs)
Functional group
Gene

Genome
Genomics
Glucagon
Glycogen
Glucogenic amino acids
Gluconeogenesis
Glycolysis
Glycosidic bond
Hormone
Hydrocarbon
Hydrogenation reaction
Hydrolysis reaction
Hydrophilic
Hydrophobic
Hydroxyapatite
Insulin
Ionic bond
Ketogenic amino acids
Ketone bodies
Linoleic acid
Lipase
Lipids
Lipoproteins
Melting point
Metabolism
Mitochondria
Molecule
Monomer
Monosaccharide
Monounsaturated fatty acid (MUFA)

Nonessential amino acids (NEAAs) or
    dispensable amino acids
Nucleic acids
Nucleotides
Nutrigenomics or nutritional genomics
Oils
Oxidation
Oxidation-reduction reactions
Oxidative phosphorylation
Peptide bond
Photosynthesis
Polymer
Polypeptide
Polysaccharide
Polyunsaturated fatty acid (PUFA)
Precursor
Protease
Proteins
Redox coenzymes
Reduction
Respiration
Side chain (R group)
Saturated fatty acids
Substrate
Sugar alcohol
trans isomer
Tricarboxylic acid cycle (TCA cycle)
Triglyceride (TG)
Unsaturated fatty acids
Vitamins

TEST YOUR NQ

1. **T/F** A condensation reaction breaks a larger molecule into two smaller molecules.
2. **T/F** Nucleotides are the building blocks of proteins.
3. **T/F** Hydrophilic molecules dissolve readily in water.
4. **T/F** Sucrose is a disaccharide containing glucose and galactose.
5. **T/F** A substrate binds the enzyme's active site and is converted into a product.
6. **T/F** When the hydrogen atoms are on opposite sides of the double bond, the structure is a *trans* isomer.
7. **T/F** An unsaturated fatty acid with 16 carbons has a lower melting temperature than a saturated fatty acid with 16 carbons.
8. **T/F** Catabolism involves the reduction of carbohydrates into carbon dioxide and water.
9. **T/F** Insulin activates glycogen degradation to regulate carbohydrate and lipid metabolism.
10. **T/F** Humans lack the enzymes to synthesize essential (indispensable) amino acids; therefore EAAs must be obtained from foods.

It is essential for dental professionals to have a basic understanding of biochemistry because it is the foundation for understanding and applying the concepts of nutrition. An overview of the biochemical concepts relevant to nutrition will serve as a useful resource as the learner goes through this textbook.

What Is Biochemistry?

Biochemistry is the study of life at the molecular level. The three major areas of biochemistry are structure, metabolism, and bioinformation. Structure describes the three-dimensional arrangement of atoms in a molecule, the smallest particle of a substance that retains all the properties of the substance. Important for life, the structure of a biomolecule determines its function. A biomolecule is any molecule that is produced by a living cell or organism, which would include carbohydrates, proteins, nucleic acids, and lipids, as well as other organic compounds found in living organisms. In contrast, a nutrient is a substance required by the body that must be supplied by an outside source, which is usually food. Metabolism involves the production and use of energy. In metabolism, energy is extracted from dietary carbohydrates, proteins, and lipids and used to create the biomolecules essential for life. This highly regulated metabolic system ensures no wastage of energy. Bioinformation involves the transfer of biological information from deoxyribonucleic acid (DNA) to ribonucleic acid (RNA) to protein. DNA stores the blueprint for life, and the resulting proteins carry out all the processes required for life.

Fundamentals of Biochemistry

Atoms in a compound are held together by two types of chemical bonds: ionic bonds and covalent bonds. An ionic bond forms between a positively charged metal ion and a negatively charged nonmetal ion. Hydroxyapatite in tooth enamel is composed of ionic bonds between calcium ions (Ca^{2+}), phosphate ions (PO_4^{3-}), and hydroxide ions (OH^-). A covalent bond forms when electrons are equally shared between two nonmetals. Nitrous oxide, commonly known as laughing gas, is a molecule containing covalent bonds between nitrogen (N) and oxygen (O) atoms. Ultimately, the biomolecules responsible for life are based on the nonmetal carbon (C) because of carbon's ability to form stable covalent bonds to itself and many other atoms, forming long chains and rings. More than 25 different elements—such as hydrogen (H), sulfur (S), and phosphorus (P)—are found in biomolecules, providing for great variety in chemical structure, properties, and reactivity in biological systems. One way to organize this variety in chemical structure is the classification of molecules into functional

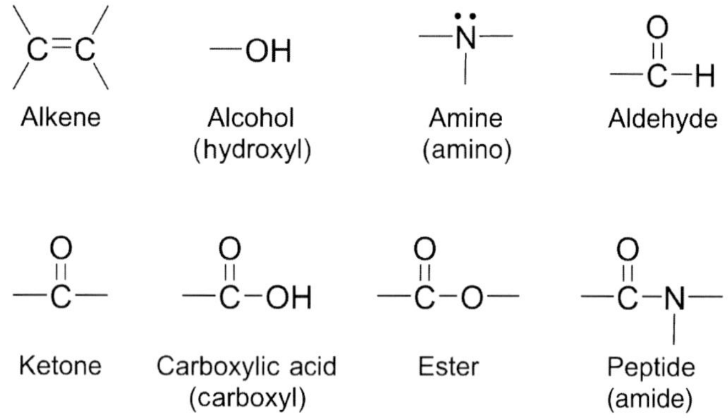

• **Fig. 2.1** Common functional groups in biochemistry.

groups. A functional group is a group of atoms that gives a family of molecules its characteristic chemical and physical properties. Molecules that have related functional groups have similar properties. Fig. 2.1 defines and exemplifies a few functional groups found in biochemistry.

Functional groups can be converted into other functional groups via chemical reactions, such as oxidation-reduction, condensation, and hydrolysis. Oxidation-reduction reactions are important in metabolism as biomolecules are degraded or synthesized. Oxidation can be defined as a loss of electrons, an increase in charge, a gain of O atoms, or a loss of H atoms. Reduction can be defined as a gain of electrons, a decrease in charge, a loss of O atoms, or a gain of H atoms. In metabolism, energy is extracted from glucose ($C_6H_{12}O_6$) by completely oxidizing it to carbon dioxide (CO_2). Condensation and hydrolysis reactions are important in digestion and metabolism. In general, a condensation reaction creates a new molecule by forming a bond between two smaller molecules, whereas a hydrolysis reaction breaks a larger molecule into two smaller molecules. When carbohydrates, proteins, and lipids are digested, these biomolecules are hydrolyzed into smaller building blocks for absorption in the digestive system.

Principle Biomolecules in Nutrition

Table 2.1 shows the four major classes of biomolecules: carbohydrates, proteins, nucleic acids, and lipids. These biomolecules are characterized by the type of polymer and monomer they contain and by their general function. A polymer is a large molecule containing numerous repeating units called monomers. A monomer is the smallest repeating unit present in a polymer.

TABLE 2.1	The Four Major Classes of Biomolecules	
Polymer	**Monomer**	**Function**
Carbohydrates (polysaccharides)	Monosaccharides	Energy source, energy storage form, and structure
Proteins	Amino acids	Structure and biocatalysts (enzymes)
Nucleic acids	Nucleotides	Genetic bioinformation transfer and energy
Lipids		Energy source, energy storage form, and biological membranes

$$6\ CO_2 + 6\ H_2O + Energy \underset{\text{degradation}}{\overset{\text{photosynthesis}}{\rightleftharpoons}} C_6H_{12}O_6 + 6\ O_2$$

• **Fig. 2.2** The carbon cycle. Plants utilize photosynthesis (use solar energy) to produce glucose ($C_6H_{12}O_6$) and oxygen (from *left* to *right*), while animals utilize respiration to degrade glucose ($C_6H_{12}O_6$) for energy (from *right* to *left*).

Carbohydrate Structure and Function

The biological function of carbohydrates involves energy metabolism and storage. As shown in Fig. 2.2, plants use photosynthesis to make oxygen (O_2) and glucose ($C_6H_{12}O_6$), the carbohydrate from which animals acquire the energy essential for life. Through the process of respiration, animals degrade glucose ($C_6H_{12}O_6$) into CO_2 and water (H_2O), and plants use these products for photosynthesis.

Carbohydrates are classified as monosaccharides, disaccharides, and polysaccharides, depending on the number of sugar monomers present (one, two, or many). Monosaccharides are composed of a single monomeric unit with the molecular formula $C_n(H_2O)_n$, where n is 3 to 8. Fig. 2.3 shows the linear structures of the most common monosaccharides. Monosaccharides undergo oxidation-reduction reactions. When a monosaccharide is reduced, the aldehyde functional group changes to a sugar alcohol (e.g., sorbitol).

In an aqueous solution, linear monosaccharides spontaneously form cyclic structures. When two monosaccharides combine, a disaccharide is formed. This involves the formation of a glycosidic bond. As shown in Fig. 2.4, two glucose monomers can combine via a condensation reaction to form maltose. Maltose is a disaccharide that results from the degradation of starch and is used in brewing alcoholic beverages. When glucose and fructose combine, the disaccharide sucrose is formed (Fig. 2.5). This disaccharide is table sugar and one of the sweetest carbohydrates. When the two monosaccharides, galactose and glucose, combine, the disaccharide lactose is formed (see Fig. 2.5). This disaccharide is found in milk and dairy products.

Many monosaccharides combine to form a polysaccharide. As shown in Table 2.2, polysaccharides can be characterized by the monosaccharide monomer present in them and their overall function. One of the most important dietary polysaccharides is starch, the storage form of energy in plants. Starch is composed of two different polysaccharides (α-amylose and amylopectin). Fig. 2.6 shows the linear structure of the polysaccharide, α-amylose.

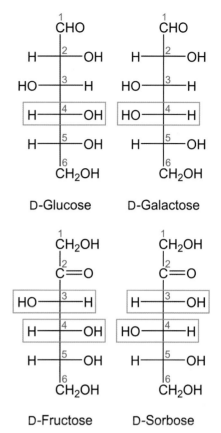

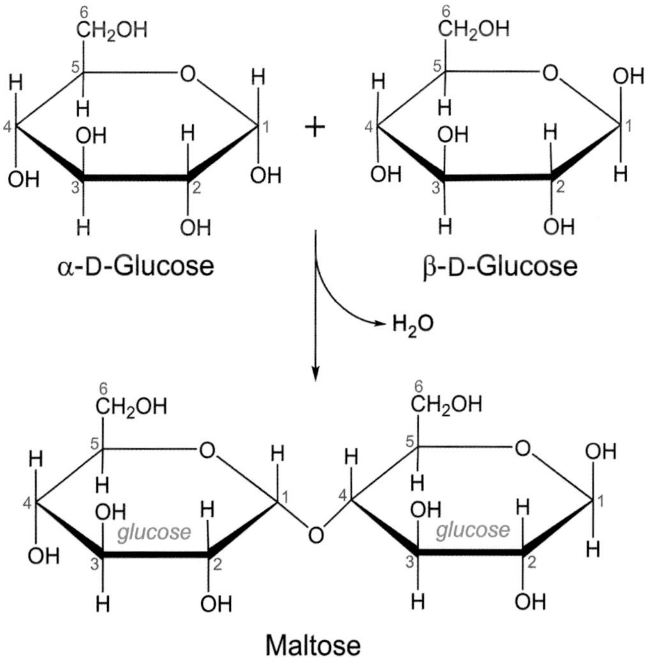

• **Fig. 2.3** The linear structures of common monosaccharides. Monosaccharides are classified as aldoses and ketoses. Aldoses contain an aldehyde functional group, while ketoses contain a ketone functional group. D-Glucose ($C_6H_{12}O_6$) is an aldohexose because it contains an aldehyde (represented by CHO at carbon 1) and six carbons. D-Fructose ($C_6H_{12}O_6$) is a ketohexose because it contains a ketone (at carbon 2) and six carbons.

• **Fig. 2.4** Formation of the disaccharide maltose from two glucose molecules. Water (H_2O) is released as a product in this condensation reaction.

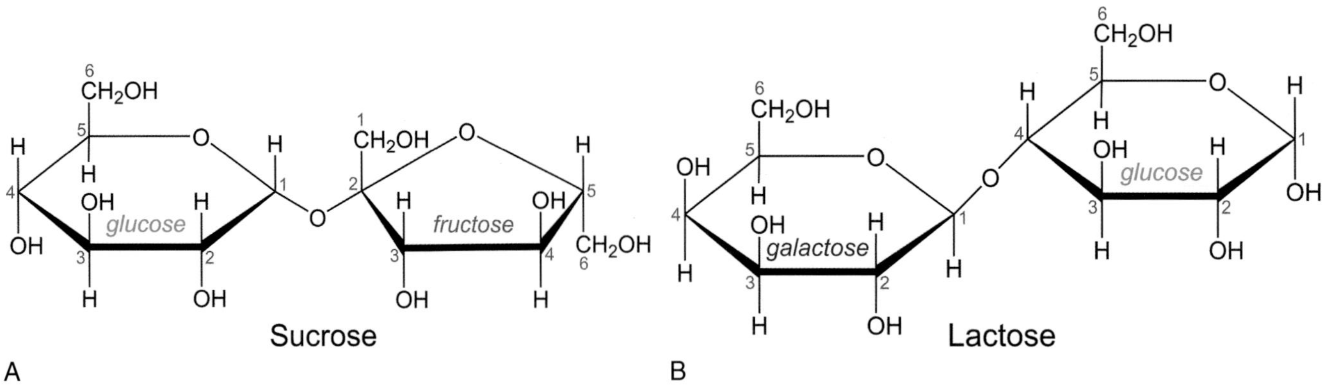

• **Fig. 2.5** The structures of the disaccharides (A) sucrose and (B) lactose.

TABLE 2.2	**Summary of Common Polysaccharides**	
Name	**Monomer**	**Biological Function**
Amylose (in starch)	Glucose	Nutrient storage (plants)
Amylopectin (in starch)	Glucose	Nutrient storage (plants)
Glycogen	Glucose	Nutrient storage (animals)
Dextran	Glucose	Nutrient storage (yeast and bacteria)
Inulin	Fructose	Nutrient storage (plants)
Cellulose	Glucose	Structure in plants
Pectin	Galacturonic acid	Structural rigidity in plants and gelling agent in yogurt and jelly
Lignin	Coniferyl alcohol	Structural rigidity in plant cell walls

Fig. 2.7 shows the branched structure of the polysaccharide, amylopectin. Important for the storage of energy in animals, **glycogen** is another branched polysaccharide containing glucose monomers. The highly branched structure of glycogen allows its rapid degradation into glucose when energy is needed.

Protein Structure and Function

In an organism, **proteins** are essential for almost every physiological function, such as providing structure, helping muscles contract, transporting and storing substances, catalyzing reactions, regulating metabolism, and supporting the immune system. Proteins are composed of building blocks or monomer units called **amino acids**. As shown in Fig. 2.8, the general structure of an amino acid consists of an amino group ($-NH_3^+$), a carboxyl group ($-COO^-$), and a **side chain (R group)** that varies from one amino acid to another. The classification of the 20 common amino acids is based on the structure of their side chain. Amino acids polymerize to form long chains called **polypeptides** linked by strong covalent **peptide bonds**. Proteins can consist of as few as

50 to as many as millions of amino acid monomers in one or more polypeptides arranged in a biologically functional way. As shown in Fig. 2.9, a protein will become biologically active when it folds into its distinct, compact three-dimensional structure.

Enzymes Catalyze Biochemical Reactions

Enzymes catalyze all biochemical reactions. Enzymes begin the process of digesting dietary proteins (**proteases**), carbohydrates (**amylases**), and lipids (**lipases**). They also execute all the metabolic reactions involving the degradation and biosynthesis of the biomolecules essential for life.

As shown in Fig. 2.10, enzymes catalyze reactions by specifically binding a **substrate** and converting it into a product. This chemical transformation takes place in a region of the enzyme called the **active site**. Many enzymes need additional help to complete a specific biochemical reaction. **Coenzymes** are nonprotein organic substances that assist enzymes and are regenerated at the end of a reaction. Many vitamins are converted into these important biologically active coenzymes.

Vitamins or "vital amines" are essential nutrients required in the diet because they cannot be synthesized by the organism itself. Many water-soluble vitamins are **precursors** of coenzymes. As shown in Table 2.3, water-soluble vitamins obtained from foods may need to be converted into a biologically active form (a coenzyme) before binding an enzyme's active site. Lipid-soluble or fat-soluble vitamins accumulate in fat deposits and cell membranes in the body. Lipid-soluble vitamins obtained from dietary sources are not involved as coenzymes, but they are converted into a biologically active form.

Nucleic Acid Structure and Function

The biological functions of **nucleic acids**, such as DNA and RNA, are to store and transfer genetic information. The genetic information in an organism, the **genome**, contains all the information needed for the complete development of a living organism. The central dogma shown in Fig. 2.11 describes bioinformation transfer within cells (DNA→RNA→Protein). Messenger RNA carries the message from DNA to the ribosome, the site of protein synthesis. The ribosome is composed of protein and ribosomal RNA. Transfer RNA carries an amino acid to the ribosome for incorporation into the growing polypeptide chain.

Nucleic acids are composed of building blocks called **nucleotides**. As shown in Fig. 2.12, the general structure of a nucleotide

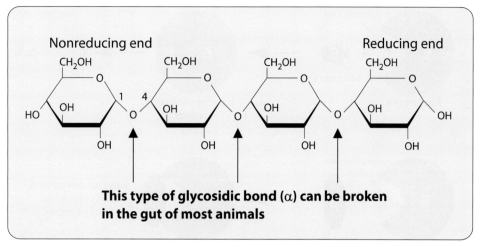

• **Fig. 2.6** The linear structure of the polysaccharide α-amylose, a component of starch-containing glycosidic linkages that are easily digested. (Reproduced with permission from Batmanian L, Worral S, Ridge J. *Biochemistry for Health Professionals*. Elsevier Australia; 2011.)

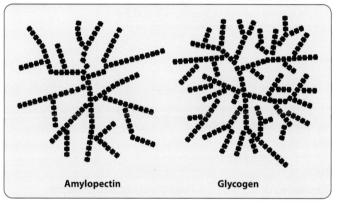

• **Fig. 2.7** The branched structures of the polysaccharides amylopectin and glycogen. Amylopectin is a component of starch (the storage form of energy in plants) containing glucose monomers. Glycogen is the storage form of energy in animals containing glucose monomers. (Reproduced with permission from Batmanian L, Worral S, Ridge J. *Biochemistry for Health Professionals*. Elsevier Australia; 2011.)

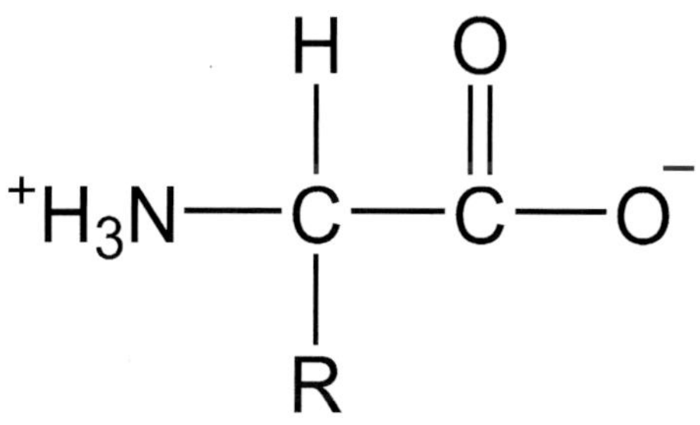

• **Fig. 2.8** Structure of an amino acid. At neutral pH, the amino group ($-NH_3^+$) is positively charged, while the carboxyl group ($-COO^-$) is negatively charged.

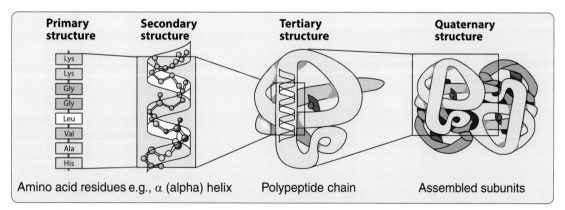

• **Fig. 2.9** The four levels of protein structure. The primary (1°) structure is the sequence of amino acids in a protein; it holds the information necessary to form the secondary (2°) structure. The secondary structure is characterized by localized regions of repeating ordered structure that leads to the formation of the compact, biologically active tertiary (3°) structure. The tertiary structure describes the positions of all atoms in the protein or the overall three-dimensional, compactly folded, biologically active structure. The association and organization of two or more protein subunits is the quaternary (4°) structure. (Reproduced with permission from Batmanian L, Worral S, Ridge J. *Biochemistry for Health Professionals*. Elsevier Australia; 2011.)

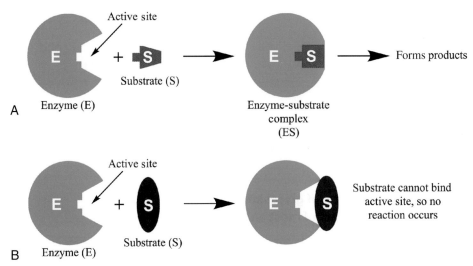

• **Fig. 2.10** Enzyme active sites bind substrate and help convert it into product. When substrate binds the active site, an intermediate enzyme-substrate (ES) complex forms and provides the greatest possibility for the reaction to occur and form products. A substrate that neither fits nor induces a fit in the active site cannot undergo reaction by the enzyme. In (A) both the substrate (S) and the active site of the enzyme (E) are flexible and adjust their shape for optimum binding between the active site and the substrate. In (B) the substrate (S) does not fit the enzyme (E) active site; thus a reaction will not occur and product will not form.

TABLE 2.3   Common Vitamins and Coenzymes

Vitamin Type	Coenzyme	Function
Water Soluble		
Thiamin (vitamin B_1)	Thiamin pyrophosphate	Decarboxylation
Riboflavin (vitamin B_2)	Flavin adenine dinucleotide and flavin mononucleotide	Redox coenzymes (electron transfer)
Niacin (vitamin B_3)	Nicotinamide adenine dinucleotide; nicotinamide adenine dinucleotide phosphate	Redox coenzymes (electron transfer)
Pantothenic acid (vitamin B_5)	Coenzyme A	Acetyl group transfer
Pyridoxine (vitamin B_6)	Pyridoxal phosphate	Transamination
Cobalamin (vitamin B_{12})	Methylcobalamin	Methyl group transfer
Ascorbic acid (vitamin C)	Ascorbic acid (vitamin C)	Collagen biosynthesis; healing of wounds
Biotin	Biocytin	Carboxylation
Folic acid	Tetrahydrofolate	Methyl group transfer
Lipid Soluble—Biologically Active Form		
Vitamin A	Retinal	Formation of visual pigments
Vitamin D	1,25-Dihydroxycholecalciferol	Absorption of calcium and phosphate, bone development
Vitamin E	α-Tocopherol	Antioxidant; prevents oxidation of vitamin A and unsaturated fatty acids
Vitamin K	Phylloquinone (vitamin K_1) and menaquinone (vitamin K_2)	Synthesis of prothrombin for blood clotting

consists of sugar attached to a nitrogenous base and phosphate. The sugar is ribose in RNA or deoxyribose in DNA.

Nutrigenomics is an emerging field which studies the interaction between nutrition and the genome. Some **bioactive** molecules found in food can influence how DNA encodes proteins, leading to changes in one's health and wellness. Eventually, personalized diets based on a patient's genetic makeup may help prevent or treat disease (see Health Application 2).

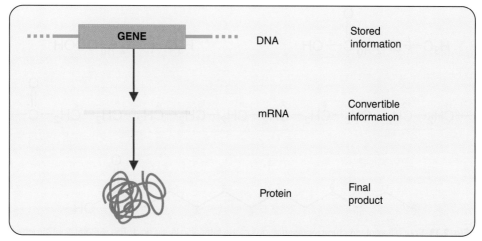

• **Fig. 2.11** The central dogma of bioinformation transfer. DNA is composed of genes that are transcribed into messenger RNA (mRNA) and translated into protein. (Reproduced with permission from Batmanian L, Worral S, Ridge J. *Biochemistry for Health Professionals*. Elsevier Australia; 2011.)

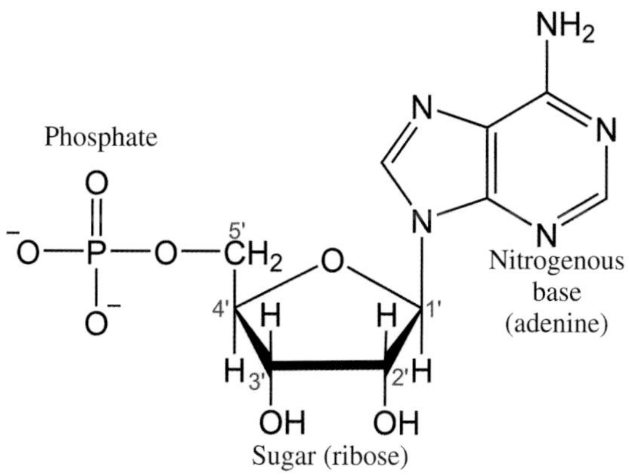

• **Fig. 2.12** The structure of the nucleotide adenosine 5'-monophosphate (AMP). AMP consists of the sugar ribose, the nitrogenous base adenine, and a phosphate group.

Lipid Structure and Function

Lipids have many different structures and biological functions. They are involved in energy metabolism and storage, serve as structural components of biological membranes, provide insulation and protection, act as **hormones** that regulate the body's major systems, serve as vitamins, and act as detergents in digestion. In contrast to **hydrophilic** ("water-loving") biomolecules, lipids are **hydrophobic** ("water-fearing") compounds that do not readily dissolve in water.

Fatty acids (FAs) are a structural component present in more complex lipids. FAs are **amphiphilic** ("loving at both ends"), possessing a hydrophilic carboxyl group "head" and hydrophobic **hydrocarbon** chain "tail" containing only carbon and hydrogen atoms. The structure of an FA (e.g., lauric acid has 12 carbon atoms) can be represented in a number of different ways, but the most common is the skeletal (line) structure, as shown in Fig. 2.13.

FAs can be classified according to the presence or absence of C=C (double) bonds. **Saturated fatty acids**—such as lauric acid, shown in Fig. 2.13—contain only C–C (single) bonds, while **unsaturated fatty acids** are alkenes that contain one or more C=C bonds. As shown in Fig. 2.14, **monounsaturated fatty acids (MUFAs)** such as oleic acid—contain just one C=C bond, while **polyunsaturated fatty acids (PUFAs)** such as **linoleic acid**—contain more than one C=C bond.

FAs have common names and systematic names, but they also utilize an abbreviated symbol notation that depends on the total number of carbons and C=C bonds present. Table 2.4 summarizes the number of carbon atoms, common name, abbreviated symbol notation, and typical lipid source for many common FAs. In contrast to the delta (Δ) numbering system, the omega (ω) numbering system indicates the position of a C=C bond by numbering the carbon chain from the methyl (–CH_3) end. Fig. 2.15 shows how the omega (ω) numbering system is used in the PUFAs linolenic acid and linoleic acid.

In MUFAs and PUFAs, the C=C bond can either be a *cis* isomer or *trans* isomer. As shown in Fig. 2.16, the ***cis*** isomer of oleic acid has the H atoms on the same side of the C=C bond, so there exists a significant bend, or "kink," in the long hydrocarbon tail. In the ***trans*** isomer of oleic acid, the H atoms are on opposite sides of the C=C bond and the long hydrocarbon tail remains straight and extended. *Cis* isomers predominate in nature.

The characteristics, properties, and reactivity of an FA can be understood in terms of its structure. One of these properties is the **melting point**, the temperature at which a substance changes from a solid to a liquid, or melts. As the number of carbon atoms increases, the melting point of the FA increases because of stronger attractive forces. Moreover, the melting points of saturated FA are higher than unsaturated FAs. Saturated FAs exhibit stronger attractive forces as a result of the compact, tight packing of their long, extended hydrocarbon tails; thus they are solids at room temperature. As shown in Fig. 2.16, unsaturated FAs have "kinks" at the *cis* C=C bonds that prevent compact packing, resulting in weaker attractive forces and lower melting points; thus they are liquids (**oils**) at room temperature.

Triglycerides (TGs), also referred to as triacylglycerols, are the storage forms of FAs and considered the metabolic fuel for cells stored in **adipose tissue** or fat. As shown in Fig. 2.17, a TG consists of a three-carbon glycerol backbone with three FAs attached.

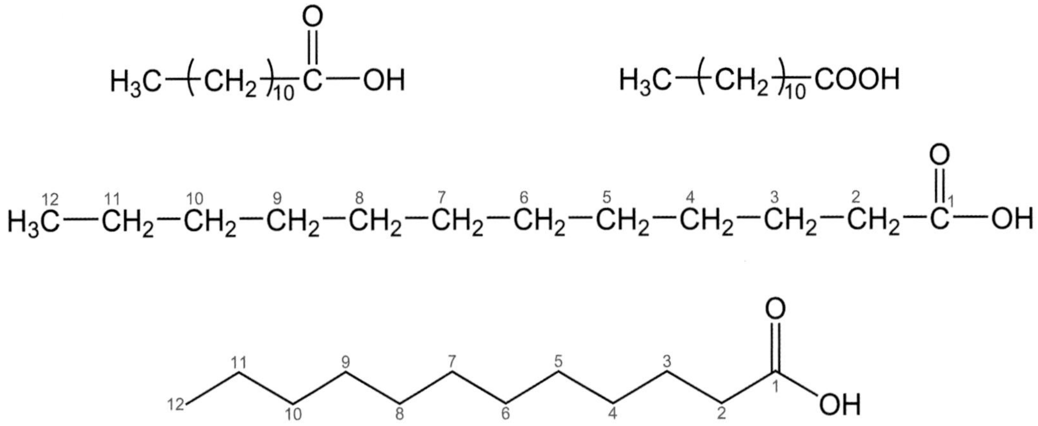

• **Fig. 2.13** Four different structural representations of the fatty acid lauric acid. The skeletal (line) structure at the bottom is the most efficient way of representing the numerous carbon atoms in the long hydrocarbon chain.

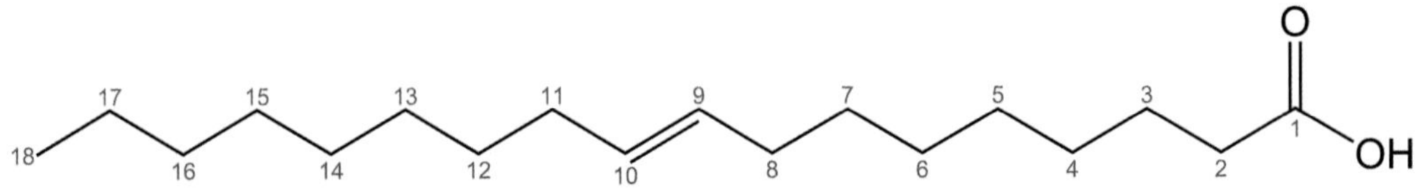

Oleic acid

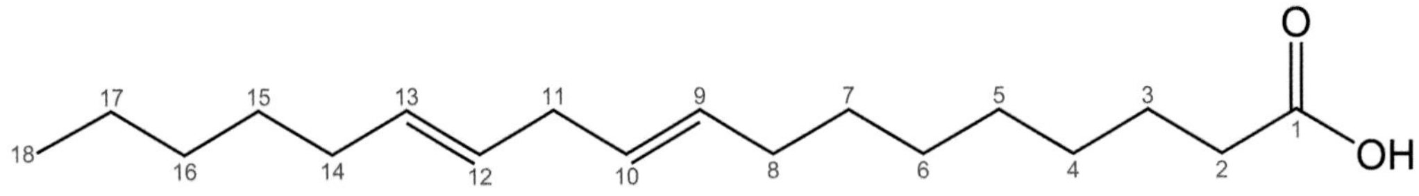

Linoleic acid

• **Fig. 2.14** Structure of unsaturated fatty acids. Oleic acid is a monounsaturated fatty acid with a C=C bond at carbon 9, while linoleic acid is a polyunsaturated fatty acid with C=C bonds at carbon 9 and carbon 12. For oleic acid the abbreviated symbol notation is $(18:1)^{\Delta 1}$ for which the first number corresponds to the total number of carbons (18), the second number corresponds to the total number of C=C bonds (1), and the superscript corresponds to the delta (Δ) locations of the C=C bonds between carbons 9 and 10 in the long carbon chain numbered starting from the carboxyl (–COOH) end. For linoleic acid, the abbreviated symbol notation is $(18:2)^{\Delta 1,2}$.

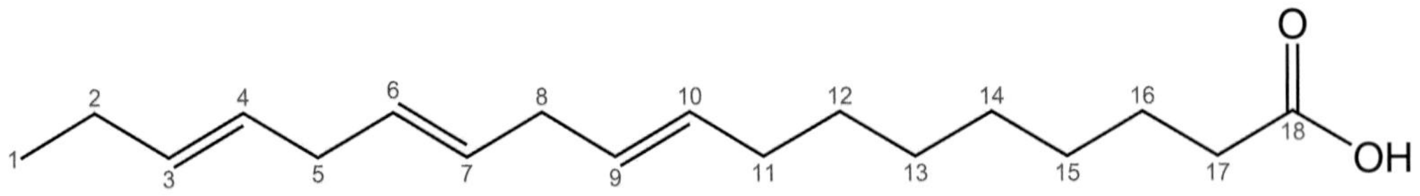

Linolenic acid (ω-3 Fatty acid)

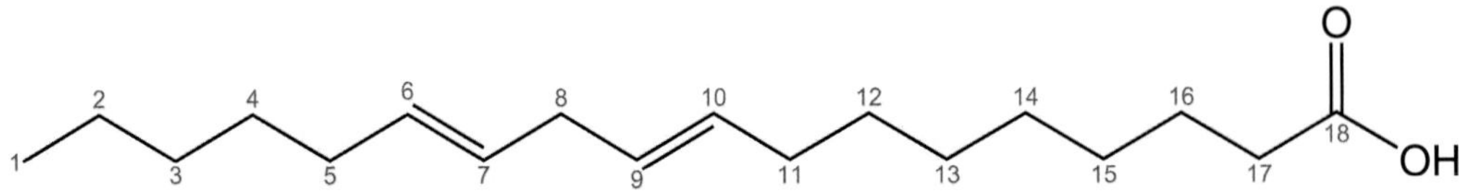

Linoleic acid (ω-6 Fatty acid)

• **Fig. 2.15** The omega (ω) numbering system for fatty acids. Linolenic acid is an ω-3 polyunsaturated fatty acid, while linoleic acid is an ω-6 polyunsaturated fatty acid.

TABLE 2.4   Summary of Common Fatty Acids

No. of Carbon Atoms	Common Name	Abbreviated Symbol Notation	Typical Lipid Source
4	Butyric acid	(4:0)	Butterfat
8	Caprylic acid	(8:0)	Coconut oil
12	Lauric acid	(12:0)	Coconut oil, palm kernel oil
14	Myristic acid	(14:0)	Butterfat, coconut oil
16	Palmitic acid	(16:0)	Palm oil, animal fat
16	Palmitoleic acid	$(16:1)^{\Delta 1}$	Some fish oils, beef fat
18	Stearic acid	(18:0)	Cocoa butter, animal fat
18	Oleic acid	$(18:1)^{\Delta 1}$	Olive oil, canola oil
18	Linoleic acid	$(18:2)^{\Delta 1,2}$	Most vegetable oils; safflower, corn, soybean
18	Linolenic acid	$(18:3)^{\Delta 1,2,3}$	Soybean oil, canola oil, walnuts, wheat germ oil
20	Arachidic acid	(20:0)	Peanut oil
20	Arachidonic acid	$(20:4)^{\Delta 4,5,6,7}$	Lard, meats
20	Eicosapentaenoic acid	$(20:5)^{\Delta 4,5,6,7,8}$	Fish oils, shellfish
22	Docosahexaenoic acid	$(22:6)^{\Delta 9,10,11,12,13,14}$	Fish oils, shellfish

Adapted from Mahan LK, Escott-Stump S, Raymond JL. *Krause's Food and The Nutrition Care Process*. 13th ed. Elsevier/Saunders; 2012.

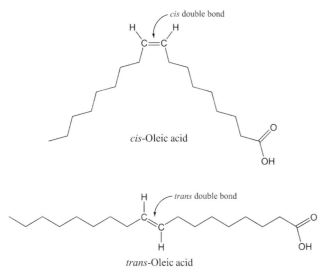

• **Fig. 2.16** Structure of *cis-trans* isomers in monounsaturated fatty acids (MUFAs). Oleic acid is an MUFA with a C=C bond at carbon 9.

The alcohol functional groups of the glycerol backbone react with the carboxylic acid functional groups of three FAs to form the three ester functional groups of a TG. The properties of a TG mirror those of the FAs present. A TG that is solid at room temperature is called a fat, whereas a TG that is liquid at room temperature is called an oil. TGs that are predominantly composed of saturated FAs are solid fats at room temperature, whereas those that are predominantly composed of unsaturated FAs are liquid oils at room temperature.

In TGs, unsaturated FAs that have C=C bonds can be the site of many different types of chemical reactions. A **hydrogenation reaction**, shown in Fig. 2.18, involves the addition of a hydrogen molecule (H_2) to a C=C bond to form a saturated FA with C–C bonds. By controlling the amount of H_2 gas added, it is possible to control how many C=C bonds are converted into C–C bonds, thereby controlling the melting point of the resultant product. Partial hydrogenation of a liquid vegetable oil can be used to create soft semisolid fat products, such as spreadable tub margarines and solid shortening. Partial hydrogenation of vegetable oil results in a small amount of the *cis* C=C bonds being converted into unwanted *trans* C=C bonds. Another common, but unwanted, reaction involving C=C bonds is oxidation. Oxidation of unsaturated fats leads to rancidity; thus **antioxidants**—such as vitamins C and E, butylated hydroxyanisole, and butylated hydroxytoluene—are added to vegetable oils.

Another class of lipids includes steroids. Steroids are a family of lipids containing a hydrophobic nucleus of four rings fused together. As shown in Fig. 2.19, **cholesterol** is the most abundant steroid and is an important stabilizing component of biological membranes. Cholesterol is also the precursor of steroid hormones (progesterone, estradiol, and testosterone), bile acids, and lipid-soluble vitamin D.

Lipids must be transported through the bloodstream to be stored, to be used for energy, or to make hormones. However, lipids do not readily dissolve in blood. Therefore they are transported via water-soluble complexes called lipoproteins. As shown in

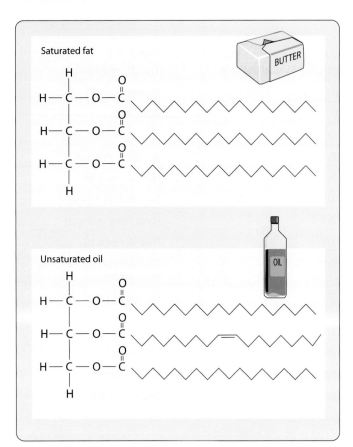

• **Fig. 2.17** Comparison of TGs containing saturated fatty acids (FAs) and unsaturated FAs. The solid fat found in butter is predominantly composed of triglycerides (TGs) containing saturated FAs. The extended hydrocarbon tails of the saturated FAs pack together better, leading to stronger attractive forces. The liquid oil found in vegetable oils is predominantly composed of TGs containing unsaturated FAs. The "kinked" hydrocarbon tails of the unsaturated FAs do not pack well, leading to weaker attractive forces. (Reproduced with permission from Batmanian L, Worral S, Ridge J. *Biochemistry for Health Professionals*. Elsevier Australia; 2011.)

Fig. 2.20, **lipoproteins** are spherical particles with a hydrophilic surface and a hydrophobic interior that can transport TGs, FAs, and cholesterol in the bloodstream (see Ch. 6 for further discussion).

Summary of Metabolism

Metabolism is how cells acquire, transform, store, and use energy. It is the sum total of all chemical reactions (organized into pathways) in an organism. It also includes the coordination, regulation, and energy requirements of those reactions. The three characteristics of **catabolism** are the production of energy, the degradation of more complex molecules into smaller molecules, and the oxidation of metabolites. In contrast, the three characteristics of

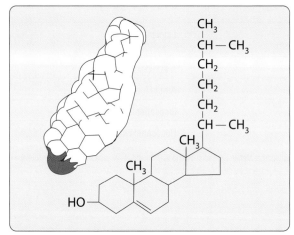

• **Fig. 2.19** Structure of cholesterol. Cholesterol consists of a hydrophobic fused ring structure with a single hydrophilic alcohol (–OH) at one end (indicated in *red* in the globular structure of cholesterol). (Reproduced with permission from Batmanian L, Worral S, Ridge J. *Biochemistry for Health Professionals*. Elsevier Australia; 2011.)

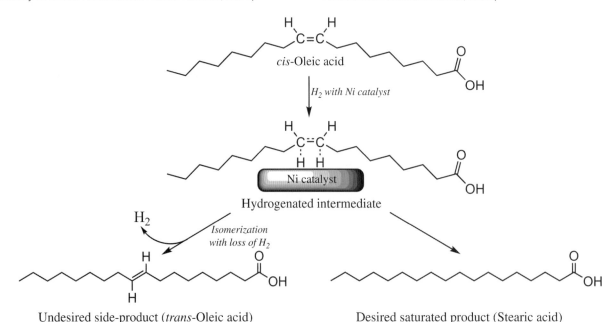

• **Fig. 2.18** Hydrogenation of unsaturated fatty acids (FAs) to form saturated FAs. In these hydrogenation reactions, a nickel (Ni) catalyst speeds up the reaction by providing a location for the H atoms to more easily react with the C=C bond. In the hydrogenation process, a slight possibility exists for the two H atoms to react with themselves and not the C=C bond. If this occurs, an undesired *trans* C=C bond results.

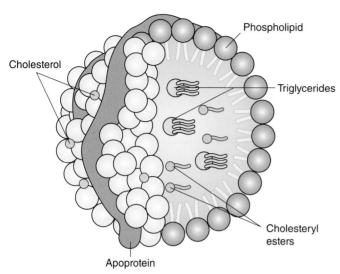

Cholesterol

Phospholipid

Triglycerides

Cholesteryl esters

Apoprotein

• **Fig. 2.20** Structure of a lipoprotein. The hydrophilic surface is composed of protein and membrane phospholipids (or glycerophospholipids) while the hydrophobic core is composed of triglycerides and cholesterol esters. (From Baynes J, Dominiczak M. *Medical Biochemistry*. 3rd ed. Mosby; 2009.)

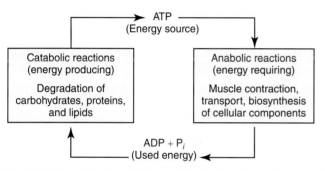

ATP
(Energy source)

Catabolic reactions
(energy producing)

Degradation of
carbohydrates, proteins,
and lipids

Anabolic reactions
(energy requiring)

Muscle contraction,
transport, biosynthesis
of cellular components

ADP + P$_i$
(Used energy)

• **Fig. 2.21** Energy flow in catabolism and anabolism. Energy is captured in catabolism to synthesize adenosine 5′-triphosphate (ATP) from adenosine diphosphate (ADP) and phosphate (P$_i$). Energy for this process is extracted from the catabolism of carbohydrates, lipids, and proteins. ATP is used as an energy source in anabolism by being hydrolyzed to ADP and P$_i$. Muscle contraction, transport, and the biosynthesis of cellular components require energy in the form of ATP.

anabolism are the requirement of energy input, the biosynthesis of more complex biomolecules from simple precursors, and the reduction of metabolites. Fig. 2.21 summarizes the flow of energy in the form of **adenosine 5′-triphosphate (ATP)** within catabolism and anabolism.

Fig. 2.22 summarizes the complex processes involved in catabolism of proteins, carbohydrates, and lipids obtained in the diet into their simpler building blocks. Dietary protein is broken down into amino acids, dietary carbohydrates into monosaccharides such as glucose, and dietary lipids into glycerol and FAs. Next, amino acids, glucose, and FAs are converted into a common intermediate called acetyl-CoA. Acetyl-CoA then enters the **tricarboxylic acid cycle (TCA cycle)**, the central metabolic pathway also known as the citric acid cycle or Krebs cycle, and is oxidized to CO_2. As nutrients are oxidized in catabolism, electrons are released from the metabolic pathways of glycolysis and the TCA cycle. **Redox coenzymes** capture and transfer these electrons, leading to the

conversion of O_2 into H_2O and the synthesis of ATP in the metabolic process called **oxidative phosphorylation**. Two of the redox coenzymes essential for this reaction are derived from the vitamins niacin and riboflwavin. Ultimately, the end products of catabolism are CO_2, H_2O, and ammonia (NH_3).

Carbohydrate Metabolism

A major source of energy for the body comes from the degradation of carbohydrates. Complete **aerobic** oxidation of glucose ($C_6H_{12}O_6$) produces CO_2, H_2O, and energy captured as ATP.

$$C_6H_{12}O_6 + 6O_2 \rightarrow 6CO_2 + 6H_2O + 36 AT$$

The digestion of dietary carbohydrates begins in the mouth as amylase enzymes hydrolyze polysaccharides into monosaccharides. These monosaccharides enter the bloodstream and are transported to the tissues that need energy. Glucose oxidation begins with **glycolysis**, entering the TCA cycle with CO_2 being produced. As glucose is oxidized, electrons are transferred by redox coenzymes to the **mitochondria**, the power source of the cell. Many coenzymes are dependent on B-complex vitamins as shown in Fig. 2.22. In oxidative phosphorylation, these electrons ultimately reduce O_2 into H_2O, and the energy is used to synthesize ATP.

Excessive amounts of dietary glucose are stored as the polysaccharide glycogen in muscles and the liver. Later, when blood glucose levels decrease and the body needs energy again, glycogen is converted back into glucose. When glycogen is depleted, **gluconeogenesis** in the liver can convert pyruvate (and other simple noncarbohydrate precursors like lactate and amino acids) into glucose for energy.

Three hormones regulate carbohydrate metabolism to maintain constant blood glucose levels (Table 2.5). **Insulin** is a signal of the "fed" state and is secreted when blood glucose levels are high. It activates glycolysis and glycogen biosynthesis-metabolic pathways that lower blood glucose levels. **Glucagon** is a signal of the "starved" state and is secreted when blood glucose levels are low. It activates gluconeogenesis and glycogen degradation-metabolic pathways that raise blood glucose levels. **Epinephrine**, the "fight-or-flight" hormone secreted for immediate energy needs, activates glycogen degradation for energy.

Protein Metabolism

The major role of dietary protein is to provide amino acids for the synthesis of new proteins for the body. Amino acids are also a source of N for the synthesis of many biomolecules, such as hormones, heme, and nitrogenous bases. Even though carbohydrates and lipids are the preferred sources of energy, proteins can be an energy source of last resort under conditions of fasting and starvation.

As shown in Fig. 2.22, the digestion of proteins begins when enzymes such as proteases hydrolyze proteins into amino acids. When amino acid levels exceed requirements, the amino group is removed, releasing free NH_3. Because high levels of NH_3 are toxic, mammals use the urea cycle to convert excess NH_3 into urea for excretion. Amino acids are further degraded, entering the TCA cycle with CO_2 being produced. The degradation of amino acids for energy can be classified as either ketogenic or glucogenic. **Ketogenic amino acids** degrade into acetyl-CoA and are converted into **ketone bodies**, soluble forms of lipids that can be used as fuel for the body. **Glucogenic amino acids** degrade into

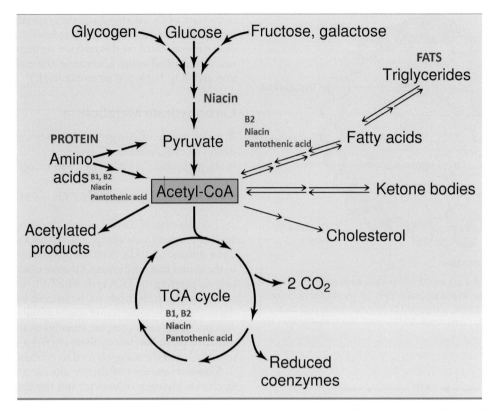

• **Fig. 2.22** Summary of the catabolism of protein, carbohydrates, and fats to create energy in the TCA (tricaroxylic acid] cycle). The diagram also shows where the B vitamins act as co-enzymes in the process of energy production. (Reproduced with permission from Meisenberg G, Simmons WH. Principles of Medical Biochemistry. © Elsevier; 2017:357.)

TABLE 2.5	Hormonal Regulation of Metabolism	
Hormone	**Increased or Stimulated**	**Decreased or Inhibited**
Insulin	Entry of glucose into cells Glycolysis Glycogen biosynthesis Triglyceride biosynthesis	Gluconeogenesis Triglyceride hydrolysis Glycogen degradation Blood glucose levels
Glucagon	Glycogen degradation (liver) Gluconeogenesis (liver) Blood glucose levels	Glycogen biosynthesis Glycolysis (liver)
Epinephrine	Glycogen degradation (muscle) Glycolysis (muscle) Triglyceride hydrolysis Blood glucose levels	Glycogen biosynthesis

TABLE 2.6	Essential (Indispensable) and Nonessential (Dispensable) Amino Acids	
Essential (Indispensable)	**Nonessential (Dispensable)**
Arginine[a]	Alanine
Histidine[a]	Asparagine
Isoleucine	Aspartic acid
Leucine	Cysteine
Lysine	Glutamic acid
Methionine	Glutamine
Phenylalanine	Glycine
Threonine	Proline
Tryptophan	Serine
Valine	Tyrosine[b]

[a]Arginine and histidine are essential (indispensable) in babies and young children but not adults.
[b]Tyrosine is synthesized from phenylalanine.

pyruvate and other TCA cycle intermediates and can be converted into glucose as a fuel for the body.

When amino acids are synthesized, they utilize common precursors found in metabolic pathways such as glycolysis and the TCA cycle. Unfortunately, humans cannot synthesize all 20 common amino acids because they lack the necessary enzymes; therefore these **essential amino acids (EAAs) or indispensable amino** acids must be obtained in the diet. The body uses enzymes to synthesize **nonessential amino acids (NEAAs) or dispensable amino acids.** Table 2.6 lists the EAAs and NEAAs.

Lipid Metabolism

Another major source of energy for the body comes from the catabolism of lipids. Because of their structure, lipids can be oxidized to produce more energy than carbohydrates or proteins. Lipids are also anhydrous ("without water"); therefore the energy per gram of lipids (9 kcal/g) is greater than that of carbohydrates (4 kcal/g). Lipids can be stored in adipose tissue in unlimited amounts.

As shown in Fig. 2.22, the digestion of dietary lipids begins when enzymes such as lipase hydrolyze TGs into free FAs and glycerol. FAs are degraded two carbons at a time, producing acetyl-CoA, which enters the TCA cycle and produces CO_2. In the degradation of FAs, electrons are captured by redox coenzymes. Subsequently, ATP is synthesized in the mitochondria via oxidative phosphorylation.

Excess dietary lipids are stored as TGs in adipose tissue. When blood glucose levels are low and glycogen stores are depleted, the utilization of TGs stored in adipose tissue is activated. As shown in Table 2.5, the hormone epinephrine activates TG hydrolysis, yielding free FAs and glycerol for energy.

Under conditions of fasting, starvation, untreated diabetes, and very low-carbohydrate diets, excessive degradation of FAs produces too much acetyl-CoA. Excessive levels of acetyl-CoA and low levels of carbohydrates result in a bottleneck at the TCA cycle. Not all the acetyl-CoA can be degraded; thus it is converted into ketone bodies and transported via the bloodstream to tissues that need energy, particularly the heart and brain, when blood glucose levels are low.

◆ Student Readiness

1. Explain how the three major areas of biochemistry (structure, metabolism, and bioinformation) are different.
2. For each of the following functional groups, find an example in the textbook of a biomolecule containing that functional group: alkene, alcohol, amine, aldehyde, ketone, carboxylic acid, ester, and peptide (amide).
3. Compare and contrast the functions of carbohydrates, proteins, nucleic acids, and lipids.
4. Differentiate between monosaccharides, disaccharides, and polysaccharides. Give an example of each.
5. Compare and contrast the structure and function of lactose and sucrose.
6. What is the difference between starch and glycogen?
7. What is the difference between enzymes and coenzymes?
8. Explain the structural reason why lipids do not readily dissolve in water.
9. What are the differences between a saturated fatty acid and an unsaturated fatty acid in terms of structure and properties?
10. In your own words, explain the central dogma of bioinformation transfer (DNA→RNA→Protein).
11. Contrast catabolism and anabolism.
12. Draw your own diagram illustrating how proteins, carbohydrates, and lipids are degraded to make energy in metabolism. Indicate on your diagram where ATP is produced. What are the three end products of catabolism containing C, H, O, or N?
13. Compare and contrast the hormones such as insulin, glucagon, and epinephrine.

◆ HEALTH APPLICATION 2

Nutrigenomics

The word genome refers to the entire DNA sequence of an organism. A gene is a region of this DNA sequence that contains instructions to produce a specific protein required for life. Human bodies have about 20,000 genes that produce proteins.[15] Mutation of a gene produces an abnormal protein, which can disrupt normal physiological processes and elicit a disease. Virtually, every disease has some basis in an individual's genes.

Genomics is the scientific discipline of mapping, sequencing, and analyzing the genome. The Human Genome Project determined the complete DNA sequence of a reference human genome from multiple anonymous people.[16,17] Over the last 20 years, genomics research has lowered the cost to sequence an individual's genome to about $100.[9] It has tailored the drug treatment of a specific cancer based on the genome of the tumor[4] and developed gene editing techniques that repair mutations in DNA.[18] This information could result in eliminating many diseases in the future.

The emergence of personalized medicine results from slight genetic variations among individuals. Single nucleotide polymorphisms, frequently called SNPs (pronounced "snips"), are the most common type of genetic variation.[10] Each SNP represents a difference in a single nucleotide and basically is an error, or typo, in DNA when it is copied and then passed on from parents to offspring. Most SNPs have no effect on health or development. However, an SNP within a gene can disrupt the function of a protein, increasing the risk of developing disease. Researchers have identified SNPs related to nutrition and health issues, such as alcohol metabolism, liver disease, diabetes, cardiovascular disease, and Crohn's disease.[5]

By integrating and applying genomics technology into nutrition research, current studies are focusing on prevention and control of chronic diseases. The scientific study of how foods or their components interact with genes,

and how individual genetic variations affect responses to nutrients (and other naturally occurring compounds), is referred to as nutrigenomics or nutritional genomics. With further research, nutrigenomics will eventually be able to characterize genetic susceptibility to diet-related chronic diseases and predict molecular responses to nutritional interventions.[1]

Genes have a powerful influence over a person's health but are not the only determinant over destiny because nutrition, emotions, age, lifestyle, and environmental factors also influence health. The scientific study of how these factors regulate gene activity without changing the underlying DNA sequence is referred to as epigenetics.[11] Epigenetic changes that switch genes on or off are required for normal development and health; however, they can also be responsible for disease.[6] These factors further complicate research by adding innumerable variables. Of the more than 25,000 bioactive (nonnutrient) food components, many have been identified as epigenetic factors. For example, a tea polyphenol reactivates epigenetically silenced genes in cancer cells.[2] Despite recent advances, there are still many unanswered questions about how epigenetic factors impact disease and the ethical and social implications of using epigenetic information in personalized medicine.[12]

A nutritionally related birth defect that has almost been cut in half by implementation of a dietary measure is a neural tube defect.[7] Folate is an example of a nutrient extensively studied because of its impact on DNA synthesis in the human genome. Epigenetic changes and SNPs that affect folate-dependent enzymes increase the risk for developmental conditions, such as neural tube defects.[3] Folate fortification in the food supply was targeted at a distinct group—females of childbearing age who are at genetic risk for having an infant with a neural tube defect—to prevent this birth defect. This public health measure has been successful in lowering the

(Continued)

◆ HEALTH APPLICATION 2

Nutrigenomics—cont'd

rate of neural tube defects. This is just one example of how a nutritional intervention might be individualized based on knowledge of nutrigenomics.

Nutritional genomics has tremendous potential to not only change the future of personal nutrition recommendations, but also dietary guidelines for the population. Health promotion advice in the *Dietary Guidelines* is based on population-based data; for example, what is statistically likely to occur with respect to risk factors and disease outcomes.[13] On the other hand, nutrigenomics research focuses on modifying this advice based on an individual's genetics.[8]

The current knowledge base for nutrigenomics is in its infancy. Nutrigenomics will someday provide the basis for personalized dietary recommendations based on the individual's genetic makeup. Chronic disease may be preventable, or delayed, by prescribing a personalized regimen of a specific nutrient based on an analysis of a person's genes. Furthermore, those individuals who are identified as having a higher disease risk through genetic testing may be more motivated to follow dietetic recommendations.[8]

Cutting-edge research is exciting and encouraging, but nutrigenomics is not ready for clinical implementation. In its most recent position paper, the Academy of Nutrition and Dietetics states that the practical application of nutritional genomics for complex chronic disease is an emerging science and that the use of nutrigenetic testing to provide dietary advice is not ready for routine dietetics practice. Most chronic diseases, such as cardiovascular disease, diabetes, and cancer, are multigenetic and

multifactorial. Therefore genetic mutations are only partially predictive of disease. Registered dietitian nutritionists (RDN) who do not have advanced genetic education may not be able to understand, interpret, and communicate complex test results in which the actual risk of developing disease may not be known.[19] Many RDNs are specializing in this field of Integrative and Functional Medical Nutrition Therapy to earn a certificate to become a functional medicine nutritionist.

As genetic analysis rapidly develops and becomes more cost effective, potential problems will result in the exploitation of the basic hypotheses. Many scientific research studies are essential when determining whether a hypothesis is true, and many of these studies will need to be long-term. A single study claiming to show a specific effect is not considered evidence-based research, ready for implementation in a clinical setting. Unscrupulous individuals will use cutting-edge research to make clinical claims that are years or decades premature by basing their work on knowledge that currently does not exist.[14] Currently, clinical claims regarding genomics and nutrition or health conditions are premature and misleading by pretending to be knowledgeable where evidence-based studies do not exist.

Already, websites are claiming to treat autism, multiple sclerosis, Parkinson disease, and other conditions using "nutrigenomics." There is currently no evidence for any nutritional treatment to prevent or cure any of these diseases, and especially not based on genetic types. Nutrigenomics is an exciting legitimate field of research, but it is an area subject to quackery.

References

1. Ferguson LR, Caterina RD, Görman U, et al. Guide and position of the International Society of Nutrigenetics/Nutrigenomics on personalised nutrition: part 1—fields of precision nutrition. *J Nutrigenet Nutrigenomics*. 2016;9(1):12–27.
2. Malcomson FC, Mathers JC. Nutrition, epigenetics and health through life. *Nutr Bull*. 2017;42(3):254–265.
3. Liew S-C, Gupta ED. Methylenetetrahydrofolate reductase (MTHFR) C677T polymorphism: epidemiology, metabolism and the associated diseases. *Eur J Med Genet*. 2015;58(1):1–10.
4. Parilla M, Ritterhouse LL. Beyond the variants: mutational patterns in next-generation sequencing data for cancer precision medicine. *Front Cell Dev Biol*. 2020;8:370.
5. Mullins VA, Bresette W, Johnstone L, et al. Genomics in personalized nutrition: can you "eat for your genes"? *Nutrients*. 2020;12(10):3118.
6. Cavalli G, Heard E. Advances in epigenetics link genetics to the environment and disease. *Nature*. 2019;571(7766):489–499.
7. Blom HJ, Shaw GM, Heijer MD, et al. Neural tube defects and folate: case far from closed. *Nat Rev Neurosci*. 2006;7(9):724–731.
8. Kohlmeier M, Caterina RD, Ferguson LR, et al. Guide and position of the International Society of Nutrigenetics/Nutrigenomics on personalized nutrition: part 2—ethics, challenges and endeavors of precision nutrition. *J Nutrigenet Nutrigenomics*. 2016;9(1):28–46.
9. Pennisi E. Upstart DNA sequencers could be a 'game changer'. *Science*. 2022;376(6599):1257–1258.
10. What are single nucleotide polymorphisms (SNPs)? *MedlinePlus Genetics*. National Library of Medicine (United States). Available at: <https://medlineplus.gov/genetics/understanding/genomicresearch/snp/>.
11. What is epigenetics? *MedlinePlus Genetics*. National Library of Medicine (United States). Available at: <https://medlineplus.gov/genetics/understanding/howgeneswork/epigenome/>.
12. Santaló J, Berdasco M. Ethical implications of epigenetics in the era of personalized medicine. *Clin Epigenet*. 2022;14:44.
13. United States Department of Agriculture and U.S. Department of Health and Human Services. *Dietary Guidelines for Americans, 2020–2025*. 9th ed. 2020. Available at: <https://www.dietaryguidelines.gov/>.
14. Novella S.. Nutrigenomics—not ready for prime time. *Science-Based Medicine*. Posted January 2, 2013. Available at: <https://sciencebasedmedicine.org/nutrigenomics-not-ready-for-prime-time/>.
15. Nurk S, Koren S, Rhie A, et al. The complete sequence of a human genome. *Science*. 2022;376(6588):44–53.
16. Lander ES, Linton LM, Birren B, et al. Initial sequencing and analysis of the human genome. *Nature*. 2001;409(6822):860–921.
17. Collins FS, Morgan M, Patrinos A. The Human Genome Project: lessons from large-scale biology. *Science*. 2003;300(5617):286–290.
18. Wang JY, Doudna JA. CRISPR technology: a decade of genome editing is only the beginning. *Science*. 2023;379(6629).
19. Camp KM, Trujillo E. Position of the Academy of Nutrition and Dietetics: nutritional genomics. *J Acad Nutr Diet*. 2014;114(2):299–312.

▶ Evolve Resources

Please visit http://evolve.elsevier.com/Mallonee/nutritional for additional practice and study support tools.

3

Digestion and Absorption

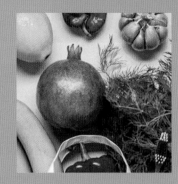

STUDENT LEARNING OUTCOMES

On completion of this chapter, the student will be able to achieve the following learning outcomes:

1. Outline the physiology of the gastrointestinal tract, including the two basic types of actions on food.
2. Related to the oral cavity:
   - Identify oral factors that influence food intake.
   - Explain to patients why saliva flow is important for oral health and overall well-being.
   - Describe the role that teeth play in digestion.
3. Related to the esophagus and gastric digestion:
   - Describe how the esophagus works.
   - Diagram the process of gastric digestion, including the two major enzymes found in gastric juice.
4. Related to the small intestine:
   - Identify the nutrients requiring digestion and the absorbable products.

- Illustrate the process of osmosis.
- Discuss with patients how digestion and absorption may affect nutritional status and oral health.
5. Related to the large intestine:
   - Differentiate the function of the large intestine from that of the small intestine.
   - Indicate the side effects of undigested residue.
   - Define the purpose of microflora.
   - Explain the role of gastrointestinal motility in digestion and absorption.
   - State the purpose of peristalsis.

KEY TERMS

Accessory organs
Active transport
Alveolar process
Anorexia
Anosmia
Autoimmune disorder
Bile
Bolus
Cancellous bone
Celiac disease
Chyme
Constipation
Demineralization
Dysgeusia
Emulsification
Gluten
Gustatory
Hypergeusia

Hypogeusia
Iatrogenic
Large intestine
Lower esophageal sphincter
Lymphatic system
Mastication
Masticatory efficiency
Microbiome
Microflora
Microvilli
Nonceliac gluten sensitivity
Olfactory nerves
Osmosis
Pancreatic enzymes
Papillae
Passive diffusion
Pathogenic
Peristalsis

Phantom taste
Portal circulation
Prebiotics
Probiotics
Proteolytic enzymes
Remineralize
Residue
Small intestinal bacterial overgrowth
Small intestine
Sphincter muscles
Symbiotics
Systemic condition
Taste buds
Trabecular bone
Umami
Valves
Wheat allergy
Xerostomia

⬡ **TEST YOUR NQ**

1. **T/F** The gastrointestinal tract is approximately 30 ft (9 m) long.
2. **T/F** Gurgling sounds in the abdomen are caused by hydrolysis.
3. **T/F** Most absorption occurs in the stomach.
4. **T/F** Fat-soluble nutrients always enter the portal circulation.
5. **T/F** Taste disorders are often the result of problems in smell rather than taste.
6. **T/F** Doorlike mechanisms between parts of the intestine are called accessory organs.
7. **T/F** The digestive process begins in the oral cavity.
8. **T/F** Villi are located in the large intestine.
9. **T/F** Missing, decayed, or poorly restored teeth can affect food intake.
10. **T/F** Saliva aids in oral clearance of food.

Foods are composed of large chemical molecules that cannot be used unless they are broken down to an absorbable form. The digestive system is designed to (1) ingest foods, (2) digest or divide complex molecules into simple, soluble materials that can be absorbed, and (3) eliminate unused residues. Only energy-providing macronutrients (carbohydrate, protein, and fat) must be digested for absorption. Most vitamins, minerals, alcohol, and water can be absorbed as eaten.

The gastrointestinal (GI) tract can also deliver complex chemical substances such as oral medications. Medications frequently affect or can be affected by foods, modifying absorption, metabolism, or excretion of either the food or the drug. They may also affect nutritional status by altering taste or salivary flow; these conditions influence the amount and types of foods consumed. The dental hygienist's knowledge of GI processes can be an asset in working with patients whose nutritional status and oral health are affected by disturbances in the GI tract.

Physiology of the Gastrointestinal Tract

The GI tract is one of the largest organs in the body and is designed for digesting and absorbing nutrients from foods. The digestive system includes the GI tract and several accessory organs (Fig. 3.1). The GI tract is a long, hollow, muscular tubular structure approximately 30 ft (9 m) long (five times the height of an average male). It extends from the mouth to the anus, comprising all the body parts through which food and nutrients pass. It includes the oral cavity, pharynx, esophagus, stomach, small intestine, and large intestine. The small intestine comprises the duodenum, jejunum, and ileum; the large intestine includes the cecum, colon, rectum, and anal tract. Accessory organs—the salivary glands, liver, gallbladder, and pancreas—provide secretions essential for digestion and absorption. Digestion involves two basic types of action on food: (1) mechanical and (2) chemical. Mechanical actions include chewing and peristalsis, which break up and mix foods, permitting better blending of foodstuffs with digestive secretions. Chemical actions involve salivary enzymes and digestive juices, reducing foodstuffs to absorbable molecules.

Chemical Action

As discussed in Chapter 2, hydrolysis reactions occur in the digestive tract for nutrients in food to be utilized. The following are basic hydrolysis reactions in food digestion:

$$\text{Protein} + H_2O \rightarrow \text{amino acids}$$

$$\text{Fat} + H_2O \rightarrow \text{fatty acids} + \text{glycerol}$$

$$\text{Carbohydrate} + H_2O \rightarrow \text{monosaccharides}$$

Enzymes produced in the GI tract allow these reactions to proceed (Table 3.1).

Mechanical Action

The wall of the GI tract is similar from the esophagus to the rectum (Fig. 3.2A). A layer of muscles encircles the tube, allowing the diameter of the tube to expand and contract. Food particles are separated and mixed by the churning action. Outer fibers of the muscular coat (longitudinal muscle) run lengthwise and are responsible for peristalsis, involuntary rhythmic waves of contraction traveling the length of the GI tract.

Doorlike mechanisms between the digestive segments, called valves or sphincter muscles, are designed to (1) retain food in each segment until completion of the mechanical actions and digestive juices, (2) allow measured amounts of food to pass into the next segment, and (3) prevent food from "backing up" into the preceding area. Regulation of these valves is complex, involving muscular function and different pressures on each side of the valve.

⬡ **DENTAL CONSIDERATIONS**

- Gurgling sounds, caused by air and fluid in the normal abdomen, indicate that peristalsis is occurring.
- If the GI tract is not functioning properly and digestion and/or absorption are affected, nutrients may not be absorbed even when ample amounts are consumed. Consequently, the patient may be prone to nutrient deficiencies or poor healing.
- Loss of motility in the stomach and small intestine, observed occasionally in diabetes mellitus, results in impaired gastric and intestinal emptying. This allows excessive growth of bacteria, which may injure the surface of the intestine, cause diarrhea, and interfere with nutrient absorption. Patients who are immobile (because of injury, trauma, or debilitating illness) or patients with uncontrolled diabetes are more prone to these disorders.
- Food-drug interactions have the potential to cause nutritional problems or erratic drug responses. Knowledge of common drugs (including over-the-counter medications, herbals, and supplements) and understanding how they interact with food is important. For example, consuming milk or milk products while taking tetracycline decreases the amount of tetracycline and calcium absorbed.

⬡ **NUTRITIONAL DIRECTIONS**

- Taking over-the-counter enzyme tablets may not be beneficial because enzymes are digested before they can be absorbed. Prescription pancreatic enzymes have a special enteric coating that prevents the enzyme from exposure to gastric juices. Lactase, a nonprescription enzyme, is effective for lactose-intolerant individuals because it is either added to or taken with lactose-containing foods, allowing conversion of lactose into two monosaccharides before gastric juices can affect the enzyme (see *Health Application 4: Lactose Intolerance* in Chapter 4).
- Patients reporting GI problems should be assessed for adequate nutrient intake using guidance tools such as the *Dietary Guidelines*. If intake is inadequate, the patient should be referred to the patient's primary care provider or a registered dietitian nutritionist (RDN).

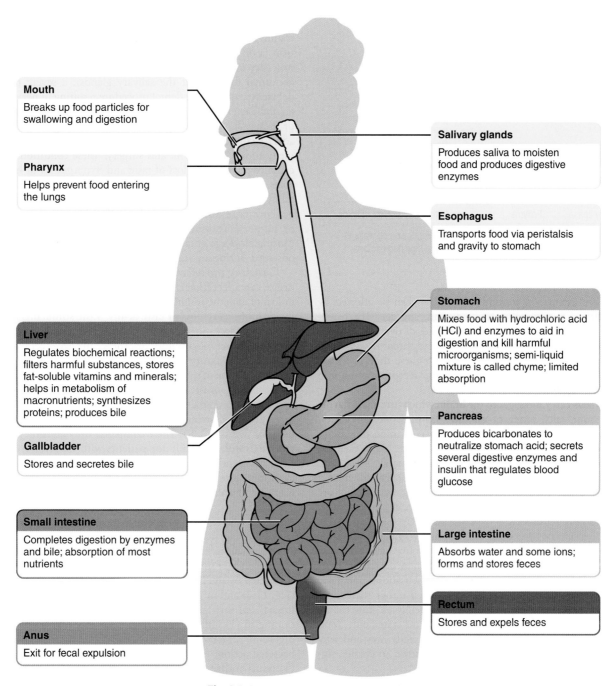

Mouth
Breaks up food particles for swallowing and digestion

Pharynx
Helps prevent food entering the lungs

Salivary glands
Produces saliva to moisten food and produces digestive enzymes

Esophagus
Transports food via peristalsis and gravity to stomach

Liver
Regulates biochemical reactions; filters harmful substances, stores fat-soluble vitamins and minerals; helps in metabolism of macronutrients; synthesizes proteins; produces bile

Gallbladder
Stores and secretes bile

Stomach
Mixes food with hydrochloric acid (HCl) and enzymes to aid in digestion and kill harmful microorganisms; semi-liquid mixture is called chyme; limited absorption

Pancreas
Produces bicarbonates to neutralize stomach acid; secrets several digestive enzymes and insulin that regulates blood glucose

Small intestine
Completes digestion by enzymes and bile; absorption of most nutrients

Large intestine
Absorbs water and some ions; forms and stores feces

Rectum
Stores and expels feces

Anus
Exit for fecal expulsion

• **Fig. 3.1** Summary of digestive organ functions.

Oral Cavity

Taste and Smell

Generally, food choices are influenced by three sensory perceptions: sight, smell, and taste. **Gustatory** (taste) sensations evoke pronounced feelings of pleasure or aversion; therefore taste is the primary determinant of food choices. Food considerations, such as healthfulness or cost, are typically rated as less important. The presentation of food, its color and aroma, may be the basis for acceptance or rejection. Food flavors are derived from characteristics of substances ingested, including taste, aroma, texture, temperature, and irritating properties. Approximately 75% of flavor is derived from odors. Taste and smell are essential for maintaining sufficient intake to meet physiologic needs.

The mouth, or oral cavity, plays an important role in the digestive system. It is the "port of entry" where receptors for sense of taste, or **taste buds**, are located. A taste bud consists of approximately 50 to 150 cells embedded in the surrounding epithelium, termed **papillae**. Taste papillae appear on the tongue as little red dots, or raised bumps, most numerous on the dorsal epithelium. For example, the circumvallate papillae have many tiny taste buds around the lateral surface. These taste buds are composed of cells that support several small hairlike nerve endings that perceive taste (Fig. 3.3). Taste buds are also located throughout the mouth—on the palate, epiglottis, and even in the proximal esophagus. These

TABLE 3.1	Digestive Functions of Saliva	
Saliva Component	Classification	Function
Mucous (mucin)	Glycoprotein	Lubricates food for easier passage and protects the lining of the gastrointestinal tract
Ptyalin (salivary amylase)	Enzyme	Initiates hydrolysis of complex carbohydrates to simple sugars
Salivary lipase	Enzyme	Initiates hydrolysis of lipids
Lysozyme (antibody)	Enzyme	Breaks down cell walls of some ingested bacteria

cells replace themselves continually, but they can be affected by disease, drugs, nutritional status, radiation, and age. The receptors that capture these tastes are distributed all over the tongue. Different parts of the tongue, soft palate, and throat have a lower threshold for perceiving specific tastes, but these differences are rather minute. As food is chewed, gustatory receptors come into contact with chemicals dissolved in saliva.

Nerve cells carry messages to the brain, which interprets flavors as sweet, sour, salty, bitter, or umami (flavorful, pleasant taste). Umami is detected in foods containing L-glutamine present in amino acids and proteins (specifically soy sauce, meat extracts, aging cheese, bacon, and monosodium glutamate). These five basic tastes reflect specific constituents of food. Genetically related differences affect food preferences, influencing what foods are consumed. Many taste buds degenerate in older adults, causing a decrease in taste sensitivity.

Food stimulates taste buds, and aromas stimulate olfactory nerves, receptors for smell. In contrast to the five basic tastes, an almost unlimited number of unique odors can be detected. Food-related aromas may be confused with taste sensations, and taste disorders often result from problems in smell rather than taste. Increasing age affects a patient's ability to smell food more than a patient's taste acuity, frequently expressed by the statement, "food just doesn't taste good." It remains unclear exactly how and why taste preferences shift, but preferences are known to change significantly with aging.

Loss of smell, or anosmia, results in limited capacity to detect flavor of food and beverages. Ability to smell food being prepared and eaten influences food selection. Smell is also a protective mechanism; odors are used to help determine whether foods are harmful or spoiled. Upper respiratory infections, nasal or sinus problems, neurologic disorders, endocrine abnormalities, aging, or head trauma may cause anosmia. A common cold often impairs a person's sense of smell, causing loss of appetite and limiting the ability to taste and enjoy food. The rate of the continuous renewal process undergone by olfactory receptor cells is depressed in malnutrition and by some antibiotics. Some of these disorders are self-limited; however, chemosensory losses from chemotherapy, upper respiratory infection, COVID-19 (coronavirus disease 2019), and aging may be irreversible.

Dysgeusia is persistent, abnormal distortion of taste, including sweet, sour, bitter, salty, or metallic tastes. Dysgeusia without identifiable taste stimuli is called phantom taste. Dysgeusia may be caused by a previous viral upper respiratory infection, head trauma, a neurologic or psychiatric disorder, a systemic condition (a disease or disorder that affects the whole body), xerostomia (dry mouth from inadequate salivary secretion secondary to abnormal function of the salivary glands), a severe nutritional deficiency, an invasive dental procedure resulting in nerve damage, an oral bacterial or fungal infection, or burning mouth syndrome, or it may have an iatrogenic causation. Iatrogenic refers to an adverse condition resulting from medical treatment, for example, medications, irradiation, and surgery. These conditions may also cause hypogeusia or loss of taste and hypergeusia or heightened taste acuity. Mouth breathing may also cause dysgeusia. The dental hygienist is frequently the first health care provider to detect a patient's taste disorder through medical history review questions or intraoral assessment. Hyperkeratinization of the epithelium causing blockage of taste buds and affecting dietary intake may be observed during an oral examination.

Gustatory and olfactory disorders, whether caused by disease or drugs, can affect food choices and dietary habits. Anorexia, a lack or loss of appetite resulting in the inability to eat, may occur when medications cause loss of taste acuity. Taste stimulants affect salivary and pancreatic secretions, gastric contractions, and intestinal motility. Therefore gustatory disorders can also affect digestion.

Because gustatory and olfactory disorders can result in deterioration of a patient's general condition or nutritional status, these abnormalities must always be considered in dental and nutritional care. Potentially adverse compensatory habits may develop (e.g., decreased sweet or salty perceptions may result in excessive usage of sweets or salt). These compensatory habits may be potentially harmful, especially for patients with diabetes or hypertension. Also, additional sugar can increase the risk of dental caries. Persistent taste distortions can lead to inadequate caloric intake, resulting in unintentional weight loss or malnutrition.

Saliva

Adequate salivary flow is essential for oral health, which includes maintenance of soft tissues in the oral cavity and taste buds. Saliva is secreted by the major (parotid, submandibular, and sublingual) (Fig. 11.2) and minor (labial, buccal, palatine, glossopalatine, and lingual) salivary glands. It is essential in taste sensations, functioning to (1) lubricate oral tissues for chewing, swallowing, and digestion; (2) remove debris and microorganisms; (3) provide antibacterial action; (4) neutralize, dilute, and buffer bacterial acids; (5) remineralize (restoration or renewal of calcium, phosphates, and other minerals to areas damaged by incipient caries, abrasion, or erosion); (6) prevent plaque accumulation; (7) facilitate taste; and (8) promote ease of speech. An average of 1 to 2 mL/min of this complex fluid helps maintain the integrity of teeth against physical, chemical, and microbial insults.

Saliva is supersaturated with calcium phosphates that allow demineralized areas of hydroxyapatite in enamel to be remineralized. Demineralization occurs when calcium, phosphate, and other minerals are lost from tooth enamel, causing the enamel to dissolve. This occurs because acids produced by fermentable carbohydrates combine with acidogenic bacteria (see Chapter 18); it is not caused by insufficient calcium. Genetic variations of saliva, especially amylase, affect food preferences and intake by influencing oral sensory properties of food.

Acidic, sour, bitter, and umami tastes stimulate salivary flow. Saliva production is also stimulated by the consumption of tasty foods and gum chewing. An increase in oral clearance rate

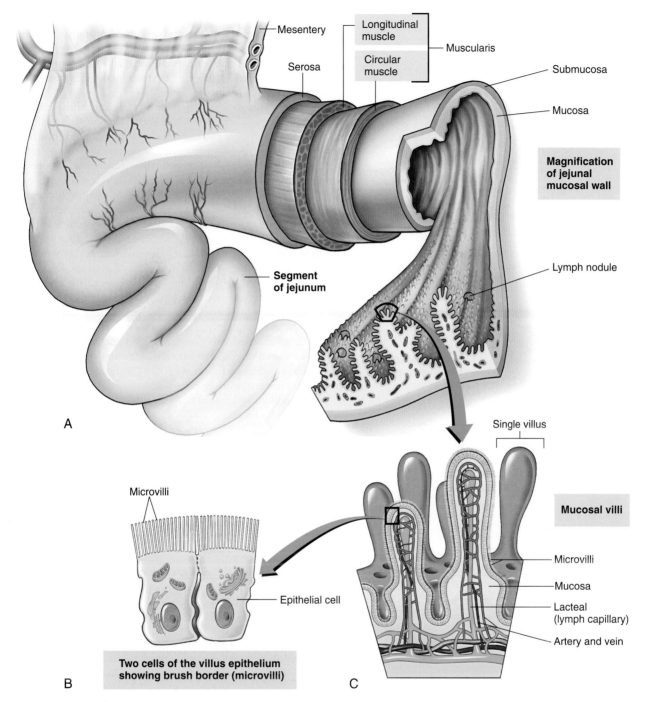

• **Fig. 3.2** Wall of the small intestine. (A) Layers composing the intestinal wall. (B) The villi covering the mucosa that absorb nutrients. (C) Further enlargement shows the brush border or microvilli enzymes that are available to further hydrolyze nutrients for absorption. (From Standring S. *Gray's Anatomy: The Anatomical Basis of Clinical Practice.* 42nd ed. Churchill Livingstone; 2021.)

decreases the risk of caries formation (see Chapter 18). Saliva moistens food particles to more easily manipulate and prepare them for swallowing.

Some chemical action or hydrolysis of nutrients begins in the mouth. Table 3.1 shows the functions of different constituents in saliva. Ptyalin, or salivary amylase, initiates starch digestion in the mouth. If a carbohydrate food, such as a cracker, is chewed and held in the mouth for a few seconds, it will begin to taste sweet, indicating hydrolysis of starch to dextrin and maltose.

Xerostomia leads to diminished gustatory function (see Chapter 20 for additional details). Xerostomia may result in frequent oral ulcerations, increased sensitivity of the tongue to spices and flavors, and increased risk of dental caries. Many drugs cause xerostomia. For example, diuretics, prescribed to help the body eliminate fluids, cause a decrease in salivary flow. Increasing fluid is important to compensate for these losses. Table 12.1 provides recommendations for the number of cups of water based on life stage and sex.

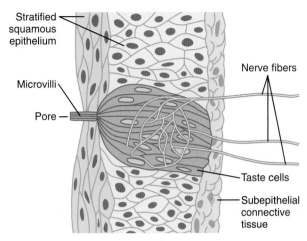

• **Fig. 3.3** Taste bud. The hairlike receptors of taste buds are located in the pore, enabling taste perception. (From Hall JE, Guyton AC. *Guyton and Hall Textbook of Medical Physiology*. 13th ed. Elsevier; 2016.)

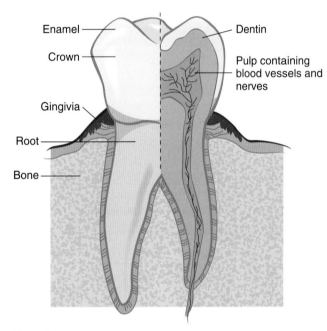

• **Fig. 3.4** Diagram of a tooth.

Teeth

Teeth play a major role in digestion by crushing and grinding food into smaller pieces, a process known as mastication. In contrast to bone, neither tooth enamel nor dentin can be repaired or replaced in significant amounts by natural processes. Only small amounts of enamel and dentin are repaired or replaced through enamel remineralization and through secondary dentin deposition around the pulp chamber of the tooth (Fig. 3.4). Mineral deposition and resorption affect the bone that supports the dentition. This supporting bone, known as alveolar bone, is primarily trabecular bone (bony spikes forming a meshwork of spaces) and cancellous bone (bone within the spaces created by the network of trabecular bone, which appears spongy and contains bone marrow in small hollows). Negative calcium balance increases susceptibility to resorption and bone loss in the alveolar process (comprising the maxillary and mandibular crest and serves as the bony investment for teeth). The maxilla and mandible to

some extent depend on the presence of teeth and occlusal forces associated with chewing to prevent calcium resorption. Chewing firm foods helps maintain proper balance between alveolar bone resorption and new bone formation. Teeth and supporting bone structures are affected by adequate nutrient intake, digestive function, and hormonal balance.

Mastication reduces food particle size. The inability to masticate food adequately may result in larger chunks of food being swallowed. These larger pieces increase the potential for obstruction in the airway. Food asphyxiation, which may result in death, may occur in individuals with defective, incomplete, or poorly fitting dentures. Patients with less than 20 teeth have a decrease in masticatory efficiency, altering their ability to adequately prepare food for swallowing. Even after patients become fully adjusted to well-fitted dentures, masticatory efficiency is rendered less than what they had with their natural teeth. Oral rehabilitation with prosthodontic treatment, including dental implants, considerably influences the well-being and quality of life of patients. Digestion of food is facilitated by increasing its surface area. It is uncertain whether food particle size affects digestibility. However, when older adults have digestive problems, masticatory efficiency is usually a factor. Frequently, when masticatory efficiency declines, people either choose foods that require less chewing or use techniques to soften foods, for example, stewing meats, steaming vegetables, or dunking cookies or toast in fluids. In many circumstances, hypersensitive, poorly restored, decayed, abscessed, or periodontally involved teeth affect food choices and limit the variety of foods chosen.

Esophagus

The swallowing reflex moves a bolus, or the swallowed mass of food, into the esophagus and is transported to the stomach by peristalsis and gravity. The esophagus is a continuous tube approximately 10 inches (25–30 cm) long connecting the pharynx with the stomach. It penetrates the diaphragm through an opening called the esophageal hiatus. The lower esophageal sphincter (LES) comprises a group of very strong circular muscle fibers located just above the stomach. The LES relaxes to permit food into the stomach but contracts tightly to prevent regurgitation, or "backwashing," of stomach contents.

⬤ DENTAL CONSIDERATIONS

- Assess the nutritional status of patients with gustatory or olfactory disorders for changes in dietary habits and appetite that may lead to a nutritional deficiency, increased use of sugar, spices (especially salt), food textures, and development of food cravings or dislikes.
- Patients commonly complain about "taste" or "flavor" of food when olfactory as well as gustatory sensations are impaired.
- Adequate salivary flow helps flush pathogenic (harmful) bacteria; enzymes are bactericidal, destroying oral bacteria, including some that cause dental caries. Without salivation, oral tissues may become ulcerated and infected, allowing caries to become rampant.
- Assess patients for possible nutritional deficiencies (niacin, vitamins A and B$_{12}$, zinc, copper, nickel) because these can be related to gustatory abnormalities.
- Loss of umami taste sensation affects quality of life and causes weight loss and health problems, particularly in older adults.
- Zinc depletion may decrease taste acuity but is not the reason for all cases of hypogeusia. Currently, no tests can accurately assess marginal zinc status.

🦷 DENTAL CONSIDERATIONS—CONT'D

- Xerostomia may compound modifications to food intake related to taste loss and make chewing and swallowing more difficult.
- Patients who are edentulous or with ill-fitting dentures should be monitored because the quality and quantity of food intake may be compromised.
- Dentures may cause alterations in taste, either caused by altered masticatory efficiency or by the appliance covering the palatal taste buds. Patients with complete dentures exhibit poorer taste and texture sensation compared to patients with partial dentures or compromised natural dentition.
- Although food intake often decreases when patients initially receive a set of dentures, after an initial adjustment period, food intake usually increases with an improved ability to chew.
- Refer patients with persistent gustatory, masticatory, or swallowing difficulties to a health care provider or RDN to determine the types of foods needed to obtain adequate nutrients.

🦷 NUTRITIONAL DIRECTIONS

- For xerostomia, increase fluid intake with meals to facilitate oral clearance. Nutrient-dense foods in a liquid or semiliquid form are beneficial for patients struggling with adequate caloric intake.
- No proven intervention enhances diminished taste acuity or ameliorates dysgeusia. Encourage experimentation with texture, spiciness, and temperature.
- To improve nutrient intake when mastication is less efficient, special cooking techniques (e.g., stewing meats), chewing longer, and choosing soft foods are preferable to pureeing foods. For example, cream-style corn can replace corn on the cob, and stewed apples can replace raw apples.
- Particularly for new denture wearers, herbs and spices and contrasting food flavor combinations (e.g., sweet and sour) can enhance taste perception.

Mumps is a viral infection of primarily the parotid gland causing pain during secretion. Because eating causes stimulation to the gland, food and fluid intake may be inhibited.[1]

Gastric Digestion

A bolus entering the stomach is mixed with gastric secretions by peristaltic contractions, producing chyme, a semifluid material produced by gastric juices on ingested food. Gastric secretions include mucus, hydrochloric acid, enzymes, and a component called intrinsic factor (Table 3.2).

The low pH of stomach contents (~1.5–3.0) is beneficial for several reasons as it (1) kills or inhibits the growth of most food bacteria, (2) denatures proteins and facilitates hydrolysis to amino acids, (3) activates gastric enzymes, (4) hydrolyzes some carbohydrates, and (5) increases solubility and absorption of calcium and iron.

Two major enzymes are found in gastric juice: pepsin and lipase. Pepsin is capable of hydrolyzing large protein molecules to smaller fragments. Gastric lipase is involved in the digestion of short- and medium-chain triglycerides (e.g., type of fat in butterfat). Mucus forms an alkaline coating in the stomach to protect it against digestion by pepsin. Intrinsic factor, secreted in the stomach, is essential for the absorption of vitamin B_{12} in the small intestine.

Normal gastric secretion is regulated by nerves and hormonal stimuli. Visual, olfactory, and gustatory senses stimulate gastric secretions. Fear, sadness, pain, and depression are generally accompanied by decreased secretions; anger, stress, and hostility may increase secretions.

An adult stomach functions as a reservoir to hold an average meal for 3 to 4 hours. The stomach empties at different rates depending on the size of the stomach and composition of the chyme. The rate of passage through the stomach (fastest to slowest) is liquids, carbohydrates, proteins, and fats. When a mixture of foods is presented, this pattern is not as well defined. The smaller the stomach capacity, the more rapidly the stomach empties. (This is exemplified in infants, who must be fed frequently until the stomach size expands.) Fats remain in the stomach longer, providing greater satiety than proteins or carbohydrates. Small amounts of chyme are released from the stomach through the pyloric sphincter to allow for adequate digestion and absorption in the small intestine.

Very little absorption occurs in the stomach because few foods are completely hydrolyzed to nutrients the body can use at this stage. Nutrients that can be absorbed from the stomach are water, alcohol, and a few water-soluble substances (e.g., amino acids and glucose).

🦷 DENTAL CONSIDERATIONS

- Dietary constituents that increase hydrochloric acid and pepsin secretions are proteins, calcium, caffeine, coffee, and alcohol; patients with ulcers or certain GI tract disorders may need to limit or omit these.
- Because gravity facilitates the movement of food down the esophagus, patients who are in a supine position may have some difficulty swallowing and may reflux gastric contents, especially after eating. Aspiration of acid reflux into the lungs is possible. To prevent an emergency situation, place the patient in a semisupine position for treatment. If possible, schedule the appointment 3 hours after a meal to minimize reflux.

🦷 NUTRITIONAL DIRECTIONS

- Vomiting is one of the body's methods of eliminating toxins from contaminated foods: it can be stimulated by rapid changes in body motion or by drugs.
- Heartburn is a result of regurgitation (reflux) of the stomach contents into the esophagus. Acidic gastric secretions produce discomfort or pain, which may be relieved if the patient remains in an upright position after eating.
- Eating in a calm, relaxing atmosphere helps reduce gastric secretions.
- Over an extended period, chronic problems with vomiting or reflux can result in sensitive teeth and varying degrees of tooth erosion, especially on lingual and occlusal surfaces.

Small Intestine

Most of the energy-providing nutrients are completely hydrolyzed and absorbed within the small intestine. Most vitamins and minerals are also absorbed in the small intestine. The small intestine is specially designed to perform these tasks with juices secreted by the accessory organs and its complex luminal wall (see Table 3.2).

TABLE 3.2 Digestive Process and Physiologic Utilization of Energy-Producing Nutrients

Site	Enzymes	Carbohydrate	Protein	Fat
Nutrient Digestion				
Mouth	Salivary amylase	Starch → maltose	No action	
	Lingual lipase			Triglycerides–diglyceride + free fatty acids
Stomach	Gastric pepsin		Proteins → peptides → amino acids	
	Gastric lipase			Emulsified fats → fatty acids + glycerol
Small intestine	Pancreatic enzyme	Starch → dextrin Dextrin → maltose		
	Pancreatic trypsin, chymotrypsin, carboxypeptidase, ribonuclease, and deoxyribonuclease		Protein → polypeptides RNA and DNA → mononucleotides	
	Pancreatic enzyme and intestinal lipase			Emulsified fats—fatty acids + glycerol
	Sucrase, lactase, maltase	Sucrose → glucose + fructose Maltose → glucose + glucose Lactose → glucose + galactose		
	Intestinal aminopeptidase and dipeptidase		Polypeptides → amino acids	
	Nucleotidase		Nucleic acids → nucleotides	
	Nucleosidase and phosphorylase		Nucleosides → purines, pyrimidines, and pentose phosphate	
Nutrients' Absorption From Small Intestine				
		Glucose, fructose, and galactose absorbed	Amino acids, mononucleotides, dipeptides, and tripeptides absorbed	Fatty acids + glycerol absorbed
Nutrient Utilization				
		Glucose oxidized for energy—$CO_2 + H_2O$	Amino acids build and repair tissue	Fatty acids + glycerol → new fat
		Unused stored as liver glycogen or changed and stored as body fat	Unused—nitrogen removed, forming urea and carbon, hydrogen, oxygen → glucose	Unused stored as body fat; some fat + phosphorus → phospholipids

DNA, Deoxyribonucleic acids; *RNA*, ribonucleic acid.

The small intestine is approximately 15 ft (4.5 m) long, and foods are retained there for 3 to 10 hours.

Digestion

Throughout the walls of the small intestine are villi, fingerlike projections rising out of the mucosa into the intestinal lumen (see Fig. 3.2B and C). These villi increase the surface area of the GI tract to approximately 3000 square feet. Each villus is also covered with a layer of epithelial cells containing microvilli, which collectively form the brush border cells. Microvilli are minute hairlike folds located on the villi, which greatly increase the intestinal absorptive surface area. The pH change and motility in the small intestine inhibit bacterial growth.

Acidic chyme entering the intestine stimulates hormones to release pancreatic juices into the duodenum. Cholecystokinin, a hormone released in response to the presence of fat in chyme, stimulates the gallbladder to contract and release bile. Bile, produced and secreted by the liver, is stored in the gallbladder. The action of bile salts allows insoluble molecules to be divided into smaller particles, a process called emulsification. This process allows greater exposure of fats to intestinal and pancreatic lipases. Peristalsis also facilitates mixing and emulsification by bile.

Pancreatic enzymes enter the duodenum through the pancreatic duct and function best in neutralized chyme. Pancreatic enzymes hydrolyze carbohydrates, proteins, and fats. Proteolytic enzymes, which hydrolyze proteins, are produced and stored in the pancreas in an inactive form.

Specific digestive enzymes lining the brush border of the microvilli are responsible for completing hydrolysis of carbohydrates, proteins, and fats. Not everything in foods can be completely digested (e.g., the human body lacks enzymes that can digest cellulose, a carbohydrate found in plants). Other factors affecting digestion and absorption that are as important to nutritional status as adequate intake include (1) amount of the nutrient consumed, (2) physiologic need, (3) condition of the digestive tract (amount of secretions, motility, and absorptive surface), (4) level of circulating hormones, (5) presence of other nutrients or drugs ingested at the same time enhancing or interfering with absorption, and (6) presence of adequate amounts of digestive enzymes.

Absorption of Nutrients

Only after absorption of the nutrient into the intestinal mucosa is it considered to be "in" the body. Generally, absorption of nutrients occurs by passive diffusion or active transport mechanisms. Passive diffusion is the passage of a permeable substance from a more concentrated solution to an area of lower concentration. Active transport occurs when absorption is from a region of lower concentration to one of a higher concentration; this mechanism requires a carrier and cellular energy. Approximately 80% to 90% of fluid intake is absorbed in the small intestine by osmosis. Osmosis is the passage of a liquid, such as water, through a semipermeable membrane to equalize osmotic pressure exerted by ions in solutions (Fig. 3.5). Water moves freely in both directions across the intestinal mucosa. Absorbable nutrients pass through the microvilli. Water-soluble nutrients enter the portal vein and fat-soluble ones enter through the lymphatic system.

Absorption into Portal Circulation

Most nutrients (monosaccharides, amino acids, glycerol, water-soluble vitamins, minerals, and short- and medium-chain fatty acids) are absorbed through the mucosa of the small intestine into the portal circulation (absorption of nutrients from the GI tract and spleen into the bloodstream to the liver through the portal vein). Metabolism of the nutrients is then initiated by the liver.

Absorption of Fat-Soluble Nutrients

The absorption process for long-chain fatty acids is complex because the molecules are large and insoluble. Long-chain fatty acids are broken apart to allow passage through the intestinal wall into the lymphatic system. The lymphatic system comprises lymph (plasmalike tissue fluid), the lymph nodes, and lymph vessels that are not connected to the blood system. Nutrients are carried through the thoracic duct and flow into the venous blood through the left subclavian vein. Absorption of the four fat-soluble vitamins—A, D, E, and K—is not as complex. Bile salts and lipases increase their water solubility by enabling absorption of these vitamins along with other fats in the lymphatic system.

> ### 🦷 DENTAL CONSIDERATIONS
>
> - An enzymatic deficiency in the GI tract results in some nutrients not being digested, thus preventing their absorption. The most prevalent enzyme deficiency is lactase deficiency, which is discussed in Chapter 4, *Health Application 4: Lactose Intolerance.*
> - Unless preventive care is taken, patients with large portions of the GI tract removed, as in bariatric surgery, may develop a nutritional deficiency because digestive secretions or absorptive areas are removed (see Fig. 3.1; Table 3.2).
> - If motility is increased, as in diarrhea, nutrients are not exposed to digestive secretions and absorptive surfaces long enough for maximum absorption. Severe or prolonged diarrhea may result in numerous deficiencies, the most rapid being a fluid deficit or dehydration.

> ### 🦷 NUTRITIONAL DIRECTIONS
>
> - The digestive process may be affected by how well food is broken apart by the teeth.
> - Dietary fat should not be eliminated entirely because it increases satiety and transports fat-soluble vitamins in the body.
> - Routine use of mineral oil as a laxative is not advisable because it reduces absorption of fat-soluble vitamins.

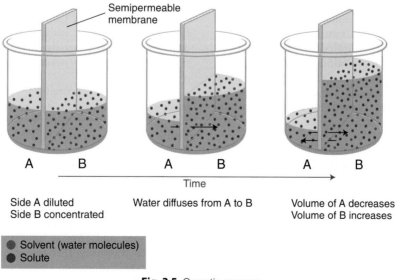

Side A diluted
Side B concentrated

Water diffuses from A to B

Volume of A decreases
Volume of B increases

🔴 Solvent (water molecules)
🔵 Solute

• **Fig. 3.5** Osmotic pressure.

Large Intestine

The cecum, colon, rectum, and anal tract constitute the large intestine, almost 5 ft (1.5 m) long. Small amounts of chyme remaining in the ileum are released through the ileocecal valve into the cecum. Only about 5% of ingested foods and digestive secretions advance to the large intestine. For most adults, it takes 16 to 24 hours for foodstuffs to travel the full length of the gut.

Functions

The large intestine, so named because of its large diameter, has little or no digestive function. Its main functions are to reabsorb water and electrolytes (mainly sodium and potassium) and to form and store the residue (feces) until defecation. Residue in the intestinal tract is the total amount of fecal solids, including undigested or unabsorbed food, metabolic (bile pigments) and bacterial products. Chyme entering the large intestine with 500 to 1000 mL of water is excreted as feces containing only 100 to 200 mL fluid. Essentially, all absorption occurs in the proximal half of the colon.

The inner lining of the large intestine is smooth, lacking the numerous villi found in the small intestine. Its only important secretion is mucus, which protects the intestinal wall, aids in holding particles of fecal matter together, and helps to control the pH in the large intestine.

Undigested Residues

Fiber, obtained from fruits, vegetables, and whole-grain products, results in increased residue and has a water-holding capacity, contributing to bulkier feces. Dietary fiber is not digestible and works as a laxative. Foods may contain other substances that increase fecal output. One example is prune juice, which yields no residue on chemical digestion but is classified as a high-residue food because inherent chemicals indirectly increase stool volume. Residue has a beneficial side effect of stimulating peristalsis, resulting in improved muscle tone.

Microflora

The body hosts microbial cells, including bacterial, fungal, protozoal, and other single-cell microorganisms, all of which constitute the microbiome. These vast numbers of microbial cells reside throughout the body, in the gut, muscles, nerves, skin, eyes, and nasal passages. The trillions of harmless microorganisms that thrive in the intestines are called microflora. These friendly bacteria are present in dozens of different strains and are essential for good health. Individuals have a microbiome as diverse and unique as fingerprints. The microbiome is not only influenced by diet and medication but also by hygiene, disease, genetics, stress, and the environment.

Types of food and medications ingested influence the type, activity, and relative numbers of bacteria. The composition of intestinal microflora is rapidly affected by food patterns, responding within 3 to 4 hours of dietary alterations. A diet rich in high-fiber foods—such as vegetables, fruits, legumes, and whole grains—is most beneficial to health-promoting gut microbes. The most common bacteria found in the gut belong to groups called *Lactobacillus* and *Bifidobacterium*.

Microflora has several important roles: (1) breaking down substances (fiber and other complex carbohydrates) that human enzymes are unable to digest, (2) synthesizing vitamins (vitamins K and B_{12}, biotin, thiamin, and riboflavin), (3) stimulating the immune system to improve protection against infection, and (4) inhibiting pathogenic bacteria. Gut microbiota cause fermentation of nondigestible carbohydrates, yielding gases and short-chain fatty acids. These short-chain fatty acids create an inhospitable environment for pathogenic bacteria. Fecal odor is a result of compounds produced by these bacteria.

Probiotics are living microorganisms that impart a health benefit to individuals when present in adequate amounts. While probiotics are essential, they are not classified as nutrients. The term *probiotics* is as general as the term *vitamin*. Each probiotic strain is unique, and the properties and effects of each strain must be assessed individually and for each health claim. Strains can differ in what they do even within the same species. In general, knowledge of probiotic strains is limited regarding which strains are needed, how much, and in what conditions.

Studies published in scientific literature report the use of probiotics in healthy patients improving numerous conditions, including inflammatory bowel diseases, digestive disorders, protection against infectious diseases, prevention of cardio-metabolic diseases, and overall promotion of well-being. In addition, antibiotic treatment frequently disturbs GI flora, sometimes resulting in *Clostridium difficile*–associated diarrhea; probiotic treatment may assist in reducing this diarrhea. Limited studies report that certain probiotics can help prevent allergies, obesity, and neurological disorders; decrease *Helicobacter pylori* colonization (a cause of ulcers) in the stomach; and improve oral health by reducing cariogenic and periodontal pathogen levels, as well as controlling oral yeast infections. *Lactobacillus acidophilus* and *Bifidobacterium*, found in some yogurts and other fermented dairy products, may help prevent pathogenic bacteria from proliferating and becoming toxic. Reported adverse effects associated with probiotic consumption include increased flatulence, abdominal bloating, brain fogginess in healthy individuals, and a longer list in patients with compromised health. Probiotics are considered a functional food or dietary supplements in the United States. They are found in fermented dairy products, such as kefir, yogurt, and cheese. New products have been introduced with probiotics added to bread, orange juice, infant formula, cereal, cookies, and even chewing gum. Probiotics are also available from nonanimal sources: coconut milk, sauerkraut, pickled or fermented vegetables or fruit (pickles, kimchi), kombucha tea, water, sourdough bread, and fermented soy products. Commercially available probiotics can be found in various forms, including capsules, tablets, and powders. These products are generally safe with few side effects, relatively inexpensive, and readily available. There is no established recommended intake.

Consumers are understandably confused about the efficacy of probiotics. The definition of probiotics, formulated by the Food and Agriculture Organization of the United Nations and World Health Organization experts, declared that probiotics are "live strains of strictly selected microorganisms which, when administered in adequate amounts, confer a health benefit on the host."[2] The US government does not test the quality of probiotics or require companies to scientifically demonstrate health benefits before labeling the product as containing probiotics. Claims to prevent or treat health problems have been approved neither by the US Food and Drug Administration nor by the European Food Safety Authority. Therefore, probiotics are not scrutinized as closely as medications and are not required to meet standards for effectiveness. With lax labeling regulations, it is difficult to know which products have proven health benefits and whether they contain what their label indicates. However, Health Canada approves several strains of probiotics for the relief of GI symptoms.[3] For example, a patented probiotic strain BLIS K12 has been approved for an oral-health claim in Canada to promote oral health.

Probiotic users may experience side effects such as impaired gastric and intestinal emptying. Individuals who take medications that affect GI motility may have developed small intestinal bacterial overgrowth (SIBO). SIBO is an excessive amount of bacteria in the GI tract causing nausea, vomiting, bloating, flatulence, and diarrhea. The American Gastroenterological Association (AGA) has provided guidelines on the role of probiotics in the management of GI disorders. In summary, they do not make recommendations for patients with a *C. difficile* infection, Crohn's disease, ulcerative colitis, and symptomatic irritable bowel syndrome; however, they find it acceptable in the context of a clinical trial. There are conditional recommendations of specific strains for patients on antibiotic treatment or a preterm or low-birth-weight infant. Finally, the AGA is against probiotic use for children with acute infectious gastroenteritis. Although they found the role of certain probiotic strains or combination strains to be a promising therapeutic intervention, they concluded there is currently not enough evidence to support a recommendation.[4]

Some probiotic products on the market do not meet established minimum criteria. Products do not usually disclose the levels or strain designations of added bacteria; thus consumers have no assurance as to whether the product has been shown to be efficacious for specific effects. Quality issues include (1) viability of organisms, (2) presence of harmful organisms, (3) protection of organisms from stomach acid, and (4) ability of a pill to properly break apart to release its ingredients.[5] Pasteurization can kill the bacteria.

Prebiotics are nondigestible food ingredients (complex carbohydrates) with beneficial effects on the health of the host by selectively providing fuel, stimulating growth or activity, or both, of beneficial colonic microorganisms present in the GI tract. Fiber, particularly fermentable fiber, is crucial for good health. Prebiotics are compounds that influence specific bacteria, their fermentation end products, and possible health effects on the host. Prebiotics increase mineral absorption (especially calcium and magnesium) from the foods containing them. Inulin and some sugars and sugar alcohols found in whole grains, legumes, onions, garlic, bananas, apples, mangoes, honey, leeks, soybeans, and artichokes are natural sources of prebiotics.

Simply put, prebiotics are food for probiotics. Probiotics together with prebiotics supporting their own growth are called symbiotics because they cooperatively promote probiotic benefits more efficiently. The benefits associated with probiotics are strain specific and benefits of prebiotics are substance specific.

The microbiome of an individual is very complex. Food provides a key factor in influencing the GI microbes and overall health. Different dietary approaches, as well as the consumption of different probiotics, prebiotics, and symbiotics, will differentially impact the human GI microbiome and health.[5] Research is expanding reliable knowledge and understanding of the health benefits of probiotics and prebiotics. Scientific research must continue to be interpreted critically.

Peristalsis

The purpose of peristalsis in the large intestine is to force feces into the rectum. These large waves occur only two to three times daily.

Constipation is a common problem for many people. The National Institute of Diabetes and Digestive and Kidney Diseases of the National Institutes of Health defines constipation as having a bowel movement fewer than three times per week with hard, dry, small, and difficult-to-pass stools.

DENTAL CONSIDERATIONS

- Bowel habits, stress, exercise, and nutritional intake (especially the amount of fiber and fluid intake) affect GI transit rate. Transit time affects the amount of harmful degradation products produced.
- Lengthy retention of feces in the large intestine allows more reabsorption of water, causing feces to become hard and dry, leading to constipation.
- Many patients may have symptoms of a chronic digestive problem, such as heartburn, abdominal pain, constipation, diarrhea, and gastroesophageal reflux disease, requiring alterations in positioning or in the dental hygiene treatment plan. Some of these problems can be addressed with dietary or lifestyle changes. Refer these patients to an RDN.
- Prebiotics pass intact into the large intestine, where they stimulate growth and activity of healthy bacteria; in contrast, probiotics influence the types of bacteria present.
- Specific probiotic strains have different biological activities and may provide various health benefits.
- For most healthy patients, microbes in probiotics are generally safe but should be consumed in moderation. However, patients who have a poor immune response, are medically compromised, older adults, children, and pregnant and lactating females should consult a health care provider or RDN before using probiotics.
- Antibiotic therapy normally kills bacteria in the colon and inhibits bacterial production of vitamins. Patients on long-term antibiotic therapy may develop deficiencies of vitamins K and B_{12} and biotin.

NUTRITIONAL DIRECTIONS

- Constipation can be treated by increasing fluid intake or by gradually increasing nondigestible food components (fiber) in the diet, or both.
- Activity affects GI mobility. Active individuals who routinely choose high-fiber foods and drink adequate amounts of liquids are less likely to become constipated than sedentary people.
- Limit processed foods, sugar, and *trans* fats. Diets containing large amounts of highly processed foods may allow pathogenic bacteria to thrive while diminishing the numbers of good bacteria and enhance growth of proinflammatory microbiota.[6]
- Fermented foods (yogurt, kefir, sauerkraut, kimchi, tempeh) may affect microflora by influencing bacteria already present.
- Look for words such as "active cultures" or "live cultures" on a food label claiming to contain probiotics in the food.
- Probiotics as a dietary supplement may be healthful in providing large amounts of beneficial bacteria if the products are responsibly formulated and stored properly.
- Purchase supplements only from reputable companies; they should bear the US Pharmacopeia (USP) or the National Formulary (NF) symbol on their packaging.
- Take probiotic supplements at least 2 hours before or after taking antibiotics.
- Caution patients with a milk allergy as some probiotics contain a trace amount of milk proteins.
- A plant-rich diet (vegetables, fruits, and legumes), high in dietary fiber, is more beneficial because it provides prebiotics as a fuel for intestinal bacteria.

◆ HEALTH APPLICATION 3

Gluten-Related Disorders

Gluten is a structural protein that is stretchy and viscous, a component of wheat, rye, barley, and triticale (a cross-bred hybrid of wheat and rye). Gluten-containing grains are not new, being introduced into the human diet approximately 10,000 years ago. Individuals with gluten-related diseases have adverse reactions to gluten. Conditions related to the ingestion of gluten can be categorized as (1) a genetically predisposed autoimmune disorder (celiac disease), (2) allergic reactions (wheat allergy), and (3) immune-mediated disorder (nonceliac gluten sensitivity [NCGS]). Although these three conditions are treated with similar diets, they are not the same conditions.

Celiac disease is an autoimmune disorder (a condition that causes the body to form antibodies to one's own tissues) caused by a permanent sensitivity to gluten in genetically susceptible individuals. If the condition is not diagnosed and treated, microvilli in the small intestine are damaged, ultimately impairing the absorption of nutrients. Microvilli normally allow nutrients to be absorbed from the small intestine into the bloodstream. Wheat allergy is another adverse immunologic reaction specific to wheat proteins. Nonceliac gluten sensitivity (NCGS) is characterized by intestinal and other symptoms related to ingesting gluten-containing foods but without celiac disease or wheat allergy. The overall clinical picture is generally less severe, and the small intestine is not impaired. Symptoms may appear within hours or days following gluten consumption.

The genes for celiac disease are present in about 30% to 40% of the general population but only a small percentage of carriers develop celiac disease.[7] Diagnosis of celiac disease begins with a blood test for specific antibodies. If this test is positive, the standard for diagnosis is a biopsy from the small intestine, unless the person is following a gluten-free diet. If the individual has been following a gluten-free diet prior to a biopsy, the lining of the small intestine may not show damage, making a definitive diagnosis difficult. The US Preventive Services Task Force determined that the effectiveness of screening for celiac disease in asymptomatic individuals is scarce, so routine screening is not recommended.[8]

Testing for wheat allergy includes a skin prick test for wheat. NCGS is diagnosed after celiac disease has been ruled out, followed by the skin prick test to determine wheat allergy. The diagnosis protocol for NCGS is based on a link between gluten ingestion and appearance of symptoms. After evaluating the response to a gluten-free diet, gluten is reintroduced and the response is assessed. NCGS can be unpleasant, but it is not harmful to long-term health; the overall clinical picture is less severe for those without concurrent autoimmune disease.

Symptoms of NCGS include abdominal pain, eczema, headache, foggy mind, fatigue, diarrhea, depression, anemia, numbness in the extremities, and joint pain. For people who suspect they have NCGS, a diagnosis to rule out celiac disease is recommended before initiating a gluten-free diet to obtain a valid diagnosis. A gluten-free diet should be the last resort when NCGS is suspected. After celiac disease and wheat allergy have been eliminated, the individual should try a gluten-free diet for at least a week, but no longer than a month, to determine if symptoms are alleviated.

Fatigue is a major symptom for most individuals with celiac disease. Other common signs and symptoms of the disease include diarrhea, abdominal pain, bloating, lactose intolerance, headaches, joint pain, skin rashes, depression, and short stature. A blistering rash, known as dermatitis herpetiformis, may be seen in patients with asymptomatic celiac disease. Without treatment, poor absorption of iron, folate, calcium, vitamin D, and other nutrients may result in anemia and osteoporosis. Other long-term serious health complications are neurologic conditions, malignancies, and lymphoid neoplasms. On the other hand, patients' health is not uniformly improved by intervention.[8]

In the oral cavity, enamel defects, recurrent aphthous stomatitis, aphthous ulcerations, geographic tongue, atrophic glossitis, and angular cheilitis (Fig. 11.5) are the most common symptoms.[9] Antibodies generated against gluten can react with a major protein causing enamel defects in developing teeth. Eruption of teeth in children with celiac disease is delayed.[10,11] Squamous cell carcinoma of the mouth, oropharynx, and esophagus is a serious long-term oral complication. People with celiac disease must permanently exclude gluten to avoid long-term adverse

consequences of this lifelong chronic condition. The only course of treatment is a strict gluten-free diet.

Many Americans who suffer from irritable bowel syndrome are probably sensitive to gluten and may benefit from a gluten-free diet. Patients with wheat allergy may also benefit from a gluten-free diet, but strict adherence may be less important. It has not been determined how strictly or for how long the diet should be followed or what complications may arise by following it.

A strict gluten-free diet can initially be an overwhelming undertaking in addition to being expensive. Gluten is a thickener; many processed foods use gluten-containing grains, additives, or preservatives. Gluten is not only in food products; beer, cosmetics, and postage stamps also contain gluten. All fresh fruits and vegetables, dairy products, and fresh meats—beef, chicken, fish, lamb, pork—are naturally gluten free. The gluten-free diet can be well balanced if foods are chosen wisely (e.g., more legumes and foods with lower energy density). Consumption of more fruits and vegetables, gluten-free whole grains, nuts, and seeds can help improve the nutritional value. A gluten-free diet may lead to reductions in beneficial gut bacteria. Probiotics may be helpful to increase gut bacteria and reduce symptoms of digestive irritation. Dietary fiber from whole foods, gluten-free sources (chia seeds, ground flaxseeds, rice bran, fruit, and vegetables) help strengthen and soothe the GI tract.

Many gluten-free foods are not fortified or enriched. Nutrients added in enrichment are lacking in whole-grain cereals. The diet may be lacking iron, calcium, fiber, thiamin, riboflavin, niacin, folate, and vitamin D. Evidence suggests that if patients are left on their own, a variety of macro- and micronutrient deficiencies can develop.[12] Gluten-free products may become healthier overall as manufacturers develop ways to fortify them. Extra sugar and fat are added to simulate the texture and fluffiness that gluten imparts, making many gluten-free products higher in fat and sugar than other products.

New high-quality gluten-free products are introduced in the market almost daily. Food manufacturers label foods "gluten-free" that are naturally free of gluten. Foods bearing "gluten-free" label cannot contain more than 20 parts per million (ppm) of gluten. (Lower amounts could not be reliably detected.)

It is believed that even gluten-containing crumbs can damage the intestinal mucosa in patients with celiac disease. Certain grains, such as oats, can be contaminated with wheat while growing and processing them. Wheat flour can remain airborne for hours (especially in bakeries) and contaminate exposed preparation surfaces and utensils, or uncovered gluten-free products such as fruits. Cross-contamination can also occur at home if foods are prepared on common surfaces or with appliances or utensils that are not thoroughly cleaned after being used to prepare gluten-containing foods, for example, the toaster, microwave, or flour sifter.

The number of Americans on a gluten-free diet increases every year. They follow a gluten-less diet believing that it is healthier or may help to lose weight. There is nothing inherently healthy about a gluten-free diet. When patients with celiac disease follow a gluten-free diet, some gain, some lose, but for most, weight remains the same. Gluten-free foods may be less nutritious than their gluten-containing counterparts, as they tend to be more heavily processed, are high in refined carbohydrates, and contain fewer vitamins and minerals and less fiber. Evidence does not indicate that gluten is harmful to healthy people without a gluten-related disorder. A significant reduction in consumption of wheat-containing products has partially been attributed to individuals choosing gluten-free or multigrain products.

For most individuals, wheat gluten may impart some healthy benefits such as (1) lower blood lipids and reduced risk of cardiovascular disease, (2) lower blood pressure, (3) improved immune system, (4) healthier composition of colonic bacteria, and (5) protection from some cancers. Because gluten-free flours, such as rice flour and cornstarch, typically cause a higher rise in blood sugars compared to wheat-based flours, a gluten-free diet may exacerbate insulin resistance, glucose intolerance, and weight gain. A gluten-free diet may adversely affect gut health in those without celiac disease or gluten sensitivity. A gluten-free diet is necessary for those with celiac disease or gluten intolerance but may not be healthy for people without those conditions.

◆ CASE APPLICATION FOR THE DENTAL HYGIENIST

Mr. A complains that he can hardly talk because his mouth is dry and sticky. Sores in his mouth make his dentures very uncomfortable. He does not leave his home often because he is unable to easily find liquids to prevent his tongue from sticking to the sides and roof of his mouth. He also has difficulty in eating. His health care provider prescribed a diuretic for his hypertension.

Nutritional Assessment
- Recent change in weight
- Dietary intake
- Preferred fluids, frequency of intake
- Food preparation techniques
- Medications taken
- Oral examination to determine the condition of the underlying tissues
- Fit of dentures
- Willingness to learn and change habits

Nutritional Diagnosis
Knowledge deficit of the effects of diuretics on hydration of the body related to lack of information and understanding.

Nutritional Goals
The patient will continue taking the diuretic. His nutrient intake will improve to prevent further weight loss, and his fluid intake will increase to 8 to 10 glasses of fluid a day.

Nutritional Implementation
Intervention: Discuss the importance of adequate salivary flow to maintain soft tissues, taste functions, and teeth. If indicated and desired, suggest products designed to relieve xerostomia to provide temporary comfort as needed.
Rationale: Xerostomia has severe deleterious effects on a patient's ability to talk and on integrity of oral tissues.

Intervention: Review the importance of meticulous oral hygiene and periodically removing dentures.
Rationale: Xerostomia promotes biofilm formation, which can lead to further gingival irritations for this patient. Removal of dentures allows underlying tissue to become healthy again.
Intervention: Discuss that although diuretics may cause this condition, they are important for his health.
Rationale: To prevent other health problems, Mr. A must continue the medication as prescribed by his health care provider.
Intervention: Discuss the ways he can increase his fluid intake to 8 to 10 glasses daily: (1) drink more fluid with meals and (2) carry fluids with him in a large covered thermal container.
Rationale: To replace fluids excreted because of the diuretic, adequate fluid intake is essential.
Intervention: Encourage increased intake of nutrient-dense liquid or semiliquid foods, such as milkshakes, cream soups, gravies, and sauces.
Rationale: These foods contain larger proportions of nutrients, which will help Mr. A to consume adequate amounts of nutrients and will prevent weight loss.
Intervention: Recommend tips to relieve the dryness in his mouth, such as ice chips or sugar-free mints and gum containing xylitol.
Rationale: The patient's comfort will be enhanced if his mouth is moist; oral complications associated with xerostomia will be minimized. The use of chewing gum or mints containing xylitol will stimulate salivary flow, reduce caries-causing bacteria, and assist with remineralization of any early carious lesions.

Evaluation
If the patient continues to take the prescribed diuretic, consumes a well-balanced diet, increases fluid intake, uses correct oral hygiene practices, maintains body weight, and can state why he acquired all these problems, dental hygiene care is effective.

◆ Student Readiness

1. Chart or diagram the GI secretions, where they are produced, and their digestive actions on nutrients present in milk. Homogenized milk contains the following: lactose (a disaccharide), proteins, emulsified fats, calcium, riboflavin, and vitamins A and D. Where are the end products absorbed?
2. Define *GI tract*, *hydrolysis*, *enzyme*, and *residue*.
3. A patient has problems secreting too much hydrochloric acid. What types of food would you recommend the patient avoid?
4. Make a small hole (1 mm in diameter) in a piece of paper. Place the tip of your tongue through the hole. Looking in the mirror, count the number of taste buds. Compare your findings with other classmates of varying ages. Observe the number of taste buds on adolescent and older patients.
5. If caloric intake were equal, which of the following breakfasts would probably delay feelings of hunger the longest? Explain your reason.
   a. Dry cereal with skim milk, toast with jelly, and coffee with sugar
   b. Egg with ham, toast with butter, and coffee with cream
6. What are absorbable products resulting from digestion of carbohydrates, proteins, and fats?
7. Within what section of the GI tract does most digestion and absorption take place?
8. Considering secretions and the functions of the GI tract, discuss the fallacy of diets that claim only one type of food (e.g., fruits) should be eaten at a given time.
9. Could constipation be called a nutrient deficiency? Defend your answer.
10. What types of problems might be encountered when a patient does not chew one's food well? Discuss dental issues that can lead to decreased ability to masticate food.
11. Bonus assignment: Read "A Review on the Gluten-Free Diet: Technological and Nutritional Challenges" found at https://www.ncbi.nlm.nih.gov/pmc/articles/PMC6213115/. Summarize the information from the article and present to the class. What information can you personally use? What information can be used when a patient declares that they are now following a gluten-free diet?

◆ CASE STUDY

An 85-year-old male reports with several new caries. He complains that his mouth is always dry because he sleeps with his mouth open due to his sinus problems. He has problems eating because the food becomes a dry lump in his mouth.
1. What information should you provide the patient to address the caries risk?
2. Do you think his problem is due to his mouth breathing or lack of fluids?
3. What information can you provide regarding his diet?
4. Can you provide some suggestions to address the dryness of meals in the mouth?
5. Discuss appropriate in-between-meal snacks to reduce risk of caries.

References

1. Brand RW, Isselhard DE, Erdman K. *Anatomy of Orofacial Structures: A Comprehensive Approach*. 8th ed. St. Louis: Elsevier; 2019.

2. Gibson GR, Hutkins R, Sanders ME, et al. Expert consensus document: the International Scientific Association for Probiotics and Prebiotics (ISAPP) consensus statement on the definition and scope of prebiotics. *Nat Rev Gastroenterol Hepatol*. 2017;14(8):491–502. https://doi.org/10.1038/nrgastro.2017.75.

3. Plaza-Diaz J, Ruiz-Ojeda FJ, Gil-Campos M, Gil A. Mechanisms of action of probiotics. *Adv Nutr*. 2019;10:S49–S66.

4. Su GL, Ko CW, Bercik P, et al. AGA clinical practice guidelines on the role of probiotics in the management of gastrointestinal disorders. *Gastroenterology*. 2020;159:697–705.

5. ConsumerLab.com. *Probiotic Supplement Review (Including Pet Probiotics)*. https://www.consumerlab.com/reviews/probiotic-supplements/probiotics/.3 Updated 24.11.20. Accessed 26.02.23.

6. Holscher HD. Diet affects the gastrointestinal microbiota and health. *JAND*. 2020;120(4):495–499.

7. Cenit MC, Codoner-Franch R, Sanz Y. Gut microbiota and risk of developing celiac disease. *J Clin Gastroenterol*. 2016;50:S148–S152.

8. United States Preventive Services Task Force Screening for celiac disease: United States Preventive Services Task Force recommendation statement. *JAMA*. 2017;317(12):1252–1257.

9. Macho V, Manso MC, Silva D, Andrade D. Does the introduction of gluten-free diet influence the prevalence of oral soft tissue lesions in celiac disease? *J Int Oral Health*. 2019;11:347–352.

10. Karlin S, Karlin E, Meiller T, et al. Dental and oral considerations in pediatric celiac disease. *J Dent Child (Chic)*. 2016;83(2):67–70.

11. Leonard MM, Weir DC, DeGroote M, et al. Value of IgA tTg in predicting mucosal recovery in children with celiac disease on a gluten free diet. *J Pediatr Gastroenterol Nutr*. 2016;64(2):286–291.

12. Vici G, Belli L, Biondi M, Polzonetti V. Gluten free diet and nutrient deficiencies: a review. *Clin Nutr*. 2016;35(6):1236–1241.

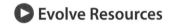

Evolve Resources

Please visit http://evolve.elsevier.com/Mallonee/nutritional for additional practice and study support tools.

4

Carbohydrate: The Efficient Fuel

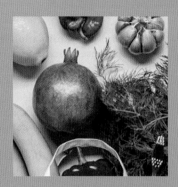

STUDENT LEARNING OBJECTIVES

On completion of this chapter, the student will be able to achieve the following learning outcomes:

1. Discuss various concepts related to the classification of carbohydrates, including:
   - Identify major carbohydrates in foods and their use in the human body.
   - Differentiate among monosaccharides, disaccharides, and polysaccharides.
   - Describe different ways in which glucose can be used by the body.
   - Summarize the functions of dietary carbohydrates.
   - Explain the importance of dietary carbohydrates.
   - Recognize dietary sources of lactose, other sugars, and starches.
   - Summarize the role and sources of dietary fiber.

2. Discuss the physiologic role of carbohydrates.
3. Discuss the acceptable macronutrient distribution range (AMDR) as related to carbohydrates, as well as sources of various types of carbohydrates.
4. Compare and contrast the concepts related to hyperstates and hypostates, such as carbohydrate excess, obesity, cardiovascular disease (CVD), carbohydrate deficiency, and dental caries. In addition, formulate recommendations for patients concerning carbohydrate consumption to reduce risk for dental caries.
5. Discuss the use of nonnutritive sweeteners and sugar substitutes.

KEY TERMS

Anticariogenic
Cariogenic
Cariostatic
Complex carbohydrates
Dental erosion
Dextrin
Dietary fiber

Fermentable carbohydrate
Functional fiber
Hyperglycemia
Hypoglycemia
Ketosis
Lipogenesis
Nondigestible

Phenylketonuria
Plaque biofilm
Resistant starch
Soluble dietary fibers
Streptococcus mutans (*S. mutans*)
Synergistic
Total fiber

⬤ TEST YOUR NQ

1. **T/F** Raw sugar is nutritionally superior to white sugar.
2. **T/F** Fructose is the principal carbohydrate in honey.
3. **T/F** All caloric sugars can be metabolized by plaque biofilm.
4. **T/F** The desire for sweetness in the diet is an acquired taste.
5. **T/F** Fiber helps regulate the rate foods pass through the gastrointestinal tract.

6. **T/F** Carbohydrates are absorbed as monosaccharides.
7. **T/F** Excessive consumption of carbohydrates is the main cause of obesity.
8. **T/F** Glucose is the same as table sugar.
9. **T/F** Eliminating sucrose from the diet prevents development of dental caries.
10. **T/F** Natural sugars in foods can be just as cariogenic as added sugars.

Carbohydrates have been the major source of energy for people since the dawn of history. Worldwide, carbohydrates are the main source of energy. Nutrition experts universally recommend that carbohydrates should represent 45%–65% of total energy intake.[1]

Carbohydrate foods add variety and palatability to the diet and are the most economical form of energy.

As discussed in Chapter 2, carbohydrates contain carbon, hydrogen, and oxygen. During photosynthesis, carbon dioxide and water result in formation of carbohydrates and release of oxygen. Because glucose and other carbohydrates are essentially hydrogen and oxygen atoms bound to a carbon backbone, a carbohydrate could also be referred to as a "hydrated carbon." Critics have labeled sugar as "toxic" and "addictive." Naturally, these unscientific statements affect food consumption patterns. Popular low-carbohydrate, high-protein weight-reduction diets have regularly caused the pendulum to swing away from choosing carbohydrate foods. Many of these diets are nutritionally unbalanced, providing inadequate amounts of nutrients known to help protect against several chronic diseases.

The first edition of the *Dietary Goals for the United States* in 1977 encouraged Americans to consume more complex carbohydrates (fruits, vegetables, legumes, and whole-grain products) to reduce their risk of various chronic diseases. Food supply data indicate that 45.9% of total calories come from carbohydrates for males, and 47.4% for females.[2] More recent, *Dietary Guidelines for Americans* recommend that people of dependent age group should consume half of the grains as whole grains. On average, Americans consume less than seven servings of grain products daily and one serving of whole grains daily.[3] Even if people are consuming an adequate number of servings of grains, the types of foods chosen need to be adjusted to improve fiber intake.

Additionally, the amount of added sugars (those added to foods during processing or by consumers) needs to be reduced to improve the quality of intake. Because most high-carbohydrate food choices are sugar-sweetened beverages (SSBs), cakes, cookies, pastries, and pies, the intake of fat as well as sugar is negatively affected. Mean intakes of sweeteners decreased for all age groups between the year 2001 to 2002 and 2017 to 2018.[4] The World Health Organization (WHO) recommends no more than 5–10 teaspoons of added sugars each day depending on age, gender, and activity level.[5] In 2017–18 the average daily intake of added sugars was 17 teaspoons for children and young adults aged 2– 19 years.[6,7] With water fluoridation, the incidence of caries has decreased in industrialized countries despite increased sugar consumption. All dental practitioners must be knowledgeable about the effect of carbohydrates on soft and hard tissues in the oral cavity and about chronic health problems caused by low-carbohydrate, high-fat diets. Dental professionals need to educate patients about ways to modify carbohydrate consumption and intake patterns that are consistent with overall good health.

Classification

Chapter 2 provides detailed information regarding the metabolism of carbohydrates. Generally, the chemical components of carbohydrates are in these proportions: $C_n(H_2O)_n$. An empirical formula such as $C_6H_{12}O_6$ or $C_{12}H_{22}O_{11}$ can readily be identified as a carbohydrate. The number of carbon atoms in the molecule is used to classify carbohydrates. Monosaccharides are simple sugars containing two to six carbon atoms. Disaccharides are composed of two simple sugars joined together and contain 12 carbon atoms. Polysaccharides are complex carbohydrates containing a minimum of 10 units of various simple sugars.

Monosaccharides and disaccharides contribute to the palatability of a food because of their sweetness. Temperature, pH,

and the presence of other substances influence the sweetness of a food. Relative sweetness of sugars is measured by subjective sensory tasting; sucrose is used as the standard of comparison (Table 4.1).

TABLE 4.1   Caloric Value and Relative Sweetness of Sugars and Sweeteners

Sugar or Sweetener	cal/g	Relative Sweetness[a]
Fructose	4	170
High-fructose corn syrup-90	4	120–160
Agave syrup	4	150
High-fructose corn syrup-55	4	120
Honey (fructose and glucose)	4	110
High-fructose corn syrup-42	4	110
Sucrose	4	100
Coconut palm sugar	4	100
Molasses (sucrose and invert sugar)	2.4	100
Brown sugar (sugar and molasses)	3.8	100
Coconut palm sugar	4	100
Dextrose	4	70–80
Lactose	4	40
Reduced Calorie Sweeteners/Sugar Alcohols		
Xylitol	2.4	100
Tagatose	1.5	92
Erythritol	0.2	70
Sorbitol	2.6	55
Mannitol	1.6	50
Hydrogenated starch hydrolysates (mixture of several sugar alcohols)	3.0	40
Nonnutritive Sweeteners		
Acesulfame K	0	200
Aspartame	0	200
Luo Han Guo (monk fruit)	0	100–250
Neotame	0	7000–13,000
Rebaudioside A (truvia, stevia)	0	200–400
Saccharin	0	200–700
Sucralose	0	600

[a]Relative to sucrose (=100).
Data from Sugar-and-Sweetener-Guide. *Sweetener Values, Including Calories and Glycemic Index.* http://www.sugar-and-sweetener-guide.com/sweetener-values.html; United States Food and Drug Administration. *Aspartame and Other Sweeteners in Foods.* https://www.fda.gov/food/food-additives-petitions/aspartame-and-other-sweeteners-food; Awuchi C. Sugar alcohols: chemistry, production, health concerns and nutritional importance of mannitol, sorbitol, xylitol, and erythritol. *Int J Adv Acad Res.* 2017;3(2):31–66.

Monosaccharides

The simplest carbohydrates, monosaccharides, are absorbed without further digestion. The monosaccharides of greatest significance in foods and body metabolism are glucose, fructose, and galactose. Fig. 2.3 in Chapter 2 identifies slight differences between these three six-carbon sugars and glucose.

Glucose

Also called dextrose or corn sugar, glucose is naturally abundant in many fruits, such as grapes, oranges, and dates, and also in some vegetables including fresh corn. It is prepared commercially as corn syrup or by special processing of starch. Glucose is the principal product formed by the digestion of disaccharides and polysaccharides. It provides energy for cells via the bloodstream. Glucose is the only sugar transported through the bloodstream that can nourish all cells in the body.

Fructose

Fructose, also known as levulose, is found naturally in honey and fruits. It is the sweetest of the monosaccharides and is a product of the digestion of sucrose. Fructose can be manufactured from glucose.

High-fructose corn syrup (HFCS) is made from corn starch; however, corn products contain only glucose molecules. HFCS is industrially produced by changing some glucose molecules into fructose, making the syrup sweeter than sucrose. It is available in several different concentrations for different products and has become a popular component of processed foods, especially soft drinks, because of its lower cost. HFCS-42 contains approximately the same amount of fructose as honey, and some natural fruit juices have twice as much fructose as glucose. The most frequently used concentrations of HFCS in foods (principally beverages) are HFCS-42 and HFCS-55. Since its introduction in the food supply in 1968, consumption of HFCS gradually increased, along with rising consumption of all sugars until 1999, when both HFCS and sugar intake began decreasing (Fig. 4.1).

Galactose

Galactose, another six-carbon sugar, is a product of lactose digestion (milk sugar). Galactose is rarely found free in nature. Physiologically, it is a constituent of nerve tissue and is produced from glucose during lactation.

Sugar Alcohols

Sugar alcohols are made from or converted to sugar. Sugar alcohols may appear naturally in foods or be added by a manufacturer. The most common polyols include sorbitol, xylitol, and mannitol.

For a given quantity, xylitol and tagatose (a naturally occurring monosaccharide) add about the same amount of sweetness as glucose but furnish fewer calories. Xylitol is found in fruits and vegetables (lettuce, carrots, and strawberries). As a food additive, it is more expensive than other sugar alcohols but has no aftertaste.

The benefit of sorbitol is that it is absorbed and metabolized more slowly than sucrose. Sorbitol, the most commonly used sugar alcohol, is the least expensive. Mannose is a six-carbon sugar found in some legumes. Mannitol, derived from mannose, is found in foods.

Incomplete absorption of sugar alcohols produces a laxative effect—soft stools or diarrhea—by causing an osmotic transfer of

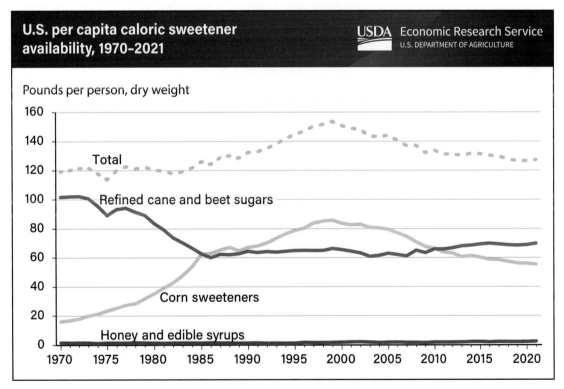

• **Fig. 4.1** United States per capita sweetener availability, 1970–2021. Notes: **Corn sweeteners** include high-fructose corn syrup, glucose syrup, and dextrose. **Edible syrups** include sorgo (sweet sorghum), maple and sugarcane syrup, edible molasses, and edible refiners syrup. (From United States Department of Agriculture. *Economic Research Service*. Food Availability (Per Capita) Data System data product.)

water into the gastrointestinal (GI) tract. Sugar alcohols are not considered sugars, and their use by food manufacturers is expected to increase to comply with the *Dietary Guidelines* for reducing sugar intake. Sugar alcohols do not cause a sudden increase in blood glucose levels and they do not contribute to tooth decay.

Disaccharides

Intact disaccharides cannot be metabolized by the body, but they contribute to body functions after digestion. As discussed in Chapter 2, monosaccharides are absorbed from the GI tract with no further action, but disaccharides and polysaccharides, or complex carbohydrates must be broken down into their constituent monosaccharides before they can be absorbed (Fig. 4.2).

Sucrose

Granulated table sugar is the most common form of sucrose, which is a combination of one molecule of glucose and one molecule of fructose, as shown in Fig. 2.4. Commercially, sucrose is produced from sugar cane or sugar beets (not to be confused with red beets). It is also found in molasses, maple syrup, and maple sugar. Some fruits (apricots, peaches, plums, raspberries, honeydew, cantaloupe) and vegetables (beets, carrots, parsnips, winter squash, peas, corn, sweet potatoes) naturally contain varying amounts of sucrose.

Lactose

The sugar found in milk is lactose. Lactose, which contains galactose and glucose (see Fig. 2.5) is unique to mammalian milk. In

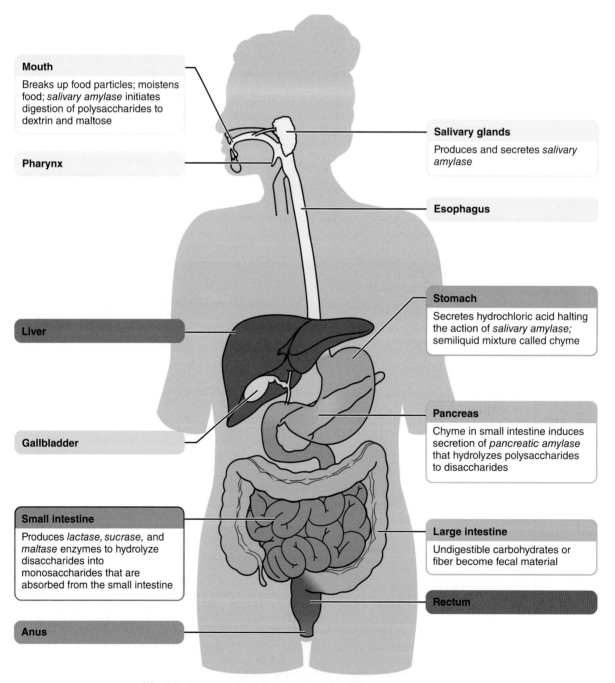

Mouth
Breaks up food particles; moistens food; *salivary amylase* initiates digestion of polysaccharides to dextrin and maltose

Pharynx

Salivary glands
Produces and secretes *salivary amylase*

Esophagus

Liver

Stomach
Secretes hydrochloric acid halting the action of *salivary amylase;* semiliquid mixture called chyme

Gallbladder

Pancreas
Chyme in small intestine induces secretion of *pancreatic amylase* that hydrolyzes polysaccharides to disaccharides

Small intestine
Produces *lactase, sucrase,* and *maltase* enzymes to hydrolyze disaccharides into monosaccharides that are absorbed from the small intestine

Large intestine
Undigestible carbohydrates or fiber become fecal material

Rectum

Anus

• **Fig. 4.2** Summary of carbohydrate digestion. Note: enzymes are in *italics*.

the fermentation of milk, some of the lactose is converted to lactic acid, giving buttermilk and yogurt their characteristic flavors.

Maltose

Maltose, shown in Fig. 2.4, contains two molecules of glucose. Also called *malt sugar*, maltose does not occur naturally. It is created in making bread and brewing beer and is present in some processed cereals and baby foods.

◆ DENTAL CONSIDERATIONS

- Assess patients with an increased risk of dental caries for frequency of sugar intake, including sources of natural and added sugars.
- Newborns exhibit a preference for sweetness; thus it is not considered an acquired taste. Although infants and young children typically select the most intensely sweet foods, the pleasure response to sweetness is observed across individuals of all ages, races, and cultures.
- A judgmental attitude or criticism by the dental hygienist is not beneficial in modifying a patient's use of carbohydrates or sugars.
- All caloric sugars and starches, whether they are naturally occurring in foods or added to foods, have some cariogenic effect.

◆ NUTRITIONAL DIRECTIONS

- Sugar alcohols are not fermented alcohols and do not need to be restricted by individuals with alcohol use disorder (AUD).
- All disaccharides contain the same caloric and nutrient content. The body cannot distinguish between natural honey, refined table sugar, or HFCS; absorption and metabolism are similar to their component sugars.
- Encourage use of hard candies and chewing gum containing sugar alcohols (xylitol and sorbitol) to prevent caries. However, inform patients that using more than three to four pieces of sugar alcohol-containing items daily may cause GI distress.

Polysaccharides or Complex Carbohydrates

Complex carbohydrates, also called polysaccharides, contain more than 10 monosaccharides (see Fig. 2.7). Some polysaccharides have a role in energy storage and are digestible. Dietary fiber is largely indigestible by intestinal enzymes in humans.

Starch

Starches are composed of many long-chain or branched glucose units. Most food sources such as cereal grains, roots, vegetables, and legumes contain complex carbohydrates in the form of starch. The amount of starch present in a vegetable increases with its maturity. For example, corn tastes much sweeter immediately after it is picked than it does several days later because the simple sugars in corn have not developed into starch. In contrast, the amount of starch in fruit decreases as it ripens—that is, complex carbohydrates are broken down into simple sugars during the ripening process. In digestion, complex carbohydrates are broken down into dextrin (long glucose chains) molecules until the end product, glucose, is absorbed (Fig. 4.3).

A cell wall, or cellulose, surrounding the starch granule causes starch to be insoluble in cold water. Cellulose is composed of long, straight chains of glucose units attached with a very strong bond to provide great mechanical strength with limited flexibility. Cooking facilitates digestion by causing granules to swell, rupturing the cell wall so that digestive enzymes have access to the starch inside the cell. In cooking, this swelling is referred to as thickening, as occurs in making gravy. Industrially, food starch is modified by chemicals to produce a better thickening agent.

Glucose Polymers

Industrially produced carbohydrate supplements are composed of glucose, maltose, and dextrins. Dextrins are intermediate products of digestive enzymes on starch molecules, or long glucose chains split into shorter ones. In the process of toasting bread, dextrins

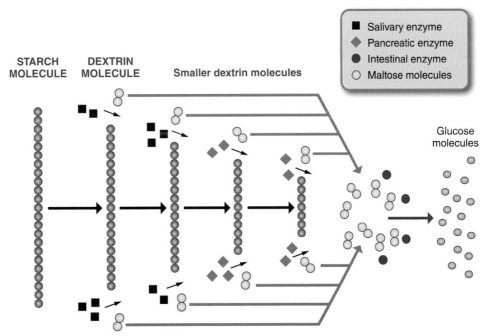

• **Fig. 4.3** The gradual breakdown of large starch molecules into glucose by digestion enzymes. (Reproduced with permission from Mahan LK, Escott-Stump S, Raymond JL: *Krause's Food and the Nutrition Care Process*. 14th ed, St Louis: Saunders Elsevier; 2017.)

are produced. Consistent with other carbohydrate products, glucose polymers provide energy equivalent to 4 cal/g.

Glycogen

Glycogen is the carbohydrate storage form of energy in humans (see Fig. 2.7). Stored in the muscle and liver, glycogen is readily available as a source of glucose and energy. Carbohydrates are frequently consumed in excess to meet immediate energy needs. Excess glucose is converted to glycogen until the limited glycogen storage capacity is filled; simultaneously, glucose is converted into fats and stored as adipose tissue. The total amount of glycogen stored is relatively small, only enough to meet energy demands for less than a day.

Dietary Fiber

Fiber refers to nondigestible components of food with desirable health effects. Nondigestible means that enzymes in the human GI tract cannot digest and absorb the substance; plant cells remain largely intact through the digestive process. Dietary fiber consists of several different types of nondigestible carbohydrates and lignin that occur naturally in plants (thus grains, fruits, and vegetables are good sources of fiber).

Dietary fiber includes polysaccharides, lignin, and associated substances in plants, such as whole grains, legumes, vegetables, fruits, seeds, and nuts (Table 4.2). Sources of dietary fiber usually contain other macronutrients, such as digestible carbohydrates and protein, normally found in foods. During food processing, many added compounds have the same physiologic effect as naturally occurring fiber but may not have other health benefits, such as vitamins and minerals.

Soluble dietary fibers become viscous (sticky, thick) in a solution. Insoluble dietary fibers, or the structural part of the plant, do not dissolve in fluids. Insoluble and soluble fibers have different physiologic functions in the body.

Resistant starch is a form of dietary fiber that cannot be digested. It delivers some of the health benefits of soluble and insoluble fibers. Resistant starches are not absorbed; thus they function as a prebiotic by providing fatty acids for bacteria in the colon. Resistant starches trap water and add bulk to the stool, helping with regularity.

Fiber added during the manufacturing process is called functional fiber. Functional fiber consists of isolated, nondigestible carbohydrates with beneficial physiologic effects in humans. Various types of fiber from carbohydrate sources are added in the manufacturing process because of their functional properties, such as thickening or emulsifying. Many of these substances, including carrageenan and guar gum, are common food additives.

Total fiber is the sum of dietary fiber and functional (added) fiber. Many fibers can be classified either as dietary fiber or functional fiber depending on whether they are a natural component of the food or added to the food during processing. Plant-based foods are a good source of dietary fiber, but commercially developed functional fibers for use in processed foods also have a beneficial role in health. Various types of fibers have distinct properties resulting in different physiologic effects (see Table 4.2). The Nutrition Facts label reflects naturally occurring dietary fiber and added isolated or synthetic fibers the Food and Drug Administration has determined have a beneficial physiologic effect on health (e.g., beta-glucans soluble fiber, psyllium husk, cellulose, guar gum, pectin, locust bean gum, and hydroxypropylmethylcellulose).

Physiologic Roles

Energy

The principal role of absorbed sugars is to provide a source of energy for (1) body functions and activity, and (2) heat to maintain body temperature. Glucose is the preferred source of energy for the brain and central nervous system, red blood cells, and lens of the eye. When carbohydrate intake is restricted, fat and protein stores may be used as an energy source. Although many organs can use fats for energy, glucose is the preferred fuel. A carbohydrate, whether it was originally from a sugar or a starch, provides 4 cal/g. Because of incomplete absorption, sugar alcohols contribute varying amounts of calories (see Table 4.1). Glycogen stores are a readily available source of glucose for tissues.

TABLE 4.2	Synopsis of Dietary Fibers	
Type of Fiber	**Dietary Fiber Sources**	**Physiologic Effects**
Insoluble Fiber		
Cellulose and hemicellulose	Whole grains, bran, plant foods (stalks and leaves of vegetables); dried beans	Laxation (increases fecal volume and decreases gut transit time); beneficial effect on serum cholesterol levels
Lignin (noncarbohydrate)	Fruits with edible seeds (strawberries, flaxseeds) mature vegetables (broccoli stems)	Antioxidant; beneficial effect on serum cholesterol levels; fermentation produces short-chain fatty acids, thus functions as a prebiotic; binds with minerals (calcium, iron, and zinc), which are then excreted
Soluble Fiber		
Gums	Oats, dried beans, legumes, barley, guar	Beneficial effect on blood glucose and serum lipids; aids satiety
Mucilages (psyllium)	Psyllium seeds, high-fiber cereals	Laxation (increases fecal volume and decreases gut transit time); binds water; beneficial effect on blood glucose and serum lipids; aids satiety
Pectin	Plant foods (apples, citrus fruits, berries, carrots)	Beneficial effect on serum cholesterol levels

Fat Storage

Sugars in the blood ensure replenishing of glycogen stores; however, excessive intake of energy from any source results in converting glucose to fats by a process known as lipogenesis. When carbohydrates are eaten in excess of needs, lipogenesis results in increased fat stores.

Conversion to Other Carbohydrates

Monosaccharides are important constituents of many compounds that regulate metabolism. Examples include heparin, which prevents blood clotting; galactolipids, which are the constituents of nervous tissue; and dermatan sulfate (a mucopolysaccharide), present in tissues rich in collagen (especially skin).

Conversion to Amino Acids

The liver can use part of the carbon framework from the sugar molecule, and part of a protein molecule contributed by the breakdown of an amino acid to produce nonessential amino acids. These are physiologically essential but are not required in the diet.

Normal Fat Metabolism

Oxidation of fats requires the presence of some carbohydrates. When carbohydrate intake is low, the body relies on energy from fat intake or stores. As detailed in Chapter 2, when fats are metabolized faster than the body can oxidize them, intermediate products called ketone bodies may accumulate. Ketones are normal products of lipid metabolism in the liver; muscles can use ketones for energy only if adequate amounts of glucose are not available. An accumulation of ketones in the blood, or incompletely oxidized fatty products, results in ketosis.

Spare Proteins

Carbohydrates, by furnishing energy in the diet, are said to be protein sparing. Energy is an essential physiologic requirement. With insufficient carbohydrate intake, the body burns protein for fuel. If carbohydrate intake is adequate, protein can be used to build and repair tissue.

Intestinal Bacteria

Dietary fiber remains in the GI tract longer than other nutrients. Undigestible fibers—such as lignin, cellulose, and hemicellulose—may be fermented by microflora in the large intestine. Fermentation produces gas and volatile fatty acids; cells lining the colon use these fatty acids for energy. Undigestible fiber functions as a prebiotic by encouraging growth of bacteria that synthesize some of the B-complex vitamins and vitamin K.

Gastrointestinal Motility

Dietary and certain functional fibers, particularly those which are poorly fermented, improve fecal bulk and laxation, ameliorate constipation, and perform various other functions (see Table 4.2). Dietary fiber and functional fibers *accelerate* transit rate (the time it takes for waste products to move through the intestine) in individuals with a slow transit time (constipation). Soluble fiber *decreases* transit rate in individuals with a rapid transit time (diarrhea). The ability of fiber to bind water in the intestine and increase bulk from nondigestible substances decreases the duration for which waste products remain in the alimentary tract. An increased transit time lengthens the duration of tissue exposure to cancer-causing nitrogenous waste products.

An added benefit of fiber is its stool-softening ability which helps prevent constipation. Fiber in the colon increases stool bulk, exercising digestive tract muscles by increasing the radius of the colon and preventing the muscle from being chronically contracted. As muscle tone is maintained and colonic pressure declines, the gut is able to resist bulging out into pouches known as diverticula (Fig. 4.4).

Soluble dietary fibers include pectins, gums, psyllium, mucilages, and algal polysaccharides; they influence the physiology of the upper GI tract. Soluble fibers are physiologically important for their gel-forming ability, resulting in increased viscosity of chyme and delayed gastric emptying. They bind bile acids, decrease serum cholesterol levels, and may improve glucose tolerance. Physiologic benefits of dietary fiber are listed in Box 4.1.

Fiber-rich foods are not energy dense and are retained longer in the stomach. They may cause one to feel full on a fewer number of calories. Whether fiber plays a significant role in weight management has yet to be determined.

Other Nutrients

Carbohydrates are normally accompanied by other nutrients. Starchy foods are especially important for their contribution of protein, minerals, and B vitamins. Whole-grain products are superior because they contain fiber plus other essential nutrients; enriched products should always be used in preference to products that are processed but not enriched.

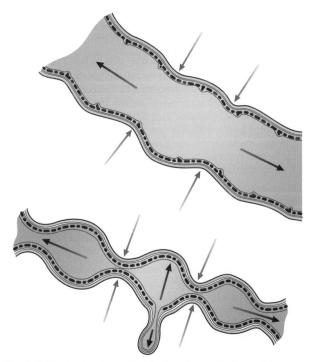

• **Fig. 4.4** Mechanism by which low-fiber, low-bulk diets might generate diverticula. Where colon contents are bulk (*top*), muscular contractions exert pressure longitudinally. If lumen is smaller (*bottom*), contractions can produce occlusion and exert pressure against the colon wall, which may produce a diverticular "blowout." (From Peckenpaugh NJ. *Nutrition Essentials and Diet Therapy*, 11th ed. Saunders Elsevier; 2010.)

• **BOX 4.1** **Benefits of a High Dietary Fiber Diet**

1. Promotes digestive health
2. Reduces mortality rate
3. Helps reduce risk of type 2 diabetes
4. Helps control weight
5. May protect against metabolic syndrome
6. Reduces risk of cardiovascular disease—lower cholesterol levels and blood pressure, and stroke
7. Reduces risk of cancer

Data from Zong G, Gao A, Hu FB, Sun Q. Whole grain intake and mortality from all causes, cardiovascular disease, and cancer. A *meta*-analysis of prospective cohort studies. *Circulation.* 2016;133:2370–2380; Aune D, Keum N, Giovannucci E, et al. Whole grain consumption and risk of cardiovascular disease, cancer, and all cause and cause specific mortality: systematic review and dose–response *meta*-analysis of prospective studies. *BMJ.* 2016;353:i2716; Chen GC, Tong X, Xu JY, et al. Whole-grain intake and total, cardiovascular, and cancer mortality: a systematic review and *meta*-analysis of prospective studies. *Am J Clin Nutr.* 2016;104(1):164–172; Dahl WJ, Stewart ML. Position of the academy of nutrition and dietetics: health implications of dietary fiber. *J Acad Nutr Diet.* 2015;115(11):1861–1870.

DENTAL CONSIDERATIONS

- Carbohydrate metabolism requires an adequate supply of B vitamins, phosphorus, and magnesium. Usually, adequate amounts of these nutrients accompany carbohydrate intake. However, this may not be true if refined sugars and breads are predominantly chosen.
- Ketosis can occur in patients with uncontrolled diabetes or in individuals who have inadequate carbohydrate intake, such as those who are ill or are following a high-protein, very-low-carbohydrate regimen because they are burning fat rather than carbohydrate. Among other concerns, ketosis creates a disturbance in a patient's acid-base balance. If a patient has acetone or fruity-smelling breath, ask them questions about their recent dietary intake.
- Increasing dietary fiber may reduce risk of gingivitis and periodontal disease.[8,9]
- Table 4.3 provides guidelines for assisting patients to increase dietary fiber.
- Some fibers added to foods by manufacturers have not been proven beneficial to human health and cannot be included in the total amount of dietary fiber, on the Nutrition Facts label.
- Increasing dietary fiber without increasing total energy intake may lead to improvements in GI health and blood pressure, reduced body fat stores, and lower risk of cardiovascular disease (CVD) and type 2 diabetes.[10,11]
- Concerns are not about consumption of individual types of sugar but rather about overconsumption of added sugar. Recommendations should focus on choosing nutrient-dense foods.

NUTRITIONAL DIRECTIONS

- Fiber tends to regulate the transit rate of foods in the GI tract. The best source of dietary fiber to relieve constipation is bran, but it must be initiated slowly to avoid severe gas and bloating.
- An excessive amount of bran (50–60 g) yields negative benefits, such as diarrhea and decreased mineral and vitamin absorption.
- Some vegetables and fruits (e.g., bananas, white potatoes, and apples) are high in pectin which binds water. They are frequently used to control diarrhea but can also help relieve constipation by softening the stool.
- Even when an individual strives to reduce caloric intake, carbohydrates are important, especially vegetables, fruits, and whole-grain breads and cereals, to provide vital nutrients.
- Carbohydrates supply 4 cal/g of energy and are a less-concentrated source of energy than fats (9 cal/g).

Requirements

The acceptable macronutrient distribution range (AMDR) for carbohydrates is based on providing energy for the body, particularly brain cells. The brain is the only organ that requires glucose. The AMDR for digestible carbohydrates is 130 g per day for adults and children. Generally, males typically consume 200–330 g per day and females consume 180–230 g per day to meet energy requirements without exceeding acceptable levels of fat and protein.

The AMDR for carbohydrates is limited to no less than 45% (to prevent excess fat intake) and no more than 65% (to ensure required nutrients from protein and fats that also provide essential micronutrients). The American diet currently furnishes approximately 50% of the calories from carbohydrates. The dietary reference intakes compiled by the National Academy of Medicine (formerly the Institute of Medicine) suggest a maximum intake of 25% or less of energy from added sugars.

As discussed in Chapter 1, the *Dietary Guidelines* recommend less than 10% of total calories for a day from added sugars. This is not due to scientific evidence that sweeteners contribute to chronic diseases but rather to meet nutrient needs within caloric limits. For most individuals, after consuming the appropriate amounts of foods from all the food groups, less than 20% of their daily calories is available for added sugars and fats. For an individual consuming 2000 cal per day, the maximum amount of added sugars, or 10% of total caloric intake, would be 11 tsp of added sugars (200 cal). Despite a sustained downward trend of caloric sweeteners available in the United States (Fig 4.1), a recent study demonstrated that many adults are consuming greater than 15% of their daily calories from added sugars.[12] Higher intake of added sugars is associated with various sociodemographic and behavioral characteristics (young age, less education, low income, less physical activity, and smoking).[12]

The comprehensive report by the WHO on nutrition recommends limiting added sugar intake to less than 10% of total energy intake (e.g., 12 tsp of added sugars for 2200 cal).[5] It further recommended that a reduction below 5% (or roughly 25 g [6 tsp] per day) would provide additional health benefits. The WHO decision was based on economic, social, and political issues—not on scientific evidence—to prevent and control chronic health problems, especially obesity.

Adequate total fiber intake is 14 g per 1000 cal per day, or 38 g for males and 25 g for females daily. That calculation is based on the amount needed to prevent CVD. Dietary fiber intake has remained relatively stable despite efforts to encourage consumers to increase intake, and a significant increase of whole-grain products in the market. Approximately 95% adults and children fall short of meeting daily fiber recommendations. Approximately 60% meet daily intake goals for total grain intake, but only 2% consume the recommended amount of whole grains and 74% exceed the limits for refined grains (Fig. 4.5).[3,13,14]

Sources

Carbohydrates are furnished by the following food groups: milk, grain, fruits, and vegetables. The only animal foods supplying significant quantities of carbohydrate are milk and milk products, which contain the disaccharide lactose. In cheese making, lactose is removed as a by-product. Consequently, most cheeses contain only trace amounts of lactose.

TABLE 4.3 Guidelines for Developing a High-Fiber Diet

Principles	Guidelines
Before recommending any changes, evaluate the patient's fiber and fluid intake. For patients ≤50-year old, the recommended level of dietary fiber is 38 g for male and 25 g for females; for patients ≥51-year old, the optimal level of dietary fiber is 30 g for male and 21 g for females.	Fiber normalizes bowel movements to once or twice a day by moderating the transit rate of food through the gastrointestinal tract. Cooking and freezing only slightly decrease fiber content; vegetables (e.g., mushrooms, peppers, onions, tomatoes) can be added to various dishes (meatloaf, spaghetti, chili, omelets, or scrambled eggs). Grinding or pureeing foods (as in smoothies) significantly decreases fiber content.
Foods containing soluble and insoluble fibers are the preferred way to increase fiber rather than fiber supplements.	Recommend choosing a rainbow of colorful foods: 2–4 daily servings of fruits, especially those with skins and edible seeds 3–5 servings of vegetables daily Combine raw vegetables with low-fat dip as appetizers or snacks, and include in brown-bag lunches. Add leafy greens, tomatoes, bell peppers, and cucumbers to sandwiches. Substitute fresh fruits and vegetables or plain popcorn for fried chips and cookies. Incorporate beans into soups, casseroles, nachos, or salads. Experiment with brown rice, rye flour, barley, buckwheat, millet, whole-wheat pasta, and bulgur. Ancient grains such as quinoa, teff, and farro may not be enriched.
Adequate fluids are important to keep the intestinal contents moving because fiber absorbs water in the intestines.	Ensure the intake of 10–12 cups of decaffeinated fluids a day to avoid problems such as fecal impactions.
Increase high-fiber foods gradually. Begin with 5- to 10-g increments to avoid adverse side effects. At least 6–8 weeks should be allowed for adaptation to prevent flatulence, abdominal cramping, and diarrhea/constipation.	Dietary fiber comes principally from whole-grain products. Choose breads and cereals with at least 2 g of fiber (5 g is ideal), but no more than 2 g of fat per serving. Add bran, bran flakes, wheat germ, chopped nuts, seeds, or oatmeal to mixed meat dishes, casseroles, salads, cooked cereal, cookies, breads, muffins, and pancake batter or for a crispy coating on meats or fish.
Increase intake of oat bran, beans, barley, and psyllium to help reduce cholesterol levels.	Use dried beans and peas as the main dish (in place of meat) at least once a week along with an overall low-fat diet.

Data from Dahl WJ, Stewart ML. Position of the academy of nutrition and dietetics: health implications of dietary fiber. *J Acad Nutr Diet.* 2015;115(11):1861–1870; Mayo Clinic. *Dietary Fiber: Essential for Health.* https://www.mayoclinic.org/healthy-lifestyle/nutrition-and-healthy-eating/in-depth/fiber/art-20043983

Other sugars are furnished from table sugar, syrups, jellies, jams, and honey. Sugars are incorporated into many popular foods (e.g., candy, beverages, cakes and desserts, chewing gum, and ice cream). About 25% of the sugar that Americans consume is added to foods in homes, institutions, and restaurants. The remainder is added to foods during processing, for example, canning; freezing; breakfast cereals; condiments and salad dressings; SSBs; cookies, crackers, and candies; flavored extracts and syrups; flour and bread products; and milk and dairy products.

Naturally occurring sugars are found in fruits, vegetables and milk. Sugars, mainly glucose and fructose, are furnished by fruits and vegetables in varying amounts that depend on their maturity (ripe bananas contain more simple sugars than green bananas) and their water content (spinach contains less carbohydrate than potatoes).

Because there is no physiologic requirement for added sugars, *MyPlate* does not include a separate section for sugars; added sugars are included in the discretionary calories. Eating sugar in moderation implies a proper balance among foods and nutrients which should be the primary consideration in food selection. Eating lower amounts does not necessarily guarantee that a diet meets nutritional requirements nor does high-sugar consumption mean a poorer-quality diet.

Complex carbohydrates, or starches, are furnished by grain products (wheat, corn, rice, oats, rye, barley, buckwheat, and millet). Some vegetables especially root and seed varieties (potatoes, sweet potatoes, beets, peas, and winter squashes) also contain considerable amounts of starch. Legumes, or dried beans and peas,

are excellent sources of complex carbohydrates. Table 4.4 shows the complex carbohydrate and sugar content of the sample menu from Fig. 1.4 in Chapter 1.

Some dietary fibers, especially hemicellulose and cellulose, and other indigestible compounds, are furnished by whole-grain breads, and cereals and legumes. Cellulose is found principally in the stems, roots, leaves, and seed coverings of plants; unpeeled fruits and leafy vegetables are good sources. Legumes are also a good source of dietary fiber (see Table 4.2). The pectin contributed by fruits and vegetables is an important source of soluble fiber. A popular American snack food, popcorn (preferably without butter and salt), is also a whole-grain food. Table 4.4 lists the fiber content of foods in the sample menu from Fig. 1.4.

The fiber in whole grains provides important contributions to health (see Box 4.1). Consumers equate whole-grain label statements with claims about fiber content and choose products containing whole grains, expecting to increase fiber intake. The fiber content of foods claiming "whole grain" varies significantly and is very low (<3 g) in many cases. "Made with whole grains" may contain principally refined flour with a small amount of whole grain. A product containing less than 3 g dietary fiber cannot be considered a good source of fiber. A product listing "whole grains" first in the ingredient list would be a healthful choice. This consumer confusion is likely caused by unclear and inconsistent labeling for whole-grain-containing products, the need for a universally accepted definition of whole-grain foods, and lack of consumer education encouraging label reading (Box 4.2).

Dietary Intakes Compared to Recommendations: Percent of the U.S. Population Ages 1 and Older Who Are Below and At or Above Each Dietary Goal

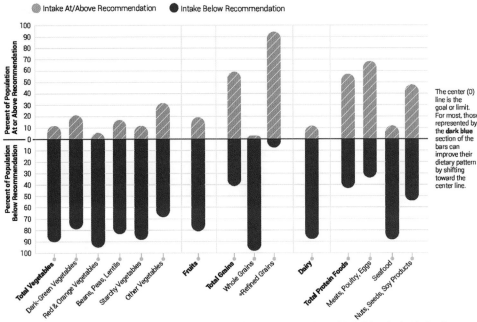

○ Intake At/Above Recommendation ● Intake Below Recommendation

The center (0) line is the goal or limit. For most, those represented by the **dark blue** section of the bars can improve their dietary pattern by shifting toward the center line.

*NOTE: Recommended daily intake of whole grains is to be at least half of total grain consumption, and the limit for refined grains is to be no more than half of total grain consumption.

Data Source: Analysis of What We Eat in America, NHANES 2013-2016, ages 1 and older, 2 days dietary intake data, weighted. *Recommended Intake Ranges:* Healthy U.S.-Style Dietary Patterns (see *Appendix 3*).

Dietary Guidelines for Americans, 2020-2025

• **Fig. 4.5** Dietary intakes compared to recommendations: percent of the United States population ages one and older who are below and at or above each dietary goal. Analysis of What We Eat in America NHANES 2013–2016, ages one and older, two days dietary intake data, weighted. Recommended intake range: healthy United States style dietary patterns. (From United States Department of Health and Human Services and United States Department of Agriculture. *2020–2025 Dietary Guidelines for Americans*. 9th ed. 2020. https://www.dietaryguidelines.gov/sites/default/files/2020-12/Dietary_Guidelines_for_Americans_2020-2025.pdf.)

⬦ DENTAL CONSIDERATIONS

- Assess total sugar intake and frequency, form, and time of day for carbohydrate intake (see Chapter 18).
- The number of teaspoons of sugar in a food product can be determined from the label (see Fig. 1.8). Four grams of sugar is equivalent to 1 tsp of sugar. A product containing 16 g of sugar is 4 tsp of sugar. Measuring the number of teaspoons of sugar in a product is a valuable visual aid for patients.
- To determine the percentage of sugar in a serving of food, (1) multiply the number of grams of added sugar in a product by 4 cal/g, (2) divide this number by the total number of calories per serving, and (3) multiply by 100 to establish the percentage of calories as sugar. Using the example of the label shown in Fig. 1.8:

$$10\,g\ sugar \times 4\,\frac{cal}{g} = 40\ cal\ from\ sugar$$

$$\frac{40\ cal\ sugar}{230\ cal/serving} = 0.17 \times 100\% = 17\%$$

- Fiber helps reduce constipation, diverticulosis, heart disease, and the risk of some cancers (see Table 4.3 for ideas to enhance fiber intake).

- A diet with adequate amounts of carbohydrate helps to maintain glycogen reserves, while a diet high in fat and very low in carbohydrate results in poor glycogen reserves. Glycogen stores in the heart are critical for continuous functioning of the heart muscle.
- Sugar increases palatability and may improve choices of certain foods otherwise disliked. Combining sugar with other nutrient-dense foods, such as milk used for pudding, may increase the variety of foods consumed and enjoyed.

⬦ NUTRITIONAL DIRECTIONS

- A tablespoon of honey has more calories than a tablespoon of sugar and only trace amounts of other nutrients. Honey is not appropriate for children younger than 1-year old because of the risk of botulism. Its retentive nature makes honey more cariogenic than refined sugar.
- Encourage patients to adhere to the *Dietary Guidelines* by discussing information from Box 4.2.

TABLE 4.4   **Carbohydrate, Dietary Fiber, and Added Sugars Content of the Sample Menu**

Sample Menu	Carbohydrate (g)	Dietary Fiber (g)	Added Sugars (g)
Breakfast			
1 cup Frosted mini-wheat cereal	41	5	12
8 oz 1% milk	12.2	0	0
12 oz black coffee	0	0	0
Mid-Morning Snack			
12 oz water	0	0	0
1 oz dry roasted almonds, unsalted	21	10	0
1 small tangerine	13	1	0
Lunch			
Sandwich with			
1 cup tuna salad	9	0	0
¼ cup thin-sliced cucumber	1	0.2	0
3 thin tomato slices	0.81	0.2	0
2 medium red leaf lettuce leaves	0.36	0.1	0
2 regular slices of 100% wheat bread	31	4.3	2
8 baby carrots	6	2	0
1 medium applesauce cookie	9	0	3
1 cup grapes	27	1	0
12 oz water	0	0	0
Mid-Afternoon Snack			
8 oz low-fat vanilla yogurt	31	0	15
12 oz herbal tea with nonnutritive sweetener	1	0	0
Dinner			
3 oz pot roast beef with	0	0	0
¼ cup sauteed mushrooms	2	1	0
1 cup white and wild rice blend with margarine	35	1	0
½ cup vegetable juice	2	0	0
2 cup tossed salad with lettuce, avocado, tomatoes, and carrots	3	1	0
¼ cup shredded low-fat muenster cheese	1	0	0
2 tablespoons vinaigrette salad dressing	4	0	3
⅛ medium cantaloupe	6	1	0
12 oz iced tea with low-calorie sweetener	1	0	0
Evening Snack			
3 cup popcorn	16	5.8	0
12 oz water	0	0	0
Totals[a]	300.36	33.1	35

[a]Totals may vary due to rounding.

From Calorie Control Council. *Nutrient Data*. https://caloriecontrol.org/healthy-weight-tool-kit/food-calorie-calculator/; USDA. *What's in the Foods You Eat Search Tool*. https://codesearch.arsnet.usda.gov/(S(xiwzrqkowqwac2dfqfeiganj))/CodeSearch.aspx.

• BOX **4.2**   Tips for Following the *Dietary Guidelines* for Carbohydrates

- Be aware of the amount of sugars in processed foods. Sugar may be identified as any of the following on food labels: sucrose, fructose, corn sweetener, cane sugar, evaporated cane juice, honey, molasses, high-fructose corn syrup, raw sugar, and maple syrup. Try to avoid foods if one of these is the first ingredient listed.
- Choose water and other beverages that contain little or no added sweeteners.
- Pay attention to nutrition labels, not only for the amount of added sugars but also for the amount of fiber in a serving. Because fiber is not absorbed, it does not contribute any calories. A product with 25 g of carbohydrate may have only 80 cal if at least 5 g of the carbohydrate is from fiber.
- Choose whole fruits in place of foods or juices with added sugars.
- Look for breads and cereals that list "whole grain" or "whole wheat" first in the ingredients list. A more promising sign is "100% whole grain." Brown color is no guarantee of whole-grain content.
- Popular whole-grain foods include black, brown, and wild rice; whole wheat, corn, barley, buckwheat, millet, oats, quinoa, rye, sorghum, and spelt. Many of the ancient grains becoming more popular are also whole-grain foods.
- Beans, lentils and dried peas are good sources of complex carbohydrates.
- Choose nutrient-dense carbohydrate food sources to provide adequate amounts of required nutrients.

From United States Department of Agriculture and United States Department of Health and Human Services. *Dietary Guidelines for Americans, 2020–2025.* 9th ed. 2020. dietaryGuidelines.gov.

Hyperstates and Hypostates

The role of carbohydrates in nutritional health and behavior continues to be misrepresented by the press and some professionals. Many stories published in the media link sugar to every practical modern-day illness, including malnutrition, hypoglycemia, diabetes mellitus, blood lipid abnormalities, hyperactivity, criminal behavior, obesity, malabsorption syndrome, allergies, gallstones, and cancer. The public's perception of sugar consumption continues to be at odds with scientific facts.

Normal physiologic conditions and disease states affect carbohydrate metabolism, which is reflected in serum glucose levels. For individuals with diabetes, a blood glucose level that is greater than 130 mg/dL before meals or greater than 180 mg/dL 2 hours after meals indicates hyperglycemia; a blood glucose level less than 70 mg/dL indicates hypoglycemia.[15] Other factors concerning too much or too little carbohydrate are discussed later.

Carbohydrate Excess

As previously mentioned, there has been a controversy regarding how much carbohydrate (mainly sucrose) is excessive. The preponderance of evidence based on scientific literature indicates that sugar consumption at the level recommended in the *Dietary Guidelines* does not directly contribute to any chronic health or behavioral problems. Avoiding excessive amounts of calories from sugars is prudent, but the scientific basis for optimal levels for preventing and controlling chronic diseases remains unsettled.[16,17] Excessive sugar consumption leading to energy imbalance may contribute to weight gain. Added sugars (>25% of total energy) may result in an inadequate intake of foods containing necessary micronutrients. Intake of nutrients at most risk for inadequacy (vitamins A, D, E, and C, and magnesium, potassium, dietary fiber, choline, and calcium)

decreases as added sugars increase above 5%–10% of total calories. But the predominant issue is the low-quality and overall high-energy intake of US diets, regardless of sweetener content. Weight gain occurs resulting from excess caloric intake, not physiologic or metabolic consequences of sucrose or any specific sugar. In the US population, added sugars account for 13% of total calorie per day, with the majority coming from SSBs, desserts and sweet snacks, sweetened coffee and tea, and candy (Fig. 4.6).[5]

A principle concern in the *Dietary Guidelines* is consumption of adequate amounts of vitamins and minerals without consuming excess energy. Sweeteners contain no other nutrients (vitamins or minerals) and, when consumed as SSBs and hard candies, provide nothing other than pleasure and energy. Consumers are drinking enormous amounts of calories in liquid form. As shown in Fig. 4.6, SSBs, fruit drinks with added sugar, and sports and energy drinks contribute 24% of all sugar intake. There has been a decline in soft drink consumption since the late 1990s, when consumption was 49.7 gallons per capita to approximately 42.9 gallons in 2022.[18]

Obesity

A common misperception is that sugar is uniquely fattening. Because the taste of sugar is so pleasant, some rationalize that sugar becomes irresistible to the point of overconsumption or addiction. However, most individuals have a limit as to how much sweet foods they can consume in a given period.

Four leading scientific and health organizations—the Food and Agriculture Organization, WHO, the National Academy of Medicine, and the Academy of Nutrition and Dietetics—have all concluded that dietary sugars are not definitively associated with causing illness or chronic diseases, including obesity. Evidence indicates that although added sugar intake may be a contributing factor to increased risk of overweight or obesity, overall diet quality must be considered.[16,17,19,20] Current findings indicate that food energy density and pleasures derived from eating promote excessive energy intake.[16,17]

Some studies indicate an association between higher intake of whole grains (minimum of three servings daily) with healthier body weights and fat stores. However, data from National Health and Nutritional Examination Surveys found no correlation between whole-grain intake and body mass index, but whole grains were related to positive nutrient profiles and chronic disease risk factors.[21] The *Dietary Guidelines* recommend a fiber-rich diet to help manage obesity as it provides bulk which may help with satiety while reducing calories consumed.

Excessive caloric intake leads to obesity, whether from carbohydrates, proteins, fats, or alcohol. Although excessive energy intake from sugar may lead to obesity, epidemiologic studies and several other studies have shown that obese patients actually consume less sugar than thin patients. Many sweet foods contain large amounts of fat. Excessive carbohydrates, including sugars, are likely to be consumed when fat is severely restricted and overall food intake is not restricted to some degree.

Altering the proportion of dietary carbohydrate is less important in weight management than the total caloric intake. Only when sugar consumption interferes with or replaces a balanced, nutrient dense eating pattern, the diet becomes inadequate. When that occurs, sugar warrants the designation of "empty calorie," indicating the diet has inadequate vitamins, minerals, and trace elements. Fortification of foods has a positive effect on nutrient density of the diet.

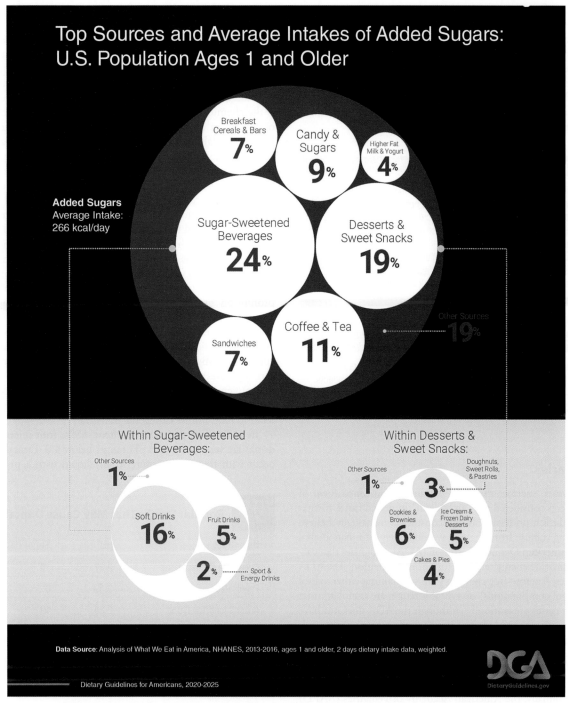

Fig. 4.6 Food category sources and added intake of added sugars in the United States population ages one year and older. (From United States Department of Agriculture and United States Department of Health and Human Services. *Dietary Guidelines for Americans, 2020–2025*. 9th ed. 2020.)

Cardiovascular Disease

The claim that sugar intake causes chronic diseases (especially diabetes and CVD) has been widely researched and continues to be controversial. Numerous studies have found an association between diets rich in added sugars (17%–21% or more of calories) or SSBs and the onset of heart disease risk factors (hypertension, stroke, and higher triglyceride levels). The biologic mechanism underlying this association is not understood.[22,23] Other systematic reviews and controlled trials using moderate amounts of sugar have not found this correlation.[24–26] Many studies focus only on consumption of SSBs; although SSBs are the most prevalent form of sugar intake, they may not be a true reflection of an individual's total sugar intake.

Carbohydrate Deficiency

Frequently, carbohydrates are eliminated in an effort to lose weight. When carbohydrates are severely restricted, protein and fat intake usually increases. Very-high-protein, low-carbohydrate diets do not necessarily lead to greater weight loss than traditional diets, and care must be taken to prevent elevated lipid levels that may accompany higher fat intake. Extremely-low-carbohydrate diets may lead to ketosis.

When complex carbohydrates are eliminated, an insufficient intake of B vitamins, iron, and fiber may occur. Vitamins and minerals are necessary for the body to use glucose, but these nutrients do not need to be present in the same foods.

DENTAL CONSIDERATIONS

- Scientific studies do not support the claim that sugars interfere with bioavailability of vitamins, minerals, or trace nutrients, or the notion that dietary imbalances are preferentially caused by increased sugar consumption. Do not assume that because a patient is obese, increased sugar intake is the culprit.
- Scientific consensus to date shows that (1) the link between sugar intake and obesity is inconsistent, (2) sugar intake alone does not cause diabetes, and (3) sugar intake is not an independent risk factor for CVD.[16,23,26]

NUTRITIONAL DIRECTIONS

- Encourage a well-balanced diet containing adequate nutrients with appropriate amounts of fruits, vegetables, and milk and dairy products.
- Several organs depend on glucose to function. A minimal-carbohydrate, high-protein, high-fat diet may result in an inadequate intake of numerous nutrients and cognitive impairment.

Dental Caries

For many years, sucrose, the most frequently consumed form of sugar, has been considered the "archvillain" in dental caries formation. Many health professionals and consumers mistakenly believe that removing sucrose from the diet would largely eliminate dental caries. The American Dental Association (ADA) recognizes that carbohydrates provide energy required for optimal nutrition. The ADA acknowledges, "sucrose-free chewing gum (containing either xylitol only or polyol combinations) or xylitol lozenges are useful adjunct therapies for caries prevention."[27] Although the ADA does not have a position statement about the use of xylitol, the most recently available executive summary of evidence based clinical recommendations from the ADA Council on Scientific Affairs Expert Panel on Nonfluoride Caries-Preventive Agents supports that xylitol may be useful as an adjunct therapy in children or adults at higher risk of caries.[27,28] Additionally, the American Academy of Pediatrics (AAPD) supports the use of xylitol and other sugar alcohols as noncariogenic sugar substitutes. However, updated AAPD policy recognizes that current evidence is inconsistent in showing a significant reduction of caries in children and that the recommended frequency (four to five times a day) may be unrealistic in clinical practice.[29]

Sucrose and other disaccharides and monosaccharides (glucose, fructose, maltose, and lactose) have unusual biochemical properties that promote bacterial growth. The presence of sucrose and other carbohydrates in the mouth increases the volume and formation rate of plaque biofilm. Even low amounts of sucrose promote production of polysaccharides (glucans) by *Streptococcus mutans (S. mutans)*, the bacteria that facilitates adherence of plaque biofilm to teeth. These glucans help provide a matrix, supporting communities of microorganisms collectively referred to as **plaque biofilm**. A **fermentable carbohydrate** (i.e., carbohydrates that can be metabolized by bacteria in plaque biofilm, including all sugars and cooked or processed starches) that can reduce salivary pH to less than 5.5 is referred to as being **cariogenic**.

Glucose, available from sucrose or any other carbohydrate food, can be used for energy by oral bacteria in plaque biofilm. These sugars lower the pH of plaque biofilm, hastening the dissolution of hydroxyapatite crystals of the enamel. **Dental erosion** is the chemical removal of minerals from the tooth structure that occurs when an acidic environment causes enamel to gradually dissolve. In laboratory tests, the rate at which fructose and glucose lower plaque biofilm pH is similar to sucrose; they are considered as cariogenic as sucrose. Therefore substituting glucose or fructose for sucrose is not significantly effective in reducing caries rates. Lactose is less cariogenic than other sugars. The kind of sugar is not significant; the concentration or quantity of sugar in a foodstuff is not critical to its cariogenic potential. The total amount of fermentable carbohydrate seems to be of less importance than the form in which it is eaten and the frequency of consumption. This may be related to variables influencing the duration for which the carbohydrate remains in contact with teeth and its potential for promoting growth of caries-forming, acid-producing bacteria. (See Chapter 18 for further discussion.)

SSBs and energy drinks contain fermentable carbohydrates and are highly acidic (Table 4.5). Despite differences in the carbohydrate content of SSBs, fruit drinks, 100% fruit juice (approximately 10% carbohydrates), sports drinks (approximately 46%–48% carbohydrates), energy drinks (approximately 9%–10% carbohydrates), flavored coffees and teas, and powdered drinks, all these beverages seem to have similar cariogenic potential.

In addition to their sugar content, SSBs, fruit juices, and sports drinks are very acidic with pH ranges below 4.0. Dental erosion can occur with frequent exposure to any liquid with a pH below 4.2.

TABLE 4.5 Popular Drinks That May Cause Dental Erosion

Beverages	pH[a]	Sugar (tsp in 12 oz)
Coca Cola Classic, 12 oz	2.37	10
Pepsi, 12 oz	2.39	0
Arizona Iced Tea, 16 oz	2.84	12
Gatorade Lemon Lime, 20 oz	2.97	9.0
Diet Coke, 12 oz	3.10	0
Diet Mountain Dew, 12 oz	3.18	0
Diet Dr. Pepper	3.20	0
Mountain Dew, 12 oz	3.22	12
Sprite, 12 oz	3.24	9.0
Apple juice, bottled, 12 oz	3.57	10
Red Bull, sugar free, 8.4 oz	3.43	0
Monster Energy Drink, 12 oz	3.48	10
V-8 Vegetable juice	4.23	less than 1.0
Starbucks, medium roast	5.11	10

[a]Neutral pH 7. Teeth erosion occurs with a pH of 2.0–4.0. Demineralization begins at critical pH of 5.5.
Data obtained from CalorieKing. https://www.calorieking.com/us/en/. Accessed August 15, 2023.

Citrus juices contain citric acid, which is especially damaging to tooth enamel; the citrate binds with calcium in saliva, reducing its potential to remineralize the tooth. Deleterious effects of 100% fruit juices may be minimized with chemical modification or calcium fortification.[30] Sour sweets and acidic products, even if they are sugar free, may increase the probability of dental erosion.[31] SSBs, acidic snack foods, natural acidic fruit, and juices increase erosion occurrence while milk and yogurt have a protective effect.[32] Research suggests the extent of enamel erosion, caused by various beverages, occurs in the following order (from greatest to least): energy drinks, sports drinks, regular soda, and diet soda.[33–35]

No definite relationship has been shown between total carbohydrate consumption and caries. Cooked starches can cause acid production in plaque biofilm due to their high retentiveness in the mouth. Some foods—such as potato chips or crackers, containing a high-carbohydrate, low-sugar content—can contribute to the caries process when salivary amylase hydrolyzes complex carbohydrate to simple sugars. Starch molecules are large and cannot penetrate into plaque biofilm. Cooked and refined cereal grains are readily hydrolyzed by salivary amylases to produce maltose, which can lower pH and demineralize enamel. Some foods high in sugar are removed more quickly. They do not lower the pH of plaque biofilm as much as starchy foods containing less sugar level. Starches, such as breads and pasta, are considered less cariogenic than sugars, but they tend to prolong the caries attack after it has been initiated (especially when sugar is added, as in sweet breads and cookies).

Some popular snack products contain sweeteners that are less cariogenic than sucrose. Sugar alcohols may decrease the risk of dental caries through any of the following mechanisms: (1) inhibiting the growth of S. mutans, (2) not promoting synthesis of plaque biofilm, or (3) not lowering plaque biofilm pH. Studies evaluating evidence for an anticariogenic effect of sugar-free chewing gum concluded that it has a caries-reducing effect, but more well-designed, randomized studies are recommended to confirm the findings.[36,37] The ADA has approved the use of its seal on sugarless gums by several gum manufacturers and has also recommended chewing gum after each meal for at least 20 minutes to reap the most benefits if oral hygiene cannot be performed.

Sorbitol causes only a slight pH decrease in plaque biofilm. Bacteria in plaque biofilm are able to ferment sorbitol and mannitol but only slowly over several weeks. After a period of adaptation, however, acid production increases.

The anticariogenic effect of xylitol has been accepted globally, as it exhibits both passive and active anticaries effects and directly inhibits the growth of S. mutans.[38] An anticariogenic substance reduces caries risk by preventing bacteria from recognizing a cariogenic food. Oral bacteria lack the enzymes to ferment xylitol; it does not lower plaque biofilm pH. The anticariogenic effect of xylitol-containing chewing gum may be enhanced by the chewing process. Xylitol stimulates secretion of saliva, which contains a large number of bicarbonate ions to neutralize acid. Additionally, xylitol promotes remineralization of early lesions on tooth enamel.

Erythritol is another sugar alcohol that may improve oral health by decreasing adherence of bacteria to tooth surfaces, inhibiting growth and activity of S. mutans, and reducing the overall number of dental caries. In studies testing the efficacy of erythritol and xylitol candy, compared with sorbitol candy, fewer dental caries developed in the erythritol group than in the xylitol or control groups.[38–40]

Lactitol cannot be metabolized by bacteria in plaque biofilm and may provide a protective effect for teeth. However, it is only about one-third as sweet as sucrose. Saccharin inhibits tooth decay in rats. Aspartame does not support the growth of S. mutans, acid production, or plaque biofilm formation.

DENTAL CONSIDERATIONS

- Approximately 90% of commonly consumed snack foods contain fermentable carbohydrates (sugars or cooked starch or both). Frequently consumed fermentable carbohydrates include chewing gum, chewable tablets, lozenges, mints, and snack foods such as gummy bears.
- Snacks contribute significantly to the nutritional intake of young children and teenagers who need larger amounts of energy for growth.
- Patients unable to tolerate adequate amounts of food at meals may require snacks to promote healing and avoid loss of lean body mass.
- Although sucrose is a major factor in caries risk, provide factual information without overemphasizing sugar's role in caries formation.
- Some foods—such as milk, yogurt, and aged cheese—actually protect teeth by increasing oral pH and inhibiting acid production.
- Assess patient's consumption of acidic beverages. Patients with frequent consumption of acidic beverages, decreased salivary flow, prolonged holding habits, or mouth breathing may be at increased risk of dental erosion.
- Excessive intake (more than 20 g per day) of sugar alcohol-containing gum and sweets may lead to unintended weight loss as a result of chronic diarrhea. One piece of sugar-free gum contains about 1.25 g sorbitol.
- Polyol-based, sugar-free products may cause dental erosion if they contain acidic flavoring.
- The association between eating and weight status is not the result of a single eating pattern but rather from a combination of food choices that are interrelated and cumulative in their effect.
- The most important cause of dental caries is frequency of consuming fermentable carbohydrates that supply substrate to caries-producing oral bacteria.
- The potential for caries risk exists every time a carbohydrate is eaten because most foods promote acid formation if no procedures are taken to remove food debris or plaque biofilm, to buffer the acid produced, or to interfere with acid production.
- The amount of carbohydrate in a food is unrelated to its caries-forming potential; all carbohydrate foods are potentially cariogenic. Proteins and fats are cariostatic, or cannot be metabolized by microorganisms in plaque biofilm, and are caries inhibiting.
- Natural sugars, primarily fructose and glucose, in unprocessed foods, such as bananas and raisins, are potentially as cariogenic as sucrose.

NUTRITIONAL DIRECTIONS

- If snacks are needed when oral hygiene cannot be performed, suggest low-fat milk products, aged cheese, or yogurt; or chew xylitol-containing gum.
- Xylitol and erythritol may cause less GI distress than other sugar alcohols.[41]
- Complete and permanent elimination of sweets is unrealistic. The best advice is to (1) use sugar in moderation, (2) limit the frequency of sugar exposure, (3) consume sweets with a meal, and (4) brush the teeth after consuming sugar-containing products. If oral hygiene cannot be performed, chew xylitol, sorbitol, or xylitol-sorbitol chewing gum.
- Encourage patients to brush their teeth before consuming acidic foods and chew sugar-free gum afterward. Brushing their teeth after consuming acidic foods may increase dental erosion.
- Sugar alcohols are less likely to promote caries; xylitol may prevent caries formation.
- Highly acidic foods may prevent bacterial fermentation but cause enamel erosion.
- Replace potentially cariogenic snacks with foods such as fresh fruits and vegetables; low-fat cottage cheese, cheese, and yogurt (flavored with nutmeg, cinnamon, or fresh fruit); peanuts; or low-fat popcorn to decrease caries risk and promote other health-conscious nutritional habits.
- Use a straw with beverages such as carbonated drinks or lemonade to reduce contact with teeth and lessen caries risk.
- Consumption of SSBs should be limited to 8 oz or less daily with a meal.
- Complex unrefined carbohydrates are high in fiber and other nutrients.

Nonnutritive Sweeteners/Sugar Substitutes

The practice of flavoring foods without additional calories is one of many approaches to the problems of excess energy intake and a sedentary lifestyle. Nonnutritive sweeteners, also called artificial sweeteners, add sweetness but contain no or minimal carbohydrates (or energy) and do not raise blood sugars. Most are synthesized compounds from fruits, herbs, or sugar itself. The use of sugar substitutes also has beneficial ramifications for dental hygiene. The desire to decrease sugar consumption is being met through widespread and increasing use of nonnutritive sweeteners. Consumption of low-caloric and noncaloric sweeteners is increasing faster than that of caloric sweeteners.[42]

Nonnutritive sweeteners are used principally due to their sweetening power, making some foods more palatable. The large variety of sweeteners is desirable because each has certain advantages and limitations. Because each sweetener has different properties, the availability of various products helps satisfy various flavor and texture requirements in foods and beverages. Sweeteners may be combined because of their synergistic effect—that is, when combined, sweeteners yield a sweeter taste than that provided by each sweetener alone.

These sweeteners have the potential to reduce sugar and energy intakes, but Americans' BMIs have risen parallel to the rise in use of nonnutritive sweeteners. Although taste buds may be fooled by their sweetness, nonnutritive sweeteners do not produce a prolonged feeling of satiety. Concerns have been expressed that nonnutritive sweeteners may promote energy intake and contribute to obesity. The preponderance of evidence from human randomized controlled studies indicates that nonnutritive sweeteners do not increase energy intake or body weight and may even reduce intake and weight.[43,44]

Currently, data is insufficient to conclusively determine whether the use of nonnutritive sweeteners replacing caloric sweeteners reduces added sugars or carbohydrate intakes, or has an effect on appetite, energy balance, body weight, or other risk factors. Nevertheless, the American Heart Association concluded that nonnutritive sweeteners could be used in a structured diet to replace added sugars, thereby resulting in decreased total energy and weight loss/weight control, and promoting beneficial effects on related metabolic parameters.[45] Individuals who use nonnutritive sweeteners may choose a healthier eating pattern and engage in better lifestyle habits.[46]

Whether use of these nonnutritive sweeteners decreases total caloric intake depends on other food choices. Making compensatory food choices, such as drinking a carbonated beverage to permit a piece of cheesecake, is ineffective in weight control, whereas replacing a high-calorie food with a low-calorie food, watching other food intake, and engaging in some form of exercise may be beneficial.

Many consumers question the safety of these products. All products on the market have been extensively researched and are safe for most people if consumed in moderation except for aspartame. Aspartame is safe in moderate amounts for everyone except individuals who have phenylketonuria, a genetic disorder characterized by an inability to metabolize the amino acid phenylalanine. Table 4.6 summarizes information regarding sugar substitutes.

DENTAL CONSIDERATIONS

- Sugar substitutes can reduce energy content and decrease cariogenicity of a product. Used in moderation, nonnutritive sweeteners are beneficial for many people, especially patients with diabetes.
- Because aspartame contains phenylalanine, aspartame-containing products are labeled to warn patients with phenylketonuria to avoid their use.
- Use of sugar substitutes is advocated for between-meal snacks to decrease tooth exposure to sugar. For individuals who do not need to decrease energy intake, sugar alcohols may be recommended.
- Nonnutritive sweeteners are not fermentable and do not promote caries formation; antimicrobial activity has not been observed. Saccharin and aspartame exhibit microbial inhibition and caries suppression.
- Dental professionals are often asked to provide advice regarding the importance of diet and the role of sugars and nonnutritive sweeteners in caries formation and weight management. A reduction of fermentable sugars and carbohydrates coupled with good oral hygiene practices will reduce incidence of dental decay.

TABLE 4.6   Noncaloric Sugar Substitutes (Nonnutritive Sweeteners)[a]

	Acesulfame K (Sweet One, Sweet & Safe, Sunette)	Aspartame[b] (NutraSweet, Equal, Sugar Twin)	Stevia (Truvia, Rebinana, PureVia, SweetLeaf, Sun Crystals)	Saccharin (Sweet and Low, Sweet Twin, NectaSweet)	Sucralose (Splenda)
Description	200% sweeter than sucrose	200% sweeter than sucrose. Made from 2 amino acids—phenylalanine and aspartic acid	200%–400% sweeter than sucrose	200%–700% sweeter than sucrose	600% sweeter than sucrose. Made from sucrose
Facts	No aftertaste. Noncariogenic. Heat stable. Works synergistically with other sweeteners	No aftertaste. Intensifies flavors. Noncariogenic	Natural, from stevia leaves. Works synergistically with other sweeteners. Readily soluble in water	Works synergistically with other sweeteners. Slight aftertaste	No aftertaste. Heat stable. Replaces sugar in equal amounts. Noncariogenic

[a]Data from Firch C, Keim KS. Position of the Academy of Nutrition and Dietetics. Use of nutritive and nonnutritive sweeteners. *J Acad Nutr Diet.* 2012;112(5):739–758.
[b]Not recommended for patients with phenylketonuria; U.S. Food & Drug Administration. *Aspartame and Other Sweeteners in Food.* https://www.fda.gov/food/food-additives-petitions/aspartame-and-other-sweeteners-food.

⬡ NUTRITIONAL DIRECTIONS

- Nonnutritive sweeteners have been deemed safe and their use is supported by many reputable health agencies.
- Although nonnutritive sweeteners may not have cariogenic potential, bulking ingredients that allow them to pour and measure more like sugar (and other constituents of a product) may have cariogenic potential if they contain fermentable carbohydrates.
- Nonnutritive sweeteners do nothing to appease the appetite, but they do provide the pleasure of sweetness. They may enable patients to choose a wide variety of foods or improve taste appeal of healthy products, such as oatmeal, while managing caloric or cariogenic intake.
- When evaluating the amount of nonnutritive sweeteners, a client (especially relevant for a child) is consuming, refer to Table 4.7.

- These acceptable daily intake limits are excessively high, but indicate amounts that may be harmful. Other nutritional requirements have not been factored into this (e.g., consuming adequate amounts of required nutrients). Remember that children need energy for growth and development.
- Combinations of sweeteners can produce a sweet taste more similar to that of sugar than can a single high-intensity sweetener.
- During pregnancy, saccharin is not recommended because it is known to cross the placenta. Refer a pregnant patient to her obstetrician for counseling about using any nonnutritive sweeteners.

◆ HEALTH APPLICATION 4

Lactose Intolerance

Some patients are unable to digest specific carbohydrates because of insufficient amounts of disaccharide-degrading enzymes. When those carbohydrates are eaten, the disaccharide is fermented by intestinal bacteria rather than being broken down into simple sugars. Lactase, an intestinal enzyme responsible for lactose digestion, is the only disaccharidase whose activity is reduced in a significant proportion of older children and adults. As per the National Institute of Diabetes and Digestive and Kidney Diseases, lactase deficiency occurs when the small intestine produces low levels of lactase and cannot digest much lactose.[47] Lactase deficiency may cause lactose malabsorption, in which undigested lactose passes to the colon, leading to lactose intolerance. Symptoms (diarrhea, abdominal cramps, flatulence, and halitosis) usually begin 30 minutes to 2 hours after consuming milk or milk products.

Not all people with lactase deficiency and lactose malabsorption have digestive symptoms. Symptoms of lactose intolerance generally do not occur until lactase production is less than 50%.

With rare exceptions, all infants of every racial and ethnic group can successfully digest the lactose in human milk and infant formulas. In most patients, the production of lactase declines following weaning (age 2 years) unless milk and milk products are consumed routinely.[48–50] Lactose intolerance primarily affects African Americans, Hispanic Americans, Native Americans, Asian Americans, Alaskan Natives, and Pacific Islanders. For most people, lactase deficiency appears to be genetically determined. It may also be a temporary condition caused by GI diseases or intestinal mucosa damage. Occasionally, an infant has a lactase deficiency at birth because of an inborn error of metabolism. Lactose intolerance can be diagnosed based on the results of a hydrogen breath test or stool acidity test ordered by a health care provider.

Nutritional Care

Lactase deficiency is easily treated by reducing lactose-containing foods in one's diet. Because milk provides significant amounts of calcium, vitamin D, phosphorus, riboflavin, and sometimes protein, elimination of milk is not advisable. The ability to digest lactose is not an all-or-nothing phenomenon; most patients with lactose intolerance can tolerate some lactose. The amount of dairy products is reduced to a patient's tolerance level (Box 4.3). Most adults and adolescents with lactose malabsorption can tolerate at least 12–18 g of lactose.[49] Larger doses may be tolerated when dairy products are ingested with other nutrients. Milk is tolerated better when taken with a meal and limited to 8 oz at a time. Whole milk is better tolerated than skim milk.

Individuals who avoid dairy products may exacerbate their risk for osteoporosis. Calcium is necessary for adequate bone accretions and optimal peak bone mass. When children's and teenagers' diets are deficient in calcium and/or vitamin D, bone accretion may be affected and optimal peak bone mass may not occur. Patients should be taught the approximate calcium composition of milk products and other calcium-rich foods (see Chapter 9) to achieve adequate intake.

Fermented dairy products—especially yogurt, buttermilk, aged cheese, and sour cream—are often better tolerated by lactase-deficient individuals than other dairy products. Because it contains active lactase and less lactose, yogurt made with the organisms *Lactobacillus bulgaricus* or *Streptococcus thermophilus* is better tolerated than nonfermented dairy products. Most commercially available unflavored yogurt can be beneficial to lactose-intolerant patients. Pasteurization of frozen yogurts decreases the lactase activity and kills lactose-producing bacteria; thus, most frozen yogurts are not well tolerated by lactose-intolerant patients.

Commercially available lactase in tablet or liquid form can be beneficial. Lactase tablets, taken with a lactose-containing food, are effective in the stomach's acidic environment for approximately 45 minutes. Liquid lactase is effective in a neutral pH and, when added to milk, the lactose is hydrolyzed before ingestion. Specialized lactose-reduced products are also commercially available.

TABLE 4.7 Acceptable Daily Intake (ADI) of Nonnutritive Sweeteners

	Saccharin	Acesulfame K	Aspartame	Sucralose	Steviol Glycosides
ADI mg/kg body weight/day[a]	15	15	50	5	4
Packets/day[a]	45	23	75	23	9

[a]Number of sweetener packets that a person weighing 60 kg (132 pound) would need to consume to meet his ADI requirement. The FDA assumed a sweetener packet is as sweet as two teaspoons (approximately 8 g) of sugar for these comparisons.

Adapted from U.S. Food & Drug Administration. *Aspartame and Other Sweeteners in Food.* https://www.fda.gov/food/food-additives-petitions/aspartame-and-other-sweeteners-food.

• BOX 4.3   Suggestions for Lactose-Intolerant Patients

- Adequate amounts of calcium are needed even when dairy products must be avoided. Because of different tolerance levels, each patient needs to experiment to determine which method is most effective for providing necessary nutrients without discomfort. Consume small amounts of lactose-containing foods with meals several times a day.
- Gradually add lactose-containing products such as dairy to the diet to test your tolerance.
- Consume fermented dairy products—yogurt,[a] kefir,[b] and buttermilk—that contain probiotics (live bacteria).
- Choose aged cheeses (e.g., Swiss, Colby, and Longhorn) that naturally contain less lactose.
- Buy lactose-reduced or lactose-free products.
- Read ingredient labels for "hidden" lactose (whey, milk by-products, nonfat dry milk powder, malted milk, buttermilk, and dry milk solids). Also, check for lactose in prescription and over-the-counter drugs.
- Drink or eat calcium-fortified foods, such as fruit juices, soy or almond milk, and cereals.

[a]Unflavored yogurt is usually best tolerated.
[b]Kefir is a fermented milk beverage that contains different bacteria than yogurt.

- Use over-the-counter lactase enzymes available in tablet or liquid form to hydrolyze the lactose in milk products or consume lactose-hydrolyzed milk available commercially.
- Increase consumption of other calcium-containing foods, such as salmon and sardines canned with bones, vegetables (collards; spinach; kale; turnip, mustard, and dandelion greens; broccoli), beans, and nuts and seeds.
- Consider commercially available nutrition supplements, such as Resource, Boost, and Sustacal (Nestle Health Science).
- If these suggestions are not feasible to maintain an adequate intake of 1000–1200 mg of calcium, consult a health care provider or registered dietitian for calcium supplements that are well absorbed. These supplements may also need to include vitamin D for optimum absorption.

Adapted from National Institute of Diabetes and Digestive and Kidney Diseases. *Eating, Diet, & Nutrition for Lactose Intolerance.* National Institute of Health. https://www.niddk.nih.gov/health-information/digestive-diseases/lactose-intolerance/eating-diet-nutrition; Mayo Clinic. *Lactose Intolerance.* https://www.mayoclinic.org/diseases-conditions/lactose-intolerance/diagnosis-treatment/drc-20374238.

◆ CASE APPLICATION FOR THE DENTAL HYGIENIST

A healthy patient needs information on how to eat less refined sugar and more complex carbohydrates. He knows that this regimen is encouraged but does not know all the health reasons. Fiber intake is also important for him, but he is not knowledgeable about the types of food needed or the benefits.

Nutritional Assessment
- Willingness/motivation to learn
- Usual dietary habits; focus especially on carbohydrate
- Basic knowledge of carbohydrate and carbohydrate principles
- Usual food/nutrient intake
- Financial status, employment status, and where most of the food is consumed
- Support system—family, friends, coworkers
- Use of community resources
- Food shopping practices

Nutritional Diagnosis
Health-seeking behavior related to lack of knowledge concerning carbohydrate and carbohydrate principles for optimal nutrition.

Nutritional Goals
The patient will consume a high-fiber food and complex carbohydrate food daily, and state three principles concerning carbohydrate.

Nutritional Implementation
Intervention: Explain (1) that the main function of carbohydrates is to provide energy for the body; (2) that excessive amounts of carbohydrates by themselves do not cause obesity but excessive overall caloric intake increases body fat (and consequently weight); and (3) the role of carbohydrates in the dental caries process and enhancing plaque biofilm formation.
Rationale: Knowledge corrects misinformation.
Intervention: (1) Follow suggestions in Table 4.3. (2) Explain the importance of fiber. Recommend 30–38 g of fiber daily and help the patient plan a diet that will provide this amount, incorporating his food preferences. Stress the importance of adequate fluid intake.

Rationale: These suggestions increase fiber in the diet. Fiber increases stool bulk, exercising digestive tract muscles and preventing them from being chronically contracted. Muscle tone is maintained, colonic pressure is diminished, and the gut is able to resist bulging out into pouches. Additionally, fiber slackens starch hydrolysis and delays glucose absorption.
Intervention: Explain sources of complex carbohydrates and fiber sources, and provide the patient with a list of these foods. Emphasize the importance of increasing fiber intake gradually and increasing noncariogenic, noncaloric fluid intake when increasing fiber.
Rationale: The patient's increased knowledge will encourage him to increase consumption of complex carbohydrate and fiber.
Intervention: (1) Recommend substituting nonnutritive sweeteners for sugar, especially at snack time. (2) Read a label with the patient to show him how to recognize sugars (they usually end in *-ose*). (3) Recommend substituting fresh fruit for juices to increase fiber. (4) Instruct him to limit products that contain complex carbohydrates and sugar, such as cookies and pastries.
Rationale: He wanted to reduce refined sugar intake; these measures will help meet this personal goal.
Intervention: Refer him to an RDN and county extension agencies.
Rationale: These will provide expert knowledge and community resources for continued compliance.
Intervention: Review labeling: (1) "no sugar added" means sugar was not added, although the product may naturally contain sugar; (2) "sugar-free" means the product contains no added sucrose but may have other sugars added, such as sorbitol; (3) a high-fiber food has been defined as containing 5 g or more per serving; (4) incorporate foods with 3 g or more fiber per serving.
Rationale: Knowing the meaning of these terms facilitates making healthy food choices.

Evaluation
The patient consumes a bran muffin, beans, or other high-fiber foods daily and verbalizes that carbohydrates provide energy and fiber, carbohydrate has several roles in maintaining gut functioning, and most sugars end in *-ose*. Other indicators of success include reading a label correctly, modifying intake of refined sugars, and using the community resources.

◆ Student Readiness

1. Differentiate between the three classes of carbohydrates.
2. Identify sources of complex carbohydrates in the diet.
3. What are the main sources of fiber in the American diet?
4. List three of your favorite foods high in added sugar. What realistic modifications can you make to your diet with respect to these high-sugar foods?
5. Explain the functions of sugars and fiber in the diet in terms a patient can understand.
6. From cereal boxes at the local grocery store, identify some of the products that claim to be high in fiber: (1) evaluate the source of fiber on the ingredient label to determine if those are soluble or insoluble fibers; and (2) rank the cereals according to the amount of dietary fiber they contain. Which would you recommend?
7. Find five breakfast cereals at the grocery store that list a whole grain as the first ingredient.
8. Role play: To a patient consuming a very-low-carbohydrate diet, discuss why this diet is not beneficial to their long-term health.
9. Role play: Advise a mother who has been told she should never give her infant anything that contains sugar because the infant will develop a sweet tooth.
10. What is the basis for the WHO's recommendation of 10% or less of calories from sugars? Why is the National Academy of Medicine recommendation of 25% or less of energy intake different?
11. Match the carbohydrates on the left with the appropriate answer in the right column.

Dextrose	Cannot be used by the body
Glycogen	Milk
Fructose	Sweetest sugar
Lactose	Glucose
Cellulose	Storage form of carbohydrate in the body

◆ CASE STUDY

A 22-year-old African American male presents with four carious lesions acquired since his last dental hygiene recare appointment. While questioning the patient, you learn that he frequently skips meals and relies heavily on snacks to get him through the day.
1. What further information about his dietary intake do you need?
2. Could the patient's snacking habits be related to the increase in his dental caries?
3. Which types of foods should be suggested as snack foods and why?
4. What other precautions could the patient practice that might be helpful in preventing further caries problems?

◆ CASE STUDY

A 22-year-old Asian female reports a history of lactose intolerance. She is concerned about her calcium intake because she has eliminated all dairy products from her diet.
1. What symptoms may the patient report that are associated with lactose intake?
2. What should be included in dietary recommendations made by the dental hygienist?
3. Which dairy products are best tolerated by lactose-deficient individuals?
4. When should lactase tablets be taken?
5. What recommendations can be provided about the intake of dairy products?

References

1. Food and Nutrition Board, Institute of Medicine. *Dietary Reference Intakes for Energy, Carbohydrate, Fiber, Fat, Fatty Acids, Cholesterol, Protein, and Amino Acids.* National Academy Press; 2002.
2. National Center for Health Statistics. *Dietary Intake for adults 20 years of age and over. Health, United States, 2015–2018 (Table McrNutr.).* 2021. https://www.cdc.gov/nchs/fastats/diet.htm.
3. United States Department of Agriculture and U.S. Department of Health and Human Services. *Dietary Guidelines for Americans, 2020–2025.* 9th ed. 2020. https://www.dietaryguidelines.gov/resources/2020–2025-dietary-guidelines-online-materials.
4. Kamil A, Wilson AR, Rehm CD. Estimated sweetness in United States diet among children and adults declined from 2001 to 2018: a serial cross-sectional surveillance study using NHANES 2001–2018. *Front Nutr.* 2021;8:777857. https://doi.org/10.3389/fnut.2021.777857.
5. World Health Organization. Guideline. *Sugars Intake for Adults and Children.* World Health Organization; 2015
6. Centers for Disease Control and Prevention. *Get the Facts: Added Sugars.* 2021. https://www.cdc.gov/nutrition/data-statistics/added-sugars.html.
7. United States Department of Agriculture, Agricultural Research Service. *Food Patterns Equivalents Intakes From Food: Mean Amounts Consumed per Individual, What We Eat in America, NHANES 2017–2018.* 2020. https://www.ars.usda.gov/ARSUserFiles/80400530/pdf/FPED/tables_1–4_FPED_1718.pdf.
8. Woelber JP, Bremer K, Vach K. An oral health optimized diet can reduce gingival and periodontal inflammation in humans—a randomized controlled pilot study. *BMC Oral Health.* 2016;17(1):28.
9. O'Connor JP, Milledge KL, O'Leary F, Cumming R, Eberhard J, Hirani V. Poor dietary intake of nutrients and food groups are associated with increased risk of periodontal disease among community-dwelling older adults: a systematic literature review. *Nutr Rev.* 2020;78(2):175–188.
10. Reynolds AN, Akerman AP, Mann J. Dietary fibre and whole grains in diabetes management: systematic review and *meta*-analyses. *PLoS Med.* 2020;17(3):e1003053.
11. Jenkins DJ, Jones PJ, Frohlich J, et al. The effect of a dietary portfolio compared to a DASH-type diet on blood pressure. *Nutr Metab Cardiovasc Dis.* 2015;25(12):1132–1139.
12. Lee SH, Zhao L, Park S, et al. High added sugars intake among United States adults: characteristics, eating occasions, and top sources, 2015–2018. *Nutrients.* 2023;15(2):265.
13. Quagliani D, Felt-Gunderson P. Closing America's fiber intake gap: communication strategies from a food and fiber summit. *Am J Lifestyle Med.* 2016;11(1):80–85.
14. Thompson HJ. The Dietary Guidelines for Americans (2020–2025): pulses, dietary fiber, and chronic disease risk—a call for clarity and action. *Nutrients.* 2021;13(11):4034. https://doi.org/10.3390/nu13114034. PMID: 34836289; PMCID: PMC8621412.
15. American Diabetes Association Professional Practice Committee. 2. Classification and diagnosis of diabetes: standards of medical care in diabetes-2022. *Diabetes Care.* 2022;45(suppl 1):S17–S38.
16. Rippe JM, Sievenpiper JL, Lê KA, et al. What is the appropriate upper limit for added sugars consumption? *Nutr Rev.* 2017;75(1):18–36.
17. Rippe JM, Angelopoulos TJ. Relationship between added sugars consumption and chronic disease risk factors: current understanding. *Nutrients.* 2016;8(11):697.
18. IBISWorld. *Per Capita Soft Drink Consumption.* 2023. https://www.ibisworld.com/us/bed/per-capita-soft-drink-consumption/1786/.
19. Boushey C, Ard J, Bazzano L, et al. *Dietary patterns and growth, size, body composition, and/or risk of overweight or obesity: a systematic review.* USDA Nutrition Evidence Systematic Review; 2020. PMID: 35129906.

20. Magriplis E, Michas G, Petridi E, et al. Dietary sugar intake and its association with obesity in children and adolescents. *Children (Basel)*. 2021;8(8):676.

21. Maki KC, Palacios OM, Koecher K, et al. The relationship between whole grain intake and body weight: results of *meta*-analyses of observational studies and randomized controlled trials. *Nutrients*. 2019;11(6):1245. https://doi.org/10.3390/nu11061245.

22. Dhurandhar NV, Thomas D. The link between dietary sugar intake and cardiovascular disease mortality: an unresolved question. *JAMA*. 2015;313(9):959–960.

23. Huang Y, Chen Z, Chen B, et al. Dietary sugar consumption and health: umbrella review. *BMJ*. 2023;381:e071609. https://doi.org/10.1136/bmj-2022-071609.

24. Angelopoulos RJ, Lowndes J, Sinnett S, et al. Fructose containing sugars at normal levels of consumption do not effect adversely components of the metabolic syndrome and risk factors for cardiovascular disease. *Nutrients*. 2016;8(4):179.

25. Kelishadi R, Mansourian M, Heidari-Beni M. Association of fructose consumption and components of metabolic syndrome in human studies: a systematic review and *meta*-analysis. *Nutrition*. 2014;30(5):503–510.

26. Tasevska N, Park Y, Jiao L, et al. Sugars and risk of mortality in the NIH-AARP diet and health study. *Am J Clin Nutr*. 2014;99(5):1077–1088.

27. Hayes C. Nonfluoride caries preventive agents show varied effectiveness in preventing dental caries. *J Evid Based Dent Pract*. 2012;12(2):79–80.

28. Rethman MP, Beltrán-Aguilar ED, Billings RJ, et al. American Dental Association council on scientific affairs expert panel on nonfluoride caries-preventive agents. Nonfluoride caries-preventive agents: executive summary of evidence-based clinical recommendations. *J Am Dent Assoc*. 2011;142(9):1065–1071.

29. American Academy of Pediatric Dentistry. *Policy on Use of Xylitol in Pediatric Dentistry. The Reference Manual of Pediatric Dentistry*. American Academy of Pediatric Dentistry; 2022:76–77.

30. Dedhia P, Pai D, Shukla SD, et al. Analysis of erosive nature of fruit beverages fortified with calcium ions: an in vitro study evaluating dental erosion in primary teeth. *ScientificWorldJournal*. 2022;2022:3756384.

31. Saads Carvalho T, Lussi A. Chapter 9: Acidic beverages and foods associated with dental erosion and erosive tooth wear. *Monogr Oral Sci*. 2020;28:91–98.

32. Salas MM, Mascimento GG, Vargas-Ferreira F. Diet influenced tooth erosion prevalence in children and adolescents: results of a meta-analysis and *meta*-regression. *J Dent*. 2015;43(8):865–875.

33. Owens BM, Kitchens M. The erosive potential of soft drinks on enamel surface substrate: an in vitro scanning electron microscopy investigation. *J Contemp Dent Pract*. 2007;8(7):11–20.

34. Shroff P, Gondivkar SM, Kumbhare SP, et al. Analyses of the erosive potential of various soft drinks and packaged fruit juices on teeth. *J Contemp Dent Pract*. 2018;19(12):1546–1551.

35. Valenzuela MJ, Waterhouse B, Aggarwal VR, Bloor K, Doran T. Effect of sugar-sweetened beverages on oral health: a systematic review and *meta*-analysis. *Eur J Public Health*. 2021;31(1):122–129.

36. Riley P, Moore D, Ahmed F, et al. Xylitol-containing products for preventing dental caries in children and adults. *Cochrane Database Syst Rev*. 2015;2015(3):CD010743.

37. Nasseripour M, Newton JT, Warburton F, et al. A systematic review and *meta*-analysis of the role of sugar-free chewing gum on *Streptococcus mutans*. *BMC Oral Health*. 2021;21(1):217.

38. Loimaranta V, Mazurel D, Deng D, Söderling E. Xylitol and erythritol inhibit real-time biofilm formation of *Streptococcus mutans*. *BMC Microbiol*. 2020;20(1).184

39. de Cock P, Mäkinen K, Honkala E, et al. Erythritol is more effective than xylitol and sorbitol in managing oral health endpoints. *Int J Dent*. 2016;2016:9868421.

40. Jain S, Mathur S. Estimating the effectiveness of lollipops containing xylitol and erythritol on salivary pH in 3–6 years olds: a randomized controlled trial. *J Indian Soc Pedod Prev Dent*. 2022;40(1):19–22.

41. Mäkinen KK. Gastrointestinal disturbances associated with the consumption of sugar alcohols with special consideration of xylitol: scientific review and instructions for dentists and other health-care professionals. *Int J Dent*. 2016;2016:5967907.

42. Center for Science in the Public Interest. *Trends in Low Calorie Sweetener Consumption in the United States Fact Sheet*. 2021. https://www.cspinet.org/sites/default/files/2022–02/LCS%20Trends%20Fact%20Sheet%20final%20copyedited.pdf.

43. Higgins KA, Mattes RD. A randomized controlled trial contrasting the effects of 4 low-calorie sweeteners and sucrose on body weight in adults with overweight or obesity. *Am J Clin Nutr*. 2019;109(5):1288–1301.

44. Laviada-Molina H, Molina-Segui F, Pérez-Gaxiola G, et al. Effects of nonnutritive sweeteners on body weight and BMI in diverse clinical contexts: systematic review and *meta*-analysis. *Obes Rev*. 2020;21(7):e13020.

45. American Heart Association. *Non-Nutritive Sweeteners (Artificial Sweeteners)*. 2018. https://www.heart.org/en/healthy-living/healthy-eating/eat-smart/sugar/nonnutritive-sweeteners-artificial-sweeteners.

46. Morze J, Danielewicz A, Hoffmann G, Schwingshackl L. Diet quality as assessed by the healthy eating index, alternate healthy eating index, dietary approaches to stop hypertension score, and health outcomes: a second update of a systematic review and *meta*-analysis of cohort studies. *J Acad Nutr Diet*. 2020;120(12):1998–2031.

47. National Institute of Diabetes and Digestive and Kidney Disease. Lactose Intolerance. 2018. https://www.niddk.nih.gov/health-information/digestive-diseases/lactose-intolerance.

48. Szilagyi A, Ishayek N. Lactose intolerance, dairy avoidance, and treatment options. *Nutrients*. 2018;10(12):1994.

49. Misselwitz B, Butter M, Verbeke K, Fox MR. Update on lactose malabsorption and intolerance: pathogenesis, diagnosis and clinical management. *Gut*. 2019;68(11):2080–2091.

50. Deng Y, Misselwitz B, Dai N, et al. Lactose intolerance in adults: biological mechanism and dietary management. *Nutrients*. 2015;7(9):8020–8035.

▶ Evolve Resources

Please visit http://evolve.elsevier.com/Mallonee/nutritional for additional practice and study support tools.

5

Protein: The Cellular Foundation

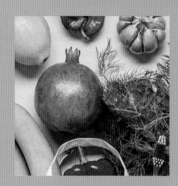

STUDENT LEARNING OUTCOMES

On completion of this chapter, the student will be able to complete the following learning outcomes:

1. Explain the role of amino acids.
2. Categorize amino acids as indispensable or dispensable, and foods as sources of high-quality or lower-quality proteins.
3. Describe the physiologic functions of proteins.
4. Formulate, discuss, and recommended the intake of protein for human health and body function.
5. Describe protein needs for individuals who consume a vegetarian or vegan diet.
6. Organize the following related to underconsumption and overconsumption of protein:

- List the problems associated with protein deficiency or excess.
- Evaluate a patient's protein consumption to determine protein inadequacy, or excess.
- Summarize how protein foods can be used to complement one another.
- Identify how protein-energy malnutrition affects oral health in children.
- Articulate how nutrition principles regarding food intake prevent a patient from consuming excessive or inadequate protein.

KEY TERMS

Bioavailability
Collagen
Complementary foods
Conditionally indispensable amino acids
Dipeptide
Dispensable amino acids (nonessential amino acids)
Erythema
Flexitarians
High-quality protein
Immune response

Immunocompromised
Immunoglobulins
Indispensable amino acids (essential amino acids)
Interstitial
Kwashiorkor
Lactovegetarian
Lacto-ovo vegetarian
Low-quality proteins
Marasmus
Necrosis

Necrotizing ulcerative gingivitis (NUG)
Nitrogen balance
Noma
Ovovegetarian
Periodontium
Protein-energy malnutrition (PEM)
Sarcopenia
Secretory immunog lobulin A (sIgA)
Vegan
Vegetarian

⬥ TEST YOUR NQ

1. **T/F** A protein deficiency during childhood may lead to increased caries susceptibility related to alterations in tooth development and diminished salivary flow.
2. **T/F** Despite poor nutrition, malnourished children have a decreased rate of caries because they do not consume much sugar.
3. **T/F** Gelatin is a good source of high-quality protein.
4. **T/F** Older patients require less protein than younger adults.
5. **T/F** High-protein intake strengthens tooth enamel.
6. **T/F** Excessive protein intake will contribute to the risk of developing diabetes.
7. **T/F** Amino acids are the building blocks of proteins.
8. **T/F** Marasmus is a protein-deficiency disorder.
9. **T/F** Protein requirements are based on the assumption that indispensable amino acids and calories are provided in adequate amounts.
10. **T/F** Positive nitrogen balance occurs during periods of growth.

Until the middle of the 19th century, many scientists thought all life was composed of a single basic chemical: protein. Protein is present in every living cell, making up almost half of the dry weight of a cell. Second to water, protein is the most plentiful substance in the body. Muscle, connective tissue and organs are examples of where proteins are found in the body. Individuals in countries such as the United States and Canada may consume high levels of protein while it is often deficient in diets of those in developing countries. High-protein diets have been increasingly popular for weight reduction and muscle strength for many years, contributing to increased protein consumption. United States total red meat commercial consumption in February 2021 was almost 4,400 million pounds while total poultry was over 3700 million pounds.[1] Considering overall protein intake, males and females consume 16.3% of the total calories in protein.[2]

Amino Acids

Individuals consume meats, eggs, milk and milk products, dried beans and peas, and nuts—all of which provide the essential nutrient, protein. As described in detail in Chapter 2, proteins are very large molecular structures containing the elements such as carbon, hydrogen, oxygen, and nitrogen. Proteins consumed are hydrolyzed by enzymes in the small intestine into individual amino acids for absorption and utilization (Fig. 5.1).

All the billions of proteins associated with life are made from combinations of 20 different amino acids. Amino acids are similar to letters of the alphabet used in different sequences and combinations to make billions of words. An amino acid contains a basic, or amino, grouping ($-NH_2$) and an acidic, or carboxyl, grouping ($-COOH$). Fig. 5.2 shows the general design of an amino acid.

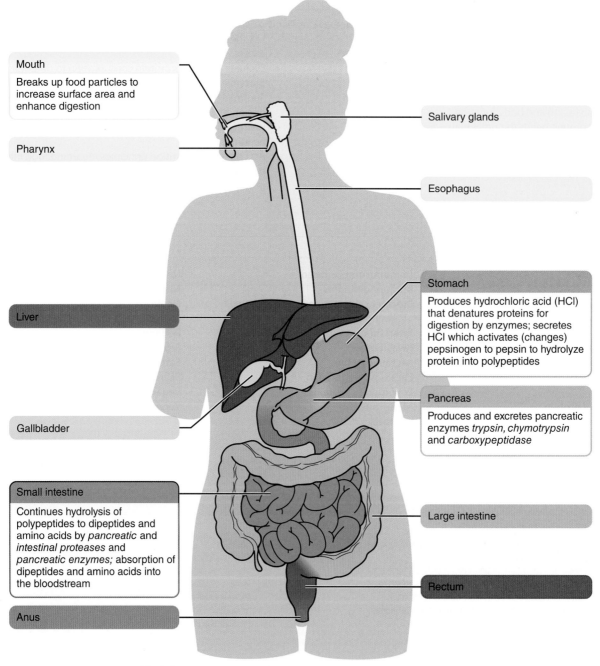

Mouth
Breaks up food particles to increase surface area and enhance digestion

Pharynx

Salivary glands

Esophagus

Liver

Stomach
Produces hydrochloric acid (HCl) that denatures proteins for digestion by enzymes; secretes HCl which activates (changes) pepsinogen to pepsin to hydrolyze protein into polypeptides

Gallbladder

Pancreas
Produces and excretes pancreatic enzymes *trypsin, chymotrypsin* and *carboxypeptidase*

Small intestine
Continues hydrolysis of polypeptides to dipeptides and amino acids by *pancreatic* and *intestinal proteases* and *pancreatic enzymes;* absorption of dipeptides and amino acids into the bloodstream

Large intestine

Rectum

Anus

• **Fig. 5.1** Summary of protein digestion. Note: active enzymes are in *italics*.

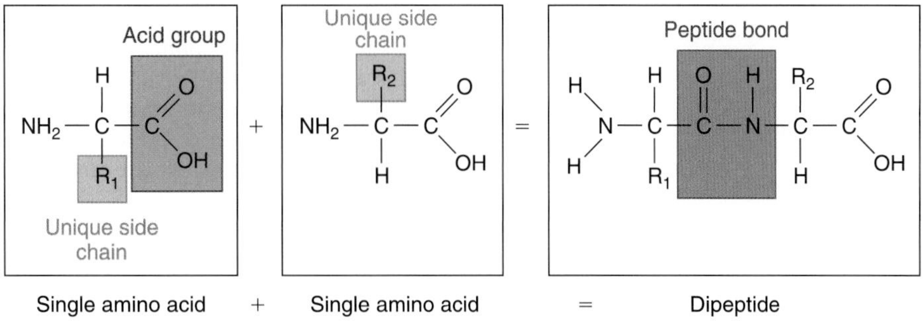

• **Fig. 5.2** Structure of amino acids. (Modified from Raymond JL, Morrow K. *Krause and Mahan's Food and the Nutrition Care Process.* 15th ed. Saunders Elsevier; 2021.)

The distinguishing feature of amino acids is the amine group, which is the body's source of nitrogen. The fundamental constituent of the protein molecule, called the side chain (R group), is the part of the structure that varies to form the many different amino acids.

Amino acids combine with each other to make long chains. As shown in Fig. 5.2, two amino acids together form a dipeptide. Several amino acids bound together form a polypeptide. Food and body proteins contain polypeptides. The number of amino acids in a protein varies greatly (from 100 to 300), but each protein has a specific number. The protein chain adopts a compact, folded, three-dimensional structure (see Chapter 2, Fig. 2.9) which is essential to perform its basic function.

Classification

A prerequisite for life and health are the 20 amino acids, the building blocks of protein. These amino acids, listed in Table 5.1, can be classified as indispensable, dispensable, or conditionally indispensable. These classifications were previously known as essential, nonessential, and conditionally essential, respectfully. Nine indispensable amino acids (essential amino acids) are required in the diet. Dispensable amino acids (nonessential amino acids) are essential for the body, but they can be produced from indispensable amino acids, and therefore are not required in normal conditions. In certain nutritional or disease states, or stages of development, several dispensable amino acids become indispensable; these are classified as conditionally indispensable amino acids.

If any one of the indispensable amino acids is not available when needed for protein synthesis, the protein cannot be produced. The body makes adequate amounts of dispensable amino acids if a sufficient amount of protein is available to furnish the nitrogen needed and enough calories are present to allow the catabolism (breakdown) of amino acids.

The amount of indispensable amino acids furnished by a food determines its ability to support growth, maintenance, and repair. A food with all the indispensable amino acids present is identified as a "complete" protein. When the nine indispensable amino acids are provided from a food in amounts adequate to maintain nitrogen balance and permit growth, the food is said to provide high-quality protein. High-quality protein foods have all the indispensable amino acids present in balanced amounts for human physiologic requirements. Foods providing high-quality proteins include meats (e.g., pork, beef, lamb, veal, goat, rabbit), poultry (chicken, turkey, duck, wild game birds), and all types of seafood.

TABLE 5.1	**Amino Acids in the Human Diet**	
Indispensable (Essential)	Dispensable[a] (Nonessential)	Conditionally Indispensable[b]
Histidine[c]	Alanine	Arginine
Isoleucine	Aspartic acid	Cysteine
Leucine	Asparagine	Glutamine
Lysine	Glutamic acid	Glycine
Methionine	Serine	Proline
Phenylalanine		Tyrosine
Threonine		
Tryptophan		
Valine		

[a]Required in the diet when the body cannot produce enough to meet metabolic needs.
[b]Required in the diet when the body is unable to synthesize adequate amounts for metabolic functions for special pathophysiologic conditions.
[c]Although histidine is considered indispensable, unlike the other eight indispensable amino acids, it does not fulfill the criteria of reducing protein deposition and inducing negative nitrogen balance promptly upon removal from the diet.
Data from Food and Nutrition Board, Institute of Medicine. *Dietary Reference Intakes for Energy, Carbohydrate, Fiber, Fat, Fatty Acids, Cholesterol, Protein, and Amino Acids (Macronutrients).* National Academy Press; 2005.

If the quantity of one or more of the indispensable amino acids in a food is insufficient for optimal protein synthesis, the food is a source of low-quality protein. Low-quality proteins, if the only protein source consumed, support life but not normal growth. These include proteins found in legumes, nuts, and grains. The amino acid in short supply relative to need is referred to as the "limiting amino acid."

Nitrogen balance refers to the balance of reactions in which protein substances are broken down or destroyed and rebuilt (Box 5.1). Healthy individuals excrete (in feces and urine, and from skin) the same amount of nitrogen as is consumed from their food. A patient with a burn or illness excretes more nitrogen than is ingested. In periods of growth, as in a child or pregnant female, the body is in positive nitrogen balance (more protein is retained than is lost daily).

• BOX 5.1   Nitrogen Balance[a]

N balance: body protein constant
N intake = N excretion
Positive N balance: increase in body protein
N intake > N excretion
Negative N balance: decrease in body protein
N intake < N excretion

Positive N Balance	Negative N Balance
Growth	Inadequate protein intake (e.g., fasting, gastrointestinal tract diseases)
Pregnancy or lactation	Inadequate energy intake
Recovery from illnesses, surgery, or trauma	Illnesses (e.g., fevers, infections, or wasting diseases)
Medications	Routine intake of glucocorticoids
Athletic training	Injury or immobilization
	Deficiency of indispensable amino acids
	Accelerated protein loss (e.g., albuminuria, protein-losing gastroenteropathy)
	Burns
	Increased secretion of thyroxine and glucocorticoids

[a]Because nitrogen is a unique component of protein metabolism, measurements of nitrogen and nitrogenous constituents in the blood and urine assess protein equilibrium in the body. Although "nitrogen balance" means that the output is equal to input, the amount of excreted nitrogen atoms is usually not the same as that ingested. For nitrogen equilibrium, not only must the diet contain the required amounts of protein, but the energy intake must also be adequate to prevent protein being used for energy.

DENTAL CONSIDERATIONS

- Inquire about the patient's use of amino acid supplements because toxicity and amino acid imbalances may occur when an excess of one amino acid is ingested. Additionally, supplements may contain toxic contaminants. For example, when large doses of tryptophan are taken, toxic metabolites build up, causing an unusual autoimmune disorder. Refer patients who take protein supplements regularly, to their health care provider or registered dietitian nutritionist (RDN).

NUTRITIONAL DIRECTIONS

- Protein from animals and fish (except for gelatin) are high-quality proteins but are not essential to an adequate diet.

Physiologic Roles

Individual indispensable amino acids act as metabolic signals influencing protein synthesis, inflammation responses and satiety, among other metabolic functions.[3] Leucine (an indispensable amino acid prevalent in animal proteins) has a unique role in stimulating skeletal muscle protein synthesis. In older adults and those experiencing physical inactivity (bed rest, surgery, trauma), efficiency of indispensable amino acids for muscle synthesis is reduced, which may increase the amount of protein needed. Resistance exercise appears to increase the efficiency of indispensable amino acids for muscle anabolism, suppress muscle protein catabolism, and promote positive nitrogen balance.[4]

Proteins are the principal source of nitrogen for the body and are fundamental components of every human cell. Although proteins are an essential part of a diet, performing many important physiologic roles, other nutrients are also essential for the body to fully utilize available protein. Proteins are necessary for many physiologic functions, which can be classified into the following seven categories:

1. *Generation of new body tissues.* Because protein is a constituent of all cells, it is necessary for growth. During periods of increased growth (infancy, childhood, adolescence, and pregnancy) and in periods of wound healing or recovery (illness, surgery, burns, or fever), the need for protein to build new tissues is increased.

2. *Repair of body tissues.* Body proteins are continuously being broken down, necessitating their replacement.

3. *Production of essential compounds.* Amino acids and proteins are constituents of regulatory enzymes, hormones, and other body secretions. The structural compound collagen is a protein substance in connective tissue that helps support body structures, such as skin, bones, teeth, and tendons. Low protein intake may affect these compounds.

4. *Regulation of fluid balance.* Protein dissolved in water forms a colloidal solution; in other words, it attracts water. Blood albumin (a protein) draws water from interstitial (space between tissue cells) fluid or cells to maintain blood volume. During protein deficiency, a decreased amount of protein in the blood causes a loss of osmotic balance, resulting in an accumulation of interstitial fluid (edema).

5. *Resistance to disease.* Antibodies, or immunoglobulins, the body's main protection against disease, are proteins. Low protein levels may negatively affect an individual's immune response, resulting in an inability to fight bacteria and other harmful organisms.

6. *Transport mechanisms.* Proteins enable insoluble fats to be transported through the blood.

7. *Energy.* After the nitrogen grouping is removed, the remaining carbon skeleton can be used for energy, furnishing 4 cal/g. Although this is not one of its main functions, protein is used in this manner when calorie intake from carbohydrate and fat is inadequate and indispensable amino acids are not available for synthesis of proteins.

Requirements

Protein requirements for health are based on body size and rate of growth. The body requires more protein during growth periods as well as for maintenance and repair of a larger body mass. To a certain extent, the better the quality of protein (amount of indispensable amino acids), the lesser the quantity required. Protein requirements are based on the assumption that indispensable amino acids and calories are provided in adequate amounts.

The recommended dietary allowances (RDAs) for protein vary proportionately for different ages and stages of life to adjust for growth rates (Table 5.2). The National Academy of Medicine determined that the daily minimum requirement of protein for adults is approximately 0.6 g/kg. Using 0.6 g/kg, a person weighing 150 lb (68.2 kg) would require 41 g of protein. Because RDAs provide a margin of safety, the National Academy of Medicine established 0.8 g/kg (0.36 g/lb) daily as the RDA. With this standard, a patient weighing 150 lb (68.2 kg) requires 56 g of protein. Ideally, protein needs are based on body weight, not energy intake. In comparison, the World Health Organization recommends 0.75 g of protein per

TABLE 5.2 Protein Recommendations

Life Stage/ Gender	Age (years)	RECOMMENDED DIETARY ALLOWANCES		
		Protein (g/kg)	Protein (g/d)	% Calories
Infants	0–6 months	1.52	9.1[a]	5–10
	7–12 months	1.2	11	5–10
Children	1–3	1.05	13	5–10
	4–8	0.95	19	10–30
Males	9–13	0.95	34	10–30
	14–18	0.85	52	10–30
	19–70	0.80	56	10–35
Females	9–13	0.95	34	10–30
	14–18	0.85	46	10–30
	19–70	0.80	46	10–35
Pregnant	All ages	1.1	71 (+25 g/day)	10–35
Lactating	All ages	1.3	71 (+25 g/day)	10–35

[a]Adequate Intake, based on 0.8 g protein/kg body weight for reference body weight. For healthy, breastfed infants, the adequate intake is the mean intake.
Data from Institute of Medicine of the National Academies. *Dietary Reference Intakes for Energy, Carbohydrates, Fiber, Fat, Protein, and Amino Acids.* National Academy Press; 2002.

BOX 5.2 Customizing Protein Intake Using the *Dietary Guidelines*

- Choose a healthy eating pattern that includes a variety of protein foods in nutrient-dense forms: seafood, lean meat, poultry, eggs, soy products, nuts and seeds, legumes (beans and peas).
- Use the recommended amounts of foods from the *Healthy Dietary Pattern* (see Table 1.1) for the appropriate calorie level to maintain a desirable weight.
- Choose the designated amount of nutrient-dense lean or low-fat meats, poultry, and fish:
  - Opt for lean meats, such as white meat of chicken or loin and round cuts of beef and pork that are trimmed, flank or strip steak, and ground beef that is 90% lean or leaner.
  - Remove visible fat from meats.
  - Remove skin from chicken.
- Limit the amounts of processed meats and poultry because of the added sodium and sugars.
- Prepare without additional fats (i.e., frying).
- Use sauces and gravies with additional fat, salt, or sugar sparingly.
- Choose unsalted nuts, seeds, and soy alternatives at least two times a week, as indicated for the appropriate calorie level.
- Choose small portions of nuts and seeds because they are high in calories.
- Choose seafood (not fried) at least twice a week in the amount indicated for the appropriate calorie level.
- Eat more beans, peas and lentils which are a natural source of fiber and protein (If counted as a protein food, do not count as a vegetable).
- Choose beans, peas, lentils or soy alternatives for the protein food at least once a week, or substitute beans for at least half of the beef, chicken, or pork in chili, burritos, pasta, or stir-fry dishes.
- Choose nonfat or low-fat dairy product in the amounts indicated for the appropriate calorie level.

kilogram of lean body weight, which translates to 45 g of protein daily for an average female and 56 g for an average male.

When any condition causes a significant protein loss, an increased protein intake (greater than the RDA) prevents excessive loss of tissue and plasma proteins. Although these conditions increase protein requirements, RDAs have not been established for them. Providing additional amounts through provision of high-quality proteins can help prevent protein malnutrition and shorten recovery periods.

Some individuals consume protein amounts close to the highest acceptable macronutrient distribution range of 35% for their age-sex group. The acceptable macronutrient distribution range (AMDR) allows a lot of flexibility in protein intake, between 10% and 35% of total calorie intake. The flexibility within the AMDR is beneficial since some literature suggests that current dietary reference intakes (DRIs) may not be sufficient to promote optimal muscle health in all populations (see the "Underconsumption and Health-Related Problems" section). Moderate evidence indicates that diets containing more than 35% of total calories from protein are generally no more effective at building muscle mass than 25% to 35%.

The *Dietary Guidelines* indicate that about 2/3 of the United States population is meeting or exceeding the protein foods recommendation.[5] The *Dietary Guidelines* encourage a healthy dietary eating pattern that includes a variety of protein-rich foods to maintain a healthy body weight. Nutrient-dense foods, within calorie limits, should be a primary focus. The foods are to be tailored to meet the preferences, culture, and budget of the individual. The message includes limiting protein foods with high amounts of fats, especially saturated fats (Box 5.2). In addition,

the *Dietary Guidelines* encourage meeting nutritional needs primarily from foods, not from protein or amino acid supplements. The *Dietary Pattern* includes oz-eq weekly recommendations for three subgroups: seafood; meats, poultry, and eggs; and nuts, seeds, soy products, beans, peas, and lentils.

Ordinarily, dietary protein is restricted only in some physiologic disease states affecting the liver and kidney because these organs are heavily involved in protein metabolism and excretion of protein waste products. If the liver and kidney are diseased, excessive amounts of protein cannot be properly handled without further organ damage.

An increasing number of Americans are becoming vegetarians (see *Health Application 5*). **Vegetarians** intentionally do not eat meat or variations of animal protein (beef, pork, poultry, seafood, other animal flesh, and sometimes by-products of animals). The *Dietary Guidelines* endorse a vegetarian diet as a healthy eating pattern. For some vegetarians, intake of protein is at the lower level than nonvegetarians at 3 ½ oz-eq/day (2000 cal/day intake).

Sources

Foods with a high-protein content are readily available in the United States. Table 5.3 lists the average protein content of some foods. Meat and milk food groups furnish most of the protein. (Although milk products are excellent sources of protein, they are not included in the protein group because of their nutrient profile—providing less iron, niacin, vitamins E or B_6 than other protein-rich foods). A variety of high-protein foods should be included, as each food has

TABLE 5.3	Protein Content of Select Foods		
Food		**Quantity**	**Protein (g)**
Chicken, light meat, cooked		1 oz	9
Edamame, cooked		½ cup	9
Milk, whole, reduced fat, or low fat		1 cup	8–9
Pork chop, lean, cooked		1 oz	8
Beef, lean cuts, cooked		1 oz	8
Beans, pinto, cooked		½ cup	8
Sunflower seeds		⅓ ¼ cup	7
Cheese, colby		1 oz	7
Egg, hard boiled		1 large	6
American processed cheese		1 oz	7
Peanut butter		2 tbsp	7
Chickpeas, canned		¼ cup	7
Milk, soy, nonfat		1 cup	6
Cottage cheese		¼ cup	6
Fish, cod, cooked		1 oz	6
Spaghetti, whole grain		1 serving	6
Oatmeal, cooked		1 cup	6
Rice, brown, cooked		1 cup	5
Walnuts		¼ cup	5
Bread, multigrain		1 slice	3
Corn, canned		½ cup	2
Milk, almond		½ cup	1
Fruits		½ cup	0.1–1

Data from Department of Agriculture (USDA), Agricultural Research Service, FoodData Central, 2020. *USDA National Nutrient Database for Standard Reference, Version 2.* http://fdc.nal.usda.gov.

Depending on sex, size, and activity level, *MyPlate* website and the *Dietary Guidelines Healthy Eating Pattern* recommend 5½ oz-eq/day (2000 calorie) of cooked lean meat, poultry, or fish daily for adults. Protein foods cover only ¼ of the plate (see Fig. 1.6A). The *Healthy Pattern* has designated the amount considered one serving (Table 5.4). About 3 tbsp of chopped/ground meat, or the size of a small matchbox, equals 1 oz of meat; a small chicken drumstick or thigh is equivalent to 2 oz of meat; and a deck of cards or the size of your palm is approximately a 3-oz; ½ cup of beans, or the amount that can fit in a cupped hand, or 1 tbsp of peanut butter (size of a ping-pong ball) can be substituted for 1 oz of meat. Not to be overlooked,

🦷 DENTAL CONSIDERATIONS

- Consuming approximately 1.0 to 1.6 g/kg (0.45–0.73 g/lb) of protein per day is above the RDA, but within the AMDR for protein. Routine consumption of 1.5 g/kg (0.68 g/lb) or more for protein is considered a high-protein diet.
- When calorie-dense protein sources (such as fried or high-fat meats) are chosen, meeting the RDAs for other nutrients is difficult.
- An inadequate protein intake could affect the physiologic functions of protein. If dietary intake seems inadequate, evaluate the patient's status in the areas described in the Physiologic Roles section and refer the patient to an RDN or health care provider.
- Assessing protein intake of patients with periodontal issues is especially important. Protein deficiencies may compromise the physiologic systemic response to inflammation and infection. Periodontal problems may increase the protein requirement to promote healing in patients with inadequate or marginal protein intake.
- Collagen is a protein substance in connective tissue that helps support body structures, such as skin, bones, teeth, and tendons.
- The DRIs indicate that protein should provide 10% to 35% of calorie intake. If protein intake seems inappropriate, determine calorie or protein intake or both. The adequacy of intake can be established by using one of the two methods. As an example of the first method, assuming consumption of 2200 cal/day, the amount of protein based on total energy intake is calculated as follows:
  2200 cal × 0.35 (maximum recommended % of total cal from protein) = 770 cal from proteins or less
  770 cal ÷ 4 (cal/g protein) = 193 g or less of protein
  An intake of 193 g protein is the highest level recommended. Because 35% is the upper limit, protein consumption above this level may jeopardize adequate intakes of nutrients.
- The second method of calculating percentage of protein intake based on actual protein intake: Protein intake of 55 g with cal intake of 2200 cal:
  55 (g protein) × 4 (cal/g protein) = 220 cal from protein
  220 (cal from proteins) ÷ 2200 (total cal intake) × 100(%) = 10% of total cal from protein
  Because 10% is the lower limit, the patient's protein may be inadequate, and professional counseling may be warranted. Refer the patient to an RDN.
- Most Americans meet or exceed consumption of meat, poultry, and eggs. It is important to expand choices, such as fish and plant-based protein.
- Animal food sources of protein are generally the most expensive. For patients with a limited income (e.g., elderly, homeless, and impoverished individuals), emphasize plant sources of protein to insure adequate intake. Complementary sources of protein (described in *Health Application 5*), which are less expensive, can provide adequate protein.
- Evaluate food intake by comparing data from the patient with the recommended servings from the *MyPlate* website for the stage of growth, and DRIs for calorie and protein requirements.

distinct nutritional contributions in addition to protein (Table 1.6). While Americans are consuming adequate or exceeding amounts of protein, they are not meeting recommendations for the subgroups within the protein foods group. As shown in Fig. 5.3, seafood is one of the least consumed protein foods. Compared to some other protein sources, seafood is nutrient dense, relatively low in calories and saturated fat, and high in beneficial fatty acids. The American Heart Association and *Dietary Guidelines* recommend that adults eat two fish meals a week, but the average intake is one 4-oz serving weekly. A seafood-rich diet is beneficial in lowering the risk of cardiovascular disease (CVD) and may help with weight control. Beans and peas are also considered a part of the protein foods group (but one serving can be counted only once—either in the protein or the vegetable group). Soy is a good source of protein and has other health benefits. Consumption of cereal products also boosts protein intake. The protein content of items from the sample menu presented in Fig. 1.4 is shown in Fig. 5.4.

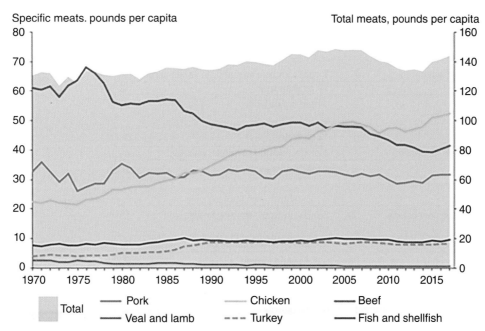

• **Fig. 5.3** United States Consumption Trends of Animal Protein. In 2017, 51% of the United States population consumed 51% red meat (beef, pork, veal and lamb), 42% poultry (chicken and turkey), and 7% fish and shellfish. Chicken and turkey had the largest gains over the past five decades. USDA, Economic Research Service using loss-adjusted food availability data form its Food Availability (Per Capita) Data System. https://www.ers.usda.gov/data-products/chart-gallery/gallery/chart-detail/?chartId=95869

NUTRITIONAL DIRECTIONS

- Regarding protein intake, according to the *Dietary Guidelines*, for those beyond the age of 2 years:
  - Limit saturated fat intake to less than 10% of the total calorie intake (i.e., a 2000 calorie intake would equate to 200 calories/day or less from saturated fat).
  - Only allow up to 5% additional total calories/day from saturated fat in protein foods (i.e., a 2000 calorie intake would equate to 100 calories/day or less from saturated fat).
  - Beans, peas, and lentils have a composition similar to that of vegetables. These can be categorized as either proteins or vegetables.
  - Fish contain varying amounts of mercury, which is a concern for pregnant and lactating females, and children. Fish with lower amounts of mercury include: salmon, anchovies, sardines, black sea bass,

  trout. tilapia, haddock, flounder, catfish, perch, light tuna, shrimp, crab, clams, scallops, oysters, and lobster.[5]
- Protein supplements are unnecessary for healthy adults participating in endurance or resistance exercise.[6] The amount of protein needed by an athlete should be determined by a Board Certified Specialist in Sports Dietetics or an RDN specializing in sports nutrition.
- Protein requirements should be met by foods from several sources (including different animal protein foods) because of other nutrients that accompany the protein. For example, pork is an excellent source of thiamin, while red meats furnish a significant amount of iron. In contrast, too many egg yolks in the diet contribute cholesterol.
- For patients with an adequate protein intake, amino acid supplements are not beneficial and could be harmful.

dairy is not optional, even though it is located above the plate where a glass is normally placed. Depending on calorie intake, the *Dietary Guidelines* recommend 1⅔ cup eq/day for toddlers to 3 cups eq/day of fat-free or low-fat milk and dairy products daily. Three cups of milk provide 24 g of protein as well as other essential nutrients.

In most cases, digestibility and nutritional value are favorably affected by cooking procedures. Proper cooking sometimes facilitates digestion and use. Cooking makes egg albumin more readily digestible, and cooking soybeans increases amino acid bioavailability. **Bioavailability** indicates the amount of nutrient available to the body after absorption. Processing affects proteins in cereal by binding lysine (an amino acid), making it unusable by the body.

Underconsumption and Health-Related Problems

Although protein foods in the United States are plentiful and protein deficiency is uncommon, several groups of individuals are susceptible to insufficient intakes: (1) older adults, (2) those with low incomes, (3) strict vegetarians or vegans, (4) people lacking education, (5) those unwilling to shop wisely, and (6) the chronically ill or hospitalized (e.g., patients with acquired immune deficiency syndrome, anorexia nervosa, or cancer).

Fewer than 10% of Americans over 70 years of age get less than the recommended 0.8 g/kg body weight per day. Lower consumption of protein by older Americans may be related to

Sample Menu	Protein (g)	lacto-ovo vegetarian Menu	Protein (g)
Breakfast			
1 ½ cup Frosted Mini-Wheat cereal	7	1 cup Complete wheat bran flakes cereal	4
12 oz skim milk	12	12 oz skim milk	12
12 oz black coffee	0	1 hard boiled egg	6
Mid-Morning Snack			
12 oz water	0	12 oz water	0
1 oz dry roasted almonds, unsalted	6	1 oz dry roasted almonds, unsalted	6
1 medium orange	1	1 medium orange	1
Lunch			
Sandwich with			
1 cup tuna salad with egg, low-calorie mayonnaise	28 0	Sandwich wrap with vegetables and rice	13
¼ cup thin-sliced cucumber		¼ cup thin-sliced cucumber	0
3 thin slices tomato	0	3 thin slices tomato	0
2 medium lettuce leaves	0	2 medium lettuce leaves	0
2 thin slices 100% wheat bread	6		
8 baby carrots	1	8 baby carrots	1
1 medium applesauce cookie	1	1 medium applesauce cookie	1
1 cup grapes	1	1 cup grapes	1
12 oz water	0	12 oz water	0
Mid-Afternoon Snack			
8 oz low-fat vanilla yogurt	11	8 oz low-fat vanilla yogurt	11
12 oz herbal tea with nonnutritive sweetener	0	12 oz herbal tea with nonnutritive sweetener	0
Dinner			
3 oz pot roast beef with	26	1 cup vegetarian baked beans	12
¼ cup sauteed mushrooms	1	½ cup sauteed mushrooms	1
1 cup white and wild rice blend cooked with cooked margarine and	4	1 cup white and wild rice blend with margarine	4
½ cup vegetable juice	1	½ cup vegetable juice	1
2 c tossed salad with lettuce, avocado, tomatoes, and carrots	2	2 cup tossed salad with lettuce, avocado, tomatoes, and carrots	2
¼ cup shredded low-fat Muenster cheese	7	¼ cup shredded low-fat Muenster cheese	7
2 tbsp vinaigrette salad dressing	0	2 tbsp vinaigrette salad dressing	0
⅛ medium cantaloupe	1	⅛ medium cantaloupe	1
12 oz iced tea with low-calorie sweetener	0	12 oz iced tea with low-calorie sweetener	0
Evening Snack			
3 cup low-fat microwave popcorn	3	3 cup low-fat microwave popcorn	3
12 oz water	0	12 oz water	0
TOTALS[a]	119		87

[a]Totals may vary due to rounding.

From Cronometer Comprehensive Nutrition Tracking. 2019.

https://cronometer.com

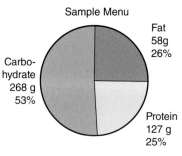

Sample Menu

Fat 58g 26%

Carbohydrate 268 g 53%

Protein 127 g 25%

Kilocalories: 2012

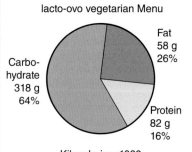

lacto-ovo vegetarian Menu

Fat 58 g 26%

Carbohydrate 318 g 64%

Protein 82 g 16%

Kilocalories: 1989

• **Fig. 5.4** Protein content of sample menu and modifications for lacto-ovo vegetarian diet. https://www.supertracker.usda.gov/default.aspx

cost, inability to prepare nutritious meals, depression, difficulty chewing, or concerns about the fat and cholesterol content of meats. A medical condition found in older adults related to inadequate amounts of dietary protein and malnutrition is sarcopenia. **Sarcopenia** is the progressive loss of muscle mass and strength with aging, increasing the risk of physical disability or poor quality of life. A moderate increase in dietary protein intake (above the RDA of 0.8 g/kg) may be beneficial to

TABLE 5.4	Portions for 1 Serving of Protein Foods
Protein Food	**Serving Size**
Seafood	1 oz
Meats	1 oz
Poultry	1 oz
Eggs	1
Nuts	½ oz
Seeds	½ oz
Soy alternatives	¼ cup
Beans, peas, lentils	¼ cup
Peanut butter	1 tbsp

maintain muscle mass and bone density in the geriatric population, while still falling within the safe and acceptable range for protein consumption.[7] According to the National Osteoporosis Foundation, dietary protein plays a valuable role in bone health. In addition, a systematic review and *meta*-analysis indicated positive trends on bone mineral density with higher protein intake in older adults.[8] When suspecting poor protein intake or malnutrition in a patient, refer to a health care provider or RDN for a nutritional assessment.

Certain physiologic conditions and impaired digestion or absorption cause excessive protein losses, especially with individuals undergoing kidney dialysis, and may precipitate protein-energy malnutrition (PEM). Although PEM is uncommon in the United States, malnutrition in these conditions is frequently unrecognized and is usually accompanied by other nutritional deficiencies. Separating effects of different nutrient deficiencies by observing clinical symptoms is often difficult. PEM affects the whole body, including every component of the orofacial complex.

The occurrence of PEM during critical developmental stages, including prenatal and postnatal periods, may affect developing tissues or lead to irreversible changes in oral tissues. During tooth development, mild-to-moderate protein deficiency results in smaller molars, significantly delayed eruption, and retardation during development of the mandible. Smaller salivary glands result in diminished salivary flow; this saliva is different in its protein composition, amylase, and aminopeptidase activity, compromising the immune function of saliva.

Poor nutrition results in poor development of the epithelium, connective tissue, and bone, along with delayed eruption and exfoliation of deciduous teeth. Although malnourished children have an increased rate of caries, the peak caries experience is delayed by approximately 2 years. The increase in caries rate may simply be related to the length of time a tooth is in the oral cavity; if the delay in exfoliation is greater than the delay in eruption, the tooth is in the mouth for longer and thus is exposed to caries-producing bacteria for longer. Children with malnutrition (e.g., in developing countries and in many urban and rural areas in developed countries) have different dietary habits that are not necessarily conducive to dental caries. However, teeth in these populations are highly susceptible to dental caries that

may be related to alterations in structure of tooth crowns and diminished salivary flow, or changes in saliva composition may be related to malnutrition issues.

The periodontium includes hard and soft tissues surrounding and supporting the teeth: gingiva, alveolar mucosa, cementum, periodontal ligaments, and alveolar bone. An insufficient intake of protein creates negative nitrogen balance, decreasing nitrogen reserves and blood protein levels, and resistance of the periodontium to infections. In addition, the ability of the periodontium to withstand the stress of injury or surgery is reduced and recovery periods are longer. In malnourished children, secretory immunoglobulin A (sIgA) levels are depressed. sIgA is the predominant immunoglobulin, or antibody, in oral, nasal, intestinal, and other mucosal secretions, providing the first line of defense in the oral cavity. Low sIgA levels in malnourished children probably play a role in their increased susceptibility to mucosal infections.

PEM may be a major reason for increased incidence of noma and necrotizing ulcerative gingivitis (NUG), conditions strongly associated with depressed immune responses caused by nutritional deficiencies, stress, and infection (see Chapter 19). Noma is a progressive necrosis (degeneration and cellular death) that usually manifests as a small ulcer on the gingiva that spreads to produce extensive destruction of lips, cheeks, and tissues covering the jaw with an accompanying foul odor. NUG is characterized by erythema (marginal redness of mucous membranes caused by inflammation) and necrosis of the interdental papilla. This painful gingivitis is generally accompanied by a metallic taste and foul oral odor. Cratered papilla often remain after treatment of the disease.

NUG occasionally occurs among college students who are under a great deal of psychological stress and have poor eating habits. It can also be observed in individuals who live in developed countries and are severely debilitated or immunocompromised (having an immune response weakened by a disease or pharmacologic agent) or in children 2 to 6 years old who live in developing countries, are malnourished, and have recently experienced a stressful event, such as viral disease.

NUG can be precipitated by emotionally stressful situations that affect eating patterns, leading to acute deficiencies and depressed immune response to bacteria normally found in the oral cavity. Decreased host resistance to infection may permit gingival lesions to spread rapidly into adjacent tissues, producing extensive necrosis and destruction of orofacial tissues, whereas in a healthy individual, the lesion is limited to the gingiva alone. Wound healing is also delayed (see Chapter 19 for further discussion).

In other areas of the world, where quantities of high-quality protein and calories are insufficient, PEM is commonly seen. Kwashiorkor develops when young children consume adequate calories and inadequate high-quality protein (Fig. 5.5). It is almost exclusively seen in association with famine in the tropics. It usually appears after the child has been weaned from breast milk. Marasmus occurs in infants when both protein and calories are deficient in the diet.

Kwashiorkor and marasmus are very serious health problems that have received much attention by the United Nations and the World Health Organization. Incaparina (a high-protein food made from maize, cottonseed and sorghum flours fortified with minerals and vitamins), skim milk powder, and the addition of lysine to cereal products have been used to improve nutritional status in developing countries.

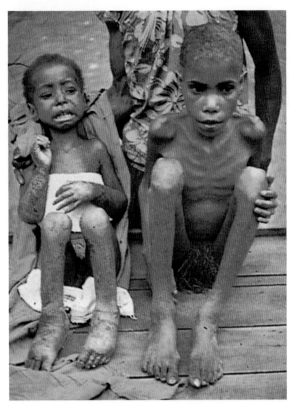

• **Fig. 5.5** Kwashiorkor and marasmus in brothers. The younger brother, on the left, has kwashiorkor with generalized edema, skin changes, pale reddish yellow hair, and an unhappy expression. The older child, on the right, has marasmus, with generalized wasting, spindly arms and legs, and an apathetic expression. From Peters W, Pasvol G, eds. *Tropical Medicine and Parasitology*, 5th ed. London: Mosby; 2002, Fig. 986.

🦷 DENTAL CONSIDERATIONS

- The protein requirement of older adults is the same as that of young adults; however, older adults are frequently less motivated or able to choose a healthy eating pattern due to physical, social, and financial reasons. Decreased protein intake is common as a result of ill-fitting dentures or edentulousness. Closely assess the protein intake of older patients.
- It would be prudent to recommend a significant proportion of protein from vegetable sources.
- Due to protein's ability to increase satiety, individuals trying to lose weight may benefit by distributing their protein intake throughout the day and include protein at breakfast. When assessing for marasmus or kwashiorkor, remember that the main difference between the two conditions is the presence of some subcutaneous fat tissue in individuals with kwashiorkor and edema, especially in the abdomen, feet, and legs. Fat stores and edema are absent in marasmus. Assess the patient's financial status because poverty is a major cause of PEM and has been identified in rural and urban inner-city areas in the United States. To assess for inadequate protein intake, look for frequent or extended periods of fasting, medications that cause anorexia, abnormal food intake, nausea and vomiting, and problems with hair (dull, dry, brittle, fragile), skin (flaky and dry), or fingernails (dry and cracked, spoon-shaped).
- Treatment of malnutrition requires referral to a health care provider or an RDN.
- Malnourished patients take longer to heal following a dental procedure and are at risk for frequent infections. Adequate infection control procedures are particularly important for these patients.
- In the United States, noma-like lesions may occur in patients with cancer whose immune systems have been severely impaired by chemotherapy or advanced acquired immune deficiency syndrome.

🦷 NUTRITIONAL DIRECTIONS

- Suggest Meals on Wheels or community senior centers for older patients with an inadequate diet and refer them to a social worker. Other ideas can be found in Chapter 16.
- Supplement dietary protein by adding skim milk powder to milk, soups, or mashed potatoes (if the patient is not lactose intolerant) and by adding cheese to foods.

Overconsumption and Health-Related Problems

An upper limit for safe levels of protein intake has not been determined, however, the Food and Nutrition Board suggests protein intake to not surpass 35% of the total calorie intake.[9] Americans frequently eat 150% to 200% of the RDA for protein. There are no additional health benefits when protein is above 35%. High-protein intakes may increase health and disease risks.

When protein intake is excessive, kidney function may be compromised. Although high-protein intake is not associated with diminished kidney function in individuals with healthy kidneys, high-protein diets may be harmful to the kidneys in individuals with preexisting metabolic renal dysfunction by overburdening the capability to excrete nitrogen waste.[10,11] When renal function is impaired but the individual is not on dialysis, the American Diabetes Association recommends limiting protein intake to 0.8 g/kg (kilogram) of body weight.[12]

In addition, fluid imbalances may increase the risk of dehydration in all age groups, but especially in infants. Metabolism of 100 cal of protein requires 350 g of water compared with 50 g of water for a similar amount of carbohydrates or fats. Water requirements are increased as well as end products of protein metabolism in the bloodstream.

Obtaining adequate protein, or within the upper range of recommended amounts, is an important dietary concern. However, if the principal source of protein is red meat and regular or high-fat dairy products, intake of saturated fat and cholesterol content is high, which raises the risk of CVD, including stroke. If carbohydrates are severely restricted by choosing primarily protein foods, high-fiber foods are limited. High-fiber plant foods help lower blood lipids. In addition, there can be a reduction of vital vitamins, minerals and phytochemicals. Restriction of plant-based carbohydrate foods limits nutrients that offer protection against cancer and other diseases and cause problems, such as constipation and diverticulosis.

🦷 DENTAL CONSIDERATIONS

- Protein intake should be fairly equally distributed throughout the day.
- Good choices of high-protein, low-fat foods include fish, skinless chicken, low-fat dairy products, and lean beef and pork.

🦷 NUTRITIONAL DIRECTIONS

- Extremely high-protein intake is especially undesirable in infants.
- Because proteins must be metabolized by the liver and filtered by the kidneys, high protein diets (above 35% of calorie intake) may result in additional work by, or stress on, these organs.

◆ HEALTH APPLICATION 5

Vegetarianism

Although there is an ample supply of protein in the United States, some people choose plant sources of protein for health reasons or because of philosophical, ecological, religious convictions or cultural and social values. Large numbers of vegetarian cookbooks and meatless "veggie" burgers and sausage-style products would lead one to believe that vegetarianism is a growing consumer movement. The Vegetarian Resource Group indicates that approximately 6% of the population are vegetarians, including vegans.[13]

Technically, variations of vegetarian diets differ in the types of foods included, as shown in Box 5.3 When milk and cheese products are included, they complement plant foods and enhance the amino acid content of the diet. If adequate quantities of eggs, milk, and milk products are consumed, all nutrients are more likely to be provided in sufficient quantities. Strict supervision is unnecessary for all types of vegetarians with the exception of vegans. The vegan diet does not include any food of animal origin (e.g., meat, milk, cheese, eggs, and butter) or any product coming from an animal (e.g., wool, silk and leather).

A *Healthy Vegetarian Dietary Pattern* was developed to provide recommendations that meet the *Dietary Guidelines* for individuals who choose to omit meat. The pattern can be adapted by vegans by substituting vitamin B_{12} fortified foods and beverages, such as soy alternatives or meat analog. The *Vegetarian Pattern* is the same as the *Healthy Pattern* except for protein foods (Table 5.5). Nutritionally, this pattern is similar to the *Healthy Pattern*, providing a little more calcium and fiber, and lower vitamin D.[5]

Textured vegetable products, or meat substitutes, are produced from vegetable proteins, usually soybeans. Protein in textured vegetable protein products is of good quality, but these products may have high sodium content. The protein in the *Dietary Guidelines Vegetarian Pattern* is provided by eggs, dairy, peas, beans, lentils, soy products, and nuts and seeds. The number of servings per week are designed to provide optimum nutrition using nutrient-dense choices.

Indispensable amino acids can be provided by plants, but larger amounts of these plant products must be consumed to match protein obtained from animal sources. Indispensable amino acids present in low levels in grains are abundant in other plants, such as beans, peas, and lentils. Beans are low in methionine and tryptophan, and corn is low in lysine and threonine. When eaten together, as in pinto beans and cornbread, they are said to be complementary foods, required in less volume.

Protein from a single source is seldom consumed alone. Foods are usually combined without awareness that they are complementary to each other (e.g., beans are usually combined with rice, bread, or crackers [wheat], or tortillas or cornbread [corn]). When a combination of plant proteins is eaten throughout the day, the amino acids provided by each complement each other; that is, the deficiencies of one are offset by the adequacies of another. Additionally, small amounts of high-quality proteins can be combined with plant foods, as in macaroni and cheese or cereal and milk, to provide adequate amounts of indispensable amino acids. If calorie intake is adequate, protein requirements are met when a variety of protein-containing foods are eaten throughout the day. Foods providing complementary amino acids do not have to be consumed simultaneously.

With some basic nutrition knowledge, patients following a vegetarian pattern are frequently healthier than those who choose to eat meat. Foods can be nutritionally balanced without meats, by providing protein from different sources. *My Vegan Plate* (Fig. 5.6) is designed specifically to address nutrient inadequacies and reduced mineral bioavailability of vegetarian and vegan diets. Table 5.5 indicates the number of servings from the food groups to meet nutrient recommendations for various calorie levels. By using a variety of unrefined and fortified foods, and enough calories to promote good health, protein quantity and other nutrients can be adequate for most individuals.

Vegetarian diets generally result in lower dietary intake of saturated fat and cholesterol, and high levels of dietary fiber, magnesium, potassium, vitamins C and E, and folate. Key nutrients that may fall short of the DRIs in the vegan diet and less often in the vegetarian diet include zinc, calcium, iron, iodine, vitamins D and B_{12}, and long-chain n-3 fatty acids.[14]

Persons following a vegan diet generally have adequate macronutrient intake (carbohydrate, protein and fat). However, vegans must pay closer attention to food choices containing riboflavin, niacin, vitamins B_1, B_2, B_{12} and D, and calcium, zinc and iodine.[15] Supplementation may be necessary. In addition, vegans may need to be concerned with higher sodium intakes.[15] Vitamin B_{12} deficiency rates are especially high for pregnant females, adolescents, older adults, and those who have adhered to a vegetarian diet since birth. Commonly available fortified foods (e.g., fortified breakfast cereals and nondairy soymilks) are emphasized to ensure good sources of vitamins B_{12} and D and calcium. Because of difficulties consuming adequate volumes of food to meet nutritional needs, the vegan diet is not recommended for infants, children, or pregnant/lactating females. During periods of rapid growth, vegans should be referred to an RDN.

Much can be said of the healthy aspects of vegetarian diets. Vegetarian diets can meet the DRIs as long as variety and amounts of foods are adequate. Vegetarian diets and lifestyles seem to be conducive to good health as exemplified by vegetarians exhibiting a lower prevalence of numerous health problems, including heart disease, type 2 diabetes, hypertension, certain types of cancer, and obesity.[14,15] It makes sense that a vegetarian diet rich in healthier plant foods is associated with substantially lower CVD risk as opposed to a vegetarian diet that includes principally less healthy plant foods.[16] Health advantages are not attributed solely to avoidance of meat products but rather benefits from phytochemical-rich plant foods. For instance, beans, peas and lentils, and whole-grain products help with blood glucose control; plant foods are associated with a lower risk of CVD.

When working with vegetarian or vegan patients, keep lines of communication open by respecting their decision, unless eating habits are potentially harmful. Patients who have an interest in pursuing a vegetarian diet should be encouraged to do so. All patients should be encouraged to have more meatless meals and to consume more plant proteins.

• BOX 5.3   Terminology for Different Types of Vegetarian Diets

Flexitarian	Do not regularly eat meat, but occasionally eat fish and poultry
Vegetarian	Plant proteins, but may or may not include egg or dairy products
Lactovegetarian	Plant proteins plus dairy products
Lacto-ovo vegetarian	Plant proteins plus milk, cheese, and eggs
Ovovegetarian	Plant proteins plus eggs
Pescatarian	Plant proteins plus fish
Vegan	Plant proteins only and abstain from using products from animals

Nutrition Tips:

*Choose mostly whole grains.
*Eat a variety of foods from each of the food groups.
*Adults age 70 and younger need 600 IU of vitamin D daily.
  Sources include fortified foods (such as some soymilks) or a vitamin D supplement.
*Sources of iodine include iodized salt (3/8 teaspoon daily) or
  an iodine supplement (150 micrograms).
*See www.vrg.org for recipes and more details.

Vegan
MY ∧ PLATE

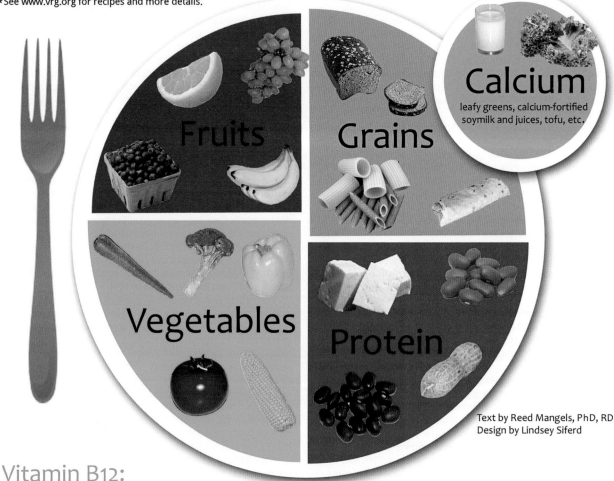

Fruits

Grains

Calcium
leafy greens, calcium-fortified
soymilk and juices, tofu, etc.

Vegetables

Protein

Text by Reed Mangels, PhD, RD
Design by Lindsey Siferd

Vitamin B12:

Vegans need a reliable source of vitamin B12. Eat daily a couple of servings of fortified foods
such as B12-fortified soymilk, breakfast cereal, meat analog, or Vegetarian Support Formula nutritional yeast.
Check the label for fortification. If fortified foods are not eaten daily,
you should take a vitamin B12 supplement (25 micrograms daily).

Note:

Like any food plan, this should only serve as a general guide for adults.
The plan can be modified according to your own personal needs. This is not personal
medical advice. Individuals with special health needs should consult a registered
dietitian or a medical doctor knowledgeable about vegan nutrition.

VRg The Vegetarian
Resource Group P.O. Box 1463 Baltimore, MD 21203 www.vrg.org (410) 366-8343

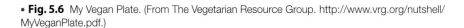

• **Fig. 5.6** My Vegan Plate. (From The Vegetarian Resource Group. http://www.vrg.org/nutshell/
MyVeganPlate.pdf.)

TABLE 5.5 Healthy Vegetarian Dietary Patterns: Recommended Amounts of Food From Each Food Group for 4 Calorie Levels

Calorie Level of Pattern[a]	1200	1800	2200	2800
Food Group	**Daily Amount**[b] of Food From Each Group (vegetable and protein foods subgroup amounts are per week)			
Vegetables (cup eq/day)	1½	2½	3	3½
Dark-green vegetables (c-eq/week)	1	1½	2	2½
Red and orange vegetables (c-eq/week)	3	5½	6	7
Beans, peas and lentils (c-eq/week)	½	1½	2	2½
Starchy vegetables (c-eq/week)	3½	5	6	7
Other vegetables (c-eq/week)	2½	4	5	5½
Fruits (c-eq/day)	1	1½	2	2½
Grains (ounce eq/day)	4	6½	7½	10½
Whole grains[c] (oz-eq/day)	2	3½	4	5½
Refined grains (oz-eq/day)	2	3	3½	5
Dairy (c-eq/day)	2½	3	3	3
Protein foods (oz-eq/day)	1½	3	3½	5
Eggs (oz-eq/week)	3	3	3	4
Beans, peas, and lentils (c-eq/week)[d]	2	6	6	10
Soy alternatives (oz-eq/week)	3	6	8	11
Nuts and seeds (oz-eq/week)	2	6	7	10
Oils (g/day)	17	24	29	36
Limit on calories for other uses, Calories/day (% of Calories)[e]	140 (12%)	150 (8%)	290 (13%)	300 (13%)

Bold indicates the food groups and the unbold are examples of foods within each group.

[a]Food intake patterns below 1400 calories are designed to meet the nutritional needs of 2- to 8-year-old children. Patterns from 1600 to 3200 calories are designed to meet the nutritional needs of children 9 years and older, and adults. If a child 4 to 8 years of age needs more calories and, therefore is following a pattern at 1600 calories or more, that child's recommended amount from the dairy group should be 2.5 cups per day. Children 9 years and older, and adults should not use calorie patterns below 1400 calories.

[b]Food group amounts shown in cup-equivalents (c-eq) or ounce-equivalents (oz-eq), as appropriate for each group, based on calorie and nutrient content. Oils are shown in grams (g).

[c]Amounts of whole grains in the pattern for children are less than the minimum of 3 oz-eq in all patterns recommended for adults.

[d]About half of total beans, peas, and lentils are shown as vegetables and half as protein foods.

[e]All foods are assumed to be in nutrient-dense forms; lean or low-fat; and prepared without added fats, sugars, refined starches, or salt. If all food choices to meet food group recommendations are in nutrient-dense forms, a small number of calories remain within the overall calorie limit of the pattern (i.e., limit on calories for other uses). The number of these calories depends on the overall calorie limit in the pattern and the amounts of food from each food group required to meet nutritional goals. Calories from protein, carbohydrates, and total fats should be within the acceptable macronutrient distribution ranges.

◆ CASE APPLICATION FOR THE DENTAL HYGIENIST

A single mother of two children comes to the clinic complaining about sensitivity to hot and cold foods and bleeding gums. She has recently lost her job and child support payments are irregular. She is very concerned about the limited amount of protein foods she is able to purchase with her food stamps. Based on her diet diary, her calorie intake is 1800 cal/day, and protein is approximately 50 g. Food intake is principally pastas, tortillas, chips, sweet pastries, and sodas.

Nutritional Assessment

- Willingness to learn
- Knowledge base of protein, carbohydrate, and fat principles for optimal nutrition
- Cultural beliefs
- Recent percentage of calories from protein (11%)

- Types of protein intake and total nutrient intake
- Overall nutrient intake
- Carbonated beverage intake

Nutritional Diagnosis

Altered health maintenance and limited nutrition knowledge related to insufficient funds to purchase foods to provide adequate nutrients.

Nutritional Goals

The patient will verbalize three principles concerning protein as well as the benefits from other nutrients. The patient will consume foods providing complementary protein and incorporate some fruits and dairy products into her menus.

(Continued)

◆ **CASE APPLICATION FOR THE DENTAL HYGIENIST—CONT'D**

Nutritional Implementation

Intervention: Discussion points: (1) the seven functions or roles of protein, (2) the difference between essential amino acids and nonessential amino acids, (3) the difference between high-quality and lower-quality protein, and (4) how to incorporate complementary proteins into menus.

Rationale: Knowledge corrects inaccurate information.

Intervention: Discuss less expensive sources of protein.

Rationale: Good sources of protein do not have to be high-priced meats.

Intervention: Encourage the use of dairy products and fortified soy alternatives.

Rationale: Dairy products and fortified soy alternatives are an excellent source of protein and provide other nutrients important to maintain health. The overall nutritional content of other plant-based "milks" (e.g., almond, rice, coconut or oat) are not similar to dairy products and fortified soy products, therefore they do not contribute to the dairy recommendations.[5]

Intervention: Encourage incorporating fruits and vegetables into the menus.

Rationale: Protein is not the only nutrient needed to maintain good oral health. In addition, consumption of adequate fruits and vegetables models healthy eating to her children.

Intervention: Refer her to a social worker

Rationale: The social worker will be knowledgeable about local and federal food programs she is eligible for and can direct her to local food banks and other resources.

Evaluation

The patient should not only understand that protein is important but also realize that it is possible to purchase cheaper sources of protein that provide all the essential amino acids. To determine this, have the patient repeat three of the principles she remembers from your teaching. The patient should also express her intention to use complementary proteins to provide adequate amounts of amino acids which will provide other nutrients necessary for health, and purchase some dairy products, fruits, and vegetables each week.

◆ Student Readiness

1. Define bioavailability, kwashiorkor, sarcopenia, nitrogen balance, high-quality protein, and complementary proteins for a patient.
2. List and explain the functions of proteins.
3. Using your desirable body weight, how many grams of protein should you consume (0.8 g/kg)?
4. Given a patient weighing 180 lb who has a calorie intake of 2500 cal, if the diet averages 15% protein, how many calories are provided by protein? How many grams of protein is this? How does this compare with the RDA for this patient?
5. What would you tell a strict vegetarian (vegan) parent about feeding her infant?
6. Due to the increased risk of protein-energy malnutrition, which patient groups may need nutritional assessments?
7. What are the oral effects of too much protein in the diet? What are the oral effects of too little protein in the diet?
8. Explain the relationship between calories and nutrition.
9. What are two methods of obtaining the indispensable amino acids from vegetarian foods? List two food combinations for each type of vegetarian diet that would provide adequate amounts of indispensable amino acids.
10. How do high-protein diets help with weight loss or maintenance?
11. Using the Internet or a reputable sports magazine, identify a professional athlete who is vegan. Note what is said about his/her health, strength, and types and amounts of foods consumed.

References

1. USDA, Economic Research Service, United States Department of Agriculture. *Livestock and Meat Domestic Data.* https://www.ers.usda.gov/data-products/livestock-meat-domestic-data.aspx.
2. Center for Disease Control. United States National Center Health Statistics. *Fast Stats-Diet/Nutrition.* 2019. https://www.cdc.gov/nchs/fastats/diet.htm.
3. Layman DK, Anthony TG, Rasmussen BB, et al. Defining meal for protein to optimize metabolic roles of amino acids. *Am J Clin Nutr.* 2015;101(6):1330S–1338S.
4. Phillips SM. The impact of protein quality on the promotion of resistance exercise-induced changes in muscle mass. *Nutr Metab (Lond).* 2016;13:64.
5. United States Department of Health and Human Services and US Department of Agriculture. *2020–2025 Dietary Guidelines for Americans.* 9th ed. 2021. https://dietaryguidelines.gov.
6. Thomas DT, Erdman KA, Burke LM. Position of the Academy of Nutrition and Dietetics, Dietitian of Canada, and the American College of Sports Medicine: nutrition and athletic performance. *J Acad Nutr Diet.* 2016;16(3):501–528.
7. Yoo JI, Choi Y, Lee J, et al. Poor dietary protein intake in elderly population with sarcopenia and osteosarcopenis: a nationwide population-based study. *J Bone Metab.* 2020;27(4):301–310.
8. Shams-White MM, Chung M, Du M, et al. Dietary protein and bone health: a systematic review and *meta*-analysis from the National Osteoporosis Foundation. *Am J Clin Nutr.* 2017;105(6):1528–1543.
9. Food and Nutrition Board of the Institute of Medicine. *Dietary Reference Intakes for Energy, Carbohydrate, Fiber, Fat, Fatty Acids, Cholesterol, Protein, and Amino Acids.* 2005. National Academies Press; 2005. https://doi.org/10.17226/10490.
10. Ko GJ, Obi Y, Tortorici AR, et al. Dietary protein intake and chronic kidney disease. *Curr Opin Clin Nutr Metab Care.* 2017;20(1):77–85.
11. Wang M, Chou J, Chang Y, et al. The role of low protein diet in ameliorating proteinuria and deferring dialysis initiation: what is old and what is new. *Panminerva Med.* 2017;59(2):157–165.
12. ElSayed NA, Aleppo G, Aroda VR, et al. 11. Chronic kidney disease and risk management: standards of care in diabetes—2023. *Diabetes Care.* 2023;46(Suppl 1):S191–S202. https://doi.org/10.2337/dc23-S011.
13. Vegetarian Resource Group. How many adults in the United States are vegan? How many adults eat vegetarian when eating out asks the vegetarian resource group in a national poll. *Vegetarian J.* 2020;39(4):28–30. https://www.vrg.org/journal/vj2020issue4/VJ_issue4_2020.pdf.
14. Posthauer MEE, Malone A, Sabate J. Position of the Academy of Nutrition and Dietetics: vegetarian diets. *J Acad Nutr Diet.* 2016;116(12):1970–1980.
15. Bakaloudi DR, Halloran A, Rippin HL, et al. Intake and adequacy of the vegan diet. A systemic review of the evidence. *J Clin Nutr.* 2020. https://doi.org/10.1016/j.clnu.2020.11.035.
16. Satija A, Shilpa NB, Spiehelman D, et al. Healthful and unhealthful plant-based diets and the risk of coronary heart disease in United States adults. *J Am Coll Cardiol.* 2017;70(4):411–422.

▶ Evolve Resources

Please visit http://evolve.elsevier.com/Mallonee/nutritional for additional practice and study support tools.

6

Lipids: The Condensed Energy

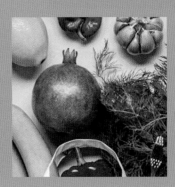

STUDENT LEARNING OUTCOMES

On completion of this chapter, the student will be able to achieve the following learning outcomes:

1. Related to the classification, chemical structure, and characteristics of lipids:
   - Describe how fatty acids affect the properties of fat.
   - Explain the function of fat in the human body.
   - Discuss the chemical structure of lipids.
   - Describe the characteristics of lipids.
2. Describe the function of various compound lipids, and identify foods that contain each of them. Also, discuss the function and sources of cholesterol.
3. List and describe the physiologic roles of lipids in the body.
4. Discuss the effects of dietary fats on oral health.
5. Related to dietary requirements of lipids:
   - Calculate the recommendation for an individual's consumption of dietary fat.
   - Evaluate a patient's food intake for appropriate amounts of saturated fats.
   - Suggest appropriate foods when dietary modification of fat intake has been recommended to a patient.
   - Compare the types of fatty acids in various fats and oils.
6. Discuss nutrition recommendations for various patient health conditions related to excess consumption and inadequate consumption of dietary fat.

KEY TERMS

Adipose tissue
α-Linolenic acid
Atherosclerosis
Calorie-dense foods
Cardiovascular disease (CVD)
Compound lipids
Docosahexaenoic acid (DHA)
Eicosapentaenoic acid (EPA)

Essential fatty acid (EFA)
Hyperlipidemia
Interesterified fats
Lipoproteins
Long-chain fatty acids
Medium-chain fatty acids
Omega-3 fatty acids
Omega-6 fatty acids

Phospholipids
Plant sterols
Protein sparing
Short-chain fatty acids
Structural lipids
Trans fatty acid

⬡ TEST YOUR NQ

1. **T/F** All foods containing more than 35% of their calories from fat are not considered healthy.
2. **T/F** Fats containing vitamin E deteriorate and become rancid rapidly.
3. **T/F** A product containing more unsaturated fatty acids than saturated fatty acids (SFAs) is a healthier food choice than one containing a higher proportion of SFAs.
4. **T/F** Dietary fat intake should be less than 20% of total calories.
5. **T/F** Bananas and avocados contain cholesterol.

6. **T/F** Oils are less fattening than solid fats.
7. **T/F** Fat intake has been linked more frequently to cancer than any other dietary factor.
8. **T/F** Nuts and cheeses are nutritious foods that can be recommended as snacks to all patients because they reduce the rate of caries.
9. **T/F** Fats contain 9 kcal/g.
10. **T/F** Omega-3 fatty acids are polyunsaturated fatty acids.

Unsweetened coconut, mayonnaise, sour cream, blue cheese, salad dressing, almonds, pecans, olives, avocados, and sausages—what do all these foods have in common? More than 50% of the calories in each of these foods come from fat, a vital nutrient in our diet.

Added fats and oils provide more calories in the average American diet than any other food group. Examination of the United States food supply trends between 1999 and 2016 showed total energy from fat increased slightly from 32% to 33.2% with intake from saturated fat accounting for 11.9% of total fat.[1] Approximately 77% of Americans consume more saturated fat than the 10% recommended in the *Dietary Guidelines 2020–2025*.[2] Changes seen in saturated fat intake may be in part due to the popularity of eating patterns in recent years that include Atkins (high in protein and low in carbohydrate) and ketogenic diets.[1] The functions of fatty acids are shown in Table 6.1.

TABLE 6.1	Common Food Sources and Physiological Actions of Fatty Acids	
Fatty Acids/Classification	**Common Food Sources**	**Physiologic Action**
SFA		
Lauric, myristic, palmitic, stearic; palmitic; carprylic, and capric acids	Animal sources (meats, eggs, butter, lard, beef tallow); processed food products containing saturated vegetable oils; coconut oil, palm and palm kernel oil; cocoa butter, fully hydrogenated vegetable oils	Raises total and LDL (except stearic acid)
MUFA		
Cis configuration (oleic and palmitoleic acid)	Olive and canola oil; avocados, almonds; macadamia nuts; lesser amounts in beef tallow, lard	Decreases total and LDL cholesterol and triglycerides; increases HDL cholesterol when substituted for SFAs and carbohydrate, but not when replacing PUFAs
Trans configuration (elaidic acid)	Partially hydrogenated vegetable oils	Raises total and LDL cholesterol similar to SFAs, decreases HDL more than SFAs. Increases CVD and diabetes risk factors
Trans configuration (vaccenic acid)	Dairy fat, meat from ruminating animals (beef, lamb)	No significant differences in blood lipids or lipoproteins observed. May have beneficial health effects, especially vaccenic acid; more research needed
PUFA		
n-6 Fatty Acids		
Linoleic acid	Soybean oil, corn oil, shortening	Decreases total and LDL cholesterol
Arachidonic acid	Meat, poultry, eggs	Precursor for important biologically active substances; substrate for synthesis of a variety of proinflammatory compounds
Conjugated linoleic acid	Ruminant meat and dairy	May help reduce body fat deposits and improve immune function
n-3 Fatty Acids		
α-Linolenic acid	Flaxseed, chia, canola oil, walnuts	Decreases cardiovascular risk
EPA; DPA; DHA	Fish and seafood	Decreases risk of sudden death from cardiovascular conditions; beneficial effects on nervous system development and health; potentially potent antiinflammatory agents

Adapted from Vannice G, Rasmussen H. Position of the Academy of Nutrition and Dietetics: dietary fatty acids for healthy adults. *J Acad Nutr Diet.* 2014;114(1):136–153.
HDL, High-density lipoprotein; *EPA,* eicosapentaenoic acid; *DPA,* docosapentaenoic acid; *DHA,* docosahaenoic acid; *LDL,* low-density lipoprotein; *MUFA,* monounsaturated fatty acid; *PUFA,* polyunsaturated fatty acid; *SFA,* saturated fatty acid.

Classification

Dietary fats should actually be called lipids. Lipids contain the same three elements as carbohydrates: carbon, hydrogen, and oxygen. Lipids contain less oxygen in proportion to hydrogen and carbon than carbohydrates. The structure of lipids is covered in detail in Chapter 2. Because of their structure, they provide more energy per gram than either carbohydrates or proteins.

The two classes of water-insoluble substances are (1) simple lipids, or triglycerides, which occur in foods and in the body; and (2) structural lipids, which are produced by the body for specific functions. The structural component of lipids is fatty acids. Triglycerides with one or more of the fatty acids replaced with carbohydrate, phosphate, or nitrogenous compounds are called compound lipids. Dietary lipids used physiologically include triglycerides, fatty acids, phospholipids, and cholesterol. Lipoproteins are found solely in the body.

Chemical Structure

Triglycerides are composed of fatty acids and glycerol, as shown:

Monoglycerides = glycerol + one fatty acid

Diglycerides = glycerol + two fatty acids

Triglycerides = glycerol + three fatty acids

A fatty acid is a chain of carbon atoms attached to hydrogen atoms with an acid grouping on one end. Glycerol is the alcohol portion of a triglyceride to which fatty acids attach. Triglycerides are the most common fat present in animal or protein foods (Fig. 6.1). Monoglycerides and diglycerides are found in the small intestine and result from the breakdown of triglycerides during digestion (Fig. 6.2). Free fatty acids, monoglycerides, and glycerol can cross cell membranes.

Three fatty acids join to glycerol in a condensation reaction to form a triglyceride.

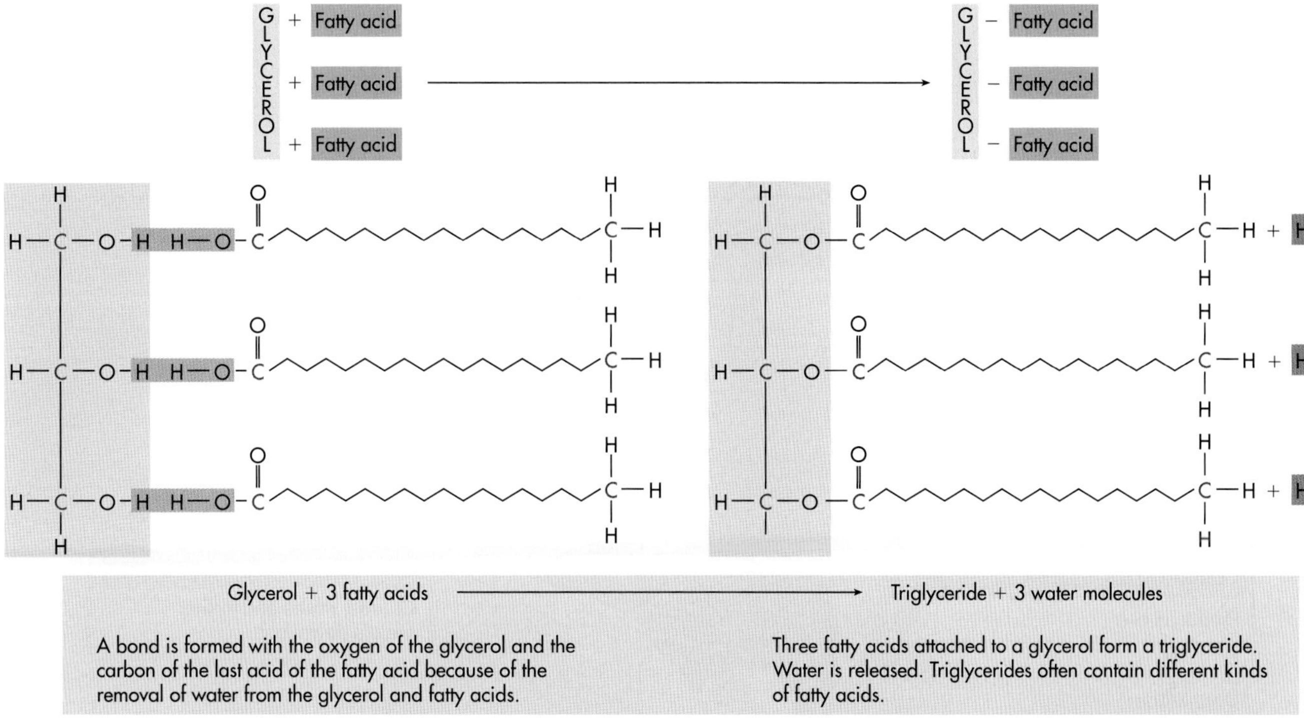

• **Fig. 6.1** Formation and structure of a triglyceride. From Grodner M, Escott-Stump S, Dorner S. *Nutritional Foundations and Clinical Applications*. 6th ed. Mosby Elsevier; 2016.

Each of the three fatty acids attached to the triglyceride can be different: they can be long, medium, or short, and saturated or unsaturated. Medium-chain and short-chain fatty acids are readily digested and absorbed, but most fats in foods (especially vegetable fats) contain predominantly long-chain fatty acids. Short-chain fatty acids contain less than six carbon atoms, medium-chain fatty acids contain 6 to 12 carbon atoms, and long-chain fatty acids contain more than 12 carbon atoms.[3]

Saturated Fatty Acids

As discussed in Chapter 2, fatty acids are classified according to their degree of saturation. Saturation of a fatty acid depends on the number of hydrogen atoms attached to the carbon chain. SFAs contain only single bonds, with each carbon atom having two hydrogen atoms attached to it (see Chapter 2). Palmitic and stearic acids (see Chapter 2), the two most prevalent SFAs, are structural components of tooth enamel and dentin.

Monounsaturated Fatty Acids

When adjacent carbon atoms are joined by a double bond because two hydrogen atoms are lacking, there is a gap between the hydrogen atoms in the chain; it is called an unsaturated fatty acid. Monounsaturated fatty acids (MUFAs) contain only one double bond (see Chapter 2). The most abundant MUFA is oleic acid. Oleic acid is also a structural component of the tooth.

Trans Fatty Acids

Hydrogenation is a commercial process in which vegetable oil is converted to a solid margarine or shortening by adding hydrogen. This process results in naturally unsaturated vegetable oils being changed to an SFA by changing unsaturated bonds to saturated bonds. The hydrogenation process not only increases the proportion of SFAs but also changes the shape of the fatty acid. When the hydrogen atoms are rotated so that they are on the opposite sides of the bond, in the "*trans*" position (see Chapter 2), the fatty acid is called a *trans* fatty acid. Partial hydrogenation results in large numbers of fatty acids having this altered shape. A common *trans* fatty acid is elaidic acid, found in partially hydrogenated vegetable oils, such as tub margarine and cooking oils. A naturally occurring *trans* fatty acid, vaccenic acid, with double bonds on adjacent carbons, is present in small amounts in human milk and the milk and meat of ruminants (cows, sheep, and deer).

Polyunsaturated Fatty Acids

When carbon atoms in a fatty acid are connected by two or more double bonds, the fatty acid is polyunsaturated (see Chapter 2). Linoleic acid and arachidonic acid are polyunsaturated fatty acids (PUFAs), also known as omega-6 fatty acids (or n-6 PUFAs). Their first double bond is on the sixth carbon atom from the omega (terminal) end.

Omega-3 fatty acids, or α-linolenic acids, make up another class of PUFAs. As shown in Chapter 2, these fatty acids are unique because the first double bond is located three carbon atoms from the omega end of the molecule; thus they are called omega-3s or *n-3s*. Omega-3 fatty acids include **α-linolenic acid** which has 18 carbon atoms and two double bonds, and **eicosapentaenoic acid (EPA)**, which has 20 carbon atoms and five double bonds.

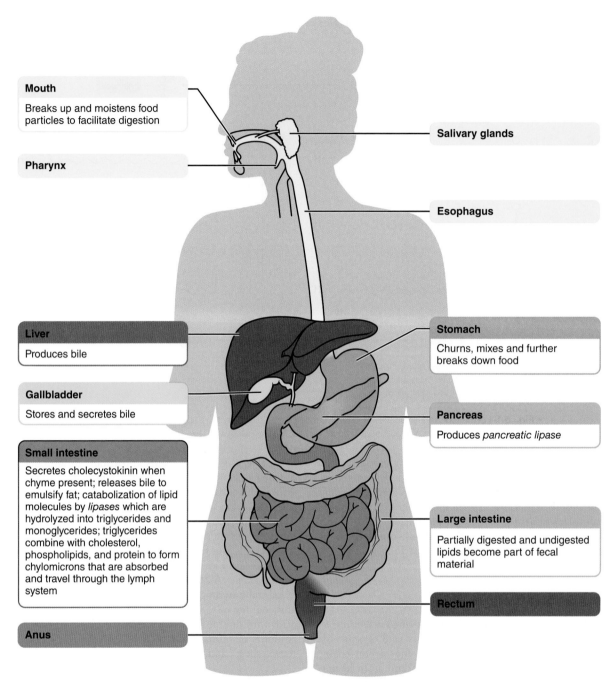

• **Fig. 6.2** Summary of lipid digestion. NOTE: Enzymes are in *italics*.

Characteristics of Fatty Acids

The carbon chain length and degree of saturation determine various properties of fats, including their flavor and hardness, or melting point (the temperature at which a product becomes a liquid). Most SFAs are solid at room temperature; for example, animal fats, being solid at room temperature, are predominantly saturated fats. Short-chain fatty acids (six carbon atoms or less), MUFAs, and PUFAs that are liquid at room temperature are oils. Milk fat contains a large amount of short-chain SFAs.

Fats with a high proportion of unsaturated fatty acids may deteriorate or become rancid, resulting in unpleasant flavors and odors. Fats become rancid when subject to high temperatures and

light, causing oxidation and decomposition of fats. The decomposition results in peroxides that may be toxic in large amounts. Vitamin E, a fat-soluble vitamin, is an antioxidant and, to some degree, protects the oil from oxidation. However, in doing so, vitamin E is inactivated and cannot be used by the body.

🦷 DENTAL CONSIDERATIONS

• Lipids are an integral part of many foods and are physiologically important.
• The primary form of fat in the body is triglyceride, not cholesterol.

⬡ NUTRITIONAL DIRECTIONS

- Frying at low temperature causes the food to absorb more oil, whereas frying at very high temperature results in less oil absorption. However, the high temperature causes an increase in oxidation and decomposition of fats that produces free radicals implicated in the development of chronic, degenerative diseases.
- The relatively small amounts of *trans* fatty acids occurring naturally in meat and dairy products do not appear to be harmful.
- Butylated hydroxyanisole and butylated hydroxytoluene are antioxidants added to processed foods to retard or prevent spoilage.

Compound Lipids

Phospholipids

Phospholipids contain phosphorus and a nitrogenous base in addition to fatty acids and glycerol. Fats from plant and animal foods contain phospholipids but are not required in the diet because the body produces adequate amounts of phospholipids. Phospholipids are not absorbed intact; they are broken down into their chemical components before absorption. As a structural component of cell membranes, tooth enamel, and dentin, they are the second most prevalent form of fat in the body. As a structural component of membranes, they are not used for energy, even in a state of severe starvation. Although the mechanism is not fully understood, phospholipids are involved in the initiation of calcification and mineralization in teeth and bones.[4] They are present in higher amounts in the enamel matrix of teeth than in dentin.

Phospholipids are important in fat absorption and transport of fat in the blood. Phospholipids mix with either fat-soluble or water-soluble ingredients to transport these products across membrane barriers. Phospholipids include lecithin, cephalin, and sphingomyelins. Phospholipids, especially lecithin, are used as additives in commercial products to act as an emulsifier to prevent fat and water components from separating.

Lecithin, the most widely distributed phospholipid, is present in all cells. Lecithin supplements have been marketed for reducing the risk of atherosclerosis (a complex disease of the arteries in which the interior lining of arteries becomes roughened and clogged with fatty deposits that hinder blood flow; Fig. 6.3), weight loss, and other chronic health conditions. However, the value of lecithin in this role is questionable because it is digested before absorption.

Cephalin is present in thromboplastin, which is necessary for blood clotting. Sphingomyelins are important constituents of brain tissue and the myelin sheath around nerve fibers.

Lipoproteins

Lipoproteins are produced by the body to transport insoluble fats in the blood. Lipoproteins are compound lipids composed of triglycerides, phospholipids, and cholesterol combined with protein (see Fig. 2.20). The liver and intestinal mucosa produce lipoproteins. Four different types of lipoproteins are present in the blood: high-density lipoproteins (HDLs), low-density lipoproteins (LDLs), very-low-density lipoproteins, and chylomicrons.

The ratio of lipid to protein in lipoproteins varies widely; these variations affect their density. Density increases as lipids decrease and protein increases. Lipoproteins can be classified according to their density and composition, as shown in Fig. 6.4. Phospholipids in lipoproteins are present in approximately the same proportions in all individuals.

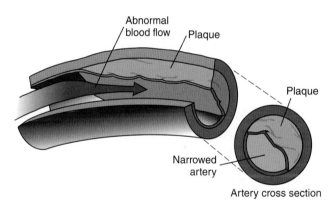

• **Fig. 6.3** Atherosclerosis. An artery narrowed by the buildup of plaque. From Workman ML, LaCharity L, Kruchko SL. *Understanding Pharmacology*. 2nd ed. Saunders; 2016.

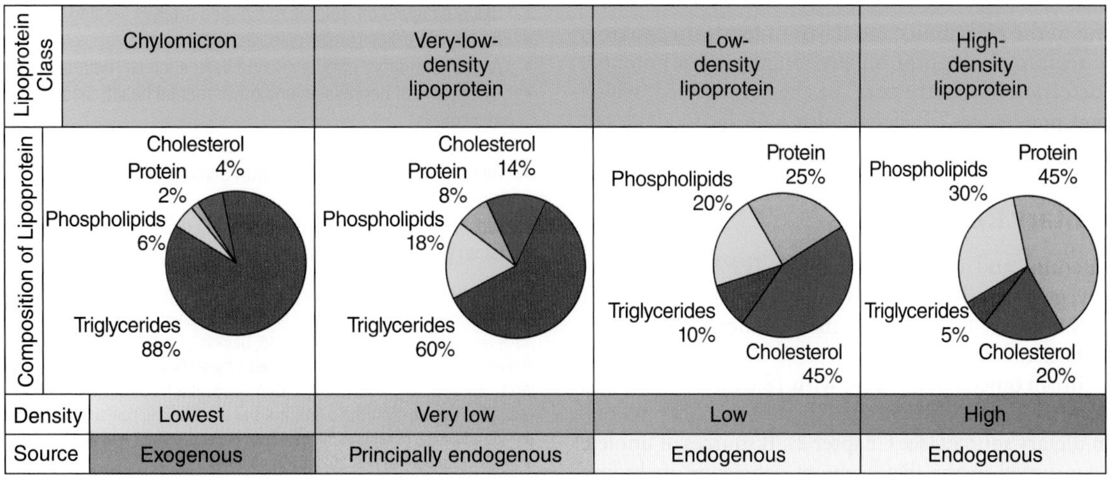

Lipoprotein Class	Chylomicron	Very-low-density lipoprotein	Low-density lipoprotein	High-density lipoprotein
Composition of Lipoprotein	Cholesterol 4%, Protein 2%, Phospholipids 6%, Triglycerides 88%	Cholesterol 14%, Protein 8%, Phospholipids 18%, Triglycerides 60%	Protein 25%, Phospholipids 20%, Triglycerides 10%, Cholesterol 45%	Protein 45%, Phospholipids 30%, Triglycerides 5%, Cholesterol 20%
Density	Lowest	Very low	Low	High
Source	Exogenous	Principally endogenous	Endogenous	Endogenous

• **Fig. 6.4** Characteristics of lipoproteins.

HDLs contain greater amounts of protein and less lipid. LDL cholesterol typically constitutes 60% to 70% of the total blood cholesterol and is considered the main agent in elevated serum cholesterol levels, or the "bad" cholesterol. Serum LDL is causally related to CVD morbidity and mortality,[5] as discussed in *Health Application 6*.

Cholesterol

Cholesterol is a fat-like, waxy substance classified as a sterol derivative with a complex ring structure (see Chapter 2. Because the body frequently produces more cholesterol than it absorbs, cholesterol intake is not essential. Cholesterol has important functions as a constituent of the brain, nervous tissue, and bile salts; a precursor of vitamin D and steroid hormones; and a structural component of cell membranes and teeth. Lipoproteins transport cholesterol in the blood.

Physiologic Roles

Energy

Dietary fats are a concentrated source of energy, furnishing 9 calories per gram. Foods high in fats are generally referred to as "calorie dense," a beneficial quality in some cases. Calorie-dense foods are high in fats (or fat and sugar) and low in vitamins, minerals, and other nutrients. A characteristic of calorie-dense foods is that less volume of food is needed to furnish energy requirements. As an energy source, fats are also referred to as protein sparing because they allow protein to be used for the important functions of building and repairing tissues.

Satiety Value

Dietary fats are important for their satiety value. Fats have a higher satiety value than carbohydrates or proteins because digestion of high-fat meals is slower than other energy-containing nutrients. The higher the fat content of a meal, the longer the food remains in the stomach. Nevertheless, approximately 95% of ingested fats are absorbed. Soft fats that are liquids at body temperature (e.g., margarine) are digested more quickly than solid fats (e.g., meat fats).

Palatability

Fats contribute to the palatability and flavor of foods. In cooking, they improve texture. A receptor on the tongue and a potential pathway for detection of a "fatty taste" has been identified, which may affect food preferences.[6] Preference for high-fat foods develops at an early age and persists through adulthood.

Complementary Relationships

Fat-soluble vitamins and essential fatty acids (EFAs) are generally found in vegetable oils, nuts, and fatty fish. The absorption of fat-soluble vitamins is facilitated by the presence of fats in the gastrointestinal tract.

Linoleic acid, an omega-6 fatty acid with 18 carbon atoms and two double bonds, cannot be synthesized by the body and must be supplied from dietary sources (see Chapter 2). If sources of linoleic acid are not consumed in the diet, signs of deficiency, including growth retardation, skin lesions, and reproductive failure, result.

For this reason, linoleic acid is an EFA. Linoleic acid may be a protective factor against heart disease.

Arachidonic acid (18 carbon chain with four double bonds) and linolenic acid (18 carbon chain with three double bonds) are also considered EFAs, but healthy individuals can produce them from sufficient quantities of linoleic acid (see Chapter 2). Linolenic acid can be converted into omega-3 fatty acids in the body, but the process is affected by numerous factors, including genetics, dietary, and lifestyle factors. Studies are inconsistent and suggest that 8% to 20% of linolenic acid is converted to the omega-3 fatty acids, EPA, and docosahexaenoic acid (DHA).[7] Omega-3 fatty acids are very important, participating in many interactions in the body to improve health, as shown in Box 6.1. Because of their importance in building and maintaining a healthy body, omega-3 fatty acid supplements have become popular. However, in a Cochrane systematic review, supplementation was not associated with either lower risk of all-cause mortality or major cardiovascular disease (CVD) outcomes.[8] Yet, research indicates that dietary intake of fatty fish is associated with lower risk for coronary heart disease and death.[9] Food sources of nutrients come with many added benefits when compared to supplements.

Fat Storage

Adipose tissue, or body fat, has several roles: (1) it provides a concentrated energy source, (2) protects internal organs, and (3) maintains body temperature.

• BOX 6.1   Health Effects of Omega-3 Fatty Acids

Omega-3 fatty acids (eicosapentanoic acid and docosahexanoic acid) serve many purposes.

Produce compounds that:
- Regulate blood pressure
- Improve immune response
- Regulate gastrointestinal inflammation
- Prevent heart arrhythmias
- Promote development of brain and nerve tissues in fetal and neonatal development, and ongoing cognitive and visual development in children
- Protect neurons in neurodegenerative conditions

Reduces or ameliorates:
- Blood pressure
- Elevated triglyceride levels (leads to coronary heart disease)
- Blood coagulation (relates to clogged arteries leading to atherosclerosis)
- Reduces cardiovascular disease risk
- Antiinflammatory effects in conditions such as rheumatoid arthritis
- Symptoms of depression and other mental health disorders in some individuals
- Serious eye problems, such as macular degeneration
- Risks/symptoms associated with dementia, Parkinson, and Alzheimer disease
- Aids in CAL (clinical attachment level) gain and pocket depth reduction as an adjunct to non-surgical periodontal therapy.

Data from Musazadeh V, Kavyani Z, Naghshbandi B, Dehghan P, Vajdi M. The beneficial effects of omega-3 polyunsaturated fatty acids on controlling blood pressure: an umbrella *meta*-analysis. *Front Nutr.* 2022;9:98545; Djuricic I, Calder PC. Beneficial outcomes of omega-6 and omega-3 polyunsaturated fatty acids on human health: an update for 2021. *Nutrients.* 2021;13(7):2421; Castro Dos Santos NC, Furukawa MV, Oliveira-Cardoso I, et al. Does the use of omega-3 fatty acids as an adjunct to non-surgical periodontal therapy provide additional benefits in the treatment of periodontitis? A systematic review and *meta*-analysis. *J Periodontal Res.* 2022;57(3):435–447.

Energy

Excess dietary carbohydrates and proteins are converted to fat and stored in adipose tissue. Fatty acids can be used as an energy source by all cells except red blood cells and central nervous system cells. People can survive total starvation for 30 to 40 days with only water to drink.

Protection of Organs

Fatty tissue surrounds vital organs and provides a cushion, protecting them from traumatic injury and shock.

Insulation

The subcutaneous layer of fat functions as an insulator that preserves body heat and maintains body temperature. Excessive layers of fat can also deter heat loss during hot weather.

Dietary Fats and Dental Health

Dietary fats are essential for oral health because they are incorporated into the tooth structure and may be involved in reducing caries risk and improving periodontal health. In regard to dental caries, studies indicate that fats may have a cariostatic effect.[10,11] Dietary fats probably have local rather than systemic influence on cariogenicity. Precisely how fats reduce the caries risk is unknown; however, several possible mechanisms are emerging, as follows:

1. Higher fatty acid content is associated with a higher pH which reduces caries risk.[10]
2. Some fatty acids, specifically oleic and linoleic acid, reduced demineralization when *Streptococcus mutans* were exposed to sucrose.[10,11]
3. Short- and medium-chain fatty acids like formic, capric, and lauric acid inhibit oral bacteria like *S. mutans*.[12]
4. Dietary fat delays gastric emptying and enhance fluoride absorption.[13]

Dietary fats like omega-3 fatty acids found in oily fish may have beneficial effects on periodontal disease and treatment.[14,15]

🦷 DENTAL CONSIDERATIONS

- Although some types of dietary fat intake may have a positive effect on dental health, patient's medical history needs to be considered when providing nutrition education.
- Lipids as a source of energy provide 9 cal/g, whereas carbohydrates and proteins provide 4 cal/g.
- While evidence does not support use of omega-3 or omega-6 fatty acids to reduce cardiovascular events,[8,18] fish consumption may have a favorable effect on blood platelets and other blood-clotting mechanisms, reducing the risk of clot formation and risk of heart disease.[9,19]
- Because omega-3 fatty acids may be beneficial to oral and general health, determine the patient's frequency of fish consumption and supplement use. An increase in fish consumption is recommended for most patients, but some fish, especially mackerel and tuna, should be consumed in moderation because of their mercury content.
- Krill oil (a type of fish oil) contains omega-3 fatty acids and may be better absorbed than other fish oils.[20] Studies have not provided convincing evidence for health benefits of krill oil in reducing cholesterol and more research is needed to determine its impact on cardiovascular outcomes.
- Both saturated and *trans* fats have an undesirable effect on heart health. Encourage patients with periodontal disease to include *more* fish and foods containing MUFA and PUFA (and less saturated fat) to improve oral and overall health status.

🔵 NUTRITIONAL DIRECTIONS

- Fats act as a lubricant in the intestines, decreasing constipation.
- Fatty fish and some oils contain omega-3 fatty acids and should be included in the diet one or two times a week as part of a healthy diet.[21] The amount varies by age so consult with guidelines.
- Intake of more than 3 g of omega-3 fatty acid supplements should be supervised by a health care provider.
- The potential relationship between periodontal disease and heart disease emphasizes important health reasons for good oral self-care and following the *Dietary Guidelines for Americans*.

Omega-3 fatty acid supplements were also shown to benefit periodontal health.[16]

The research has identified an association, but not a cause-and-effect relationship between dietary fats and dental health. However, overall health may be promoted by reducing saturated fat intake and increasing MUFA and PUFA.[17]

Dietary Requirements

A certain amount of fat is needed to provide adequate amounts of fat-soluble vitamins and EFAs. The acceptable macronutrient distribution range for fat is between 20% and 35% of energy intake for adults (see). The lower limit for fat intake was established to minimize the increase in blood triglyceride levels and decrease in HDL cholesterol levels that occur with higher intakes of refined carbohydrates. The upper limit of 35% calories from fat was based on information indicating that higher fat intake is associated with a greater intake of energy and SFA, which may be detrimental to health. Box 6.2 shows a method for calculating the National Academy of Medicine (formerly the Institute of Medicine) recommendation for dietary fat. The World Health Organization

---

● BOX 6.2 Calculating Total Daily Fat Recommendations for Specific Calorie Levels[a]

To calculate dietary fat:
1. Determine calorie level of the diet (see Dietary Reference Intake for Energy for Active Individuals, p. ii) (e.g., patient needs 2000 cal).
2. Multiply the calories by 0.35 to determine the number of calories of fat the diet can contain (e.g., 2000 cal×0.35 [% of total calories]=700 cal from fat).
3. Divide the answer by 9 to determine the grams of fat allowed daily (e.g., 700 cal from fat÷9 cal/g of fat=77.7 g of fat).

Calorie Level	Grams of Fat per Day
1200	<46
1500	<58
1800	<70
2000	<78
2200	<86
2400	<93

[a] Total fat intake limited to less than 35% of the total daily calories.

Institute of Medicine. Dietary Reference Intakes for Energy, Carbohydrate, Fiber, Fat, Fatty Acids, Cholesterol, Protein, and Amino Acids. Washington, DC: The National Academies Press; 2005.

recommends a total fat intake of less than 30% of total calories to avoid excess weight gain.[22]

The *Dietary Guidelines* do not indicate a specific amount of fat but rather indicate that fat intake should be limited based on an individual's calorie requirement to achieve/maintain a healthy weight. The *Dietary Guidelines* and dietary reference intakes (DRIs) also recommend that SFA and *trans* fatty acid intakes be as low as possible while consuming a diet providing an adequate intake of all essential nutrients. The *Dietary Guidelines* recommend less than 10% of calories from saturated fats, replacing them with MUFAs and PUFAs. Currently, approximately 11% of the calories from fats consumed by Americans are saturated.[2] Studies do not support substituting saturated fats with refined carbohydrate foods, but modifying the type of fat seems to provide better protection against CVD.[23,24]

The recommendation for oils in the United States for a 2000-calorie intake is 27 g (about 5 tsp) daily.[2] Average intakes of oils is approximately 23 g daily.[25]

Adequate intake established for linoleic acid is 0.6% of energy intake or 17 g/day for males and 12 g/day for females between 19 and 50 years, and 14 g/day for males and 11 g/day for females older than 51 years. A dietary reference intake has not been established for omega-3 fatty acids (EPA and DHA); more information is needed to establish an amount necessary to maximize cardiac health.[26] Dietary guidelines recommend 8 ounces of fish/seafood weekly which would provide approximately 250 mg/day of EPA and DHA[2]; current daily intake is around 52 to 88 mg/day from food and supplements.[27,28]

An adult can produce all the cholesterol needed; thus no dietary requirement is necessary. On the other hand, the National Academy of Medicine recommends individuals eat as little dietary cholesterol as possible without compromising an adequate dietary intake.[2]

Sources

As already discussed, foods contain a combination of fatty acids; each of the fatty acids attached to the glycerol may be different, resulting in different proportions of SFA, MUFA, or PUFA. The *Dietary Guidelines* emphasize that rather than attempting to reduce fat intake, the focus should be on fewer calories and less saturated fat intake. Fig. 6.5 compares the types of fatty acids in

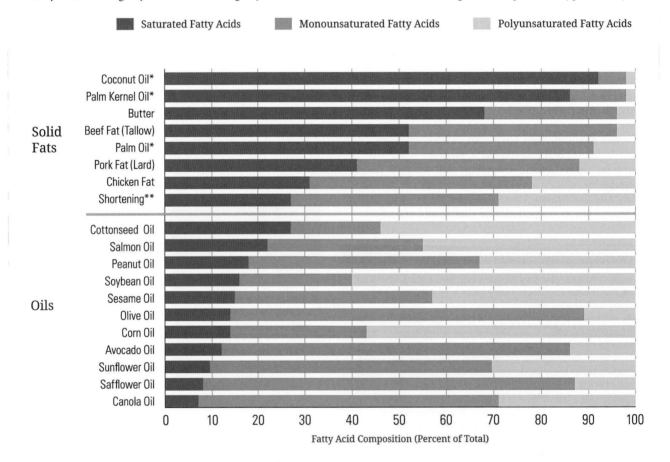

* Coconut, palm kernel, and palm oil are called oils because they come from plants. However, they are solid or semi-solid at room temperature due to their high content of short-chain saturated fatty acids. They are considered solid fats for nutritional purposes.

** Shortening may be made from partially hydrogenated vegetable oil, which contains *trans* fatty acids.

DATA SOURCES: U.S. Department of Agriculture, Agricultural Research Service, Nutrient Data Laboratory. USDA National Nutrient Database for Standard Reference. Release 27, 2015. Available at: http://ndb.nal.usda.gov/. Accessed August 31, 2015.

• **Fig. 6.5** Fatty acid profiles of common fats and oils.

various fats and oils; consumptions of vegetable oils with PUFA and MUFA should be encouraged. For example, olive oil, with approximately 9% PUFA, 69% MUFA, and 15% SFA, is considered a good source of MUFA. On the other hand, coconut and palm kernel oil (technically solids at room temperature, thus they are not an oil) contain more than 83% SFA and negligible amounts of PUFA and MUFA.

Table 6.2 itemizes selected animal products containing SFAs, MUFAs, and PUFAs. Of the food groups (excluding fats and oils), animal products (meat and milk) contribute the largest proportion of saturated fat, although their share has been declining. SFAs are found in animal fats, butter fat, coconut oil, cocoa butter, coffee creamers, and fully hydrogenated vegetable oils. As shown in Fig. 6.6, the biggest food contributors of saturated fat consumed by Americans are sandwiches containing cheese, meat, or both—including burgers, tacos, burritos; desserts and sweet snacks; and

pasta, rice, and grain-based mixed dishes.[2] Animal products, canola, and olive oils supply approximately 50% of MUFAs. Oleic acid, the most prevalent MUFA, is present in most fats, oils, nuts, seeds, and avocados.

PUFAs from the n-6 series are derived from land plants, especially foods from the grain group, and additional fats and oils (see Fig. 6.5). Linoleic acid is the most prevalent PUFA in the food supply.[7,29] Cottonseed, soybean, and corn oils provide the most PUFA; food sources are leafy greens, nuts and seeds.[7] Most oils are consumed in packaged foods, such as salad dressings, mayonnaise, prepared vegetables, snack chips, and nuts and seeds. More than 65% of all vegetable oil consumed in the United States is soybean oil.[30] It is also the principal source of omega-3 fatty acids in the American diet. Conjugated linoleic acids are natural components of beef, lamb, and dairy products. Linolenic acid is present in plant products—flaxseed, canola, and soybean oils; soybeans; walnuts;

TABLE 6.2 Fatty Acids and Cholesterol Content of Selected Foods (per 100 g)

Food	Total Fat (g)	SFA (g)	MUFA (g)	PUFA (Total) (g)	Cholesterol (mg)
Cheese, cheddar	33.3	18.9	9.3	1.4	99
Cheese, Monterey	30.3	19.1	8.8	0.90	89
Cottage cheese, 2%	2.3	1.2	0.5	0.08	12
Cream cheese	34.4	20.2	8.9	1.48	101
Ice cream, vanilla	11.0	6.8	3.0	0.45	44
Yogurt, low fat	1.3	0.8	0.3	0.04	5
Greek yogurt, low fat	4.7	3.01	1.19	0.186	24
Milk, 1%	1.0	0.63	0.3	0.04	5
Milk, 2%	1.98	1.23	0.6	0.07	8
Milk, whole, 3.7%	3.25	1.86	0.8	0.20	10
Milk, soy	5	0.07	0.9	2.69	0
Milk, oat	3.92	2.07	0.08	0.25	12
Milk, almond, unsweetened	2.98	0.25	1.78	0.67	0
Beef, lean ground (85%/15%)	15.3	5.81	6.6	0.48	89
Chicken breast, skinless	3.2	1.0	1.2	0.79	116
Chicken breast, with skin	7.8	2.2	3.0	1.7	84
Chicken thigh, skinless	15.8	4.4	6.2	3.5	91
Egg, large whole	9.51	3.1	3.71	1.91	372
Egg white	0.2	0	0	0	0
Pork chop, center loin, lean only	11.1	3.5	4.2	1.4	84
Salmon, canned	5.0	0.9	1.2	1.42	55
Salmon, chinook	13.4	3.2	5.7	2.7	84
Shrimp, mixed species	1.7	0.52	0.4	0.6	211
Veal loin, lean only	4.4	1.7	2.1	0.26	78

Data from United States Department of Agriculture (USDA), Agricultural Research Service, Nutrient Data Laboratory. *USDA National Nutrient Database for Standard Reference, Release 28.* http://www.ars.usda.gov/nea/bhnrc/mafcl.
MUFA, Monounsaturated fatty acid; *PUFA,* polyunsaturated fatty acid; *SFA,* saturated fatty acid.

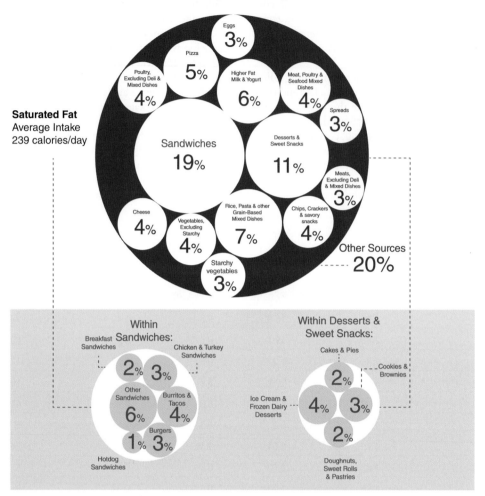

• **Fig. 6.6** Top sources and average intakes of saturated fats in the United States population ages 1 and older. From What We Eat in American (WWEIA), NHANES, 2013–2016, ages 1 and older, 2 days dietary intake data, weighted. From United States Department of Health and Human Services and United States Department of Agriculture. *2020–2025 Dietary Guidelines for Americans.* 9th ed.; 2020. https://www.dietaryguidelines.gov/.

flaxseed; and wheat germ.[7] Table 6.3 indicates the amount of saturated fat, monounsaturated fat, and polyunsaturated fat in the sample menu introduced in Fig. 1.4.

Long-chain omega-3 fatty acids (EPA and DHA), obtained from seafood, include fatty fish such as mackerel, salmon, herring, and albacore tuna, and fish oils.[2] Most shellfish contain very little omega-3s except the rich source found in oysters. These foods are also low in saturated fat. The *Dietary Guidelines* and American Heart Association (AHA) recommend consumption of fish at least two times a week or at least 6 to 8 oz-eq/week.[2,31] Well-controlled studies substantiate that fish intake containing EPA and DHA is associated with reducing CVD.[9]

The Food and Drug Administration required *trans* fat, related to hydrogenation of fats, be eliminated as a food additive in 2018.[32] The World Health Organization's goal was to remove added *trans* fats in the food supply by 2023. Efforts are continuing to complete this initiative by 2025.[33] However, some trans fats occur naturally in foods. Box 6.3 details how to limit the total amount of fat in the diet, focusing on reducing

foods high in saturated and *trans* fats and choosing more foods containing unsaturated fats.

Only animal products contain cholesterol; it is not found in egg whites or plant foods (e.g., vegetable oils). Cholesterol is highest in egg yolks, liver, and other organ meats. Since foods higher in saturated fats also contain cholesterol, when saturated fats are within the recommended lower amounts, cholesterol will be limited. The average amount of cholesterol intake in the United States is slightly below 300 mg.[34] Recommendations for cholesterol intake were removed from the dietary guidelines, but it remains controversial whether recommendations are needed for limiting cholesterol intake. A new *meta*-analysis suggested that high dietary cholesterol intake is associated with the risk for CVD and mortality.[35]

Food Choices

The percentage of fat by weight is widely marked on food labels and in advertising. Although this information is correct, it is

TABLE 6.3   **Saturated Fat, Monosaturated Fat, and Polyunsaturated Content of the Sample Menu**

Sample Menu	Saturated Fat (g)	Monounsaturated Fat (g)	Polyunsaturated Fat (g)
Breakfast			
1½ cup frosted mini-wheat cereal	0	0	1
12 oz skim milk	0	0	0
12 oz black coffee	0	0	0
Mid-morning snack			
12 oz water	0	0	0
1 oz dry roasted almonds, unsalted	1	9	4
1 medium orange	0	0	0
Lunch			
Sandwich with			
1 cup tuna salad with egg, low-calorie mayonnaise	2	3	4
¼ cup thin-sliced cucumber	0	0	0
3 thin slices tomato	0	0	0
2 lettuce leaves	0	0	0
2 thin slices 100% wheat bread	0	0	1
8 baby carrots	0	0	0
1 medium applesauce cookie	1	1	0
1 cup grapes	0	0	0
12 oz water	0	0	0
Mid-Afternoon Snack			
8 oz low-fat vanilla yogurt	2	1	0
12 oz herbal tea with nonnutritive sweetener	0	0	0
Dinner			
3 oz pot roast beef with	4	5	0
¼ cup sauteed mushrooms	0	0	0
1 cup white and wild rice blend with margarine and cooked in	1	2	1
½ c vegetable juice	0	0	0
2 c tossed salad with lettuce, avocado, tomatoes, and carrots	0	0	0
¼ cup shredded low-fat Muenster cheese	3	1	0
2 tbsp vinaigrette salad dressing	1	2	3
⅛ medium cantaloupe	0	0	0
12 oz iced tea with low-calorie sweetener	0	0	0
Evening Snack			
3 cup low-fat microwave popcorn	0	1	1
12 oz water	0	0	0
Totals[a]	15	25	15

From nutrient data MyPlate Tools.https://www.myplate.gov/resources/tools. Accessed April 8, 2023.
[a]Totals may vary due to rounding off.

misleading and confusing. The recommendation limiting fat to 35% refers to the percentage of fat based on total calories in the total diet. As shown in Table 6.4, the percentage of fat in whole milk is 48% of the total calories, not 3.25% as the label indicates.

The Nutrition Facts label on foods (see Chapter 1) indicates the grams and % Daily Value for fat, saturated fat, and *trans* fats in a serving. All *trans* fats, including those from ruminant animals, are included on the Nutrition Facts label. Since 2006, when the United States Food and Drug Administration (FDA) began requiring the amount of *trans* fats on the Nutrition Facts label, the amount of *trans* fats in foods has declined significantly. In 2013, the FDA determined that partially hydrogenated oils (the major source of commercially produced *trans* fats) were no longer "generally recognized as safe" based on its being a contributing factor to CVD.[32] The FDA allowed food manufacturers a 3-year compliance period to eliminate *trans* fatty acids from their products with a final timeline of January 1, 2021.[32] Only naturally occurring *trans* fatty acids remain in the foods of animal origin including meat and dairy.

For most people, a decrease in high-fat meat and whole dairy product consumption is recommended by the Dietary Guidelines replacing them with lean meat and lower fat cheese options.[2] In recent years, through improvements in breeding and feeding livestock, these products have become lower in fat, saturated fat, calories, and cholesterol. Important nutrients are present in beef, pork, and lamb; moderate consumption

TABLE 6.4 Analysis of Fat Content of Milk

Type of Milk	Calories per 245 g (1 cup)	Total Fat (g)	Percentage of Fat by Weight	Percentage of Fat by Calories
Whole milk (3.25%)	149	7.9	3.3	48
Low-fat milk (2%)	125	4.7	1.9	34
Low-fat milk (1%)	105	2.4	1	21
Skim milk	83	0.20	0.1	2

Data from United States Department of Agriculture (USDA), Agricultural Research Service, Nutrient Data Laboratory. *USDA National Nutrient Database for Standard Reference, Release 28.* http://www.ars.usda.gov/nea/bhnrc/mafcl.

• BOX 6.3 Wise Choices of Dietary Fats

Purchasing and Planning

- Read nutrition labels on foods to determine the amount of fat and saturated fat in a serving. Low fat is less than 3 g fat per serving.
- Choose fats and oils with 2 g or less saturated fat per tablespoon, such as tub margarines and vegetable oils (e.g., canola, corn, safflower, sunflower, and olive oil). Liquid vegetable oil should be listed as the first ingredient. Avoid saturated fats such as butter, lard, palm, and coconut oils.
- Substitute plain low-fat Greek-style yogurt for mayonnaise or sour cream. Consider light sour cream (compare fat content on labels) as a substitute for full-fat sour cream.
- Purchase fresh fruits, vegetables, and nuts for snacks rather than sugar-sweetened beverages, chips, pastries, and high-calorie baked goods (e.g., muffins, doughnuts).
- Choose two or three servings of lean meat, skinless poultry, or fish, with a daily total of about 6 oz.
- Choose a vegetarian entree (e.g., dry beans and peas) at least once a week.
- Include fish (not fried) at least twice a week.
- Include a variety of fresh lean meats (not processed).
- Choose "select" grade beef rather than "choice" because it contains fewer calories as a result of less fat marbling. Fat content of meats also depends on the type of cut; leaner cuts include flank steak, sirloin or tenderloin, loin pork chops, and 85% or greater lean ground beef.
- Choose lean turkey or chicken sausage, or turkey bacon.
- Use low-fat ground turkey or extra-lean ground beef in casseroles, spaghetti, and chili.
- Moderate the use of egg yolks (maximum of four egg yolks weekly) and organ meats (liver, brain, and kidney).
- Choose tuna packed in water, not in oil (compare fat content on labels).
- Select fat-free or low-fat milk and dairy products. Choose cheese with 6 g or less of fat per ounce (90% of the calories in cream cheese are from fat).

Food Preparation

- Use fats and oils (e.g., olive, canola, corn, sunflower, or cottonseed) sparingly in cooking (roast, bake, grill, or broil when possible). Baste meats with broth or stock.

- Use nonstick cookware and an aerosol cooking spray.
- Prepare and eat smaller portions.
- Use the paste method for making gravy or sauces: add flour or cornstarch to cold liquids slowly and blend well.
- Season with herbs, lemon juice, or stock rather than lard, bacon, ham, margarine, or fatty sauces.
- Remove skin from poultry and visible fat from beef and pork products.
- Skim fat from homemade soups or stews by chilling and removing the fat layer that rises to the top.
- Include olives and healthful fats, such as flaxseed oils, nuts, and avocados.
- Rely on mustard, salad greens, shredded carrots, tomato slices, sweet peppers, and red onions to add moisture to sandwiches rather than high-fat spreads.
- Top a baked potato with salsa and a dollop of fat-free Greek yogurt instead of butter or sour cream.
- Substitute two egg whites for one whole egg.
- Prepare broth-based chicken, vegetable, or bean-based soups rather than cream soups made with high-fat dairy products.
- Marinate leaner cuts of meat in lemon juice, flavored vinegars, or fruit juices.
- Sauté with olive oil instead of butter.
- Sprinkle slivered nuts, flaxseed, or sunflower seeds on salads instead of bacon bits.
- Choose a handful of nuts rather than chips or crackers.
- Place meat or poultry on a rack to allow the fat to drain.
- Steam, simmer, boil, broil, bake, grill, air fry, or microwave foods rather than frying them in oil.
- Use smaller servings of oil-based or low-fat salad dressings.
- Use whole-grain flours to enhance the flavor of baked goods made with less fat.
- Choose nonhydrogenated peanut butter or other nut-butter spreads on celery, banana, or rice or popcorn cakes.
- Add avocado slices rather than cheese to a salad or sandwich.

DENTAL CONSIDERATIONS

- Use Box 6.2 when determining fat recommendations.
- Interview the patient to evaluate fat intake within the context of their overall diet. Everyone needs adequate amounts of fat to provide EFAs and aid the absorption of fat-soluble vitamins. However, excess intake may lead to overweight and obesity that is a risk factor for many chronic health conditions.
- Assess patients' intake of dairy and meat products; they frequently consume more fat than they realize because of the inherent "hidden" fats. Foods having a higher fat content are more calorie dense. For example, 1 oz of peanuts and 45 medium-size baby carrots have the same number of calories (160 cal). Carrots have only a trace of fat; peanuts contain 14 g of fat per 1 oz (28 g). Knowledge of fat content in food is necessary to assess fat intake.
- Have patients read a Nutrition Facts label to determine whether the product is a healthy choice with regard to fat.
- Foods such as nuts and certain cheeses (cheddar, Monterey Jack, Swiss) may protect teeth against acid attack, especially when consumed after fermentable carbohydrates.[36,37] Even though they are generally considered nutritious foods, they have a relatively high-fat content and may not be appropriate for all people.
- Teach patients to read labels and understand that the percentage of fat should be determined based on the total calories, not the weight of the food. To determine fat content, use either of the following formulas:
  - Grams of fat×9=calories provided by fat, or
  - Calories of fat÷total calories of the product×100=% fat content of the product.
- Encourage intake of fruits and vegetables, whole-grain foods, and low-fat dairy products, and discourage intake of fatty meats, fried foods, and processed foods that are low in fiber and high in saturated and *trans* fats.

NUTRITIONAL DIRECTIONS

- Butter contains more saturated and *trans* fats along with cholesterol than most margarines.
- Purchase processed foods that contain more PUFAs and MUFAs than SFAs. If the food label only lists the total fat, saturated fat, and *trans* fat content, subtract the total number of grams of saturated fat and *trans* fat from the total fat. For example, if the product contains 8 g of fat with 2 g of saturated fat and 1 g of *trans* fat, the 5 g of MUFAs and PUFAs is more than the 3 g of saturated and *trans* fats. This product is acceptable, but if there is another similar product that contains less than 3 g of saturated and *trans* fats, that product would be a wiser choice.
- Fully hydrogenated fats contain almost no *trans* fats.
- Tropical oils—including palm, palm kernel, and coconut oils—have high levels of saturated fats and their consumption should be limited. Tropical oils raise total cholesterol levels, but their effect on the risk for CVD[38] remains unclear.
- Fruits, vegetables, and whole-grain foods are good choices to replace high-fat foods.
- A few fruits and vegetables (plants) contain a small amount of fat (actually considered an oil). Bananas contain a trace of fat (0.55 g or 0.5% fat by weight and 6% of the calories); avocados contain 31 g of fat (15% by weight and 86% of the calories). Over 75% of the fat in avocados is MUFA with a small amount being PUFA. Both bananas and avocados are good sources of several vitamins and minerals.
- Increasing intake of dietary sources of omega-3 fatty acids is recommended versus taking supplements.
- Fats and oils (100% fat) are necessary to provide adequate EFAs and fat-soluble vitamins; fat consumption is averaged over time, such as the day or week, to avoid exceeding the maximum intake of 35% fat.
- Children younger than 2 years of age grow rapidly; fat restriction is potentially unsafe for this age group because of uncertainties about the amounts of energy, cholesterol, and EFAs required for growth. After age 6 months, the *Dietary Guidelines* are applicable.[2]

of these products is encouraged for everyone. Loin (sirloin, tenderloin, or center loin) and round cuts (top, bottom, eye, or tip) and lean or extra-lean ground beef contain the least amount of fat. More important than the fat content of any product is the SFA content and relationship to CVD.

Overconsumption and Health-Related Problems

Some conditions related to fat intake are encountered in patients seen in dental hygiene practice. The following conditions may suggest alteration of the type or possibly the amount of dietary fat: obesity, diabetes mellitus, hyperlipidemia (elevated concentrations of any or all of the blood lipids, especially triglycerides and LDL cholesterol), fatty infiltration of the liver, and certain types of cancer.

Obesity

Excessive fat stores are a common disorder in the United States (as discussed in Chapter 1, *Health Application 1*). Although the cause is usually overconsumption of all energy nutrients, calories from fat are concentrated, therefore small amounts can rapidly increase calorie intake.

Blood Lipid Levels

Hyperlipidemia (elevated blood lipids) along with other risk factors is associated with CVD.[39] Many factors can affect blood lipid levels; the strongest dietary determinants of blood cholesterol are saturated and *trans* fats. Reduction of total dietary fat content helps to reduce saturated fat content. Decreasing saturated fat intake reduces cardiovascular events by 17%.[40] There is moderate quality evidence to encourage PUFAs to reduce the risk of CVD.[40] Evidence suggests that medium-chain fatty acids like lauric acid may have a neutral effect on CVD risk, but more research is needed to establish this conclusion.[41]

Since the FDA regulations banned *trans* fats coming from processed foods, a new industrial process called interesterified fats is being used in the food industry. Highly saturated fats like stearic and palmitic acid are blended with oils to produce fats with intermediate characteristics. Early research on the health effects of interesterified fats suggests that they did not seem to affect blood lipids, but more research is needed to identify their effect on CVD risk.[42] Factors and dietary modifications influencing serum lipid levels are discussed in more detail in *Health Application 6*.

Coconut oil recently has been touted as being "near miraculous," protecting against preventing the heart disease and melting away excess body fat. Despite all the hype, these claims—especially for improving conditions such as dementia, Alzheimer disease, autism, cancer, diabetes, or thyroid dysfunction—have not been supported by large, well-controlled human studies published in peer-reviewed journals demonstrating their health benefits.[43] Coconut oil, containing 60% medium-chain triglycerides, is a solid at room temperature and does not deteriorate rapidly. Natural coconut products and virgin coconut oil affect blood lipid levels differently even though they contain the same saturated fats. More importantly, SFAs in processed coconut oil (refined, bleached, and deodorized) are shown to increase total and LDL cholesterol (unhealthy) as well as HDL levels (beneficial).[44] However, epidemiologic studies with indigenous populations that consume coconut flesh or coconut cream as part of a traditional diet have found low rates of CVD.[45] The difference may be the unprocessed form of coconut along with a high fiber diet low in added sugar among these populations. One tablespoon of virgin coconut oil contains 13.6 g of saturated fat, contributing a significant portion of the recommended total daily saturated fat limit of less than 7% of energy. Thus it must be used sparingly, especially by patients who would benefit from reductions in total and LDL-cholesterol levels.

Cancer

A large portion of deaths caused by cancer in the United States each year can be attributed to diet and physical inactivity. Research continues to examine whether the association between high-fat diets and various cancers is attributable to the total amount of fat, the particular type of fat, the calories contributed by fat, or some other factor associated with high-fat foods. Saturated fat and PUFA intake have not been associated with an increased risk for breast cancer, however, increased intake of MUFAs may reduce risk.[46] However, we know that fatty acids are consumed within the context of the diet and dietary patterns higher in saturated fat, red meat, and processed meats are associated with a higher risk of cancer.[47] Thus experts agree that it is best to limit total fat intake by increasing the consumption of fish and lean meat, fruits, vegetables, and whole-grain products while decreasing high-fat meats and foods, especially those high in saturated fats. These are important concepts of the Mediterranean Diet that have been shown to reduce the risk of postmenopausal breast cancer.[48]

🦷 DENTAL CONSIDERATIONS

- Inquire about a family history of CVD and other risks associated with heart disease such as high blood pressure, diabetes, and cholesterol level.
- Teach patients to read Nutrition Facts label to identify saturated fat content to encourage healthier choices.
- Guide patients toward a whole food–based diet that focuses on the food choices proven to have health benefits.
- Coconut oil cannot be assumed to have the same health effects as other oils, and should not replace other plant oils.
- Coconut oil is not low in calories nor can it be considered a healthy food (does not contain less than 15% of calories from fat).

🦷 NUTRITIONAL DIRECTIONS

- Ten percent of total calorie intake should be from linoleic acid. Serum cholesterol can be reduced by increasing intake of MUFAs and PUFAs (see Table 6.1 and Fig. 6.5).
- Limit dietary cholesterol intake to around 300 mg daily by limiting high-fat meats and whole milk and cheese.
- "Low cholesterol" on a food label can be misleading. A cholesterol-free product, such as stick margarine, can still be high in SFAs that elevates blood cholesterol.
- Choosing foods containing soluble fibers may decrease serum cholesterol.
- Wise food choices to prevent heart disease include unsaturated fats found in liquid vegetable oils, nuts, and seeds; and omega-3 unsaturated fats from fatty fish, such as salmon, sardines, and shellfish.
- Interesterified fat may be listed on food labels as fully hydrogenated oil.

Underconsumption and Health-Related Problems

Overconsumption of fat is a primary concern in health care, whereas underconsumption of fats is rare in the United States. However, clinical symptoms of fat deficiency may occur, especially in patients with malabsorption syndromes such as cystic fibrosis. EFA deficiency results in poor growth, dermatitis, reduced resistance to infection, and poor reproductive capacity.

When overall food intake, including fats, is poor, patients lose weight, depleting subcutaneous fat stores needed to maintain body temperature. Patients with anorexia nervosa are of special concern (see Chapter 17).

🦷 DENTAL CONSIDERATIONS

- If a patient appears underweight with a BMI below 18.5, it may indicate low amounts of subcutaneous fat and these patients may be unable to regulate body temperature.
- A patient with inadequate fat intake is thin, has dry skin and dull hair, and is sensitive to cold temperatures. If these signs and symptoms are noted, suggest an examination by a health care provider.

🦷 NUTRITIONAL DIRECTION

- Although much attention is given to the problems with fat consumption, fats have important physiologic functions, therefore a certain amount of fat must be provided in the diet.

Fat Replacers

As a result of health concerns regarding dietary fats, numerous foods are being manufactured containing less fat. Fat replacers may be helpful in reducing fat and energy consumption. Most of the formulations to replace fat are carbohydrate and protein based, but lipid-based materials are available. Each of these fat replacers possess diverse sensory, functional, and physiologic properties that affect their incorporation into various types of products (Table 6.5). Low-calorie salad dressing, low-fat yogurt, and imitation margarine are made by using modified starches and gums to reduce oil or fat in a product.

By substituting fat replacers for fats, total fat intake can be reduced, and some weight loss may be achieved. However, an overall attention to portion size, making healthy choices, and physical activity are needed to achieve a healthy weight. By consuming large portions of lower fat products, an individual can potentially negate the calorie and fat savings of the replacement foods. Fat substitutes seem to pose little risk to health, but data are sparse regarding possible benefits under conditions of normal consumer use.

DENTAL CONSIDERATIONS

- Assess the use of fat replacers.
- Evaluate overall dietary habits because a patient may think that using fat replacers will make a desirable change in health without considering other aspects of the diet.
- If a patient exhibits symptoms such as gastrointestinal distress after consuming a product containing a fat substitute, recommend avoidance of that fat substitute.

NUTRITIONAL DIRECTIONS

- Patients allergic to eggs or cow's milk could be at risk for an allergic reaction to Simplesse because it is made from egg white and milk protein.
- Intake of fat replacers needs to be balanced with variety and moderation in food choices to achieve an overall healthy, nutritious diet.

TABLE 6.5   Fat Replacers

Generic Name (Trade Name)	kcal/g	Appropriate Uses
Carbohydrate Based		
Cellulose	0	Dairy-type products, sauces, frozen desserts, salad dressings
Dextrins	4	Salad dressings, puddings, spreads, dairy-type products, frozen desserts
Fiber	0	Baked goods, meats, spreads, extruded products
Gums	0	Salad dressings, desserts, processed meats
Inulin	1–1.2	Yogurt, cheese, frozen desserts, baked goods, icings, fillings, whipped cream, dairy products, fiber supplements, processed meats
Maltodextrin	4	Baked goods, dairy products, salad dressings, spreads, sauces, frostings, fillings, processed meats, frozen desserts
Nu-Trim	4	Baked goods, milk, cheese, ice cream
Oatrim	1–4	Baked goods, fillings and frostings, frozen desserts, dairy beverages, cheese, salad dressings, processed meats, confections
Polydextrose	1	Baked goods, chewing gums, confections, salad dressings, frozen dairy desserts, gelatins, puddings
Polyols	1.6–3	Bulking agent
Starch and modified food starch	1–4	Processed meats, salad dressings, baked goods, fillings and frostings, sauces, condiments, frozen desserts, dairy products
Z-Trim	0	Baked goods, burgers, hot dogs, cheese, ice cream, yogurt
Protein-based		
Microparticulated whey protein (simplesse)	1–2	Dairy products (e.g., ice cream, butter, sour cream, cheese, yogurt), salad dressings, margarine- and mayonnaise-type products, baked goods, coffee creamers, soups, sauces
Modified whey protein concentrate		Milk and dairy products (e.g., cheese, yogurt, sour cream, ice cream), baked goods, frostings, salad dressings, mayonnaise-type products
Fat Based		
Emulsifiers	9	Cake mixes, cookies, icings, vegetable dairy products
EPG[a]		Formulated products, baking and frying
Salatrim	5	Confections, baked goods, dairy products
Sorbestrin[a]	1.5	Fried foods, salad dressings, mayonnaise, baked goods
Modified plant-based oil (Epogee)	1	Chocolate candies, nut butters, nutrition bars, plant-based proteins, meal replacement beverages, frozen dairy products

[a]May require United States Food and Drug Administration approval.
EPG, Esterified propoxylated glycerol.
Data from Calorie Control Council. *Glossary of Fat Replacers*. Calorie Control Council; 2023. http://www.caloriecontrol.org/glossary-of-fat-replacers/.

Hyperlipidemia

Despite years of research and copious studies, CVD is still a major concern in the United States. Costs for CVD are expected to double from $555 billion in 2016 to $1.1 trillion in 2035.[49] *Healthy People 2020* established 50 objectives for heart disease and stroke. CVDs include hypertension, heart disease, stroke, congenital cardiovascular defects, myocardial ischemia, congestive heart failure, and many other anomalies. Dietary issues were addressed, that is, obesity and types of fats consumed. CVD prevalence in the United States has declined overall;[50] mortality has decreased because of improvements in treatment and a reduction in risk factors. One of the *Healthy People 2030* objectives to lower the rate of deaths from heart disease from 90.0 per 100,000 in 2021 shows improvement from 2018 when the rate was 90.9 per 100,000, but has not reached the target of 71.1 per 100,000.[51] The most common kind of CVD is coronary atherosclerosis, the leading cause of death in the United States. Heart disease remains the number one leading cause, and stroke is the fifth leading cause of death.[52]

Hyperlipidemia, or increased plasma cholesterol and LDL levels, appears to be a major risk factor for CVD. The American Heart Association and American College of Cardiology routinely re-evaluate guidelines and update recommendations for health care professionals to help prevent CVD. Continual scientific research provides more information allowing refinement of recommendations on detection and management of established risk factors, including evidence of the safety and efficacy of interventions previously considered promising. The leading risk factor for death and disability is poor diet quality globally, which contributed to 11 million deaths in 2017.[53] Most CVDs are preventable through the adoption of healthy diet and lifestyles, basically adhering to the *Dietary Guidelines* and choosing more fruits and vegetables, nuts/seeds, whole grains, and seafood, and reducing sodium intake.

The AHA and American College of Cardiology encourage a fasting lipoprotein profile screening (total cholesterol, LDL and HDL cholesterol, and triglycerides) for all adults older than age 20 years every 5 years along with an assessment of risk factors. More than 93.9 million Americans over age 20 years have total cholesterol levels greater than 200 mg/dL and almost 28 million greater than or equal to 240 mg/dL.[54] Average blood cholesterol values have declined since about 1960. LDL levels less than 100 mg/dL throughout life are associated with a very low risk for CVD; LDL greater than 100 mg/dL is the primary target of therapy. Reducing LDL cholesterol at early stages produces favorable outcomes for coronary lesions and reduces the likelihood of acute coronary syndromes.[54] Table 6.6 shows levels that are considered desirable or optimal. Higher levels of HDL have been thought to be a protective factor for CVD, however, many other factors need to be considered. The AHA recommends *Life's Essential 8* to support heart health including: physical activity; avoiding tobacco/nicotine use; healthy diet choices; reaching and maintaining a healthy weight; adequate sleep; and maintaining cholesterol, blood pressure, and glucose at or below normal levels.[54,55] Patients could go to AHA's My Life Check https://mlc.heart.org/ for their "heart score." This might be something a clinician could include in the nutrition assessment for their patient.

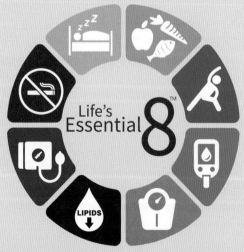

• Life's Essential 8 (From https://www.heart.org/en/healthy-living/healthy-lifestyle/lifes-essential-8)

Beginning in 1988, the National Heart, Lung, and Blood Institute introduced two diets designed to lower blood cholesterol based on the individual's lipoprotein profile. AHA currently supports a healthy diet consistent with a DASH-type eating plan (Box 6.4).[54] Maintaining a healthy diet and lifestyle offers the greatest potential for reducing the risk of CVD in the general public.

Specific dietary recommendations are similar to those mentioned in Box 6.3. Natural food sources generally are recommended for nutrients rather than supplements. Other diets and lifestyle changes recommended in the *Dietary Guidelines* include the Mediterranean diet which promotes vegetables, monounsaturated fats, nuts (Fig. 6.7), healthy vegetarian (plant-based) dietary pattern, and Dietary Approaches to Stop Hypertension (DASH) eating pattern (see Chapter 12). All of these dietary patterns may reduce the risk of CVD and have benefits for overall health.[56–58]

Many other dietary factors have been proposed to help reduce the risk of CVD. Some of these are generally unproven or have uncertain effects on CVD. Although naturally occurring antioxidants in foods seem to prevent CVD, vitamin and mineral supplements are inconclusive and have not shown major benefits in CVD prevention.[59] Phytochemicals found in fruits and vegetables may be important in reducing the risk of atherosclerosis. Foods containing antioxidants from a variety of fruits and vegetables, whole grains, and vegetable oils, and spices such as turmeric, garlic, and cinnamon, are recommended. Until more is known about the mode of action of these compounds, the most prudent practice to ensure optimum consumption of bioactive compounds is by increasing intake of fruits and vegetables and replacing salt with spices.

Plant sterols (also called phytosterols) are bioactive compounds found in all vegetable foods, which inhibit cholesterol absorption. Small quantities of sterols are present in a variety of foods, including fruits, vegetables, nuts, seeds, cereals, and legumes. Consumption of soy protein–rich foods, a source of plant sterols, may indirectly reduce CVD risk if they replace products containing saturated fat and cholesterol. Plant sterols may lower LDL-C up to 12%.[60] In the United States, sterols are added to margarine spread, orange juice, and other products. Plant sterols need to be in combination with a healthy diet and physical activity.

The AHA recommends patients without CVD eat a variety of fish, preferably fatty fish, at least twice a week. Some individuals who already have CVD may be advised to consume at least 1 g of EPA and DHA daily, preferably from fatty fish. Fish oil supplement purity is unknown so primary care providers may recommend a prescription form of purified EPA. Of all the dietary changes recommended, cholesterol intake probably has the least effect on plasma cholesterol concentrations in most individuals because of less endogenous cholesterol production in response to cholesterol absorption. Consuming one large egg daily with less than 200 mg cholesterol does not increase risk for CVD. AHA recommendations do not limit the number of eggs as long as total dietary cholesterol is about 300 mg/day.[61] However, the *Dietary Guidelines* no longer provide a specific target for dietary cholesterol and instead recommend healthy eating patterns to reduce total dietary fat that also reduce dietary cholesterol intake. However, a low-cholesterol, low-fat diet only modestly reduces total and LDL cholesterol so medications may be needed to reach blood lipids targets to reduced risk for CVD.[62] By replacing some SFAs with MUFAs and some PUFAs, and decreasing total fat, LDL can be lowered without decreasing HDL concentrations. These changes result in a more palatable diet that is better received by Americans.

Because of Americans' high intake of added sugars, which exceeds discretionary calorie allowances, especially in the form of sugar-containing beverages, concurrent with the *Dietary Guidelines*, the AHA recommends reducing added sugar intake.[2] A high intake of refined carbohydrates negatively affects lipid profile (decreases HDL, increases triglyceride and LDL).[63] A prudent upper limit of the discretionary calorie allowance from added sugars is 140 cal for an 1800-cal diet and 250 cal for a 2200-cal diet, consistent with the United States-Style Dietary Pattern.[2]

One of the most important factors in decreasing the risk of CVD is the types of foods chosen to replace saturated fat intake. When a decrease in saturated fats is recommended, suggestions should be made regarding what types of foods/fats should be chosen to replace those calories. Overall dietary quality includes (1) carbohydrate quality (whole vs refined grains, and dietary fiber); (2) intake of specific individual fatty acids; (3) inclusion of a variety of healthful foods such as fruits, vegetables, nuts, fish, dairy products, and vegetable oils; (4) limited amounts of added sugars and processed meats and foods; and (5) energy balance. Recommendations will continue to change as research leads to knowledge about the effects of specific fatty acids on lipid profiles and CVD.

TABLE 6.6 Desirable/Optimal Blood Lipid Levels

Lipid	Desirable/Optimal Level (mg/dL)
Total cholesterol	<200
LDL	<100
HDL	40 (men) >50 (females)
Triglyceride	<150

Data from Grundy SM, Stone NJ, Bailey AL, Beam C, Birtcher KK, Blumenthal RS, et al. 2018 AHA/ACC/AACVPR/AAPA/ABC/ACPM/ADA/AGS/APhA/ASPC/NLA/PCNA guideline on the management of blood cholesterol: a report of the American College of Cardiology/American Heart Association Task Force on Clinical Practice Guidelines. *Circulation.* 2019;139(25):e1082–e1143; Centers for Disease Control. *What is Cholesterol?* 2022. https://www.cdc.gov/cholesterol/about.htm#optimal. *HDL*, High-density lipoprotein; *LDL*, low-density lipoprotein.

• BOX 6.4 Lifestyle Management Guidelines

The optimal goal for all Americans, regardless of risk for CVD, is to follow these recommendations:

- Consume a dietary pattern that emphasizes intake of vegetables, fruits, and whole grains; this includes low-fat dairy products, poultry, fish, legumes, nontropical vegetable oils and nuts; and limits intake of added sugars, sodium, processed foods, and red meats.
  - Adapt this dietary pattern to appropriate calorie requirements, personal and cultural food preferences, and nutrition therapy for other medical conditions (including diabetes mellitus).
  - Achieve this pattern by following plans such as the Mediterranean pattern, DASH dietary pattern, and the USDA MyPlate.
- Reduce the percentage of calories from saturated fat.
- Avoid tobacco, nicotine, and secondhand smoke.
- Engage in aerobic physical activity of moderate to vigorous intensity for at least 150 min/week.

Data from American Heart Association. *The American Heart Association Diet and Lifestyle Recommendations.* 2021. https://www.heart.org/en/healthy-living/healthy-eating/eat-smart/nutrition-basics/aha-diet-and-lifestyle-recommendations.

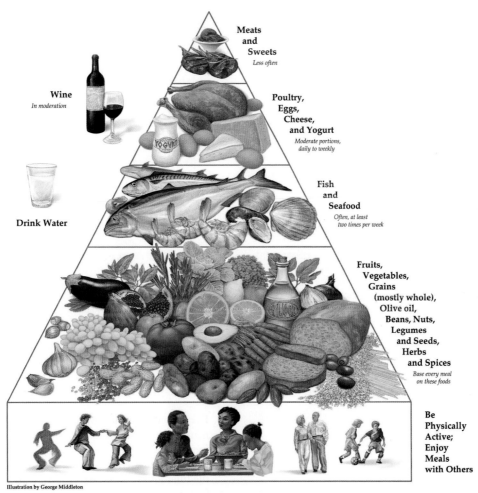

Mediterranean Diet Pyramid
A contemporary approach to delicious, healthy eating

Meats and Sweets
Less often

Wine
In moderation

Poultry, Eggs, Cheese, and Yogurt
Moderate portions, daily to weekly

Drink Water

Fish and Seafood
Often, at least two times per week

Fruits, Vegetables, Grains (mostly whole), Olive oil, Beans, Nuts, Legumes and Seeds, Herbs and Spices
Base every meal on these foods

Be Physically Active; Enjoy Meals with Others

Illustration by George Middleton

© 2009 Oldways Preservation and Exchange Trust • www.oldwayspt.org

• **Fig. 6.7** Mediterranean Diet Pyramid. The Traditional Healthy Mediterranean Diet Pyramid. Courtesy Oldways Preservation and Exchange Trust. http://www.oldwayspt.org.

◆ CASE APPLICATION FOR THE DENTAL HYGIENIST

A 50-year-old patient complains to his dental hygienist that he has recently been having chest pain. A recent testing at his grocery store indicated his blood cholesterol level to be elevated. A health care provider told him several years ago that his cholesterol was slightly elevated and that he probably should lower his fat intake. No formal medical nutrition treatment was ordered and no follow-up work has been done. His blood pressure is 145/90 mm Hg.

He continues to eat anything he wants. He realizes that some foods are high in fat and should be avoided, but he is unable to identify these foods. When questioned about fat requirements and different types of fat, he says that he does not understand all of those big medical terms. He also indicates that his parents ate what they wanted without all these problems and concerns.

Nutritional Assessment

- Readiness/willingness to change
- Knowledge level concerning fat principles and how these relate to his overall health
- Total amount of fat intake
- Typical foods eaten
- Type of dietary habits: who purchases and prepares the food, where he lives, and where most meals are eaten
- Food preferences
- Blood pressure
- Serum lipids, if known
- Family medical history (if parents are still alive, if not, cause of death)

Nutritional Diagnosis

Lack of regular medical care; low health literacy; lack of nutrition knowledge; and how diet relates to the condition that places patient at increased risk for CVD.

Nutritional Goals

The patient will identify and implement strategies to reduce total and saturated fat in his diet; be able to list healthy choices lower in fat that will fit in his diet; and be able to describe the effect of diet changes on his cholesterol.

Nutritional Implementation

Intervention: Emphasize the importance of having a thorough examination annually by a health care provider and a confirmation of laboratory work with a complete fasting lipid profile.

Rationale: Dietary changes and lifestyle changes are probably indicated; however, the best individuals to diagnose and prescribe treatment are a health care provider and RDN.

Intervention: Explain how diet and lifestyle affect his condition focusing on the AHA Life's Essential 8: (1) make healthy food choices with whole grains, lean meats, vegetables, fruit, and lower fat dairy products; (2) be more physically active; (3) if overweight, modest weight loss can help reduce blood pressure and CVD risk; (4) tobacco cessation to reduce the risk of heart disease; and (5) adequate sleep. If the patient is technology savvy, direct them to the AHA website https://www.heart.org/en/healthy-living/healthy-lifestyle/lifes-essential-8 for more information.

Rationale: When patient is ready for change, health literacy and intention to make behavioral change support success.

Intervention: Explain the difference between dietary fats such as PUFAs and SFAs and create a list of foods low in SFA along with sources of PUFAs in collaboration with the patient.

Rationale: Educating patient and identifying healthy options from his preferred foods may help reduce the risk for CVD.

Intervention: Teach the patient how to read nutrition labels (use an actual food label for teaching); use a margarine brand that lists the first ingredient as liquid oil: (1) identify the total and SFA along with cholesterol in the food; (2) explain AHA recommendation to limit daily cholesterol intake to 300 mg or less; and (3) explain how the fat percentage in a food identifies it as being lower in fat (see Box 1.4).

Rationale: Educating the patient on reading food labels may aid in making healthy choices and reduce serum cholesterol levels to help reduce the risk for CVD.

Intervention: Inquire at each recare appointment about progress on making lifestyle changes and monitoring of blood lipid levels to support patient in making long-term change.

Rationale: Seeing evidence of improvement can provide motivation for compliance.

Intervention: Monitor blood pressure values at each recare appointment. Inform the patient that hypertension is another risk factor for heart disease and both are associated with periodontal disease. Refer to the health care provider for elevated values.

Rationale: If the patient is aware of his blood pressure and the harmful effects of blood pressure elevation, he may make lifestyle modifications to improve his overall health and reduce not only blood pressure, but also the risk for CVD.

Intervention: Discuss ways the patient can decrease the amount of dietary fat and saturated fats: advise him to (1) eat smaller servings of meat; (2) trim visible fat from meats; (3) choose lean meats, skinless poultry, and fatty fish; (4) avoid fried foods; and (5) use less salad dressing, change the type of fat (use olive oil), or reduce the amount of fat in the salad dressing (fat free or low fat).

Rationale: These all are ways to decrease fat intake, thereby decreasing the progression of atherosclerosis. The use of more fish increases intake of omega-3 fatty acids.

Evaluation

Evaluation includes making an appointment with the primary care provider and following through with assessment of blood lipids and blood pressure, this is the first step in addressing the patient's overall health. Ideally the dental hygiene nutrition counseling with the patient to identify strategies to reduce fat and saturated fat intake, results in the patient beginning to make better healthy food choices. Progress needs to be celebrated at each appointment. In addition, attention to lifestyle modifications to increase physical activity and setting a quit date for tobacco cessation should be revisited at each visit to provide ongoing support. Outcomes may include improvement in (1) blood cholesterol, (2) blood pressure is within normal values, and (3) the patient has begun a tobacco cessation program.

◆ Student Readiness

1. Describe the following terms: lipoproteins, hyperlipidemia, structural lipids, and EFA.
2. A patient wants to know which foods to consume to (1) increase PUFAs, (2) increase MUFAs, and (3) decrease SFAs. Name three sources of each.
3. In observing physical properties of fats, how could you estimate the polyunsaturated and saturated fat content of a food?
4. What unsaturated fatty acid is essential in the diet? What are the functions of unsaturated fatty acids in the body?
5. Compare the Nutrition Facts labels of three brands of stick margarine, three brands of tub margarine, two brands of diet margarine, and two brands of spray margarine. How do they

differ in their polyunsaturated-to-saturated fat ratio? List the first ingredient of each.

6. Describe the functions of fat in the diet.

7. Evaluate one day of your intake for types of foods consumed and amounts of cholesterol, trans fatty acid, and saturated fat. If that day represented your average cholesterol and saturated fat intake over an extended period, determine whether the cholesterol or saturated fat content of intake should be reduced. List some simple, realistic suggestions for decreasing their intake.

8. Describe the role of cholesterol in the body.

9. Calculate the caloric value of the following items:
   2 slices bacon (8 g of fat, 4 g of protein)
   1 tbsp margarine (12 g of fat)
   1 tbsp whipped margarine (8 g of fat)
   1 tbsp mayonnaise (6 g of fat)
   1 tbsp lard (13 g of fat)

10. Calculate the grams of fat a patient could consume on (1) a 1500-cal diet and (2) a 2000-cal diet to meet the *Dietary Guidelines*.

11. List five points you think a patient should know about fats in general.

References

1. Shan Z, Rehm CD, Rogers G, et al. Trends in dietary carbohydrate, protein, and fat intake and diet quality among United States adults, 1999–2016. *JAMA*. 2019;322(12):1178–1187.

2. United States Department of Agriculture and U.S. Department of Health and Human Services. *Dietary Guidelines for Americans*. 9th ed. 2020. dietaryguidelines.gov

3. Schönfeld P, Wojtczak L. Short- and medium-chain fatty acids in energy metabolism: the cellular perspective. *J Lipid Res*. 2016;57(6):943–954.

4. Anada R, Hara ES, Nagaoka N, Okada M, Kamioka H, Matsumoto T. Important roles of odontoblast membrane phospholipids in early dentin mineralization. *J Mater Chem B*. 2023;11:657–666.

5. Mattiuzzi C, Sanchis-Gomar F, Lippi G. Worldwide burden of LDL cholesterol: implications in cardiovascular disease. *Nutr Metab Cardiovasc Dis*. 2020;30(2):241–244. https://doi.org/10.1016/j.numecd.2019.09.008.

6. Zhou X, Shen Y, Parker JK, Kennedy OB, Methven L. Relative effects of sensory modalities and importance of fatty acid sensitivity on fat perception in a real food model. *Chemosens Percept*. 2016;9:105–119.

7. Linus Pauling Institute. *Essential Fatty Acids*. Linus Pauling Institute; 2019. https://lpi.oregonstate.edu/mic/other-nutrients/essential-fatty-acids.

8. Abdelhamid AS, Brown TJ, Brainard JS, et al. Omega-3 fatty acids for the primary and secondary prevention of cardiovascular disease. *Cochrane Database Syst Rev*. 2018;7(7):CD003177.

9. Zhang B, Xiong K, Cai J, Ma A. Fish consumption and coronary heart disease: a *meta*-analysis. *Nutrients*. 2020;12(8):2278.

10. Giacaman RA, Jobet-Vila P, Muñoz-Sandoval C. Fatty acid effect on sucrose-induced enamel demineralization and cariogenicity of an experimental biofilm-caries model. *Odontology*. 2015;103(2):169–176.

11. Giacaman RA, Valenzuela-Ramos R, Muñoz-Sandoval C. In situ anticariogenic activity of free fatty acids after sucrose exposure to oral biofilms formed on enamel. *Am J Dent*. 2016;29(2):81–86.

12. Huang R, Li M, Gregory RL. Bacterial interactions in dental biofilm. *Virulence*. 2011;2(5):435–444. https://doi.org/10.4161/viru.2.5.16140.

13. McGown EL, Kolstad DL, Suttie JW. Effect of dietary fat on fluoride absorption and tissue fluoride retention in rats. *J Nutr*. 1976;106(4):575–579.

14. Castro Dos Santos NC, Furukawa MV, Oliveira-Cardoso I, et al. Does the use of omega-3 fatty acids as an adjunct to non-surgical periodontal therapy provide additional benefits in the treatment of periodontitis? A systematic review and *meta*-analysis. *J Periodontal Res*. 2022;57(3):435–447.

15. Chatterjee D, Chatterjee A, Kalra D, Kapoor A, Vijay S, Jain S. Role of adjunct use of omega 3 fatty acids in periodontal therapy of periodontitis. A systematic review and *meta*-analysis. *J Oral Biol Craniofac Res*. 2022;12(1):55–62.

16. Heo H, Bae JH, Amano A, Park T, Choi YH. Supplemental or dietary intake of omega-3 fatty acids for the treatment of periodontitis: a *meta*-analysis. *J Clin Periodontol*. 2022;49(4):362–377.

17. Varela-López A, Giampieri F, Bullón P, Battino M, Quiles JL. Role of lipids in the onset, progression and treatment of periodontal disease. A systematic review of studies in humans. *Int J Mol Sci*. 2016;17(8):1202.

18. Mazidi M, Shekoohi N, Katsiki N, Banach M. Omega-6 fatty acids and the risk of cardiovascular disease: insights from a systematic review and *meta*-analysis of randomized controlled trials and a Mendelian randomization study. *Arch Med Sci*. 2022;18(2):466–479.

19. Adili R, Hawley M, Holinstat M. Regulation of platelet function and thrombosis by omega-3 and omega-6 polyunsaturated fatty acids. *Prostaglandins Other Lipid Mediat*. 2018;139:10–18.

20. Ulven SM, Holven KB. Comparison of bioavailability of krill oil versus fish oil and health effect. *Vasc Health Risk Manag*. 2015;11:511–524. https://doi.org/10.2147/VHRM.S85165.

21. Environmental Protection Agency, Food and Drug Administration. Stay Healthy by Eating Fish and Shellfish Wisely. 2022. https://www.epa.gov/choose-fish-and-shellfish-wisely/stay-healthy-eating-fish-and-shellfish-wisely.

22. World Health Organization. *Healthy Diet: Key Facts*. https://www.who.int/news-room/fact-sheets/detail/healthy-diet.

23. Li Y, Hruby A, Bernstein AM, et al. Saturated fats compared with unsaturated fats and sources of carbohydrates in relation to risk of coronary heart disease: a prospective cohort study. *J Am Coll Cardiol*. 2015;66(14):1538–1548.

24. DiNicolantonio JJ, Lucan SC, O'Keefe JH. The evidence for saturated fat and for sugar related to coronary heart disease. *Prog Cardiovasc Dis*. 2016;58(5):464–472.

25. Statista. *United States Edible Oils Consumption Per Capita 2014–2027*. Statista. https://www.statista.com/forecasts/1291634/edible-oils-market-per-capita-consumption-united-states.

26. Flock MR, Harris WS, Kris-Etherton PM. Long-chain omega-3 fatty acids: time to establish a dietary reference intake. *Nutr Rev*. 2013;71(10):692–707.

27. Zhang Z, Fulgoni VL, Kris-Etherton PM, Mitmesser SH. Dietary intakes of EPA and DHA omega-3 fatty acids among United States childbearing-age and pregnant women: an analysis of NHANES 2001–2014. *Nutrients*. 2018;10(4):416.

28. Thompson M, Hein N, Hanson C, et al. Omega-3 fatty acid intake by age, gender, and pregnancy status in the United States: National Health and Nutrition Examination Survey 2003–2014. *Nutrients*. 2019;11(1):177.

29. Orsavova J, Misurcova L, Vavra Ambrozova J, Vicha R, Mlcek J. Fatty acids composition of vegetable oils and its contribution to dietary energy intake and dependence of cardiovascular mortality on dietary intake of fatty acids. *Int J Mol Sci*. 2015;16(6):12871–12890.

30. Statista. *U.S. Consumption of Edible Oils by Type 2022*. Statista. 2023. https://www.statista.com/statistics/301044/edible-oils-consumption-united-states-by-type/.

31. American Heart Association. *Fish and Omega-3 Fatty Acids*. 2021. https://www.heart.org/en/healthy-living/healthy-eating/eat-smart/fats/fish-and-omega-3-fatty-acids.

32. Food and Drug Administration. *Trans Fat*. FDA. 2018. https://www.fda.gov/food/food-additives-petitions/final-determination-regarding-partially-hydrogenated-oils-removing-trans-fat.

33. World Health Organization. *REPLACE Trans Fat*. 2021. https://www.who.int/teams/nutrition-and-food-safety/replace-trans-fat.

34. Xu Z, McClure ST, Appel LJ. Dietary cholesterol intake and sources among U.S adults: results from National Health and Nutrition Examination Surveys (NHANES), 2001–2014. *Nutrients.* 2018;10(6):771.

35. Zhao B, Gan L, Graubard BI, Männistö S, Albanes D, Huang J. Associations of dietary cholesterol, serum cholesterol, and egg consumption with overall and cause-specific mortality: systematic review and updated *meta*-analysis. *Circulation.* 2022;145(20):1506–1520.

36. Lorenzini EC, Lazzari B, Tartaglia GM, et al. Oral ecological environment modifications by hard-cheese: from pH to microbiome: a prospective cohort study based on 16S rRNA metabarcoding approach. *J Transl Med.* 2022;20(1):312.

37. Kashket S, DePaola DP. Cheese consumption and the development and progression of dental caries. *Nutr Rev.* 2002;60(4):97–103.

38. Unhapipatpong C, Shantavasinkul PC, Kasemsup V, et al. Tropical oil consumption and cardiovascular disease: an umbrella review of systematic reviews and meta analyses. *Nutrients.* 2021;13(5):1549.

39. Alloubani A, Nimer R, Samara R. Relationship between hyperlipidemia, cardiovascular disease and stroke: a systematic review. *Curr Cardiol Rev.* 2021;17(6): e051121189015.

40. Hooper L, Martin N, Jimoh OF, Kirk C, Foster E, Abdelhamid AS. Reduction in saturated fat intake for cardiovascular disease. *Cochrane Database Syst Rev.* 2020;8(8):CD011737.

41. Perna M, Hewlings S. Saturated fatty acid chain length and risk of cardiovascular disease: a systematic review. *Nutrients.* 2022;15(1):30.

42. van Rooijen MA, Mensink RP. Palmitic acid versus stearic acid: effects of interesterification and intakes on cardiometabolic risk markers—a systematic review. *Nutrients.* 2020;12(3):615.

43. Sankararaman S, Sferra TJ. Are we going nuts on coconut oil? *Curr Nutr Rep.* 2018;7(3):107–115.

44. Neelakantan N, Seah JYH, van Dam RM. The effect of coconut oil consumption on cardiovascular risk factors. *Circulation.* 2020;141(10):803–814.

45. Eyres L, Eyres MF, Chisholm A, Brown RC. Coconut oil consumption and cardiovascular risk factors in humans. *Nutr Rev.* 2016;74(4):267–280.

46. Guo F, Wang M, Guo X, et al. The association between fatty acid intake and breast cancer based on the NHANES and Mendelian randomization study. *Cancer Epidemiol.* 2021;73:101966. https://doi.org/10.1016/j.canep.2021.101966.

47. Dandamudi A, Tommie J, Nommsen-Rivers L, Couch S. Dietary patterns and breast cancer risk: a systematic review. *Anticancer Res.* 2018;38(6):3209–3222.

48. van den Brandt PA, Schulpen M. Mediterranean diet adherence and risk of postmenopausal breast cancer: results of a cohort study and *meta*-analysis. *Int J Cancer.* 2017;140(10):2220–2231.

49. American Heart Association, American Stroke Association. *Cardiovascular Disease—A Costly Burden for America Projections Through 2035*; 2018:15. https://www.heart.org/-/media/Files/About-Us/Policy-Research/Fact-Sheets/Public-Health-Advocacy-and-Research/CVD-A-Costly-Burden-for-America-Projections-Through-2035.pdf.

50. Centers for Disease Control and Prevention, National Center for Health Statistics. *Heart Disease Prevalence—Health, United States 2020–2021.* 2022. https://www.cdc.gov/nchs/hus/topics/heart-disease-prevalence.htm.

51. United States Department of Health and Human Services, Office of Prevention and Health Promotion. *Healthy People 2030: Reduce Coronary Heart Disease Deaths.* https://survey.alchemer.com/s3/6526245/HP2030-Data-Survey.

52. Centers for Disease Control and Prevention. Leading Causes of Death. 2022. https://www.cdc.gov/nchs/fastats/leading-causes-of-death.htm.

53. Afshin A, Sur PJ, Fay KA, et al. Health effects of dietary risks in 195 countries, 1990–2017: a systematic analysis for the Global Burden of Disease Study 2017. *The Lancet.* 2019;393(10184):1958–1972. https://doi.org/10.1016/S0140-6736(19)30041-8.

54. Tsao CW, Aday AW, Almarzooq ZI, et al. Heart disease and stroke statistics-2022 update: a report from the American Heart Association. *Circulation.* 2022;145(8):e153–e639.

55. American Heart Association. *My Life Check®.* https://mlc.heart.org/.

56. Rosato V, Temple NJ, La Vecchia C, Castellan G, Tavani A, Guercio V. Mediterranean diet and cardiovascular disease: a systematic review and *meta*-analysis of observational studies. *Eur J Nutr.* 2019;58(1):173–191.

57. Jeong SY, Wee CC, Kovell LC, et al. Effects of diet on 10-year atherosclerotic cardiovascular disease risk (from the DASH trial). *Am J Cardiol.* 2023;187:10–17. https://doi.org/10.1016/j.amjcard.2022.10.019.

58. Gan ZH, Cheong HC, Tu YK, Kuo PH. Association between plant-based dietary patterns and risk of cardiovascular disease: a systematic review and *meta*-analysis of prospective cohort studies. *Nutrients.* 2021;13(11):3952.

59. O'Connor EA, Evans CV, Ivlev I, et al. Vitamin and mineral supplements for the primary prevention of cardiovascular disease and cancer: updated evidence report and systematic review for the United States Preventive Services Task Force. *JAMA.* 2022;327(23):2334–2347.

60. Turini E, Sarsale M, Petri D, et al. Efficacy of plant sterol-enriched food for primary prevention and treatment of hypercholesterolemia: a systematic literature review. *Foods.* 2022;11(6):839.

61. Carson JAS, Lichtenstein AH, Anderson CAM, et al. Dietary cholesterol and cardiovascular risk: a science advisory from the American Heart Association. *Circulation.* 2020;141(3):e39–e53.

62. Chawla S, Tessarolo Silva F, Amaral Medeiros S, Mekary RA, Radenkovic D. The effect of low-fat and low-carbohydrate diets on weight loss and lipid levels: a systematic review and *meta*-analysis. *Nutrients.* 2020;12(12):3774.

63. Marshall S, Petocz P, Duve E, et al. The effect of replacing refined grains with whole grains on cardiovascular risk factors: a systematic review and *meta*-analysis of randomized controlled trials with grade clinical recommendation. *J Acad Nutr Diet.* 2020;120(11):1859–1883.e31. https://doi.org/10.1016/j.jand.2020.06.021.

▶ Evolve Resources

Please visit http://evolve.elsevier.com/Mallonee/nutritional for additional practice and study support tools.

7

Use of the Energy Nutrients: Metabolism and Balance

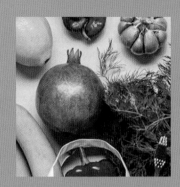

STUDENT LEARNING OBJECTIVES

On completion of this chapter, the student will be able to achieve the following learning outcomes:

1. Discuss the roles of the liver and the kidneys in metabolism. In addition, describe carbohydrate metabolism.
2. Discuss protein metabolism.
3. Discuss lipid metabolism, alcohol metabolism, metabolic relationships, and metabolic energy.
4. Identify factors affecting the basal metabolic rate.
5. Calculate energy needs according to a patient's weight and activities.
6. Discuss physiological and psychological factors affecting energy balance.

7. Discuss the following related to inadequate energy intake:
   - Summarize the effects of inadequate energy intake.
   - Explain the principles for and importance of regulating energy balance to a patient.
   - Individualize dental hygiene considerations to patients regarding energy metabolism.
   - Relate nutritional directions to meet patients' needs regarding energy metabolism.

KEY TERMS

Appetite
Basal energy expenditure
Basal metabolic rate (BMR)
Calorimeter
Catecholamines
Cofactor
Glycemic index

Glycogenesis
High-energy phosphate compounds
Hunger
Indirect calorimetry
Ketoacidosis
Ketonuria
Kilocalorie (kcal)

Lipolysis
Normoglycemic
Pedometer
Postabsorptive state
Renal failure
Thermic effect

TEST YOUR NQ

1. **T/F** Insulin is a hormone that decreases blood glucose levels.
2. **T/F** Even during sleep, the body requires energy.
3. **T/F** BMR stands for BMR.
4. **T/F** A malnourished patient would have a low BMR.
5. **T/F** The hypothalamus controls hunger and satiety.
6. **T/F** Hunger is the same as appetite.

7. **T/F** Fats are a good source of quick energy.
8. **T/F** The kidneys play an important role in maintaining nutrient balance within the body.
9. **T/F** Ketoacidosis can occur as a result of strict carbohydrate restriction.
10. **T/F** Vitamins are a source of energy.

After foods are chewed and digested, the macronutrients (carbohydrate, protein, fat, and alcohol) supplying physiologic energy for the body are converted to glucose, fatty acids, and amino acids. These basic nutrient units are delivered to cells where, at the direction of specific enzymes, they can be used.

Recall from earlier chapters that no single nutrient can be isolated from the others because nutrients are concurrently distributed in foods and share many points of interaction in digestion, absorption, and metabolism. Metabolism encompasses the continuous processes whereby living organisms and cells convert nutrients into energy, body structure, and waste.

Metabolism

In metabolic activity the two major chemical reactions are catabolism and anabolism. Catabolism is splitting complex substances into simpler substances; anabolism is using absorbed nutrients to build or synthesize more complex compounds (see Chapter 2 for more detail). Anabolism and catabolism are continuous reactions in the body. Cells in the epithelial lining of the oral and gastrointestinal mucosa are replaced approximately every 3 to 7 days. Despite this rapid turnover, the rate of catabolism is usually equal to that of anabolism in a healthy adult. During certain stages of life, such as growth periods or pregnancy, more anabolism is occurring than catabolism. Conversely, when illness or stress occurs, catabolism exceeds anabolism.

Other phases of metabolism include delivery of nutrients to the cells where they are needed and delivery of waste products to sites where they can be excreted. After absorption of the macronutrients in the body, glucose, fatty acids, and amino acids can be used to yield energy through a common pathway within the mitochondria of cells (Fig. 7.1). The catabolic end products of carbohydrates, proteins, and fats are carbon dioxide, water, and energy. Nitrogen is an additional end product of protein.

The Krebs cycle (also called citric acid cycle or tricarboxylic acid [TCA] cycle) converts glucose, fatty acids, and amino acids to a usable form of energy, requiring many enzymes. Additional information on the TCA cycle can be found in Chapter 2. For activation of some enzymes, vitamins or minerals or both must be available. An enzyme needing vitamins for activation is called a coenzyme. Thiamin, riboflavin, and niacin are B vitamins essential as coenzymes in the TCA cycle. An enzyme may also require a cofactor. A cofactor functions in the same way as coenzymes, but the molecule required is a mineral or electrolyte.

Anabolic processes require energy. Examples of anabolism are the building of new muscle tissue or bone and the secretion of cellular products such as hormones. Hormones are "messengers" produced by a group of cells that stimulate or retard the functions of other cells. Hormones principally control different metabolic functions that affect secretions and growth. Anabolism involves the use of glucose, amino acids, fatty acids, and glycerol to build various substances needed for proper functioning of the body which includes proteins, carbohydrates, lipids, and nucleic acids. All nutrients are intertwined in this process. For instance, dispensable amino acids are ordinarily used to build proteins, but glucose can also be converted to amino acids and fatty acids.

Role of the Liver

The liver plays a major regulatory role by controlling the kinds and quantities of nutrients in the bloodstream. All monosaccharides are converted to glucose in the liver to provide an energy supply for the cells. Glycogen, a polysaccharide, also can be broken down to glucose and released into the circulating blood as needed. Other end products of digestion may be oxidized to provide energy; converted to glucose, protein, fat, or other substances; or released to circulate at prescribed levels in the blood for use by all the cells.

Role of the Kidneys

Kidneys perform the important metabolic task of removing waste products from the blood and, along with the liver, control the levels of many nutrients in the blood. Metabolic end products from cells, unnecessary substances absorbed by the gastrointestinal tract, potentially harmful compounds that have been detoxified by the liver, and drugs are removed from the blood by the kidneys.

Kidneys accomplish this task by a process of filtration and reabsorption. Glucose, amino acids, vitamins, water, and various minerals are reabsorbed or excreted by the kidneys depending on the body's need. Excess nitrogen from protein catabolism also is excreted by the kidneys. Kidneys help maintain nutrient balance within the body. Other routes of excretion of waste products are through the bowel; the skin, which excretes water and electrolytes; and the lungs, which remove carbon dioxide and water.

⬡ DENTAL CONSIDERATIONS

- The goal of nutrition in a dental setting is to promote anabolism for growth or healing.
- Uncontrolled blood glucose levels may cause numerous complications, such as poor wound healing and increased risk of infection for patients with diabetes.
- The kidneys' ability to reabsorb nutrients may be altered by certain medications, especially diuretics, or a kidney disorder. Function also depends on fluid balance.

⬡ NUTRITIONAL DIRECTIONS

- The liver is a vital organ for metabolism of food and drugs.
- The kidneys help the body dispose of waste products and drugs. Adequate fluid intake (9–11 cups per day) facilitates this process.
- If the kidneys are not working properly, drugs and nutrients may be retained or lost. Both are undesirable.

Carbohydrate Metabolism

Monosaccharides are transported through the portal vein to the liver for glycogenesis, a process of glycogen formation. During this process, sugars—including fructose, galactose, sorbitol, and xylitol—may be stored as glycogen. Glucose, the circulating sugar in the blood, is the major energy supply for cells. The level of circulating glucose is closely monitored by the liver and is constantly maintained at a normoglycemic level (normal blood glucose range), between 70 and 100 mg/dL. Insulin is a hormone that

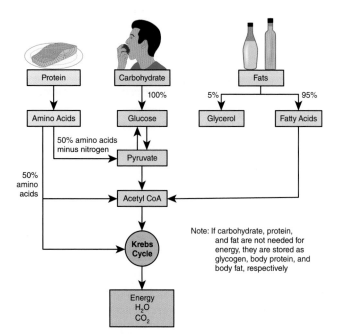

• **Fig. 7.1** Metabolic pathways. (Modified from Peckenpaugh NJ. *Nutrition Essentials and Diet Therapy.* 11th ed. Saunders; 2010.)

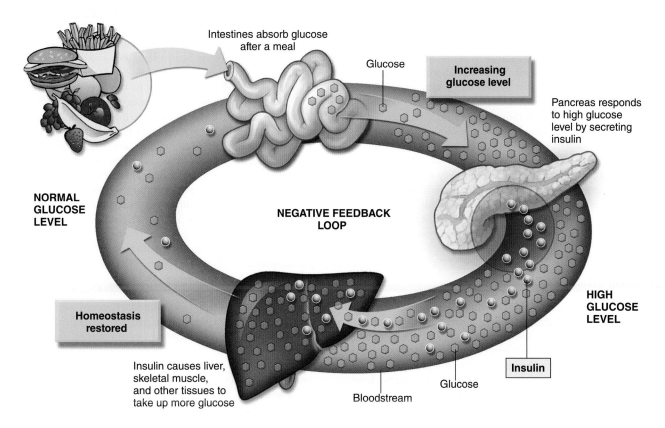

• Fig. 7.2 Role of insulin. Insulin operates in a negative feedback loop that prevents blood glucose concentration from increasing too far above the normal (or setpoint) level. Insulin promotes uptake of glucose by all cells of the body, enabling them to catabolize or store it, or both. The liver and skeletal muscles are especially well-adapted for storage of glucose as glycogen. Excess glucose is removed from the bloodstream. If the glucose level falls below the setpoint level, hormones such as glucagon promote the release of glucose from storage into the bloodstream. (Reproduced with permission from Thibodeau GA, Patton KT. *Anatomy and Physiology*. 9th ed. St. Louis, MO: Mosby Elsevier; 2016.)

lowers blood glucose levels. Blood glucose levels peak at 140 mg/dL 30 to 60 minutes after a meal and return to normal within 3 hours in individuals with normal secretion and use of insulin. This consistent blood glucose level is significant, indicating the necessity of a certain amount of glucose in the blood for normal functioning of body tissues (Fig. 7.2). Hyperglycemia (elevated blood glucose) and hypoglycemia (decreased blood glucose) are very serious conditions that can be fatal; the precipitating cause for either should be identified. Many patients with diabetes who take insulin or an antidiabetic medication, or both, that can cause hypoglycemia may exhibit symptoms related to hypoglycemia, particularly if they have not eaten within a 4- to 5-hour time span. These patients need to be treated with a carbohydrate source before continuing treatment (see *Health Application 7*).

Carbohydrate foods and beverages are digested and absorbed at different rates. Individuals with diabetes often respond differently to different carbohydrate sources. Glycemic index (GI) measures the effect of different carbohydrate foods on blood glucose levels. The thought is that a food with a high GI will raise blood glucose to a greater extent than a food with a low GI. In general, dairy products, legumes, pasta, fruits, and sugars have a low GI. Breads, cereals, and rice can have either a low or high GI. There is no standardized definition for low-, high-, or moderate-GI foods.[1,2] The American Diabetes Association reports mixed findings and limited evidence regarding consumption of low GI and high GI foods for glycemic control.[1] For weight loss measures, the Academy of Nutrition and Dietetics recommends a low-GI diet to be most effective when there is a reduction in overall energy intake.[3] The recommendation for all individuals, including those with diabetes, includes increasing intake of whole grains, legumes, fruits, and vegetables while limiting intake of refined carbohydrates and added sugars.

A complex hormonal system maintains a constant blood glucose level. Insulin is the primary hormone that lowers blood glucose levels. When hyperglycemia occurs, insulin is secreted to decrease blood glucose levels. Conversely, hypoglycemia elicits the secretion of several hormones (thyroid, epinephrine, glucagon, and growth hormone) to increase blood glucose levels. The liver can elevate blood glucose levels by converting amino acids from protein and glycerol from fats to glucose. The process of synthesizing glucose from noncarbohydrate sources is known as gluconeogenesis (see Chapter 2 for additional details).

Dietary carbohydrates ensure optimal glycogen stores and are digested faster than other energy nutrients. The liver can degrade glycogen to glucose. The amount of energy available from glycogen stores is generally less than a day's energy expenditure or approximately 1200 to 1800 cal. Red blood cells and cells in the heart, brain, and renal medulla prefer glucose as their energy source.

Protein Metabolism

Amino acids are transported through the portal vein into the liver. The liver has a central role monitoring the intake and breakdown of most of the amino acids. Individual amino acids are released by the liver to enter the general circulation at specific levels so that each amino acid is available as needed to synthesize each individual protein. Amino acids transported in the blood are rapidly removed for use by cells. If individual amino acids increase above a specific level in the blood, they are removed and oxidized for energy.

Protein metabolism is in a constant dynamic state, with catabolism and anabolism occurring continuously to replace worn-out proteins in cells. Even during anabolic periods, such as growth, muscle catabolism is elevated as each cell remodels itself. Anabolic and catabolic processes are controlled by the liver and hormones. Insulin, thyroxine, and growth hormone stimulate protein synthesis.

Anabolism

A small reservoir of amino acids, which is called the *amino acid metabolic pool*, is available for anabolism and to maintain the dynamic state of equilibrium. Increasing muscle size is considered an increase in body mass, not protein storage. High-protein diets are neither safe nor effective as a means to increase muscle mass without physical activity or exercise to promote muscle development. To maintain a satisfactory protein status, a daily supply of essential amino acids obtained from the diet is necessary.

Anabolism depends on the presence of all essential amino acids simultaneously. It is not a stepwise process in which the synthesis of a protein can be started at one point and completed when the needed amino acid appears later.

Protein synthesis is also affected by calorie intake. If calorie intake is inadequate, tissue proteins are used for energy, resulting in increased nitrogen excretion. This process requires pyridoxine, a form of vitamin B.

Catabolism

Amino acids are catabolized principally in the liver, but metabolism also occurs to some extent in the kidneys and muscles. Removal of the nitrogen grouping from amino acids, a process requiring the B vitamins pyridoxine and riboflavin, yields carbon skeletons and ammonia. The carbon skeletons can be (1) used to make nonessential amino acids, (2) used to produce energy via the TCA cycle, or (3) converted to fats and stored as fatty tissue. Not all ingested protein is used to build muscle.

Excess amino acids not needed for protein anabolism or energy are converted to fat and stored in the body. If calorie intake is inadequate, proteins are used for energy rather than to build or repair lean body mass or produce essential protein-based compounds.

Urea is the major waste product of protein catabolism. Ammonia is a toxic substance that the liver converts to urea to be excreted by the kidneys. The levels of urea and ammonia vary directly with dietary protein levels.

Lipid Metabolism

Hormones involved in carbohydrate metabolism also control fat metabolism. Insulin increases fat synthesis, whereas thyroxine, epinephrine, growth hormone, and glucocorticoids increase fat mobilization. The liver is the principal regulator of fat metabolism and lipoprotein synthesis. Fatty acids can be hydrolyzed or modified by shortening, lengthening, or adding double bonds before their release from the liver into the circulation. The liver produces cholesterol, removes it from the blood, and uses it to make bile acid.

Metabolism of chylomicrons in the liver results in triglycerides being transported to the tissues for energy or other uses, or carried to adipose tissue to be stored. Serum triglycerides are the result of not only absorption from foods but also the conversion of carbohydrates and proteins into fats. Triglycerides can be synthesized in the intestinal mucosa, adipose tissue, and liver. Fats are synthesized in the process of lipogenesis and broken down during lipolysis (the splitting or decomposition of fat). These continual processes are in equilibrium when energy needs are balanced.

The process of hydrolyzing triglycerides into two-carbon entities to enter the Krebs cycle for energy production is known as oxidation. A detailed discussion on oxidation can be found in Chapter 2. During oxidation, 1 lb of fat results in the release of 3500 cal of energy. When excessive amounts of fats are oxidized for energy, the liver is overwhelmed, and acidic metabolic products, or ketones, are formed. Ketones are not oxidized in the liver but rather are carried to the skeletal and cardiac muscles, where, under normal circumstances, they are rapidly metabolized.

If the glucose supply is reduced, the capacity of the tissues to use ketone bodies may be exceeded. Accumulation of ketone bodies is known as ketosis. Ketosis may lead to ketoacidosis (acidic condition due to accumulation of large quantities of ketone bodies in the blood). The signs and symptoms of ketoacidosis include nausea, vomiting, and stomach pain. Ketoacidosis can be a dangerous condition for several reasons. Bases must neutralize these strong acids (ketones) to maintain acid-base balance in the blood. Ketones are excreted in the urine, a condition known as ketonuria, along with sodium. If adequate amounts of base are not available, acidosis may result. In addition to the loss of sodium ions, large amounts of water are lost, which can lead to dehydration (or rapid weight loss for an individual reducing calorie intake). When blood glucose levels remain low for several days, brain and nerve cells adapt to use ketones for some of their fuel requirements.

Carbohydrates play a predominant role in heavy physical activity or exercise when the muscle's oxygen supply is limited, but triglycerides provide about half the energy with continued exercise. Although fats can be stored as adipose tissue in virtually inexhaustible amounts, their slower rate of metabolism makes them a less efficient source of quick energy.

Alcohol Metabolism

Although alcohol is considered a drug, the amount of calories it provides can be used by the body for energy, providing approximately 7 cal/g. When consumed in excessive amounts, alcohol is a toxin. Caloric content of alcoholic beverages can be calculated by using the equations given in Box 7.1. Alcoholic beverages contain negligible nutrients.

Alcohol is metabolized primarily by the liver. Alcohol provides an alternative fuel that is oxidized instead of fat; this may result in accumulation of lipids in the liver.

A well-balanced diet accompanied by habitual consumption of alcoholic beverages in excess of energy needs can be a risk factor for weight gain. However, excessive amounts of alcohol in a person with alcohol use disorder may result in poor appetite for

---

• BOX 7.1 | **Calculation of Energy Value of Alcoholic Beverages**

The equation for determining energy (caloric) value of liquors is as follows:

Ounces of beverage × proof × 0.8 cal/proof/1 oz

Example: 1.5 oz × 86 proof × 0.8 cal/proof/1 oz = 103.2 cal

The equation for determining energy (caloric) value of beer and wines is as follows:

Ounces of beverage × % of alcohol × 1.6

Example: 12 oz × 5% × 1.6 = 96 cal

From Gastineau CF. Nutrition note: alcohol and calories. *Mayo Clin Proc.* 1976;51(2):88.

---

food leading him to weight loss and malnutrition. In addition to causing liver damage, alcohol can interfere with the transport, activation, catabolism, and storage of vital nutrients.[4] In individuals without liver disease, there may be protective effects of low to moderate alcohol consumption on cardiovascular events; however, heavy use has a marked effect so limited consumption should be encouraged.[5]

The *Dietary Guidelines* advise moderation in alcohol consumption: one drink a day for females and no more than two drinks a day for males. An alcoholic beverage is defined as 12 oz of regular beer, 5 oz of wine, or 1.5 oz of 80-proof distilled spirits. Females who are breastfeeding, pregnant, or planning to get pregnant, should avoid alcoholic beverages.

Metabolic Interrelationships

The body is an overwhelmingly complex system. Whether excessive food intake is in the form of protein, carbohydrate, fat, or alcohol, most excess energy intake is stored as adipose tissue (Fig. 7.3). Glycogen is another storage form of energy; however, the amount of glycogen stored in the body is limited.

Protein from the metabolic pool of amino acids and in lean muscle mass, is generally not considered a good source of energy, but it can be used for energy if calorie intake is below calorie expenditure. Fat is a good source of energy, but carbohydrate is the preferred fuel to meet body's energy needs. However, the body cannot metabolize excessive quantities of fat without some side effects—ketoacidosis, hyperlipidemia, and accumulation of fat in the liver.

Carbohydrates can be used in forming nonessential amino acids. Proteins contribute to synthesis of some lipids (e.g., lipoproteins). Although lipids do not contribute significantly to the synthesis of amino acids, glycerol from triglycerides can be used

for the synthesis of carbohydrates. Fatty acids and some amino acids can be converted to glucose.

Catabolism of all classes of foodstuffs involves oxidation through the TCA cycle to produce energy. The quantity of calories in the diet from carbohydrate or lipids, influences protein metabolism. In some situations, one nutrient can be substituted for another because of their interrelationship. For example, a decrease in carbohydrate intake increases lipolysis; protein excess can be used for energy requirement. In view of body's adaptability to easily shift from carbohydrate to fat and vice versa to get the main source of energy, and substantial body fat stores, the body can well tolerate large variations in macronutrient intake (energy sources) and energy expenditure.

In addition to energy-providing nutrients, vitamins and minerals are essential for digestion, absorption, and metabolism of carbohydrate, protein, and fat. Although vitamins and minerals are

---

🦷 DENTAL CONSIDERATIONS

- Glycogen stores are depleted with a carbohydrate-poor diet even when high levels of fat and protein are eaten. A patient who ingests a carbohydrate-poor diet has decreased energy reserves and is prone to prolonged healing periods and fatigue.
- Insulin deficiency can cause slow glycogenesis, low glycogen storage, decreased glucose catabolism and increased blood glucose.
- Blood glucose concentrations are increased only slightly when fructose, sorbitol, or xylitol is given because these sugars are absorbed more slowly; less insulin is required for their metabolism. Caution with portion size is still a consideration for individuals with diabetes.
- Patients with compromised liver or renal function may postpone progression of their condition by avoiding excessive amounts of protein.
- Ketoacidosis does not result from rapid breakdown of adipose tissue alone; severe curtailment of carbohydrate intake must occur simultaneously. Ensure that patients consume an adequate amount of carbohydrate.
- Ketoacidosis is a risk in patients with uncontrolled diabetes mellitus (see *Health Application 7*) or those fasting (due to illness or weight loss). In these cases, the body starts burning fat for energy rather than carbohydrates, leading to a build up of ketones in the blood. Question patients with fruity-smelling breath about recent food and fluid intake, weight loss, and conditions such as diabetes mellitus.
- High ketone levels may be associated with starvation or high-protein, low-carbohydrate, and low-calorie diets. These result in decreased appetite and occasional nausea which can worsen patient's condition.
- Symptoms of hypoglycemia include weakness or light-headedness; confusion; irritability; pale color; sweating; and rapid, shallow breathing. Or the patient may experience hypoglycemic unawareness, yet have low blood glucose levels.

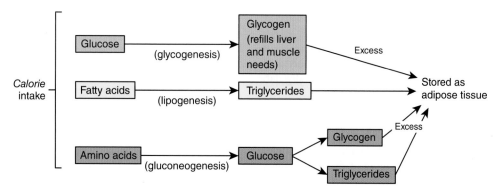

• **Fig. 7.3** Metabolic pathways of excess energy. (Modified from Nix S. *Williams' Basic Nutrition and Diet Therapy*. 15th ed. St Louis, MO: Mosby Elsevier; 2017.)

NUTRITIONAL DIRECTIONS

- A diet high in protein without limiting total energy intake may convert excess protein to fat stores.
- Increasing protein intake does not necessarily (or may not) increase muscle tissue and may lead to dehydration.
- High-protein, low-carbohydrate diets have been promoted as an effective way of reducing calories by creating a state of ketoacidosis to lose weight. The amount of calories lost may be insignificant when considering the risk involved.
- The National Institute on Alcohol Abuse and Alcoholism defines binge drinking as four drinks for females and five drinks for males within 2 hours. The Substance Abuse and Mental Health Services Administration (SAMHSA) defines binge drinking as five or more alcoholic beverages for males, or four or more alcoholic beverages for females on the same occasion on at least 1 day in the past month. SAMHSA defines heavy drinking as binge drinking on five or more days in the past month.[6]

not required in as large quantity as macronutrients are required in, their presence as cofactors in the metabolic process is important. When a deficiency occurs, reactions do not proceed normally. For example, although protein may be consumed alone (as in liquid protein supplements), many other nutrients including vitamins and minerals must be present for the protein to be used by cells. Each nutrient has its specific function; all nutrients must be present simultaneously for optimal benefits.

A detailed discussion on metabolic interrelationships is beyond the scope of this text. These interrelationships are important, and for optimal use of nutrients, food sources of all the nutrients should be consumed. The best way to obtain optimal nutrition is to include a variety of food from all the food groups.

Metabolic Energy

Without energy from chemical reactions, people cannot blink their eyes, wiggle their toes, or fully process their thoughts. Energy is required for all these physiologic functions. Energy from food is converted into forms which the body can use: electrical energy for the brain and nerves, mechanical energy for muscles, thermal energy for body heat, and chemical energy for the synthesis of new compounds.

The potential energy value of foods and energy exchanges occurring within the body are expressed in terms of "kilocalorie." A kilocalorie (kcal) is the amount of heat required to increase the temperature of 1 kg of water to 1°C. A kilocalorie is 1000 times larger than a calorie. Although kilocalorie is the proper term, it is commonly used interchangeably with calorie (cal) or Calorie (Cal).

Carbohydrate, fat, protein, and even alcohol provide energy for humans. Vitamins and minerals are not energy sources but are necessary for energy-producing reactions. The commonly used physiologic energy values are 4 cal/g carbohydrate, 9 cal/g fat, 4 cal/g protein, and 7 cal/g alcohol.

Measurement of Potential Energy

The amount of energy, or calories, available in a food may be precisely calculated by placing a weighed amount of food inside a device used to measure calories, called a calorimeter (Fig. 7.4). As a food is burned, an increase in water temperature indicates the heat given off or potential (free) energy of that food.

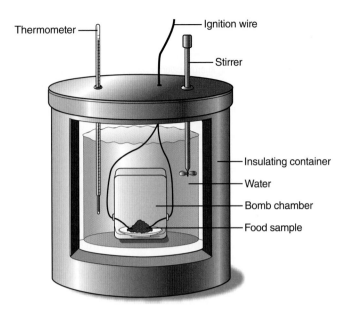

• **Fig. 7.4** Cross section of a bomb calorimeter. To determine energy, a dried portion of food is burned inside a chamber charged with oxygen that is surrounded by water. As the food is burned, it gives off heat. The heat raises the temperature of the water surrounding the chamber. The increase in water temperature indicates the number of calories contained in the food. One calorie equals the amount of heat needed to raise the temperature of 1 kg of water by 1°C. (Reproduced with permission from Grodner M, Escott-Stump S, Dorner S. *Nutritional Foundations and Clinical Applications. A Nursing Approach*. 6th ed. St. Louis, MO: Mosby Elsevier; 2016.)

Energy Production

The metabolism of basic nutrients results in the production of cellular energy which is stored as adenosine triphosphate (ATP). ATP is an instant source of cellular energy for mechanical work, transport of nutrients and waste products, and synthesis of chemical compounds generated from the Krebs cycle. ATP units, also called high-energy phosphate compounds, are the currency, or "money," that the body uses for energy. Because ATP can be metabolized without oxygen, the reaction is classified as anaerobic. The body must always have a supply of ATP, and several systems ensure a constant supply in the body. A more detailed discussion on ATP can be found in Chapter 2.

Increasing calorie intake from carbohydrates and fats would not produce optimal energy without adequate protein intake. Energy use is remarkably sensitive to the quantity and the quality of dietary protein.

Basal Metabolic Rate

Even during sleep, the body requires energy for the basic minimum tasks of respiration and circulation and for many intricate activities within each cell. Basal metabolic rate (BMR) indicates energy required for involuntary physiologic functions to maintain life, including respiration, circulation, and maintenance of muscle tone and body temperature. The BMR is lowest while lying down, awaking, resting, and relaxing in a comfortable environment, not having eaten for 12 to 15 hours. The BMR can be measured in a clinical setting using indirect calorimetry, which indirectly measures the rate of oxygen used while the person is resting. Because digestion and absorption require energy, the BMR is the amount of energy required when the body is in a postabsorptive state (the state in which digestion and absorption are minimal).

Factors Affecting the Basal Metabolic Rate

Various factors can increase or decrease the BMR which determines energy needs.

Sleep

Metabolic rate is the lowest after a few hours of sleep because muscles then become more relaxed. Approximately 10% less energy is needed for the BMR during this relaxed state.

Age

From birth through age 2 years, growth results in the highest BMR, which then decreases until the pubertal growth spurt and is followed by a gradual decline for the rest of the life cycle (Fig. 7.5).

Pregnancy and Lactation

During the last trimester of pregnancy, the BMR increases approximately 15% to 30%. The amount of energy necessary to produce milk for lactation can increase the BMR as much as 40%.

Surface Area and Size

The more the body surface area, the greater the BMR. Because of greater surface area, a tall, thin person requires more energy than a short one of similar weight.

State of Health

Illnesses and diseases may increase or decrease the BMR. Patients recovering from a wasting illness require extra energy to build new tissue. Additionally, the activity level may be influenced by such conditions as lack of sleep, exhaustion, tenseness, fatigue, or depression.

Body Composition and Gender

In adults, lean body mass is the best single predictor of the BMR. Because cells in muscles and glands are more active than cells in bone and fat, body composition influences the BMR. The amount of muscle versus fat tissue in adults is a distinguishing factor; normally, females have more fat tissue and use fewer calories than males. Differences in the BMR may be primarily related to typical variations in body composition rather than directly related to sex.

Muscle tone is an important factor in metabolism; the state of tension or relaxation also has an effect. An athlete having better muscle tone requires more calories than a sedentary individual of similar size and shape.

Endocrine Glands: Chemical Messengers

Thyroxine, the iodine-containing hormone secreted by the thyroid gland, has a greater influence on the rate of metabolic processes than secretions from any other gland.

Adrenal glands affect metabolism to a lesser degree. Stimulations by fright, excitement, or even joy can cause a temporary increase in the BMR by releasing catecholamines, particularly epinephrine. Catecholamines are obtained from tyrosine or phenylalanines. The pituitary gland accounts for about 15% to 20% increase in the BMR during the growth of children and adolescents.

Temperature

The BMR can be affected by body temperature or climate. The BMR is slightly higher in cooler climates to maintain normal body temperature. A fever will increase the BMR.

Fasting and Starvation

Individuals who are undernourished or have been fasting for long periods have a lower than normal BMR. This is a result of decreased muscle mass and an adaptive body process to conserve energy. Numerous studies indicate that the body responds to dieting the way it does to fasting, by decreasing the BMR.

Total Energy Requirements

Basal energy expenditure includes calories necessary to maintain BMR plus additional calories needed for thermic effect, voluntary activities, and any increased needs from catabolic processes (e.g., disease states or fever) or anabolic processes (e.g., growth or pregnancy) for a 24-hour period. The thermic effect of food refers to increased energy expenditure resulting from the consumption of food or the number of calories needed for digestion.

BMR can be estimated using several methods based on a patient's age, sex, and body size. For most individuals, the BMR accounts for 65% to 70% of the body's total energy requirement. Calculations determining a patient's BMR are inexact, but many general guidelines have been formulated to obtain closely precise BMR value by calculation. One quick guideline for adults is as follows:

$$10 \times \text{ideal weight (lb)} = \text{calories needed for BMR daily}$$

Food digestion requires energy. The thermic effect of a mixed diet is estimated to be approximately 10% of the energy required for BMR. Many times, this factor is omitted in calculations determining total energy expenditure.

Physical Activity

The most variable factor affecting total energy needs, is muscle activity which is influenced by the physical activity level (Table 7.1). Energy expenditure may range from as low as 15% for sedentary individuals and increase to 50% for those individuals that are more physically active.[7]

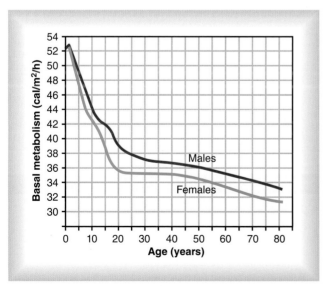

• **Fig. 7.5** Normal basal metabolic rates at different ages for each sex. (Reproduced with permission from Guyton AC, Hall JE. *Textbook of Medical Physiology.* 13th ed. Philadelphia, PA: Elsevier; 2016.)

TABLE 7.1	Energy Expenditure During Various Activities		
Activity (1 h)	130 lb	155 lb	180 lb
Aerobics, low impact	295	352	409
Aerobics, high impact	413	493	572
Cycling, 14–15.9 mph, vigorous bicycling	590	704	817
Cycling, <10 mph, leisure bicycling	236	281	327
Diving, springboard or platform	177	211	245
Downhill snow skiing, moderate	354	422	490
Downhill snow skiing, racing	472	563	654
Fishing, general	177	211	245
Football or baseball, playing catch	148	176	204
Football, competitive	531	633	735
Football, touch, flag, general	472	563	654
Frisbee playing, general	177	211	245
Golf, walking and carrying clubs	266	317	368
Handball	708	844	981
Hiking, cross-country	354	422	490
Horseback riding	236	281	327
Housework, light	148	176	204
Judo, karate, jujitsu, martial arts	590	704	817
Marching band, playing instrument	236	281	327
Mowing lawn, walk, power mower	325	387	449
Pushing stroller, walking with children	148	176	204
Racquetball, playing	413	493	572
Raking lawn	254	303	351
Rowing machine, light	207	246	286
Rowing machine, vigorous	502	598	695
Running, 5 mph (12-min mile)	472	563	654
Running 6 mph (9-min mile)	590	704	817
Running, 7 mph (8.5-min mile)	679	809	940
Stationary cycling, light	325	387	449
Walking 2.0 mph	177	211	245
Walking 3.0 mph, moderate	195	232	270
Walking 4.0 mph, very brisk	295	352	409

Adapted from NutriStrategy Software. Calories are calculated based on research data from *Med Sci Sports Exercise*. 2015 by NutriStrategy. http://www.nutristrategy.com/activitylist4.htm.

physical activity help with reversing heart disease, weight control and physical strength, but reductions in mortality risks and blood pressure are observed with even small increase in activity.[9,10] The American Cancer Society supports regular physical activity for cancer prevention.[11] The exercise or activity should be the one that an individual enjoys to enhance the likelihood of consistent participation in exercise. Inactive individuals may need to gradually increase the duration and intensity of exercise.

Estimated Energy Requirements

The estimated energy requirements established by the National Academy of Medicine (formerly the Institute of Medicine) indicate the daily calorie intake needed to maintain energy balance in healthy individuals of a specific age, sex, weight, height, and level of physical activity. These levels are recommended to sustain body weights in the desired range for good health (body mass index [BMI] 18.5–25 kg/m^2), while maintaining a lifestyle with adequate levels of physical activity. A Recommended Dietary Allowance was not established because energy intakes greater than the estimated energy requirement could result in weight gain. Weight gain resulting in a BMI greater than 25 kg/m^2 is associated with an increased risk of early mortality. Numerous studies substantiate a morbidity risk of type 2 diabetes, hypertension, CVD, stroke, gallbladder disease, osteoarthritis, and some types of cancer for BMIs greater than 25 kg/m^2. The National Academy of Medicine suggests that at the end of adolescence, BMI should be around 22 kg/m^2 to allow for a moderate weight gain in midlife without exceeding the 25 kg/m^2 threshold.[12]

DENTAL CONSIDERATIONS

- Encourage intake of adequate amounts of the macronutrients and energy to spare protein for growth or healing, as needed. If energy is insufficient, healing is prolonged.
- Low-carbohydrate diets are not as effective in supporting high activity levels as a high intake of complex carbohydrates. For athletic patients, advise increased intake of complex carbohydrates.
- For healthy males, the BMR usually ranges from about 1580 to 1870 cal daily, whereas approximately 1150 to 1440 cal is needed for females. If energy intake is inadequate, physical status may deteriorate. A referral to a health care provider or registered dietitian nutritionist (RDN) is needed to improve nutrient intake.
- Increased thyroxine activity (hyperthyroidism) may double the BMR and can cause vitamin deficiencies because the quantity of many enzymes is increased. Unless physical activity is above average, the BMR represents the largest proportion of a patient's energy requirement. Determination of the BMR can be used to evaluate adequacy of calorie intake.
- Encourage inactive adults to engage in some leisure time while carrying out physical activity and do not discourage adults who already participate in high activity levels.

NUTRITIONAL DIRECTIONS

- The BMR may be elevated or depressed. A high BMR requires more calories; fewer calories are needed for a low BMR.
- Because the BMR decreases about 2% every 10 years after age 25 years, many patients gain weight because previous eating habits are maintained without increasing activity.
- A naturally higher BMR is a reason why children and pregnant females do not feel as cold as adults under the same weather conditions. Do not overdress children based on an adult's perception.

The *Dietary Guidelines* address the need for regular physical activity. Along with these sources, the Physical Activities Guidelines from the United States Department of Health and Human Services recommend 2.5 hours per week of moderate intensity activities for substantial health benefits.[8] Not only does

Energy Balance

The proper energy balance for stable weight is maintained when calorie intake equals the amount of energy needed for body processes and physical activities (Fig. 7.6). Energy balance is maintained when the calorie intake equals the amount of energy needed for body processes and physical activities. This statement sounds simple, but very few Americans are able to maintain energy balance at an appropriate body weight. Many factors help create this unbalanced equation; because it is a complex system, there are no easy answers. The government recommendation is 1600 cal/day for females and 2200 cal/day for males. Dental professionals, in collaboration with dietetic professionals, can play a role in health promotion efforts to educate patients in the prevention and management of obesity.

Many healthy patients are able to control energy intake to balance energy output with little effort; their appetite, or desire to eat, controls food intake to balance energy expenditure. Hunger, or the physiologic drive to eat, is regulated by a complex network of factors (see Fig. 7.6). Appetite is frequently used in the same sense as hunger, but it usually implies desire for specific types of food and is related to the pleasurable sensation of eating.

Hunger and appetite greatly affect weight balance. When more calories are consumed than the body needs, the excess is stored inside body as fat, resulting in weight gain. One pound of body fat is equivalent to 3500 cal. Overweight patients have a very difficult time losing extra pounds and maintaining their energy balance to keep off unwanted pounds. Weight control can be approached by either decreasing the number of calories consumed or increasing physical activities. A combination of both is most effective (Box 7.2).

Intake is generally regarded as the key to weight regulation. A patient's weight tends to remain stable for long periods with only a 1- to 5-lb gain or loss of adipose tissue over a year. Even small daily deviations can result in gradual yet significant fluctuations in fat stores. For instance, an additional 100 cal daily would result in a 10-lb weight gain over 1 year and a 100-lb gain over 10 years.

Physiologic Factors

The hypothalamus, located in the middle of the brain, is especially important in controlling hunger. A satiety center and a hunger (or feeding) center are present within the hypothalamus.

Stimulation of the hunger center causes insatiable hunger; damage to this area results in no desire for food. Stimulation of the satiety center results in complete satiety. If the satiety center of the hypothalamus is destroyed, the appetite becomes voracious, resulting in obesity. The feeding center stimulates the drive to eat, whereas the satiety center inhibits the feeding center.

Usually, the body discerns food characteristics such as sweetness and viscosity to gauge intake. The body may use this information to determine how much food is needed to meet its caloric requirements. High intensity sweeteners may reduce calorie intake in the short term, but whether they are effective as a long-term weight management strategy is unknown.[13] Several mechanisms affect the amount eaten at a particular meal. Distention of the stomach results in inhibitory signals that suppress the feeding center, reducing the desire to eat. Cholecystokinin in response to fat in the duodenum has a strong direct effect on the feeding

---

> ### • BOX 7.2 Equation for Weight Loss
>
> The total energy expenditure for a sedentary individual 67 inches tall who weighs 191 lb (BMI = 30) is 2235 cal.
>
> For 1 lb weight loss per week, decrease calorie intake by 500 cal/day:
> 2235 − 500 = 1735 cal/day
>
> The result of a 500-cal deficit in 1 week:
> 500 × 7 = 3500 cal
>
> A calorie reduction combined with exercise to lose 2 lb/week can be accomplished by increasing calorie expenditure by 500 cal/day.
>
> Cycling at a rate of 15 mph or running at a rate of 10 min/mile for 45 min = 525 cal:
> 525 × 7 = 3675 cal
>
> This would result in a weight loss of 2 lb/week or 8 lb/month.

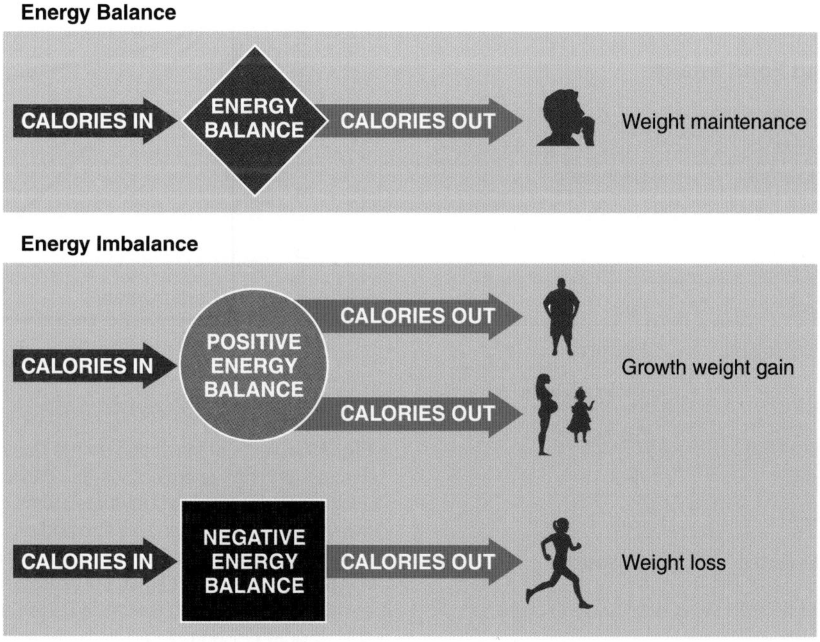

• **Fig. 7.6** Factors affecting energy balance.

center, causing the person to stop eating. Food in the stomach and duodenum causes the secretion of glucagon and insulin, both of which suppress the feeding center.

The hypothalamus is also responsive to body temperature. Cold temperatures lead to increased food intake, resulting in a higher metabolic rate and more fat stores for insulation.

The relationship between physical activity and food intake is unclear. Physical activity has been reported to increase, decrease, or have no effect on appetite. These findings cannot be explained but may be related to the timing or duration of the activity, individual metabolic differences, or some unknown reason. Generally, acute exercise decreases food intake after the activity, but regular physical activity promotes increased energy intake.

Nutritional and hormonal signals affect the brain and liver to stimulate satiety and feeding centers (Table 7.2).

Psychological Factors

Appetite is affected by the fact that eating is rewarding or pleasurable and makes us feel good. Eating behavior of individuals can be influenced by external factors—including time, taste, smell, and sight of food. Greater weight usually means that the individual is responding to feelings and emotions rather than actual hunger. Boredom and stress are factors that frequently affect eating habits of overweight individuals.

Energy Expenditure

Contrary to popular opinion, obese females have a similar or higher metabolic rate than thinner females. The effect of this is a less weight gain for a given increase in calorie intake. Genetics may also play a role in the BMR. Some families have low metabolic rates, but not all individuals with a low BMR are obese.

Physical activity tolerance of obese individuals is less than normal, but any activity uses more calories because of the amount of additional mass to be moved. Not all inactive patients are obese; thus activity level does not seem to be a principal determinant in

the development of obesity. Because of differences in body composition (percentage of muscle and fat), the BMR affects energy expenditure for various activities. Weight loss resulting from a specific energy deficit is invariably smaller than expected. Conversely, overconsumption fails to produce anticipated weight gains. Adjustments in energy expenditure seem to be adaptive.

Because food is abundant in the United States and most Americans enjoy eating, increased physical activity is needed to balance energy intake. Walking is a physical activity that has been emphasized because it is inexpensive and convenient, and most individuals are physically able to walk, even if they initially need to walk slowly. Numerous studies have shown that using a pedometer (a small meter worn at the waist that monitors the number of steps a person takes) results in a significant increase in the number of steps per week.[14-16] Usually, the goal is 10,000 steps a day, but individuals are encouraged to start at a comfortable pace and distance, gradually increasing intensity and distance.

Inadequate Energy Intake

A deficiency in energy intake may result in a depressed rate of growth in children and weight loss in adults. Intentional weight loss may be helpful or harmful, depending on the methods used for losing weight. Decreased fat stores are normally the goal, but loss of muscle may be an undesirable side effect (Fig. 7.7).

Inadequate energy intake may result in malnutrition and become a serious problem in the face of a physiologically stressful situation. Inadequate intake may be intentional, as in the case of anorexia nervosa (discussed in Chapter 17), a psychological disorder in which undernourishment is not perceived by the individual. Inadequate intake causes a vicious downward spiral in which metabolic imbalances decrease hunger and may become life-threatening without proper treatment.

TABLE 7.2	**Stimuli Affecting Food Intake**	
	FOOD INTAKE	
Signal	**Increased**	**Decreased**
Food odors	Pleasant	Repulsive
Taste	Desirable	Offensive
Climate (temperature)	Cold	Hot
Gastrointestinal	Hunger pains	Distention
		Cholecystokinin
		Glucagon
Glucose level	Low	High
Lipoprotein	High	Low
Nutrient stores	Decreased	Increased

From Davis JR, Sherer K. *Applied Nutrition and Diet Therapy for Nurses.* 2nd ed. Saunders; 1994.

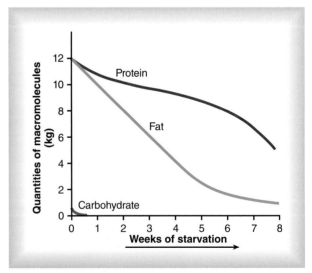

• **Fig. 7.7** Effects of starvation on the body. Three major macromolecules serve as primary energy sources: carbohydrates, fats, and proteins. During starvation, the carbohydrate stores (glycogen) are rapidly depleted. However, stored lipids can mobilize and provide much of a person's energy needs for several weeks. Eventually, lipid stores run low and the body starts using proteins as a major source of energy, causing the breakdown of muscle and other protein-rich tissues. Muscle damage during starvation usually leads to death. (Reproduced with permission from Guyton AC, Hall JE. *Textbook of Medical Physiology.* 13th ed. Philadelphia, PA: Elsevier; 2016.)

● DENTAL CONSIDERATIONS

- Observe emotional factors. Depression and stress as well as other emotional factors result in overeating and decreased activity in some patients. Referral to a health care provider may be indicated.
- A positive energy balance is desirable during the periods of growth; a proportionately larger amount of energy is needed by pregnant and lactating females, and by children.
- Be aware of the complexities of maintaining energy balance and encourage healthy eating patterns consistent with the *Dietary Guidelines*.

- If calories are underestimated, the body must use stored energy (fat and protein), putting the patient at risk for undernutrition. If excessive calories are consumed, the body converts excess calories to fat.
- It is acceptable for the dental professional to promote a healthy dietary pattern based on the *Dietary Guidelines* to maintain a healthy weight. It is out of the scope of practice for the dental hygienist to assess and counsel patients on weight loss. Refer patients to an RDN.

● NUTRITIONAL DIRECTIONS

- Exercise or physical activity may enhance the BMR by increasing the amount of lean body mass, which uses more energy than fat.
- To gain 1 lb of fat, a patient must consume 3500 cal more than the number of calories used.
- To lose 1 lb of weight, energy intake must be 3500 cal less than the number of calories used.
- A decrease from prior activity level or additional calorie intake may result in weight gain.

- Although quitting smoking is linked to an increased risk of weight gain, encourage patients who smoke to enroll in a smoking cessation program along with a weight loss program. Remind the patient that the benefits of not smoking outweigh the potential risk factors of weight gain associated with quitting smoking (see *Health Application 19* in Chapter 19).

◆ HEALTH APPLICATION 7

Diabetes Mellitus

Diabetes mellitus is a heterogeneous group of metabolic abnormalities in which carbohydrates, proteins, fats, and insulin are ineffectively metabolized, leading to disturbances in fluid and electrolyte balances (Fig. 7.8). It is a chronic, lifelong disease. Diabetes mellitus is specifically related to hormonal pancreatic secretions but involves the entire endocrine system.

Diabetes mellitus is presently one of the most common disorders, with rates increasing at an alarming pace, especially in children and adolescents. African Americans, Hispanic Americans, and Native Americans have the highest incidence of diabetes mellitus of all cultural population groups. In addition to metabolic complications secondary to diabetes mellitus, life expectancy is approximately 70% to 80% that of the general population. The Centers for Disease Control and Prevention estimates that more than 28 million individuals in the United States have diabetes mellitus, 96 million have prediabetes, and an additional 8.5 million have diabetes but are not aware of it.[17] Type 2 diabetes mellitus (T2DM) can be prevented or delayed by changes in lifestyles by high-risk individuals. Physical activity improves the body's sensitivity to insulin and helps the body metabolize glucose better, preventing development of diabetes in individuals who are at high risk.

Prediabetes occurs when blood glucose levels are higher than normal, but not high enough to be diagnosed as diabetes. Comparison of diagnostic values can be found in Table 7.4. It is also known as impaired glucose tolerance or impaired fasting glucose, depending on the test used when it was detected. The individuals with prediabetes are at risk of the long-term complications associated with T2DM. Changes to lifestyle behaviors, such as weight reduction, watching portion sizes, and regular physical activity, can return blood glucose levels to normal ranges. Research looking at long-term effects of lifestyle interventions demonstrated a 27% reduction in the development of diabetes in the group that incorporated health minded behavior changes.[18] Dental hygienists can partner with their patients during routine preventive appointments by encouraging healthy dietary patterns and physical activity.

The two most prevalent types of diabetes mellitus are characterized by different metabolic defects. These two can appear to be very different conditions (Table 7.3). Type 1 diabetes mellitus (T1DM), which affects 5% to 10% of individuals, is distinguished by little or no endogenous insulin production and autoimmune β-cell destruction. Diagnostic values can be found in Table 7.4. This condition most commonly manifests in young people but can occur at any age. T1DM was formerly known as juvenile or insulin-

dependent diabetes; the name was changed because adults also develop type 1 diabetes and those with T2DM can be on insulin. Onset is sudden, with all the clinical symptoms associated with this condition. Patients are prone to ketosis and must receive exogenous insulin for their entire lives.

Approximately 90% to 95% of Americans with diabetes have T2DM, which results from insulin resistance, usually with a relative insulin deficiency. Family history, age, history of gestational diabetes, obesity (BMI > 27 kg/m²), and sedentary lifestyle are the risk factors associated with diabetes. For obese patients, increased fat stores cause some degree of insulin resistance. In many cases, insulin is secreted in adequate or higher-than-normal amounts, but glucose uptake by body cells (except for the brain) is decreased.

Abnormalities in insulin levels precipitate clinical manifestations. Insulin deficiency or defects in insulin action or both result in hyperglycemia, the main manifestation of T2DM. Diagnostic values can be found in Table 7.4. Symptoms of hyperglycemia include thirst, frequent urination, hunger, blurry vision, fatigue, frequent infections, and dry, itchy skin; or the patient can be asymptomatic.

Treatment should be implemented as soon as possible after diagnosis to prevent complications of metabolic alterations secondary to diabetes mellitus. Elevated blood glucose levels can damage almost every major organ of the body. Early, tight control of diabetes can postpone and minimize many of these severe complications. Chronic complications develop slowly over long periods as body tissues are adversely exposed to hyperglycemia and hypoglycemia. Hyperglycemia in T2DM causes macrovascular and microvascular disease (involving large and small vessels) and can damage almost every major organ of the body. Patients with uncontrolled diabetes experience slow wound healing, frequent abscesses, periodontal disease, a predisposition to bacterial infections, a compromised immune system, skin irritations, pruritus (itching), numbness and tingling of the extremities, and visual disturbances. The American Diabetes Association defines uncontrolled blood glucose levels as three consecutive readings of 200 mg/dL or greater and/or an A$_{1c}$ of 9% or greater.[19] Because of the increased risks of infection and slow wound healing in hyperglycemia, consultation with the primary care provider is needed for the patient with an A1c above normal to determine if blood glucose level management needs to be better controlled before continuing with treatment.

Obtaining a blood glucose level using a glucometer (a meter used to monitor capillary blood glucose levels) and a fingerstick to obtain a blood

(Continued)

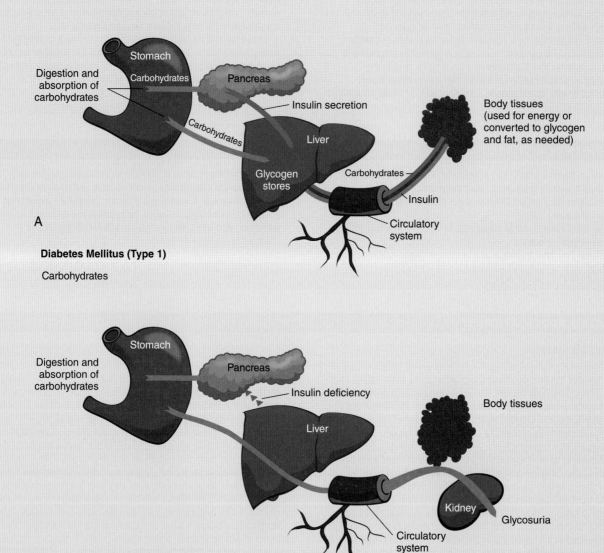

Normal

Carbohydrates

Stomach

Digestion and absorption of carbohydrates

Carbohydrates

Pancreas

Insulin secretion

Carbohydrates

Liver

Glycogen stores

Carbohydrates

Insulin

Circulatory system

Body tissues (used for energy or converted to glycogen and fat, as needed)

A

Diabetes Mellitus (Type 1)

Carbohydrates

Stomach

Digestion and absorption of carbohydrates

Pancreas

Insulin deficiency

Liver

Body tissues

Kidney

Glycosuria

Circulatory system

B

• **Fig. 7.8** Comparison of carbohydrate use in patients without diabetes (A) and patients with diabetes (B). (Adapted from *What Is Diabetes?* Eli Lilly & Co.; 1973.)

sample provides a "snapshot" of the blood glucose level at the time it is taken. However, patients may be using a continuous glucose monitoring (CGM) system and glucose values can be seen in a cell phone app without the need for a fingerstick. This valuable information should be obtained prior to a dental procedure to identify either very high (>200 mg/dL) or very low (<70 mg/dL) blood glucose levels. It is measured in milligrams per deciliter (mg/dL) or millimoles per liter (mmol/L). For patients not diagnosed with diabetes but with multiple risk factors, the American Diabetes Association suggests that screening be carried out in a health care setting. However, research suggests the feasibility and effectiveness of screening for undiagnosed T2DM in a dental environment.[20]

Another valuable reading is the glycosylated hemoglobin (A₁C) assay, a widely accepted and reliable measure of a blood glucose average level over the past 3 months. It provides a guide for long-term planning and possible adjustments to diabetes treatment. This reading helps evaluate metabolic control and determines whether the target range is maintained.[19]

Changes in capillary membranes can occur with uncontrolled blood glucose levels and result in renal complications (leading to renal failure, the inability of kidneys to excrete toxic waste materials), obstruction of circulation in the extremities (leading to gangrene), and progressive blood vessel damage in the retina of the eye (leading to blindness). Neuropathy, or deterioration of nervous tissue, also is frequently seen in patients with diabetes mellitus.

Abnormalities of the gastrointestinal tract causing nausea, early satiety, and frequent vomiting interfere with food intake and absorption.

Hypoglycemia, or low blood glucose levels (<70 mg/dL) can occur when a patient is taking insulin or an antidiabetic medication whose side effect is hypoglycemia. Symptoms include rapid heartbeat, hunger, shakiness, blurry vision, sweating, fatigue, dizziness, and irritability. However, the patient may be unaware of these symptoms (hypoglycemia unawareness); as a precautionary measure, obtain blood glucose readings before treatment to prevent a medical emergency. A patient whose blood glucose level is less than 70 mg/dL should be treated with 15 g of a carbohydrate source, such as 3 to 4 glucose tablets (amount per instructions), glucose gel (usually 1 tube, amount per instructions), 1 tablespoon of sugar or honey, hard candies (see food label for amount to consume), 4 oz of regular soda, or 4 oz of fruit juice. Wait 15 minutes and retest. If the blood glucose level is still less than 70 mg/dL or symptoms remain, repeat. When the blood glucose level is greater than 70 mg/dL, continue with treatment, and offer a meal or snack within 30 minutes.[21] If the patient is experiencing severe hypoglycemia (e.g., being uncooperative, unable to take fluids, or unconscious), administer glucagon to bring the blood glucose value into an appropriate range. In addition to the traditional intramuscular injection, new options for glucagon administration include a nasal spray (Baqsimi) and ready to use auto-injector (Gvoke HypoPen). Call 911 for assistance.[21]

TABLE 7.3 Comparison of Type 1 and Type 2 Diabetes Mellitus

	Type 1	Type 2
Prevalence	Approximately 5%–10% of cases	90%–95% of cases (1 in 5 adults >65 years old)
Age at onset	Most frequently during childhood or puberty, but may occur at later ages	Frequently >40 years, but occurring more frequently in overweight children and adolescents
Precipitating cause	Genetic, autoimmune destruction of the pancreatic cells that produce insulin	Obesity and inactivity
Type of onset	Sudden, but may develop slowly in adults	Usually gradual; may go undetected for years
Family history of diabetes	Frequently positive	Usually positive
Nutritional status at the time of onset	Normal weight with recent weight loss, but occasionally obese	Usually overweight (BMI > 25) with increased percentage of body fat predominantly in the abdominal region
Symptoms	Polydipsia, polyphagia, ketoacidosis, weight loss	Glycosuria without ketonuria; absent or mild polyuria and polydipsia
Blood glucose stability	Fluctuates widely in response to changes in insulin, diet, exercise, infection, and stress	Fluctuations less marked
Control of diabetes	Difficult	Easy, especially if diet is followed
Ketosis	Frequent	Seldom
Plasma insulin	Negligible or absent	May be low (not absent) or high, with insulin resistance
Vascular complications and degenerative changes	Occurs after diabetes is present for approximately 5 years	Increased risk of macrovascular and microvascular complications
Medical nutrition therapy	Required	May eliminate need for hypoglycemic agents or insulin or both
Medication	Insulin required for all	Usually can be controlled with hypoglycemic agents; insulin may be necessary for some

TABLE 7.4 American Diabetes Association Comparison of Diagnostic Values

Result	Fasting Plasma Glucose (mg/dL)	2-h Plasma Glucose (mg/dL)	A_{1c} (%)
Normal	<100	<140	<5.7
Prediabetes	100–125	140–199	5.7–6.4
Diabetes	126 or higher	200 or higher	6.5 or higher

Diabetes is diagnosed based on the plasma glucose levels.
From ElSayed NA, Aleppo G, Aroda VR, et al., American Diabetes Association. 2. Classification and diagnosis of diabetes: Standards of Medical Care in Diabetes—2023. *Diabetes Care.* 2023;46(suppl. 1):S19–S40.

Medical nutrition therapy is the cornerstone for preventing hyperglycemia and hypoglycemia and decreasing chronic complications. No single dietary plan can be appropriate for all individuals with different personalities and lifestyles. The objective of a meal plan is to empower patients to maintain good control of their diabetes or to promote near-normal blood glucose, lipid, and blood pressure levels. Additionally, food choices should promote overall health by providing optimal nutrition and allowing physical activity; achieving or maintaining an ideal body weight; and preventing or delaying development or progression of periodontal disease, cardiovascular, renal, retinal, neurologic, and other complications associated with diabetes, insofar as these are related to metabolic control. The meal plan should be flexible to allow personal and cultural preferences and lifestyles, while respecting the individual's wishes and willingness to make changes. Table 7.5 lists some of the specific nutrition recommendations by the American Diabetes Association.

Not only are food choices important to the diabetes meal pattern, but spacing of meals and portion sizes also are important concepts to consider.

Carbohydrate consumption during the day should be spaced to every 4 to 5 hours, allowing the addition of nutrient-dense snacks throughout the day. The use of food scales plus measuring cups and spoons will help with portion size. Dental professionals need to understand and respect the role that nutrition plays in diabetes in order to support the patient's efforts and emphasize healthful eating patterns.

Carbohydrate counting, consistent with the *Dietary Guidelines* and *MyPlate*, focuses on total carbohydrate consumption. Because carbohydrate is the major factor in blood glucose fluctuations, the given amount of carbohydrate affects insulin requirements more than the protein and fat content.

For individuals with a healthy weight and normal lipid profile, the American Diabetes Association recommends the same guidelines as advocated by the National Cholesterol Education Program, discussed in Chapter 6. Because many patients with diabetes have undesirable lipid levels, a moderate increase in monounsaturated fat with a moderate intake of carbohydrate is recommended. [22]

Certified Diabetes Care and Education Specialist

All individuals with diabetes or at risk of diabetes should be referred to a certified diabetes care and education specialist (CDCES). A CDCES is the diabetes expert. As defined by the credentialing organization, the Certification Board for Diabetes Care and Education Specialists, a CDCES is "a health professional who possesses comprehensive knowledge of and experience in prediabetes, diabetes prevention, and management. The CDCES educates and supports people affected by diabetes to understand and manage the condition. A CDCES promotes self-management to achieve individualized behavioral and treatment goals that optimize health outcomes." [23] Physicians, registered nurses, pharmacists, and dietitians are included in the examples of health professionals who are eligible to complete the rigorous requirements needed to attain this certification. There is a Unique Qualifications Pathway (UQ) for healthcare professionals that do not meet the discipline requirement of those listed that may pursue the CDCES. At present, the guidelines don't clearly specify this as a pathway for dental hygienists. Further information can be found on the CDCES website https://www.cbdce.org/.

◆ **HEALTH APPLICATION 7—CONT'D**

TABLE 7.5 American Diabetes Association Medical Nutrition Therapy Recommendations

ABC Rating[a]	Recommendation
Effectiveness of Nutrition Therapy	
A	An individualized nutrition program, preferably provided by a registered dietitian, is recommended for all people with T1DM, T2DM, prediabetes, and gestational diabetes.
Energy Balance	
A	Individuals with diabetes should use behavior modification to achieve and maintain a minimum 5% weight loss.
Protein	
B	In individuals with T2DM, ingested protein appears to increase insulin response without increasing plasma glucose concentrations. Therefore carbohydrate sources high in protein should not be used to treat or prevent hypoglycemia.
Carbohydrates	
B	Encourage avoiding highly and ultra-processed foods with a focus on whole grain, high fiber (at least 14 grams per 1,000 kcal) and more nutrient dense sources of carbohydrates.
B	Minimize consumption of sugar-sweetened beverages to help manage high blood glucose and reduce CVD risk.
A	Choose nutrient dense foods and minimize foods and beverages with added sugars.
B	Educate the patient about the impact of carbohydrates on blood glucose.
B	For those using fixed insulin doses, educate on consistent patterns of carbohydrate intake to reduce risk for hypoglycemia.
Dietary Fat	
B	Whereas data on the ideal total dietary fat content for people with diabetes are inconclusive, an eating plan emphasizing elements of a Mediterranean-style diet rich in monounsaturated fats may improve glucose metabolism and lower cardiovascular disease risk and can be an effective alternative to a diet low in total fat but relatively high in carbohydrates.
Eating Patterns and Macronutrient Distribution	
B	As there is no single ideal dietary distribution of calories among carbohydrates, fats, and proteins for people with diabetes, macronutrient distribution should be individualized while keeping nutrient quality, total calorie, and metabolic goals in mind.
B	Carbohydrate intake from whole grains, vegetables, fruits, legumes, and dairy products, with an emphasis on foods with higher fiber and lower glycemic load, should be advised over other sources, especially those containing sugars.
B	Minimize the overall consumption of carbohydrate intake that have the capacity to displace healthier, more nutrient-dense food choices.
Micronutrients and Herbal Supplements	
C	There is no clear evidence that dietary supplementation with vitamins, minerals, herbs, or spices can for glycemic benefits and there may be safety concerns regarding the long-term use of antioxidant supplements.
Alcohol	
C	Adults with diabetes who drink alcohol should do so in moderation (no more than one drink/day for adult females and no more than two drinks/day for adult males).
B	Alcohol consumption may place people with diabetes at increased risk for delayed hypoglycemia, especially if taking insulin or diabetes medications in which hypoglycemia is a side effect. Education and awareness regarding the recognition and management of delayed hypoglycemia are warranted.
Sodium	
B	As for the general population, people with diabetes should limit sodium consumption to <2300 mg/day, although further restriction may be indicated for those with both diabetes and hypertension.
Nonnutritive Sweeteners	
B	The use of nonnutritive sweeteners has the potential to reduce overall calorie and carbohydrate intake if substituted for caloric sweeteners and without compensation by the intake of additional calories from other food sources. Nonnutritive sweeteners are generally safe to use within the defined acceptable daily intake levels.

[a]ABC rating—evidence based on research criteria: A, strong supporting evidence; B, some supporting evidence; C, limited supporting evidence. Data from: American Diabetes Association Professional Practice Committee. 5. Facilitating positive health behaviors and well-being to improve health outcomes: Standards of Care in Diabetes—2024. Diabetes Care 2024;47(Suppl. 1): S77–S110.

Data from ElSayed NA, Aleppo G, Aroda VR, et al., American Diabetes Association. 5. Facilitating positive health behaviors and well-being to improve health outcomes: Standards of Care in Diabetes—2023. *Diabetes Care.* 2023;46(suppl 1):S68–S96.

◆ CASE APPLICATION FOR THE DENTAL HYGIENIST

On a routine recare appointment, Ronnie, who is 10 years old, reports that he was diagnosed with type 2 diabetes about a year ago. He appears to be about 100 lb overweight. After talking with him, you learn that he does not want to be labeled as "different" from his friends, so he eats when and what they eat. Typically, they eat cheeseburgers, pizza, French fries, shakes, and regular sodas throughout the day. He says that he does not have time to eat breakfast. He does not floss his teeth, has numerous caries, and has bleeding on probing.

Nutritional Assessment
- Observe height, weight, BMI, and age
- Knowledge of diabetes guidelines
- Motivation level
- Food/nutrient intake
- Eating habits
- Support from family and friends
- Activity level

Nutritional Diagnosis

Given the age of the patient and the complexity of nutrition guidance needed for T2DM, this is beyond the scope of practice for the dental hygienist.

Nutritional Goals

Support the patient in following a healthy eating pattern as outlined in the *Dietary Guidelines* and being physically active.

Nutritional Implementation

Intervention: Give Ronnie and his parents the reference of a CDCES or an RDN who can provide individualized nutritional counseling based on the patient's unique needs.

Rationale: Nutrient-dense food choices, rather than high-calorie foods, are needed to maintain his health and promote growth. The knowledge of nutrition and expertise of an RDN or CDCES in counseling is recommended to address the obesity and T2DM without affecting his linear growth.

Intervention: Explain that some of his food choices are not good for his overall physical or oral health.

Rationale: Consuming too many carbohydrates at meals and snacks affects his blood glucose level and increases the risk of caries.

Intervention: Explain that carbohydrates, proteins, and fats, all provide calories, but fats are the most concentrated source of energy.

Rationale: To maintain his weight while still growing, wise food choices are advisable. Foods high in fat and sugar will not help him in his attempts to look his best and may worsen his diabetes status.

Intervention: Stress the importance of consuming complex carbohydrate and fiber, and reducing intake of fat and calories.

Rationale: Complex carbohydrate and fiber intake are effective in helping maintain a lower calorie intake without excessive hunger. Fat reduction enhances weight maintenance because a lower fat intake may help reduce energy intake and decrease risk of developing heart disease.

Intervention: Discuss the benefits of eating at routine times.

Rationale: This is important for controlling his diabetes and may allow him time to brush his teeth after eating, reducing his risk of caries.

Intervention: Discuss the importance of a plan incorporating diet, physical activity, and behavior change.

Rationale: This combination of therapies has proven more effective for long-term weight control.

Intervention: Explain that good oral hygiene is very important for patients with diabetes because of an exaggerated response to plaque biofilm.

Rationale: Knowledge may help increase compliance.

Intervention: Identify physical activities he enjoys. Encourage him to use a fitness watch or cell phone app to track his steps and set goals for gradually increasing steps. Ways to be more active might include: walking to school and friend's home instead of having his mom or dad drive him; taking the dog for a walk; or walking with his family after dinner.

Rationale: Weight and diabetes control are improved when energy expenditure is increased along with decreased calorie intake. Additionally, physical activity helps increase muscle mass and improves strength.

Evaluation

The patient consulted with the RDN and reduced the number of sodas he was drinking before the next recall visit. Also, he had no new caries.

◆ CASE STUDY

Jay G. is a 16-year-old high school athlete on the football and baseball teams. He recently developed three dental caries. His classmates have encouraged him to eat a high-protein, low-carbohydrate diet. His mother is concerned about this and talks to her best friend who is a dental hygienist.

1. What points do you think the dental hygienist should mention to this mother?
2. For increased energy expenditure, what should be the primary source of nutrients?
3. Would decreasing dietary carbohydrate content have a positive effect on the rate of dental caries?
4. What is the effect of high-protein intake?
5. On a high-protein, low-carbohydrate diet (approximately 120 g of protein, 80 g of carbohydrate, 2800 cal), where would most of his energy requirements come from? Is this good or bad?
6. Which vitamins are important in the production of energy?

3. Assuming that height and weight are the same, is the BMR higher or lower in:
   A male or a female?
   An athlete or a sedentary person?
   A 40-year-old or a 20-year-old?
   A female who is not pregnant or a female who is pregnant?
4. How many calories of protein, fat, and carbohydrate, are in 1 cup of homogenized milk that contains 8.5 g of protein, 8.5 g of fat, and 12 g of carbohydrate?

References

1. ElSayed NA, Aleppo G, Aroda VR, et al. American Diabetes Association. 5. Facilitating positive health behaviors and wellbeing to improve health outcomes Standards of Care in Diabetes—2023. *Diabetes Care.* 2023;46(suppl 1):S68–S96.
2. Comerford KB, Papanikolaou Y, Jones JM, et al. Toward an evidence-based definition and classification of carbohydrate food quality: an expert panel report. *Nutrients.* 2021;13(8):2667. https://doi.org/10.3390/nu13082667.
3. Raynor HA, Champagne CM. Position of the Academy of Nutrition and Dietetics. Interventions for the treatment of overweight and obesity in adults. *J Acad Nutr Diet.* 2016;116(1):129–147.
4. Butts M, Sundaram VL, Murughiyan U, Borthakur A, Singh S. The influence of alcohol consumption on intestinal nutrient absorption:

◆ Student Readiness

1. Define the terms energy, thermogenic effect, basal metabolism, and basal energy expenditure.
2. Calculate your total caloric needs for 1 day (BMR plus estimated voluntary energy expenditures plus thermogenic effect).

a comprehensive review. *Nutrients*. 2023;15(7):1571. https://doi.org/10.3390/nu15071571.

5. Krittanawong C, Isath A, Rosenson RS, et al. Alcohol consumption and cardiovascular health. *Am J Med*. 2022;135(10):1213–1230.e3.

6. National Institute on Alcohol Abuse and Alcoholism. *Drinking Levels Defined*. https://www.niaaa.nih.gov/alcohol-health/overview-alcohol-consumption/moderate-binge-drinking.

7. National Academies of Sciences, Engineering, and Medicine. *Dietary Reference Intakes for Energy*. The National Academies Press; 2023. https://doi.org/10.17226/26818.

8. United States Department of Health and Human Services. *Physical Activity Guidelines for Americans*. 2nd ed. 2018. https://health.gov/sites/default/files/2019–09/Physical_Activity_Guidelines_2nd_edition.pdf.

9. Williams B, Mancia G, Spiering W, et al. ESC Scientific Document Group. 2018 ESC/ESH Guidelines for the management of arterial hypertension. *Eur Heart J*. 2018;39(33):3021–3104.

10. Sanchez-Lastra MA, Ding D, et al. Physical activity and mortality across levels of adiposity: a prospective cohort study from the UK biobank. *Mayo Clin Proc*. 2021;96(1):105–119.

11. Rock CL, Thomson C, Gansler T, et al. American Cancer Society guideline for diet and physical activity for cancer prevention. *CA Cancer J Clin*. 2020;70(4):245–271.

12. Institute of Medicine (IOM), National Academy of Sciences. *Dietary Reference Intakes for Energy, Carbohydrates, Fiber, Fat, Protein and Amino acids (Macronutrients)*. National Academy Press; 2002.

13. Wilk K, Korytek W, Pelczyńska M, Moszak M, Bogdański P. The effect of artificial sweeteners use on sweet taste perception and weight loss efficacy: a review. *Nutrients*. 2022;14(6):1261. https://doi.org/10.3390/nu14061261.

14. Belanger-Gravel A, Godin G, Bilodeau A, et al. The effect of implementation intentions on physical activity among obese older adults: a randomized control study. *Psychol Health*. 2013;28(2):217–233.

15. Hall KS, Hyde ET, Bassett DR, et al. Systematic review of the prospective association of daily step counts with risk of mortality, cardiovascular disease, and dysglycemia. *Int J Behav Nutr Phys Act*. 2020;17(1):78. https://doi.org/10.1186/s12966-020-00978-9.

16. Feig EH, Harnedy LE, Celano CM, Huffman JC. Increase in daily steps during the early phase of a physical activity intervention for type 2 diabetes as a predictor of intervention outcome. *Int J Behav Med*. 2021;28(6):834–839.

17. Centers for Disease Control and Prevention. *National Diabetes Statistics Report Website*. https://www.cdc.gov/diabetes/data/statistics-report/index.html.

18. Diabetes Prevention Program Research Group Long-term effects of lifestyle intervention or metformin on diabetes development and microvascular complications over 15-year follow-up: the Diabetes Prevention Program Outcomes Study. *Lancet Diabetes Endocrinol*. 2015;3(11):866–875.

19. ElSayed NA, Aleppo G, Aroda VR, et al. American Diabetes Association. 2. Classification and diagnosis of diabetes: Standards of Medical Care in Diabetes—2023. *Diabetes Care*. 2023;46(suppl 1):S19–S40.

20. Chinnasamy A, Moodie M. Prevalence of undiagnosed diabetes and prediabetes in the dental setting: a systematic review and *meta*-analysis. *Int J Dent*. 2020;2020 2964020.

21. Centers for Disease Control and Prevention. *How to Treat Low Blood Sugar (Hypoglycemia)*. https://www.cdc.gov/diabetes/basics/low-blood-sugar-treatment.html

22. Quin F, et al. Metabolic effects of monounsaturated fatty acid-enriched diets compared with carbohydrate or polyunsaturated fatty acid-enriched diets in patients with type 2 diabetes: a systematic review and *meta*-analysis of randomized controlled trials. *Diabetes Care*. 2016;39(8):1448–1457.

23. Certification Board for Diabetes Care and Education. Thinking about earning the CDCES? 2024. http://www.ncbde.org/.

 Evolve Resources

Please visit http://evolve.elsevier.com/Mallonee/nutritional for additional practice and study support tools.

8

Vitamins Required for Calcified Structures

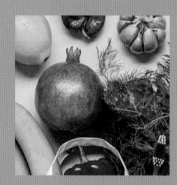

STUDENT LEARNING OUTCOMES

On completion of this chapter, the student will be able to achieve the following learning outcomes:

1. Discuss the following points related to vitamins:
   - Discuss the requirements and deficiencies of vitamins.
   - List the fat-soluble vitamins, as well as the water-soluble vitamins.
   - Compare the characteristics of water-soluble vitamins with those of fat-soluble vitamins.

2. For vitamin A, C, D, E, and K:
   - Identify functions, deficiency, toxicity, and oral symptoms associated with each vitamin.
   - Identify foods that are good sources of each vitamin.
   - Customize nutrition recommendations for these vitamins to meet patient's needs.
   - Counsel a patient on individual nutrition recommendations to meet needs for these vitamins.

KEY TERMS

Alopecia
Ameloblasts
Anticoagulant
Calcitonin
Collagen
Diplopia
Enamel hypoplasia
Epiphyses
Fibroblasts
Follicular hyperkeratosis
Hematopoiesis
Hypercarotenemia

Hypervitaminosis A
Leukoplakia
Lysosomes
Meta-analysis
Night blindness
Odontoblasts
Osteoblasts
Osteocalcin
Osteoclasts
Osteodentin
Osteomalacia
Petechiae

Prothrombin
Retinoic acid
Rhodopsin
Scorbutic
Secondary deficiency
Tocopherols
Tocotrienols
Xeroderma
Xerophthalmia

⬡ TEST YOUR NQ

1. **T/F** Fat-soluble vitamins are stored in the body.
2. **T/F** Vitamins do not provide energy.
3. **T/F** Vitamin E is found in vegetable oils and green leafy vegetables.
4. **T/F** Fat-soluble vitamins include A, D, E, and K.
5. **T/F** Animal foods are the principal dietary source of beta-carotene.
6. **T/F** Xerophthalmia occurs with a deficiency of vitamin A.

7. **T/F** The liver and kidney help convert vitamin D to its active form.
8. **T/F** An excess of vitamin D causes rickets.
9. **T/F** Vitamin K is essential for regulating blood calcium and phosphorus levels.
10. **T/F** Vitamin C is needed for wound healing.

Overview of Vitamins

Nutrients never work alone but rather in partnership with each other. Vitamins are catalysts for all metabolic reactions using proteins, fats, and carbohydrates for energy, growth, and cell maintenance. Because only small amounts of these chemical substances are obtained from food and facilitate millions of processes, they may be regarded as "miracle workers."

Eating fats, carbohydrates, and proteins without enough vitamins means that the energy from these nutrients cannot be used. The opposite is also true. Vitamins do not provide energy, and they cannot be used without an adequate supply of fats, carbohydrates,

• BOX 8.1   **Vitamins Required for Calcified Structures**

Fat-Soluble Vitamins
Vitamin A
Vitamin D
Vitamin E
Vitamin K

Water-Soluble Vitamins
Vitamin C

proteins, and minerals. Most vitamins come in several forms; each form may perform a different task. Vitamins are easily destroyed by the heat, oxidation, and chemical processes used in their extraction. In this text, water-soluble vitamins, fat-soluble vitamins, and minerals are presented based on their function in calcified structures (teeth and periodontium) or their role in oral soft tissues (oral mucous membranes and salivary glands) to familiarize the dental hygienist with nutrients that might be involved when oral changes are observed. Most dental hygiene students are well aware of the role of several minerals in calcified structures in the oral cavity, but vitamins presented in this chapter are also important for healthy teeth and the periodontium (Box 8.1).

Most nutrients have various functions; some are involved in both calcified and soft oral tissues. Oral physiologic roles for these nutrients are presented in appropriate chapters, but information such as requirements and food sources are found only when the vitamin is first discussed. Fat-soluble and water-soluble vitamins differ in many ways, but a basic understanding of their fundamental similarities can facilitate learning.

Requirements

Although vitamins are vital to life, they are required in minute amounts. Vitamins are similar to hormones because of their potent effects, but they must come from an outside source because they either cannot be produced by the body or cannot be produced in adequate amounts to meet physiologic needs. Each vitamin is essential, although the amount needed may vary from 2.4 µg per day (for vitamin B_{12}) to 550 mg per day (for choline).

The dietary reference intakes (DRIs) are the amounts of vitamins for healthy populations and may differ by age, period of growth (e.g., adolescence, pregnancy, and lactation), and sex.[1] Personal factors (e.g., smoking; use of alcohol, caffeine, or drugs; medical conditions; and stress) modify an individual's requirements and may lead to increased nutrient needs.

Deficiencies

If adequate amounts of the nutrient are unavailable to sustain biochemical functions, a nutritional deficiency occurs. A nutritional deficiency as a result of decreased intake is called a primary deficiency. A vitamin deficiency caused by inadequate absorption or use, increased requirements, excretion, or destruction is called a secondary deficiency. Nutrients are codependent; a deficiency of one may cause deficiency symptoms of another.

A CDC report suggests less than 10% of individuals in the United States had a nutrient deficiency in 2012,[2] although several groups are at risk (Box 8.2). Vitamin levels in the blood are often unmeasurable; thus a nutritional deficiency may be identified on

• BOX 8.2   **Groups at Potential Risk of Nutritional Deficiencies**

- Older adults
- Impoverished, low income
- Vegans
- Chronic disease states
- Alcoholics
- Inadequate dietary intake
- Smokers
- Excessive caffeine use
- Polypharmacy
- Physiologic stress
- Periods of rapid growth
  - Pregnancy
  - Lactation
  - Infants, children, adolescents
- Medical conditions causing
  - Inadequate absorption
  - Inadequate use
  - Excessive excretion
  - Destruction
- Surgery
- Burns
- Fever

the basis of clinical signs and symptoms and their response to vitamin supplementation. However, one of the peculiarities of vitamins is that the symptoms of a deficiency frequently resemble the symptoms caused by excessive intake (toxicity), making definitive diagnosis difficult.

Nutrition deficiencies in the U.S. population

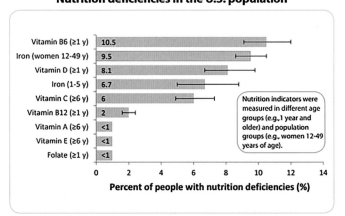

Nutrition indicators were measured in different age groups (e.g., 1 year and older) and population groups (e.g., women 12-49 years of age).

• The graph shows prevalence estimates of nutrition deficiencies among people who live in the U.S. (NHANES 2003-2006). Of all the nutrients listed, the most people had vitamin B6, iron, and vitamin D deficiencies, and the fewest people had vitamin A, vitamin E, and folate deficiencies. (From https://www.cdc.gov/nutritionreport/pdf/4page_%202nd%20nutrition%20report_508_032912.pdf)

Characteristics of Fat-Soluble Vitamins

Although the four fat-soluble vitamins (A, D, E, and K) differ in function, use, and sources, they have several similar characteristics: (1) they are soluble in fat or fat solvents; (2) they are fairly stable to heat, as in cooking; (3) they are organic substances (contain carbon); (4) they do not contain nitrogen; (5) they are absorbed in the intestine along with fats and lipids in foods; and (6) they require bile for absorption.

Fat-soluble vitamins are different from water-soluble vitamins mainly because larger amounts can be stored in the body. Vitamins A and D are stored for long periods; thus minor shortages may not be identified until drastic depletion has occurred. For example, vitamin A can be stored in the liver to meet basic needs for at least 1 year. Observable signs and symptoms of a dietary deficiency are often not identified until they are in an advanced state. Dietary deficiencies occur when foods consumed do not provide necessary amounts of a nutrient.

International units (IU) reflect this biologic activity in animal studies and do not always represent absorption rates in humans. Because of this, the retinol activity equivalents (RAEs) standard was created for vitamin A. The recommended dietary allowances (RDAs) for vitamins A and E were determined based on the biologic effectiveness of each form because the different forms of these vitamins have varying activity levels. After the measurement of all active forms of the vitamins, the quantity is converted to micrograms or milligrams and totaled to indicate the amount of vitamin in that food. RAEs reflect vitamin A activity of foods. Although previous food tables listed IUs, more accurate weight measurements in micrograms or milligrams are now used.

Characteristics of Water-Soluble Vitamins

B-complex vitamins and vitamin C are water soluble and are organic substances. In contrast to vitamin C and fat-soluble vitamins, B-complex vitamins contain nitrogen. Water-soluble vitamins have vital roles as coenzymes, which are necessary for almost every cellular reaction in the body (Figure 2–22). Vitamin C is discussed in this chapter with the fat-soluble vitamins because of its vital role in collagen synthesis which serves as a structural component of teeth[3]; it is also important in oral soft tissues. B-complex vitamins are discussed in Chapter 11.

Most water-soluble vitamins are readily absorbed in the jejunum. High concentrations of these vitamins result in decreased absorption efficiency. The body stores very small amounts of each of these vitamins; few water-soluble vitamins produce toxic symptoms. Because of their limited storage, daily intake is important.

● DENTAL CONSIDERATIONS

- Assessment is crucial to determine nutrient needs. Assess for the following: smoking, alcohol use, excessive caffeine use, medications, physiologic stress, chronic conditions, or surgery. If any of these is present, vitamin requirements in the diet may need to be altered.
- Dietary and physical assessments are more diagnostic for vitamin deficiencies than laboratory values. A combination of the three assessments provides the greatest amount of information on an individual's nutrition status.
- Patients with mobile teeth, missing teeth, ill-fitting dentures and/or partials, and those who do not wear dentures are at greater risk of malnutrition.[4]
- Evaluate nutrient intake of groups at high risk for developing nutritional deficiencies, such as older adults, impoverished/low-income patients, patients with chronic diseases, and those with physiologic disorders that interfere with food consumption. If indicated, refer the patient to a registered dietitian nutritionist (RDN).

● NUTRITIONAL DIRECTIONS

- No vitamin contains calories, but some vitamins, especially the B-complex vitamins, are essential to the production of energy.

Vitamin A (Retinol, Carotene)

Retinol is the dietary source of vitamin A from animal sources, and beta-carotene is the principal carotenoid present in plant pigments. Retinoic acid is the most biologically active form of vitamin A.

Physiologic Roles

Vitamin A has many hormone-like roles in the body. It is also required for vision, immune function, integrity of the epithelium, reproduction, normal growth and development (e.g., bone), and facilitating the transcription of DNA into RNA.[5,6]

Vision

Retinol is converted to retinal in the eye. Retinal combines with opsin, a protein in the eye, to form the visual pigment, rhodopsin.[5,6] Night blindness may result from inadequate vitamin A to permit rhodopsin production.[6] This condition takes years to develop in adults, but occurs much sooner in children because they have fewer body stores.

Growth

Vitamin A is necessary for growth and repair of soft tissues and bones. In skeletal tissue, vitamin A is necessary for resorption of old bone and synthesis of new bone.[6] Retinoic acid, produced by the body from retinal, is the form of vitamin A involved in the development of bone and teeth, especially in the formation of ameloblasts (enamel-forming cells) and odontoblasts (dentin-forming cells) along with growth and maintenance of bone. Vitamin A deficiency during preeruptive stages of tooth development leads to enamel hypoplasia and defective dentin formation.[7]

Cancer

Vitamin A and carotene have consistently been associated with cancer prevention because of their importance in the development and integrity of cells. The antioxidant role of vitamin A is discussed in *Health Application 8*. Antioxidants prevent cell membrane damage by free radicals that are produced by cells and tissues using free oxygen. Unchecked by an antioxidant, free radicals can damage the structure and impair the function of cell membranes. Studies suggest that vitamin A and beta-carotene may resolve oral leukoplakia, but relapse is common.[8] Leukoplakia (see Figs. 17.11 and 17.16) is a white plaque that forms on oral mucous membranes that cannot be wiped away. It has the potential to become cancerous. Whether beta-carotene or some other components in fruits and vegetables can help to resolve leukoplakia has not been determined. Increasing consumption of fruits and vegetables is recommended because some studies show an increased risk of lung cancer among smokers using beta-carotene supplements.[9] The American Cancer Society does not support vitamin A supplementation for cancer prevention, but recommends getting the vitamin through food sources.[10]

Requirements

As shown in Table 8.1, the RDA for vitamin A is 900 µg RAE for males and 700 µg RAE for females (1 RAE = 1 µg = 12 µg

TABLE 8.1 Dietary Reference Intakes for Vitamin A

Life Stage	EAR (µg/day) Male	EAR (µg/day) Female	RDA (µg/day) Male	RDA (µg/day) Female	AI (µ/day)	UL (µg/day)[a]
0–6 months					400	600
7–12 months					500	600
1–3 years	210	210	300	300		600
4–8 years	275	275	400	400		900
9–13 years	445	420	600	600		1700
14–18 years	630	485	900	700		2800
>18 years	625	500	900	700		3000
Pregnancy						
14–18 years		530		750		2800
19–50 years		550		770		3000
Lactation						
14–18 years		885		1200		2800
19–50 years		900		1300		3000

[a]Preformed vitamin A.

AI, Adequate intake; *EAR*, estimated average requirement; *RDA*, recommended dietary allowance; *UL*, upper intake level.

Data from Institute of Medicine (IOM), Panel on Micronutrients. Dietary Reference Intakes for Vitamin C, Vitamin K, Arsenic, Boron, Chromium, Copper, Iodine, Iron, Manganese, Molybdenum, Nickel, Silicon, Vanadium, and Zinc. National Academies Press; 2001.

beta-carotene = 3.3 IU). The tolerable upper intake level (UL) is 3000 µg RAE per day. The need for vitamin A is increased during periods of rapid growth, when gastrointestinal problems affect its absorption or conversion (e.g., cystic fibrosis, celiac disease, Crohn's disease, or chronic diarrhea), and in hepatic diseases that limit vitamin A storage or conversion of beta-carotene to its active form. Although no UL has been established for beta-carotene, the National Academy of Medicine (formerly the Institute of Medicine) does not advise supplements for healthy people.[11]

Average intake in the United States meets the RDA,[2,12] and because vitamin A can be stored in the liver, most adults have sufficient quantities to maintain health. Inadequate intake occurs in lower socioeconomic groups as a consequence of inadequate vegetable and fruit intake.

Sources

Vitamin A, as preformed retinol, is found in organ meats, such as liver. It is also found in milk, cheese, butter, eggs, cod liver oil, and fortified foods (e.g., breakfast cereals). Sometimes retinol is added to skim milk and margarine. Beta-carotene or provitamin A is also present in yellow, orange, and green leafy vegetables (e.g., spinach, turnip greens, broccoli; Table 8.2). Although not as well absorbed as from animal sources and fortified foods, beta-carotene is still a valuable source of vitamin A. Beta-carotene is deep red in pure form and derives its name from carrots from which it was first isolated. Chlorophyll disguises carotenoids in green vegetables. Most yellow, orange, and dark-green fruits and vegetables are high in carotene or vitamin A content. The deeper the color, the more vitamin A activity is present in a fruit or vegetable.

Absorption and Excretion

Absorption is optimal when body stores are depleted and when adequate amounts of other interrelated nutrients are present. The presence of vitamin E and the hormone thyroxine also enhances the use of vitamin A.

The liver stores approximately 90% of vitamin A, while smaller quantities are stored in the kidneys, lungs, and adipose tissue. Adequate serum proteins are necessary to mobilize vitamin A from the liver. Vitamin A is not readily excreted by the body, but a small amount is lost in urine.

Hyper States and Hypo States

Extreme levels of vitamin A (high or low) can cause serious problems, even resulting in death (Fig. 8.1).

Toxicity

When present in high concentrations, unbound vitamin A causes damage to cell membranes, especially in red blood cells and lysosomes (small bodies occurring in many types of cells). Large amounts of vitamin A supplements can exceed the storage capacity of the liver. If this occurs, free vitamin A enters the bloodstream and exerts toxic effects on cell membranes. High levels of vitamin A in the body are referred to as hypervitaminosis A.

Maternal consumption of vitamin A supplements before conception and during the first trimester of pregnancy has been associated with fetal birth defects (see Table 13.3 for effects of vitamin A toxicity during pregnancy).[5,13] Toxicity is evident in infants by bulging of the fontanel as a result of increased cerebrospinal fluid

TABLE 8.2	Food Sources of Vitamin A	
Food	**Portion**	**Vitamin A (µg RAE)**
Beef liver, cooked	1 slice	6531
Cod liver oil	1 tbsp	4080
Pumpkin, canned	1 cup	1879
Sweet potato, baked	1 medium	1436
Spinach, cooked	1 cup	614
Carrots, baby	5	418
Butternut squash, baked	½ cup	292
Turnip greens, cooked	½ cup	274
Cantaloupe	1 cup	270
Milk, 2% fortified	1 cup	203
Collard greens, cooked	½ cup	166
Apricots, dried	½ cup	144
Romaine lettuce, shredded	1 cup	130
Red pepper	½ cup	118
Margarine	1 tbsp	115
Butter	1 tbsp	106
Egg, hard boiled	1	90
Cheddar cheese	1 oz	90
Spinach, raw	1 cup	71
Broccoli, cooked	½ cup	6

RAEs, Retinol activity equivalents.
Data from United States Department of Agriculture (USDA), Agricultural Research Service.
What's in the Foods You Eat Search Tool. 2019–2020. https://www.ars.usda.gov/northeast-area/beltsville-md-bhnrc/beltsville-human-nutrition-research-center/food-surveys-research-group/docs/whats-in-the-foods-you-eat-search-tool/.

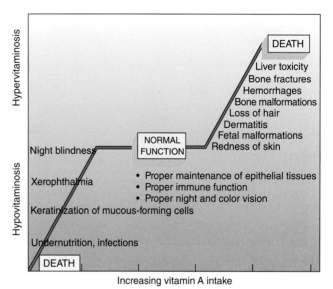

• **Fig. 8.1** Vitamin A intake. This chart shows how changing the amount of vitamin A in the diet can lead to hypovitaminosis A or hypervitaminosis A. In the extreme, either condition can lead to death. (From Patton KT, Thibodeau GA. *Anatomy and Physiology*. 9th ed. Mosby Elsevier; 2016.)

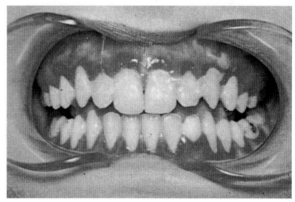

• **Fig. 8.2** Hypervitaminosis A. Bright-red marginal discoloration of the gingiva shown here is characteristic. (Courtesy Dr M. D. Muenter. From McLaren DS. *A Colour Atlas and Text of Diet-Related Disorders*. 2nd ed. Mosby–Year Book; 1992.)

pressure. Other clinical symptoms include severe headache; nausea and vomiting; **diplopia** (double vision); lethargy and irritability; **alopecia** (hair loss); dryness of the mucous membranes; reddened gingiva (Fig. 8.2); thinning of the epithelium; cracking and bleeding lips; and increased activity of **osteoclasts** (cells associated with bone resorption), which leads to decalcification; desquamation of oral mucosa, and liver abnormalities.[5,13]

Excess vitamin A (primarily in the form of retinol) may have a negative impact on bone health. Excess intake of vitamin A in the long term could contribute to osteoporosis and risk for fracture.[13] How this change in bone mineral density may affect alveolar bone is unknown.

Toxicity from excessive intake of vitamin A food sources occurs occasionally, but most cases are a result of too much supplementation. Beta-carotene is much less toxic than vitamin A. The body converts only the amount of carotenoids it needs into vitamin A. Although beta-carotenes are not toxic, overconsumption may result in **hypercarotenemia**, yellow pigmentation of the skin occurring first on the palms of the hands and soles of the feet, which is caused by carotene storage in fatty tissue (Fig. 8.3).[5] This condition subsides when ingestion of beta-carotene is reduced.

Deficiency

Groups most at risk for deficiency include premature infants, infants, children, pregnant and lactating females in low and middle-income countries along with those who may have fat malabsorption conditions such as cystic fibrosis, celiac disease, Crohn's disease, and ulcerative colitis.[5] Mild vitamin A deficiency may contribute to a depressed immune response.

Inadequate vitamin A intake results in degeneration of epithelial cells in the eye and cessation of tear secretion. Lids become swollen and sticky with pus, and eyes become sensitive to light in **xerophthalmia**, sometimes resulting in permanent blindness. The first symptom of xerophthalmia is night blindness,[13] followed by the occurrence of xerotic, keratinized spots on the conjunctiva, called Bitot spots. Bitot spots can generally be reversed with vitamin A supplementation to prevent the development of permanent blindness (Fig. 8.4).[14]

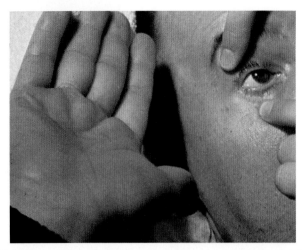

• **Fig. 8.3** Hypercarotenosis. The face, eye, and palm of the hand. The sclerae remain clear, distinguishing the condition from jaundice. (Courtesy Dr I.A. Abrahamson, Sr. From McLaren DS. *A Colour Atlas and Text of Diet-Related Disorders*. 2nd ed. Mosby–Year Book; 1992.)

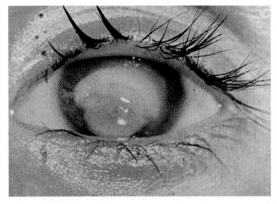

• **Fig. 8.4** Xerophthalmia. (From McLaren DS. *A Colour Atlas and Text of Diet-Related Disorders*. 2nd ed. Mosby–Year Book; 1992.)

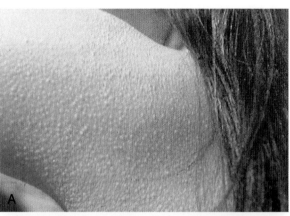

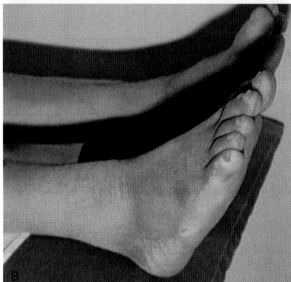

• **Fig. 8.5** (A) Follicular hyperkeratosis caused by vitamin A deficiency. (B) Hyperkeratosis. The skin over parts of the body is thickened, dry, and wrinkled, associated with vitamin A deficiency. (From McLaren DS. *A Colour Atlas and Text of Diet-Related Disorders*. 2nd ed. Mosby–Year Book; 1992.)

Degeneration of epithelial cells results in an inability to produce mucus. This occurs not only in epithelial cells, but also in the intestines and lungs. Xeroderma can progress until the whole body is covered with dry, flaky, scaly skin that is similar to dandruff. It is followed by follicular hyperkeratosis, in which the skin is thickened, dry, and wrinkled (Fig. 8.5).[15] Keratinization may also affect the oral mucosa, and the respiratory and gastrointestinal tracts. In these areas, degeneration of epithelial cells results in increased risk of infection and delayed or impaired wound healing.

Severe vitamin A deficiency may result in enamel hypoplasia and defective dentin formation in developing teeth. Enamel hypoplasia involves defects in the enamel matrix and incomplete calcification of the enamel, thereby inhibiting enamel formation. Odontoblasts lose their ability to arrange themselves in normal parallel linear formation, resulting in degeneration and atrophy of ameloblasts. The result is small pits or grooves in the crown (Fig. 8.6).

DENTAL CONSIDERATIONS

- A deficiency of vitamin A is associated with increased risk of infection and poor wound healing.
- Vitamin A or beta-carotene supplements are not recommended for most healthy adults unless specifically advised to do so by a health care provider or RDN.
- Assess for signs of vitamin A deficiency and toxicity as symptoms may be similar and refer to a health care provider or RDN for further evaluation.
- In contrast to vitamin A, beta-carotene is not toxic, but large amounts can cause a temporary change in skin color. Hypercarotenemia may be distinguished from jaundice because the sclera retains its normal white color.
- Any disorder affecting fat absorption such as cystic fibrosis or Crohn's disease also affects fat-soluble vitamin absorption, making these patients prone to vitamin A deficiency.
- A patient with alcohol use disorder, cirrhosis, or fatty liver may be deficient in vitamin A because of impaired liver function.[16–18]

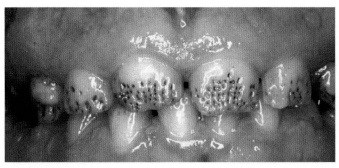

• **Fig. 8.6** Enamel hypoplasia. Pitting occurred on the surfaces of the maxillary central and lateral incisors where the enamel is thin. (From Nelson SJ. *Wheeler's Dental Anatomy: Physiology and Occlusion.* 10th ed. Saunders; 2014.)

⚙ NUTRITIONAL DIRECTIONS

- Vitamin A from animal or fortified foods is used better by the body than beta-carotene.
- Encourage patients to consume dark-green, yellow, and orange fruits and vegetables daily to receive the recommended amount of vitamin A. MyPlate recommends 3 to 4 cups per day for males and 2 to 3 cups per day for females.
- Fortified foods and vitamin supplements should be used judiciously to prevent toxicity.
- Recommend storing vitamin supplements in a cool, dark place to prevent deterioration.
- Females of childbearing age need to limit intake of preformed vitamin A (retinol, retinyl, and retinoyl acetate)—found in liver, fortified foods (breakfast cereals), and dietary supplements—to 100% of the Daily Value because of the increased risk of birth defects during pregnancy.

Vitamin D (Calciferol)

Although vitamin D has been called a vitamin, it is more appropriately classified as a hormone (a compound secreted by one type of cell that acts to control the function of another type of cell). Skin cells are able to make vitamin D when the precursor 7-dehydrocholesterol, present in the skin, is exposed to ultraviolet (UV) light or sunshine.[19] Vitamin D from food, ergocalciferol (vitamin D_2), or cholecalciferol (vitamin D_3) are biologically inert.[19] Further metabolism occurs in the liver with conversion of vitamin D_2 or vitamin D_3 into 25-hydroxycholecalciferol (calcidiol), and a final change to the active form of 1,25-dihydroxycholecalciferol (calciferol) primarily by the kidney.[19] A special enzyme in the kidney, α-1-hydroxylase, activates calcidiol to produce calcitriol, the active form of vitamin D (Fig. 8.7). Individuals with liver and kidney disease are often unable to convert vitamin D to its active form.[20]

Until recently, vitamin D was viewed primarily as a protective agent against bone disease, such as rickets. Research has shown, however, that thousands of vitamin D receptors binding sites are present in different types of cells, and the hormone is involved in the regulation of hundreds of human genes.[19] A flurry of reports from many nations have highlighted a variety of vitamin D insufficiency and deficiency diseases.[21] Research also suggests that vitamin D deficiency is a significant concern in racial and ethnic groups.[21]

Physiologic Roles

Vitamin D is intricately related to calcium and phosphorus, each being required for optimal use of the other. Vitamin D helps the body absorb and regulate calcium. The primary role of vitamin D is mineralization of bones and teeth, and regulation of blood calcium and phosphorus levels. It functions with the parathyroid and thyroid (calcitonin) hormones to regulate intestinal absorption of calcium and phosphorus, enhance renal calcium and phosphorus reabsorption, and regulate skeletal calcium and phosphorus reserves (see Fig. 8.7).

Vitamin D may also be involved in the functioning of cells involved in hematopoiesis (formation of red blood cells), the skin, cardiovascular function, and immune responses. Its regulatory role helps keep serum calcium in the appropriate range to maintain cardiac and neuromuscular function.[22] Calciferol (1,25-dihydroxycholecalciferol) interacts with osteoblasts (cells that help produce collagen and build and reform new bone) to increase the withdrawal of osteocalcin (calcium-binding noncollagen protein in bone) and other bone-building compounds, or interacts with parathyroid hormone to mobilize calcium stores from the skeleton when calcium is needed.

Requirements

The vitamin D requirement is difficult to determine, and there are widely varying recommendations. When sufficient sunlight is available, people may not require an exogenous dietary source of vitamin D. Because many people worldwide live in northern latitudes or in areas where weather conditions limit exposure to the sunlight and because many factors can interfere with UV light–dependent synthesis of vitamin D in the skin, vitamin D is considered an essential dietary nutrient.[21] Vitamin D is measured in micrograms (mcg or μg) or IU. One microgram is equivalent to 40 IU.

The National Academy of Medicine determined that an adequate intake of vitamin D for ages 1 to 70 years is 15 μg (600 IU); the recommended amount increases to 20 μg (800 IU) after age 70 (Table 8.3).[22] The US Preventive Services Task Force found inconclusive evidence to support supplementation of vitamin D and hence does not recommend daily vitamin D supplements for healthy individuals.[23]

The estimated average requirement to prevent rickets is 10 μg or 400 IU. In 2008, the American Academy of Pediatrics recommended 10 μg (400 IU) of vitamin D for infants to prevent rickets with the National Academy of Medicine supporting this recommendation in 2011.[23,24] Therefore, supplementation is needed for infants who are breastfed or consuming less than 1 L/day of formula. Despite this recommendation, in 2020 only 27% of infants were meeting the guideline.[25]

For adults with osteoporosis, there is no consensus on vitamin recommendations with the International Osteoporosis Foundation recommending 20 to 25 μg (800–1000 IU) and the American Association of Clinical Endocrinologists/American College of Endocrinology (AACE/ACE) recommending 25 to 50 μg (1000–2000 IU).[26] To reach this level of vitamin D, supplementation is necessary because obtaining it from food sources is difficult.[26] Beginning in 2018, the nutrition label includes the actual amounts of vitamin D in micrograms as well as the percent of the daily value (DV).[27]

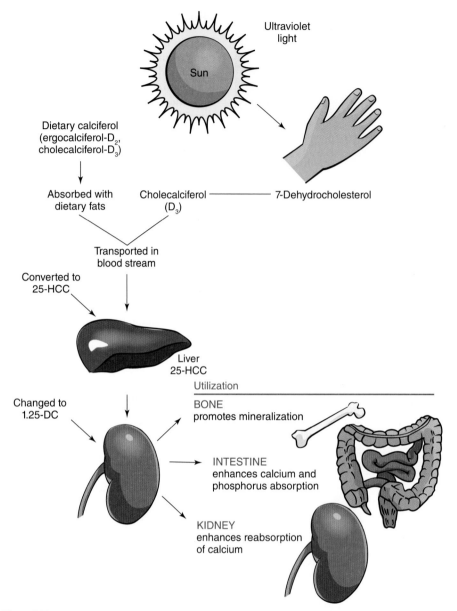

• **Fig. 8.7** Vitamin D metabolism. *1.25-DC*, [dihydroxycholecalciferol (calciferol)]; *25-HCC*, 25-hydrocalciferol [hydroxycholecalciferol (calcidiol)]. (Adapted from Kumar V, Abbas A, Aster J. *Robbins Basic Pathology*. 10th ed. Saunders; 2017.)

Sources

Sunlight

The body's ability to produce adequate amounts of vitamin D from sunlight is why the sun has been considered a source of health. UV radiation is the principal cause of sunburn and cellular damage that leads to skin cancer. UV radiation penetrates uncovered skin and converts a precursor of vitamin D to previtamin D₃, which becomes the active form of vitamin D₃, or calcitriol (see Fig. 8.7). However, the melanin pigment provides a natural protection against UV rays, therefore dark-skinned individuals have lower production of vitamin D.[28] Most people experience an increase in vitamin D levels during summer because changes in the angulation of the sun occur throughout the year. During summer, 10 to 15 minutes a day of midday sun (without sunblock)

can replete the body's supply depending on the latitude where one lives and time of the year.[29]

Many people in the northern hemisphere (above a line approximately between the northern border of California and Boston), especially older adults and darker-skinned individuals, may lack sufficient exposure to UV radiation[28,30] from mid-October through mid-March. Cloud cover, fog, haze, shade, and pollution can reduce the UV energy needed for vitamin D. UVB radiation does not penetrate glass. A broad spectrum sunscreen is protective from both UVA and UVB rays and interferes with the formation of vitamin D₃. Dermatologists continue to advise sunscreen and clothing protection for anyone in the sun to prevent skin cancer. Although sunscreen inhibits vitamin D production, its use and moderation in sun exposure are important to protect against skin cancer. With

TABLE 8.3 Dietary Reference Intakes for Vitamin D

Life Stage[a]	AI µg/day (IU)	EAR µg/day (IU)	RDA µg/day (IU)	UL µg/day (IU)
0–6 months	10 µg/day (400 IU)			25 (1000)
7–12 months	10 (400)			38 (1500)
1–3 years		10 (400)	15 (600)	63 (2500)
4–8 years		10 (400)	15 (600)	75 (3000)
9–13 years		10 (400)	15 (600)	100 (4000)
14–18 years		10 (400)	15 (600)	100 (4000)
19–30 years		10 (400)	15 (600)	100 (4000)
31–50 years		10 (400)	15 (600)	100 (4000)
51–70 years		10 (400)	15 (600)	100 (4000)
>70 years		10 (400)	20 (800)	100 (4000)
Pregnant and Lactating				
19–50 years		10 (400)	15 (600)	100 (4000)

[a]All groups except pregnancy and lactation are males and females.

EAR, Estimated average requirement; *RDA*, recommended dietary allowance; *UL*, upper intake level.

Data from Institute of Medicine, Committee to Review Dietary Reference Intakes for Vitamin D and Calcium, Ross AC, Taylor CL, Yaktine AL, Del Valle HB, eds. *Dietary Reference Intakes for Calcium and Vitamin D*. National Academies Press; 2011.

TABLE 8.4 Food Sources of Vitamin D

Food	Portion	Vitamin D (mcg)
Salmon, cooked	3 oz	8.2
Sardines, canned in oil, drained	1 can	3.6
Raisin bran	1 cup	2.9
Milk (skim, 1% or 2%), fortified with vitamin D	1 cup	2.7
Chocolate milk, low-fat, fortified with vitamin D	1 cup	2.7
Orange juice, fortified with vitamin D	1 cup	2.5
Milk, almond	1 cup	2.2
Yogurt, nonfat, fortified with vitamin D	6 oz	2
Milk, soy	1 cup	1.7
American cheese, fortified with vitamin D	1 oz	1.5
Egg	1 large	1.2
Tuna fish, canned in water, drained	3 oz	1.2
Margarine, fortified	1 tbsp	0.5

Data from United States Department of Agriculture (USDA), Agricultural Research Service. *What's in the Foods Your Eat* Search Tool. 2019–2020. https://www.ars.usda.gov/northeast-area/beltsville-md-bhnrc/beltsville-human-nutrition-research-center/food-surveys-research-group/docs/whats-in-the-foods-you-eat-search-tool/.

increasing age, vitamin D production by the skin is reduced about 13% per decade.[31]

Food

Although adequate quantities of vitamin D may be derived from exposure to sunlight, additional food sources are necessary in most cases. Naturally occurring vitamin D content in foods is variable; food tables do not normally list vitamin D content. This information has been added to the National Nutrient Database for Standard Reference (available at https://data.nal.usda.gov/dataset/usda-national-nutrient-database-standard-reference-legacy-release). Natural sources include oily fish such as salmon, trout, sardines, and tuna, as well as cod liver and fish oils (Table 8.4).

Because vitamin D deficiencies are prevalent in the United States, the United States Food and Drug Administration allows vitamin D fortification of milk, milk alternatives (e.g., soy, almond, and coconut "milk"), orange juice and other foods.[32] Other foods, such as margarine, infant cereals, prepared breakfast cereals, cereal bars, chocolate beverage mixes, and yogurt, also may be fortified with vitamin D (see Table 8.4).[33] The food additive regulations were amended to allow companies to effectively double the amount of vitamin D to a maximum level of 200 IU/cup milk, 200 IU/cup plant-based milk alternatives (e.g., soy, almond beverage), and 151 IU/6 oz for plant-based yogurt alternatives.[32]

Vitamin D fortification of milk is voluntary, but most milk in the United States is fortified to provide 10 µg (400 IU) of cholecalciferol per quart. Vitamin D fortification of milk enhances absorption and utilization of the calcium and phosphorus inherent in milk and vice versa. Children especially benefit from vitamin D fortification of milk for bone growth. Vitamin D from fortified regular and low-fat cheese is absorbed and metabolized well by the body. Because fortification is optional, it cannot be taken for granted.

Nutrition labels can be used to assess daily intake of vitamin D; this information plus the amount of exposure to sunlight must be considered to ensure adequate amounts of vitamin D. Vitamin D is in multivitamins, prenatal vitamins, calcium–vitamin D combinations, and individual vitamin D supplements. Most multivitamins provide 400 IU per dose. Vitamin D_3 is more effective at increasing calcifediol levels in the blood than vitamin D_2 (ergocalciferol).[22]

Absorption

As with other nutrients, optimal absorption occurs when all closely interrelated nutrients (particularly calcium and phosphorus) are present in sufficient quantities. Conversely, diets high in fiber can result in less vitamin D absorption.

Hyper States and Hypo States

Toxicity

Vitamin D has the potential to become toxic at high levels. The risk for harm increases as the intake level exceeds the UL. Because vitamin D increases calcium absorption it may result in hypercalcemia with symptoms that include: nausea, vomiting, poor appetite, loss of appetite, constipation, dehydration, polyuria, dizziness, muscle weakness, kidney stones, and tingling sensations in the mouth.[22] In extreme cases, Vitamin D toxicity can result in renal failure, confusion, heart rhythm abnormalities, and calcification of soft tissues such as coronary vessels and heart valves.[22] Unless symptoms are detected and the source of vitamin D is removed immediately, permanent damage results.

The most common reason for vitamin D toxicity has been from manufacturing errors or prolonged intake of excessive supplements or cod liver oil; otherwise, toxicity through diet is unlikely.[22] Toxicity from excessive vitamin D intake may occur when a concentrated calciferol preparation is mistakenly given. For example, an infant given a commercial formula and a vitamin supplement, can easily ingest vitamin D well above the adequate intake (AI) level.

Deficiency

Prevalence of vitamin D deficiency is estimated to be 5.9% in the United States, 7.4% in Canada, and 13% in Europe.[21] Inadequacy of vitamin D had an average prevalence of 24% in the United States, 37% in Canada, and 40% in Europe showing the widespread issue.[21] In adults, adequate intake of vitamin D has been linked in research studies to conditions as diverse as cancer, cardiovascular disease (CVD), hypertension, type 2 diabetes mellitus, depression, osteoporosis, multiple sclerosis, Alzheimer's disease, along with risk for infection and severity of coronavirus disease 2019 (COVID-19).[22,34,35]

Vitamin D deficiency affects skeletal structure in children and adults. Signs of deficiency are commonly found in children because of inadequate intake, decreased stores, decreased exposure to the sun, and/or use of sunscreen.[22] In older adult patients, deficiencies may result from inadequate intake with little exposure to the sun, reduced skin thickness and ability to synthesis vitamin D, inability of the kidney to convert vitamin D to its active form, or inadequate absorption of vitamin D from the gastrointestinal tract.[22] Plasma vitamin D is significantly lower in older patients

than among the younger population; it is consistently higher for older males than females. Despite inconsistent evidence on benefit of vitamin D supplementation for primary prevention of fracture and bone health, a health care provider may recommend vitamin D and calcium supplements to older patients to prevent osteoporosis.[22,36] When supplementation is recommended, care must be taken to prevent excess intake. Vitamin D deficiency is associated with muscle weakness, however, supplementation has not been shown to improve musculoskeletal health.[37]

Rickets

Laboratory values indicating serum calcium or phosphorus above or below normal values, the failure of bones to grow properly in length, and radiographs showing abnormal epiphyses (the terminal end or growth points of bones) indicate deficiencies (Fig. 8.8). Because vitamin D is intricately related to calcium and phosphorus functions, a change in any of these three nutrients affects the others.

The name *rickets* came from the word *wrikken*, meaning "to bend or twist." Rickets, caused by vitamin D deficiency, usually occurs in children and is characterized by weak bones and skeletal deformities. Rachitic deformities such as bowlegs or knock-knees develop (Fig. 8.9A).[38] The epiphyses of bones do not develop normally in children with this condition; thus bones are twisted and warped. Other bone changes include thickened wrists and ankles; muscle weakness; bone pain; a row of beadlike protuberances (rachitic rosary) on each side of the narrow, distorted chest (pigeon breast) at the juncture of the ribs and costal cartilage; and dental abscesses (Fig. 8.9B).[38] A narrow pelvis, making future childbearing difficult in females, is also observed.

Nutritional rickets develops during the time of extremely rapid growth when children have had only a brief period to acquire vitamin D stores. Adequate intake of vitamin D during pregnancy and lactation is important because vitamin D is passed from the

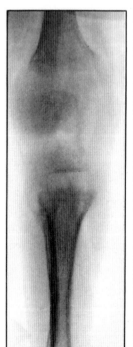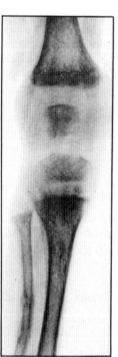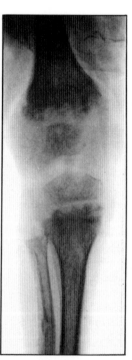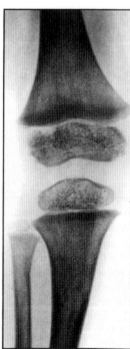

• **Fig. 8.8** Active rickets of the knees. The metaphyses of the bones are concave and irregular, and the zone of uncalcified osteoid is enlarged. These radiographs show the progressive changes over 10 months, during which healing took place in this case. (Courtesy Prof. A. Prader. From McLaren DS. *A Colour Atlas and Text of Diet-Related Disorders*. 2nd ed. Mosby–Year Book; 1992.)

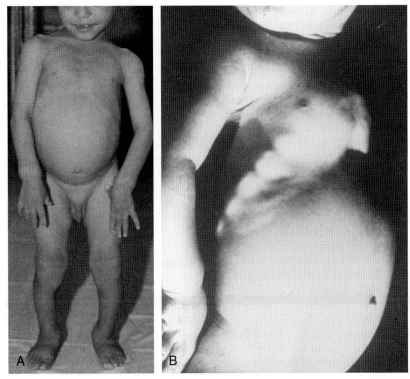

• **Fig. 8.9** (A) Bowlegs in rickets. The typical lateral curvature indicates that the weakened bones have bent after the second year as a result of standing. (B) Rachitic rosary in a young infant. (A, From McLaren DS. *A Colour Atlas and Text of Diet-Related Disorders*. 2nd ed. Mosby–Year Book; 1992. B, From Kliegman RM, Stanton BMD, St. Geme J, Schor NF. *Nelson Textbook of Pediatrics*. 20th ed. Elsevier; 2016.)

mother to the infant before birth and in breast milk. However, adequate vitamin D cannot be met solely by breastfeeding.[22] While we might think nutritional rickets is non-existent in the United States, a higher incidence was found in Minnesota in the early 2000s. The rising numbers were possibly due to inadequate vitamin D supplementation of breastfed infants; lack of sun exposure or use of sunscreens; and arrival of immigrants from countries with higher incidence.[22,39,40]

The alveolar bone is affected similar to other bones in the body when rickets occurs. The trabeculae of the alveolar bone may be affected. Higher rates of early childhood caries may also be seen in populations with rickets.[41]

Enamel Hypoplasia and Dental Decay

Enamel and dentin hypoplasia may be evident in molars, canines, and incisors in those with nutritional rickets.[42] A landmark study conducted in 1973 reported the possibility of increased risk of enamel hypoplasia in children of mothers experiencing vitamin D deficiency during pregnancy.[43] Since then research has continued to explore the association between low vitamin D levels prenatally and in childhood, finding low levels of vitamin D and nutritional rickets associated with higher rates of early childhood caries.[41,44]

Periodontitis

Lower vitamin D levels are seen in patients with periodontal disease as compared to those without periodontitis.[45] Vitamin D inadequacy may also impact the immune response, postoperative wound healing, periodontal disease progression due to alveolar bone resorption, and tooth loss.[46] Studies suggest an association between adequate vitamin D intake and less gingival inflammation and maintenance of alveolar bone health, however, the impact

of vitamin D supplementation as an adjunct to nonsurgical periodontal therapy needs more research.[45,46] However, it may be prudent to have patient's vitamin D levels evaluated prior to periodontal treatment to ensure that they are in the normal range.[45]

Osteomalacia

Vitamin D deficiency in adults can lead to osteomalacia; it is also intricately related to calcium intake.[47] Osteomalacia is characterized by decreased bone mineralization or softening of the bones, which may lead to deformities of the limbs, spine, thorax, and pelvis. The main symptoms are bone and muscle pain; fatigue; stress fractures in stress-bearing bones; and muscle weakness, resulting in kyphosis, or an uneven gait.[47] Oral manifestations may include loss of the lamina dura around the roots of the teeth, sparse trabecular bone, and thinning of cortical bone which can be seen in intraoral radiographs or CBCT (cone beam computed tomography) images.[48] The condition is more prevalent in females of childbearing age with calcium depletion because of multiple pregnancies, older adults, and other individuals with little sun exposure.

Following assessment of serum vitamin D levels, a health care provider or RDN may recommend a vitamin D supplement and/or a calcium supplement (with vitamin D to maximize absorption of calcium), especially for females who are at high risk for osteoporosis because of risk factors. Other medications may also be prescribed to prevent further deterioration of bone mineral density.

Osteoporosis

Osteoporosis was previously thought to be a calcium deficiency, but research indicates that vitamin D levels are as important as calcium intake.[26] As discussed previously, vitamin D deficiency interferes with mineralization of the skeleton, reducing bone density and increasing risk of bone fractures. Osteoporosis is a disease characterized by fragile bones and is associated with an increased incidence of bone fractures, especially the hip. Supplementation of vitamin D and calcium may lead to a reduction in the risk of future fractures and provides an even better protection to those at greatest risk of deficiency of these nutrients.[26] While there is no consensus on the vitamin D amount, the review of international scientific guidelines suggests from 800 to 2000 IU/day.[26] Osteoporosis is discussed further in *Health Application 9*.

Cancer Risk

Laboratory, animal, and epidemiologic evidence suggests that vitamin D may be protective against some cancers. Numerous studies indicate that higher vitamin levels in blood are associated with reduced mortality from prostate, colon and colorectal cancers, and breast cancer.[22] However, the relationship of vitamin D and incidence of these cancers is uncertain; evidence is based on limited data, and more studies are needed to determine optimal levels and intakes of vitamin D to reduce cancer risk.[22,49]

Cardiovascular Risk

Recent systematic review and *meta*-analysis by the United States Preventive Services Task Force found little or no benefit from Vitamin D to prevent cardiovascular disease.[49] However, in some populations such as those with kidney disease undergoing dialysis, higher levels of vitamin D have been shown to reduce risk of CVD and mortality.[50]

⬡ DENTAL CONSIDERATIONS

- Assess for vitamin D deficiency, especially in young children, pregnant and lactating females, and older adults.
- Vitamin D supplements should only be recommended if a laboratory evaluation of serum levels indicates that it is below normal levels because patients vary widely in their susceptibility to vitamin D toxicity. Do recommend patients choose a healthy diet with sources of vitamin D, but do not recommend patients take vitamin D supplements. Refer them to a health care provider or RDN for evaluation.
- Conditions leading to vitamin D deficiency include any abnormalities that (1) interfere with intestinal fat absorption (e.g., diarrhea, steatorrhea, celiac disease, Crohn's disease, and cystic fibrosis), and (2) abnormalities in calcium balance and bone metabolism caused by disease states such as renal failure. Evaluate the patient's health status for risk of vitamin D deficiency.
- Patients with minimal or no exposure to the sunlight should be monitored for adequate vitamin D intake or supplementation or both, to maintain adequate vitamin D stores. Question the patient regarding living environment or hobbies to determine exposure to the sunlight.
- Determine the use of sunscreens. Consistent use of sunscreens may contribute to vitamin D deficiency in some patients. Sunscreens with a sun protection factor of 8 or greater block the UV rays from the sun necessary to produce vitamin D.
- Medications that have the potential to interact with vitamin D supplements include corticosteroids (e.g., prednisone), used to minimize inflammation; orlistat, used for weight loss; statins used to lower cholesterol (e.g., Lipitor), corticosteroids (e.g., prednisone), and thiazide diuretics.[22]
- Calcitriol regulates the rate of calcium and phosphorus resorption from bone.
- Low skeletal bone mass may also be associated with periodontal bone loss and tooth loss.

⬡ NUTRITIONAL DIRECTIONS

- The bright sunlight between 11:00 a.m. and 2:00 p.m. offers maximum conversion. For light-skinned individuals, 10 to 15 minutes of daily sun exposure results in adequate conversion.
- Toxicity may result from excess intake of cod liver oil or from taking excessive vitamin D supplements.
- Older individuals, especially individuals living in a long-term care facility, are at high risk for vitamin D deficiency.
- Provide meal or snack ideas to include fortified cereal with fortified low-fat milk; raw vegetables with a fortified yogurt dip; or topping a salad with salmon.
- Encourage patients to consume adequate amounts of fruits and vegetables, exercise, discontinue tobacco use, and drink alcohol only in moderation for overall health.

Vitamin E (Tocopherol)

Eight different compounds are collectively called vitamin E: four tocopherols and four tocotrienols. Biologic activity of each form varies; α-tocopherol is the most active form and is the only one that will meet human requirements.[51]

Physiologic Roles

Vitamin E is the most important fat-soluble antioxidant. Vitamin E protects the integrity of normal cell membranes and effectively prevents hemolysis of red blood cells. It also protects vitamins A and C, beta-carotene, and unsaturated fatty acids from oxidation. Vitamin E is also involved in immune function. It inhibits aggregation of platelets and may impact blood clotting because of its effects on vitamin K–dependent clotting factors.[52] The role of vitamin E as an antioxidant is discussed further in *Health Application 8*.

Requirements

The DRIs for vitamin E (AI, RDA, and UL) are based solely on the α-tocopherol form because humans are unable to convert and use other forms. The RDA for vitamin E is 15 mg of α-tocopherol for healthy individuals 14 years old and older except for lactating females (Table 8.5).[53] One milligram of α-tocopherol is the same as 1.5 IU. High intakes of polyunsaturated fatty acids increase the vitamin E requirement. Most polyunsaturated oils contain vitamin E, but chemical reactions may have rendered the antioxidant ineffective. If an individual's systemic stores are low, the vitamin E requirement is increased.

The daily UL is 1000 mg of α-tocopherol (1500 IU of natural vitamin E is equivalent to 1000 IU of synthetic vitamin E)[53]. The UL was established because of the adverse health effect of excessive bleeding. Supplemental amounts in excess of the RDA should not be recommended.

Sources

Vitamin E is available from vegetable oils and margarine made from them; whole-grain or fortified cereals; wheat germ; nuts; green leafy vegetables; and some fruits. Meats, fish, and animal fats contain very little vitamin E. Table 8.6 lists the amounts of vitamin E in some foods. Because vitamin E is widely distributed in foods, dietary deficiencies seldom occur if a well-balanced, varied diet is consumed.[2,51]

TABLE 8.5 Dietary Reference Intakes for Vitamin E (α-Tocopherol)[a]

Life Stage	EAR (mg/day)	RDA (mg/day)	AI (mg/day)	UL (mg/day)
0–6 months			4	
7–12 months			6	
1–3 years	5	6		200
4–8 years	6	7		300
9–13 years	9	11		600
14–18 years	12	15		800
19–70 years	12	15		1000
>70 years	12	15		1000
Pregnancy				
≤18 years	12	15		800
19–50	12	15		1000
Lactation				
≤18 years	16	19		800
19–50 years	16	19		1000

[a]α-Tocopherol includes the only form of α-tocopherol that occurs naturally in foods and some of the forms that occur in fortified foods and supplements, but not all forms because some that are used in fortified foods and supplements have not been shown to meet human requirements.

AI, Adequate intake; *EAR*, estimated average requirement; *RDA*, recommended dietary allowance; *UL*, upper intake level.

Data from Institute of Medicine (IOM), Panel on Dietary Antioxidants and Related Compounds. *Dietary Reference Intakes for Vitamin C, Vitamin E, Selenium, and Carotenoids.* National Academies Press; 2000.

TABLE 8.6 Food Sources of Vitamin E

Food	Portion	Vitamin E (mg)
Wheat germ oil	1 tbsp	20.9
Sunflower seeds	¼ cup	9.4
Almonds	1 oz	6.7
Safflower oil	1 tbsp	6.43
Sunflower oil	1 tbsp	5.75
Hazelnuts	1 oz	4.96
Corn oil	1 tbsp	3.16
Avocado	1 medium	3.1
Peanut butter	2 tbsp	2.92
Canola oil	1 tbsp	2.42
Tomatoes, canned	1 cup	2.18
Spinach, cooked	½ cup	2.14
Peanut oil	1 tbsp	2.13
Peanuts	1 oz	1.97
Soybean oil	1 tbsp	1.71
Sweet potato, baked	1 large	1.67
Mango, fresh	1 cup	1.48
Apricot, sliced	1 cup	1.38
Margarine	1 tbsp	1.26

Data from United States Department of Agriculture (USDA), Agricultural Research Service. *What's in the Foods Your Eat* Search Tool. 2019–2020. https://www.ars.usda.gov/northeast-area/beltsville-md-bhnrc/beltsville-human-nutrition-research-center/food-surveys-research-group/docs/whats-in-the-foods-you-eat-search-tool/.

Absorption and Excretion

Absorption of vitamin E is inefficient, ranging from 10% to 33% in healthy individuals.[54] Efficiency of absorption depends on the body's ability to absorb fat and seems to decline as the amount of dietary vitamin E increases.

Hyper States and Hypo States

Vitamin E Toxicity

Higher doses of vitamin E supplementation may result in bleeding issues including hemorrhagic stroke.[51] There are inconsistent findings related to risk of death and high doses of vitamin E supplements, therefore more research is needed to clarify the relationship.[55,56]

Vitamin E Deficiency

Individuals who may benefit from vitamin E supplementation are premature and preterm infants, patient's having inflammatory bowel disease such as Crohn's disease and ulcerative colitis; cystic fibrosis; and post-bariatric surgery.[51,57–60] Typically consuming vitamin E-rich foods will meet needs, but for those with fat malabsorption conditions, a water-soluble form may be required to enhance absorption.[51]

Health Effects

While there are many claims about the benefits of vitamin E, available evidence has not shown a benefit in preventing or treating disease.[51] Research has explored vitamin E supplementation for prevention and treatment of cardiovascular disease, cancer, cognitive decline (e.g., dementia and Alzheimer's disease), and eye disorders (e.g., macular degeneration and cataracts) and the findings are inconsistent with the need for more research.[49,61–63]

🦷 DENTAL CONSIDERATIONS

- Vitamin E may help the immune system function better; thus assess the intake of vitamin E in immunocompromised patients.
- Vitamin E supplementation of 200 IU in conjunction with nonsurgical periodontal therapy may improve outcomes with a decrease in attachment loss, however, larger, long-term studies are still needed.[64,65] However, adequate intake from food sources should be encouraged.
- Vitamin E supplementation may be of special concern for patients with vitamin K deficiency or with known coagulation defects, or for patients receiving anticoagulation therapy, which interferes with vitamin K activity, because it can increase risk for hemorrhaging.
- Naturally occurring α-tocopherol from foods is twice as potent as the synthetic form, making it more desirable to obtain vitamin E from food sources.

⬡ NUTRITIONAL DIRECTIONS

- When oils are reused in frying, heavy losses of vitamin E occur.
- An increase in fruits and vegetables provides more low-fat sources of vitamin E.
- Despite the widespread media coverage of the benefits of vitamin E, advise patients to limit vitamin E supplements to the RDA unless they are instructed otherwise by their health care provider.
- Adverse effects of excessive amounts of vitamin E are associated with vitamin E supplements only; food sources of vitamin E are not associated with adverse effects.
- If vitamin E supplements are recommended by a health care provider or RDN, they should be consumed with a meal containing fat to assist with absorption.
- Vitamin E supplements cannot replace other evidence-based ways to reduce disease risks: not smoking, regular physical activity, maintaining a healthy weight, and eating a well-balanced, healthy diet.

Vitamin K (Quinone)

Three forms of vitamin K, a fat-soluble vitamin, have been identified, all belonging to a group of chemical compounds known as quinones. The naturally occurring vitamins are K_1 (phylloquinone) which occurs in green plants, and K_2 (menaquinone) which is formed by bacteria in the intestine and found in animal tissues.[66] The fat-soluble synthetic compound menadione (vitamin K_3) is two to three times as potent as the natural vitamin.

Physiologic Roles

Vitamin K–dependent proteins have been identified in bone, kidney, and other tissues. Vitamin K_2 activates vitamin K–dependent proteins, activating osteocalciun (protein required to bind calcium to the mineral matrix), thus strengthening bone and may also slacken the loss of bone.[66] Vitamin K functions as a catalyst in the synthesis of blood-clotting factors, primarily in maintaining prothrombin levels, which is the first stage in forming a clot.[66] A low prothrombin level results in impaired blood coagulation.

Requirements

The AI (Adequate Intake) is 120 µg for males and 90 µg for females. No UL for vitamin K has been established (Table 8.7).

Sources

Although limited amounts of vitamin K are stored in the body, a shortage of vitamin K is unlikely because it is derived from food and microflora in the gut. Green leafy vegetables are high in vitamin K, but meats are also a source (Table 8.8). The most common sources in the diet include spinach, kale, broccoli, iceberg lettuce, spices (e.g., parsley and marjoram), cheese, fermented vegetables (e.g., sauerkraut) and cooking oils (soybean and canola).[66,67]

Bacterial flora in the jejunum and ileum synthesize vitamin K and provide about half of the body's requirement. However, synthesis of vitamin K by intestinal bacteria does not provide adequate amounts of the vitamin; therefore a restriction of dietary vitamin K can alter clotting factors.

TABLE 8.7	**Dietary Reference Intakes for Vitamin K**	
	AI	
Life Stage	**Male (µg/day)**	**Female (µg/day)**
0–6 months	2	2
7–12 months	2.5	2.5
1–3 years	30	30
4–8 years	55	55
9–13 years	60	60
14–18 years	75	75
>18 years	120	90
Pregnancy		
≤18 years		75
19–50 years		90
Lactation		
≤18 years		75
19–50 years		90

Data from Institute of Medicine (IOM), Panel on Dietary Antioxidants and Related Compounds. *Dietary Reference Intakes for Vitamin A, Vitamin K, Arsenic, Boron, Chromium, Copper, Iodine, Iron, Manganese, Molybdenum, Nickel, Silicon, Vanadium, and Zinc.* National Academies Press; 2001.

TABLE 8.8	**Food Sources of Vitamin K**	
Food	**Portion**	**Vitamin K (µg)**
Spinach, cooked	½ cup	509.8
Collard greens, cooked	½ cup	304.6
Kale, cooked	½ cup	271.8
Mustard greens, cooked	½ cup	193.3
Brussels sprouts, cooked	½ cup	142.4
Broccoli, cooked	½ cup	82.1
Cabbage, raw	1 cup	68.4
Asparagus, cooked	½ cup	40.1
Ground beef, cooked	3 oz	1.1

Data from United States Department of Agriculture (USDA), Agricultural Research Service. *What's in the Foods Your Eat* Search Tool. 2019–2020. https://www.ars.usda.gov/northeast-area/beltsville-md-bhnrc/beltsville-human-nutrition-research-center/food-surveys-research-group/docs/whats-in-the-foods-you-eat-search-tool/.

Absorption and Excretion

Fat intake stimulates secretion of bile acids which aids in absorption of vitamin K. Vitamin K is carried by the lymphatic system in chylomicrons to the liver where they may become a component of lipoproteins and stored in the liver or sent to peripheral tissues.[67] Excretion is through bile into the feces as water-soluble metabolites or in the urine.

Hyper States and Hypo States

Deficiency

Primary vitamin K deficiency is uncommon, but disease or drug therapy may cause deficiencies. Groups most at risk of vitamin K inadequacy include newborn infants and individuals with malabsorption disorders.

Newborns may develop vitamin K deficiency bleeding (VKDB) because the gut is sterile during the first weeks after birth and breast milk is low in vitamin K.[66] Newborns are usually given a single dose of vitamin K intramuscularly immediately after birth to prevent hemorrhage, however, recent increases in parents refusing the vitamin K administration has resulted in an increase in VKDB.[68]

Vitamin K deficiency is common in conditions such as celiac disease, ulcerative colitis, cystic fibrosis, short bowel syndrome, and post-bariatric surgery as a result of malabsorption.[66,69,70] In vitamin K deficiency or in patients taking anticoagulants, blood-clotting time is delayed, increasing the risk of bleeding problems.

Toxicity

No toxicity symptoms have been documented from food or supplement intake of vitamin K.[66]

⬡ DENTAL CONSIDERATIONS

- Excessive amounts of vitamin A or E or both have a detrimental effect on vitamin K absorption.
- Vitamin K should never be confused with the symbol "K" on a food label because it is used to designate potassium or kosher foods. If information is confusing or unclear, double-check with a health care provider or RDN.
- Consultation with the medical provider is necessary prior to any invasive dental treatment for someone at risk for deficiency to determine if vitamin K supplementation is needed to prevent prolonged bleeding.
- Cholestyramine prescribed for high cholesterol binds with bile salts. The presence of bile is required for vitamin K absorption. Patients taking cholestyramine are at risk of vitamin K deficiency; thus assess for bleeding problems such as petechiae (pinpoint, flat red spots) or ecchymosis (bruising).
- Antibiotic therapy kills gut bacteria that produce vitamin K and when taking longterm, it may be a factor in vitamin K deficiency, especially with impaired hepatic or renal function.
- Patients receiving oral anticoagulants (usually warfarin) to prevent blood clots from forming may develop serious hemorrhaging problems. They should keep vitamin K intake consistent and should not consume vitamin K supplements.

⬡ NUTRITIONAL DIRECTIONS

- A lack of vitamin K may lead to bleeding problems.
- Vitamin K is stable to heat; cooking does not affect the vitamin K content of foods.

Vitamin C (Ascorbic Acid)

Physiologic Roles

As a coenzyme, vitamin C has numerous metabolic roles. It is important in the production of collagen (the primary structural protein in connective tissue, cartilage, and bone) which plays a vital role in wound healing.[71] During the development of connective tissue, bones, and teeth, vitamin C is important in the formation of fibroblasts (collagen-forming cells), osteoblasts, and odontoblasts. Vitamin C strengthens tissues and promotes capillary integrity. Vitamin C enhances iron absorption and use.[71,72] It has a coenzymatic function in the metabolism of amino acids, neurotransmitters (e.g., epinephrine and norepinephrine), regulation of gene expression, and dopamine synthesis.[72] Vitamin C can also affect immune responses because of its high concentration in white blood cells.[72]

Vitamin C functions as an antioxidant in numerous physiologic reactions. In its role as an antioxidant, it protects cells and tissues against damage caused by free radicals, toxic chemicals, and pollutants.[71] More details on the role of vitamin C as an antioxidant are found in *Health Application 8*.

Requirements

The RDA is established at 90 mg daily for males and 75 mg daily for females, increasing during pregnancy and lactation (Table 8.9). The requirement for vitamin C is increased under many situations in which it is directly involved (e.g., stress, healing, and infections). It is detrimentally affected by many drugs (e.g., tobacco, alcohol, oral contraceptives, and aspirin) which increase requirements, and is usually the first nutrient to be depleted. Smokers may benefit from an additional intake of 35 mg per day because they are more likely to experience biologic processes that damage cells and deplete vitamin C.[53] The UL is 2000 mg per day.

Sources

The RDA can usually be met by choosing at least one serving daily of foods known as an excellent source of vitamin C (e.g., citrus fruits and juices, cantaloupe, green and red peppers, broccoli, kiwi, strawberries, and papaya). Good sources include peaches, cabbage, potatoes, sweet potatoes, and tomatoes; at least two servings of these sources a day may be required to meet the RDA (Table 8.10).

Hyper States and Hypo States

Vitamin C Deficiency

Health care professionals in the United States generally consider vitamin C deficiency, or scurvy, to be a disease of historical significance only. However, the National Health and Nutrition Examination Survey (NHANES) data showed a prevalence of 8.4% with vitamin C deficiency.[73] This is higher than other high income countries like Canada where the prevalence range was generally below 3% in more recent epidemiologic studies.[73] Certain groups are at increased risk for deficiency including those who smoke, exposed to passive secondhand smoke, individuals with limited diets (e.g., substance use disorders, food fads), having low socioeconomic status with food insecurity, elderly, experiencing pregnancy/lactation, and malabsorption conditions.[74]

Scurvy, caused by vitamin C deficiency, can occur in 20 days. It is characterized by spontaneous gingival hemorrhaging

TABLE 8.9 Dietary Reference Intakes for Vitamin C

Life Stage	EAR (mg/day) Male	EAR (mg/day) Female	RDA (mg/day) Male	RDA (mg/day) Female	AI (mg/day) Male	AI (mg/day) Female	UL (mg/day)
0–6 months					40	50	
7–12 months					50	50	
1–3 years	13	13	15	15			400
4–8 years	22	22	25	25			650
9–13 years	39	39	45	45			1200
14–18 years	63	56	75	65			1800
19–70 years	75	60	90	75			2000
>70 years	75	60	90	75			2000
Pregnancy							
≤18 years	66		80				1800
19–50 years	70		85				2000
Lactation							
≤18 years	96		115				1800
19–50 years	100		120				2000

AI, Adequate intake; *EAR*, estimated average requirement; *RDA*, recommended dietary allowance; *UL*, upper intake level.
Data from Institute of Medicine (IOM), Panel on Dietary Antioxidants and Related Compounds. *Dietary Reference Intakes for Vitamin C, Vitamin E, Selenium, and Carotenoids.* National Academies Press; 2000.

perifollicular petechiae (see Fig. 8.10), follicular hyperkeratosis, diarrhea, fatigue, depression, and cessation of bone growth.[71]

Inadequate amounts of vitamin C during tooth development may cause changes in ameloblasts and odontoblasts, resulting in scorbutic changes in the teeth or changes similar to those caused by scurvy. Atrophy of ameloblasts and odontoblasts leads to a decrease in their orderly polar arrangement in a vitamin C-deficient

DENTAL CONSIDERATIONS

- Older patients (especially those who live alone or who avoid acidic foods to control gastroesophageal reflux), patients undergoing peritoneal dialysis or hemodialysis, smokers, and individuals with substance use disorder are at greatest risk to develop vitamin C deficiency symptoms. Assess for deficiency: red to purple gingiva; shiny and hyperkeratotic; bleeding on probing or may bleed spontaneously; nosebleeds; generalized pain; melena (stools containing blood), dyspnea; fatigue; and petechiae (especially lower legs and back).[78]
- At this time, the evidence does not support supplementation of amounts above the RDA of vitamin C to reduce the frequency or severity of a cold.[79]
- Corticosteroids, such as prednisone, and salicylates can increase excretion of vitamin C.
- Evaluate intake of vitamin C as inadequacies may increase gingival bleeding and the patient should be referred for further evaluation and treatment with a health care provider. Typically with vitamin C intake, the gingival bleeding will begin to improve in one to two weeks.[80]

NUTRITIONAL DIRECTIONS

- Vitamin C requirements are readily available from small amounts of food. One cup of orange juice contains approximately 70 mg of vitamin C which meets the RDA for adult females, but males would require an additional serving.
- Patients who smoke need an additional 35 mg of vitamin C daily; a male who smokes should consume 125 mg instead of 90 mg of vitamin C each day. (Refer patients who smoke to a smoking cessation program, as discussed in Chapter 19, *Health Application 19*.)
- Deficiency symptoms may develop within 8 to 12 weeks after dietary elimination of vitamin C.[81]
- Vitamin C is sensitive to temperature, light, and oxidation. Proper storage is important to retain vitamin C.[82]
- Cut fruits and vegetables in as large pieces as possible to decrease the surface area minimizing nutrient loss. The pieces should be stored in a tightly covered container in the refrigerator. Minimize the duration for which they remain exposed to air.
- Packaged salad mixes that have been chopped or shredded, lose vitamin C.[82]
- Cook fruits and vegetables for a limited amount of time in a limited amount of water in a tightly covered device. An alternative is to steam vegetables in a basket with the water below. The more water added for cooking, the more ascorbic acid leaches out of the fruit or vegetable.
- Use quick cooking methods, such as stir frying or a microwave to preserve vitamin C content.[82]
- Ascorbic acid is another name for vitamin C.
- Acidic fruits and vegetables retain their ascorbic acid content better than nonacidic foods.
- Megadoses of vitamin C (2000 mg or greater per day) can interfere with vitamin B_{12} metabolism.

TABLE 8.10	Food Sources of Vitamin C	
Food	**Portion**	**Vitamin C (mg)**
Papaya	1 fruit	201
Red sweet pepper, raw	1 regular	153.2
Tomato juice, canned	1 cup	123.5
Guava	1	125.6
Orange juice	1 cup	71.2
Mango	1	76.4
Strawberries, sliced	1 cup	84
Grapefruit	1/2	48
Orange	1	86.5
Pineapple, chunks	1 cup	18.2
Kiwi	1	56
Cantaloupe	1 cup	16.9
Broccoli, cooked	½ cup	62.5
Brussels sprouts, cooked	½ cup	58.1
Potato, baked	1 large	50.8
Sweet potato, baked	1 large	45.8
Cauliflower, cooked	½ cup	26.5
Cabbage, raw	1 cup	32.9
Tomato	1 large	20.4
Turnip greens, cooked	½ cup	19.8
Tomato sauce, canned	1 cup	1.7

Data from United States Department of Agriculture (USDA), Agricultural Research Service. *What's in the Foods You Eat* Search Tool. 2019–2020. https://www.ars.usda.gov/northeast-area/beltsville-md-bhnrc/beltsville-human-nutrition-research-center/food-surveys-research-group/docs/whats-in-the-foods-you-eat-search-tool/.

environment. Any new dentin deposits forming at this time are similar to osteodentin (dentin that resembles bone); the pulp also atrophies and is hyperemetic. Dentin deposits completely cease in severe vitamin C deficiency, with hypercalcification of predentin. Dentinal tubules also lack their normal parallel arrangement. In scorbutic adults, the dentin reabsorbs and is porotic.

Vitamin C deficiency has been associated with periodontal disease; supplementation has been shown to reduce gingival bleeding, but it has not been shown to impact attachment level or pocket probing depth in the short term although long-term scurvy may result in tooth mobility (Fig. 8.11).[75,76] Despite this finding, a dietary pattern high in fruits and vegetables has been shown to reduce pocket probing depths so it is important to encourage a healthy diet.[77]

Vitamin C Toxicity

Intakes exceeding the UL of 2000 mg may result in stomach upset and diarrhea, and interfere with vitamin B_{12} absorption.

• **Fig. 8.10** Perifollicular petechiae. Minimal bleeding in hair follicles is often one of the earliest clinical manifestations of vitamin C deficiency. (Courtesy Dr. H. H. Sandstead. From McLaren DS. *A Colour Atlas and Text of Diet-Related Disorders*. 2nd ed. Mosby–Year Book; 1992.)

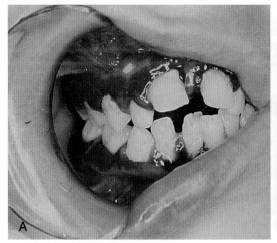
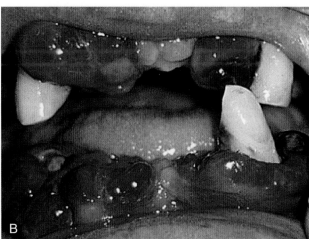

• **Fig. 8.11** (A) Ascorbic acid deficiency. The gingiva is bright red and edematous. The earliest changes involve the interdental papillae which swell and tend to bleed easily. (B) Effects on the periodontium in the long term can result in tooth mobility (Note the bluish red gingiva). (From Swartz MH. *Textbook of Physical Diagnosis: History and Examination*. 7th ed. Saunders Elsevier; 2014.)

HEALTH APPLICATION 8

Antioxidants

Free radicals are highly unstable and reactive molecular fragments. They contain one or more unpaired electrons, which try to gain electrons to become more stable. During this process, the free radicals oxidize (damage) body cells. UV radiation from the sun, air pollution, ozone, and smoking are just a few conditions that can generate free radicals in the body. Antioxidants donate electrons to the free radicals to make them stable. This protects body cells from damage. The antioxidant is oxidized and destroyed. In some situations, an antioxidant can regain or regenerate an electron to allow it to function.

Although antioxidants have some properties in common, each one has unique properties. The best sources of antioxidants are beans (specifically small red, kidney, pinto, and black beans), fruits (particularly blueberries, cranberries, blackberries, plums and prunes, raspberries, strawberries, apples, cherries, grapes, pears, bananas, kiwi, mangoes, pomegranates, and pineapple), vegetables (especially potatoes, artichokes, okra, kale, and bell peppers), nuts (walnuts, pecans, pistachio, and almonds), dark chocolate, coffee and tea, and red wine.

Much has been learned about the functions of vitamins C and E, beta-carotene, and other phytochemicals (biologically active substances found in plants), and the minerals selenium, zinc, copper, and manganese in their roles as antioxidants. Numerous studies have suggested that antioxidants may be important in preventing CVD, cancer, age-related eye disease, and other chronic conditions associated with aging. Ascorbic acid is one of the strongest antioxidants and radical scavengers, serving as a primary defense against free radicals in the blood. However, the connections between vitamin C and these processes have yet to be established. Research has shown vitamin C and other antioxidants in amounts greater than the RDA may be desirable, particularly from food sources.

Increased serum antioxidant concentrations are associated with a reduced risk of periodontitis. Research studies with antioxidant supplementation have indicated conflicting conclusions in regard to reduction of CVD and prevention of cancers. A systematic review and *meta*-analysis found no evidence to support the claim that antioxidant supplementation prevents mortality in healthy people or patients with CVD, cancer, or all-cause mortality.[83] However, higher dietary intake of fruits and vegetables containing antioxidants were associated with a reduced risk of CVD, cancer, and all-cause mortality reinforcing the role of the dental hygienist to encourage intake of a healthy diet pattern like those in the Dietary Guidelines.[83]

Polyphenols are antioxidants that are naturally occurring compounds found in fruits (grapes, apples, pears, cherries, and berries), vegetables, cereals, legumes, chocolate, and beverages (red wine, coffee, black and green tea). There has been much interest in the potential health benefits of plant polyphenols. Diets rich in polyphenols over a period of time may contribute to a reduction in the risk of certain cancers, CVD, diabetes, osteoporosis, and neurodegenerative diseases.[84–87] More research is needed to determine an optimal level of polyphenols' intake and their association with health benefits.

Apparently, the image of antioxidants as valiant warriors protecting the body from rampaging free radicals is too simplistic. The American Heart Association does not recommend antioxidant supplements, waiting for more convincing data.[88] Because of the lay press publicity surrounding the potential health benefits, many Americans are taking some form of antioxidant supplement to prevent chronic diseases.

High-intake levels of some antioxidants are well tolerated by most individuals, but several known factors must be considered before recommending supplements. Toxic effects occur with vitamin A; organ damage and deaths have been reported. Vitamin E supplements can antagonize vitamin K activity, enhance the effect of anticoagulant drugs, and be associated with adverse CVD outcomes.[89] Adverse effects of vitamin C include diarrhea, increased risk of kidney stones, and decreased absorption of vitamin B_{12}. Although vitamin C increases iron absorption, large amounts decrease availability of vitamin B_{12}. Erosion and hypersensitivity of tooth enamel may be adverse effects of chewable vitamin C tablets. Simultaneous intake of carotenoids with α-tocopherol may inhibit the absorption of vitamin E. Possibly unexplored interactions may occur between large amounts of antioxidants and other nutrients. If a patient chooses to take vitamin C supplements, there is no benefit in taking more expensive products containing bioflavonoids when compared to simple ascorbic acid.

Antioxidants may counteract the effects of cell damage produced by metabolic reactions and environmental factors such as pollution, smoking, and toxic chemicals in the diet. However, the health toll of a smoking habit is not corrected by making healthy eating choices or taking vitamins (see Chapter 19, *Health Application 19*). Recommendations for supplemental amounts of these nutrients should be reserved for claims that have been well substantiated by clinical trials showing cause and effect with identification of related side effects. Patients should also be cautioned against taking megadoses of vitamins and minerals because side effects, nutrient-nutrient interactions, and drug-nutrient interactions can occur. Individuals who are seriously ill with cancer, CVD, or other conditions, should talk with their health care provider about everything they put into their bodies, including vitamins, supplements, or herbs.

The *Dietary Guidelines* emphasize consumption of a varied diet to help prevent several chronic diseases. Dietary patterns high in fruits and vegetables are associated with a lower risk of disease. Advise patients to eat a healthy diet that includes many fruits and vegetables, especially those that are high in vitamins C and E, and beta-carotene. A pill cannot provide what is available from a healthful diet—thus the bottom line is to "eat your fruits and veggies." Antioxidant supplements cannot be expected to undo an unhealthy living of a lifetime. Adequate intake ideally should be in the form of improving food choices rather than supplements because as yet unidentified components present in food may be beneficial and protective. Beyond diet, decreased exposure to free radicals and increased physical activity are essential.

CASE APPLICATION FOR THE DENTAL HYGIENIST

A healthy patient asks your advice about taking vitamin C supplements to prevent periodontal disease. She is unaware of what foods to eat, or the symptoms of an excess or deficiency.

Nutritional Assessment
- Income
- Living arrangements, cooking and storage facilities
- Dietary assessment
- Tobacco and other drug use
- Knowledge level about vitamin C
- Beliefs about water-soluble vitamins
- Knowledge level about periodontal disease

- Physical status, especially any bleeding problems
- Use of over-the-counter or health care provider-prescribed supplements or medications
- Emotional state

Nutritional Diagnosis
Health-seeking behavior related to inadequate/insufficient knowledge about vitamin C and periodontal disease.

Nutritional Goals
The patient will consume foods high in vitamin C and state beliefs/information about vitamin C and periodontal disease.

◆ CASE APPLICATION FOR THE DENTAL HYGIENIST—CONT'D

Nutritional Implementation

Intervention: Teach the patient, the following about vitamin C: (1) functions, (2) requirements, and (3) sources. Teach the following about periodontal disease: (1) causes and (2) preventive factors.

Rationale: This provides the patient with a sound knowledge base about vitamin C and periodontal disease.

Intervention: Explain hyper- and hypo-vitamin C states.

Rationale: Large amounts of vitamin C decrease absorption of vitamin B_{12} and cause diarrhea, gastrointestinal distress, and kidney stones. Because vitamin C helps maintain capillary integrity, a vitamin C deficiency results in bleeding problems. Encourage food sources rather than supplements for increasing vitamin C.

Intervention: Provide oral hygiene education.

Rationale: The primary cause of periodontal disease is plaque biofilm. Providing education to effectively remove the plaque biofilm is essential. A vitamin deficiency does not cause periodontal disease, but it could exacerbate existing periodontal issues.

Evaluation

A patient states that she consumes citrus fruits, strawberries, cantaloupes, and mangoes. Additionally, she states that supplements are unnecessary for vitamin C, and large doses may interfere with the absorption of other nutrients. She further states if she does develop any bleeding problems, she will seek help. Last, the patient should verbalize information concerning excesses and deficiencies of vitamin C.

◆ Student Readiness

1. How do water-soluble vitamins differ from fat-soluble vitamins? What do these differences mean as you choose foods for your own menu? What do these differences mean as you teach patients about nutrition?
2. A patient asks why so many foods are now fortified with vitamin D. How would you respond?
3. Keep a record of your food intake for one day. Use a table of nutrient values of foods (https://www.ars.usda.gov/northeast-area/beltsville-md-bhnrc/beltsville-human-nutrition-research-center/food-surveys-research-group/docs/main-service-page/) or a nutrient analysis apps (MyFitnessPal) or Nutritrac to determine your vitamin A intake. Was intake adequate? What are some wiser food choices to enhance intake if below the RDA?
4. Prepare a menu for one day that provides adequate amounts of vitamins A and D. Use the menu you developed and eliminate all milk products and canned fish. How does this impact the vitamin D intake? Now, remove various types of egg products, green leafy vegetables, and dark-yellow vegetables, and see the effect on the vitamin A content of the meal plan.
5. Justify the rationale of vitamin D supplementation of milk products in the United States. What age groups do benefit the most from vitamin D supplementation in milk?
6. Name the deficiency and toxicity conditions associated with vitamins A, D, K, and C.
7. Name five foods other than oranges that are good sources of vitamin C.

References

1. Institute of Medicine. *DRI Dietary Reference Intakes: Applications in Dietary Assessment.* National Academies Press; 2000. https://www.ncbi.nlm.nih.gov/books/NBK222871/.
2. Pfeiffer CM, Sternberg MR, Schleicher RL, Haynes BMH, Rybak ME, Pirkle JL. The CDC's second national report on biochemical indicators of diet and nutrition in the United States population is a valuable tool for researchers and policy makers. *J Nutr.* 2013;143(6):938S–947S.
3. Murererehe J, Uwitonze AM, Nikuze P, Patel J, Razzaque MS. Beneficial effects of vitamin C in maintaining optimal oral health. *Front Nutr.* 2022;8 805809.
4. Meguro A, Ohara Y, Iwasaki M, et al. Denture wearing is associated with nutritional status among older adults requiring long-term care: a cross-sectional study. *J Dent Sci.* 2022;17(1):500–506.
5. Office of Dietary Supplements, National Institutes of Health. *Vitamin A and Carotenoids: Fact Sheet for Health Professionals.* 2022. https://ods.od.nih.gov/factsheets/VitaminA-Consumer/
6. Carazo A, Macáková K, Matoušová K, Krčmová LK, Protti M, Mladěnka P. Vitamin A update: forms, sources, kinetics, detection, function, deficiency, therapeutic use and toxicity. *Nutrients.* 2021;13(5):1703.
7. Gutierrez Gossweiler A, Martinez-Mier EA. Chapter 6: vitamins and oral health. *Monogr Oral Sci.* 2020;28:59–67. https://doi.org/10.1159/000455372.
8. Lodi G, Franchini R, Warnakulasuriya S, et al. Interventions for treating oral leukoplakia to prevent oral cancer. *Cochrane Database Syst Rev.* 2016;7(7): CD001829.
9. Kordiak J, Bielec F, Jabłoński S, Pastuszak-Lewandoska D. Role of beta-carotene in lung cancer primary chemoprevention: a systematic review with *meta*-analysis and *meta*-regression. *Nutrients.* 2022;14(7):1361.
10. Rock CL, Thomson C, Gansler T, et al. American Cancer Society guideline for diet and physical activity for cancer prevention. *CA.* 2020;70(4):245–271.
11. Institute of Medicine Panel on Micronutrients. *Dietary Reference Intakes for Vitamin A, Vitamin K, Arsenic, Boron, Chromium, Copper, Iodine, Iron, Manganese, Molybdenum, Nickel, Silicon, Vanadium, and Zinc.* National Academies Press; 2001. http://www.ncbi.nlm.nih.gov/books/NBK222310/.
12. Bird JK, Murphy RA, Ciappio ED, McBurney MI. Risk of deficiency in multiple concurrent micronutrients in children and adults in the United States. *Nutrients.* 2017;9(7):655.
13. Olson JM, Ameer MA, Goyal A. *Vitamin A toxicity.* In: StatPearls. StatPearls Publishing; 2022. http://www.ncbi.nlm.nih.gov/books/NBK532916/.
14. Imdad A, Mayo-Wilson E, Haykal MR, et al. Vitamin A supplementation for preventing morbidity and mortality in children from six months to five years of age. *Cochrane Database Syst Rev.* 2022;3(3). https://doi.org/10.1002/14651858.CD008524.pub4.
15. Nosewicz J, Spaccarelli N, Roberts KM, et al. The epidemiology, impact, and diagnosis of micronutrient nutritional dermatoses part 1: zinc, selenium, copper, vitamin A, and vitamin C. *J Am Acad Dermatol.* 2022;86(2):267–278.
16. Clugston RD, Blaner WS. The adverse effects of alcohol on vitamin A metabolism. *Nutrients.* 2012;4(5):356–371.
17. Nagel M, Labenz C, Dobbermann H, et al. Suppressed serological vitamin A in patients with liver cirrhosis is associated with impaired liver function and clinical deteriotation. *Eur J Gastroenterol Hepatol.* 2022;34(10):1053–1059.
18. Saeed A, Dullaart RPF, Schreuder TCMA, Blokzijl H, Faber KN. Disturbed vitamin a metabolism in non-alcoholic fatty liver disease (NAFLD). *Nutrients.* 2017;10(1):29.

19. Bikle DD. Vitamin D metabolism, mechanism of action, and clinical applications. *Chem Biol.* 2014;21(3):319–329.

20. Parizadeh SM, Rezayi M, Jafarzadeh-Esfehani R, et al. Association of vitamin D status with liver and kidney disease: a systematic review of clinical trials, and cross-sectional and cohort studies. *Int J Vitam Nutr Res.* 2021;91(1–2):175–187.

21. Cashman KD. Vitamin D deficiency: defining, prevalence, causes, and strategies of addressing. *Calcif Tissue Int.* 2020;106(1):14–29.

22. Office of Dietary Supplements, National Institutes of Health. *Vitamin D.* 2022. https://ods.od.nih.gov/factsheets/VitaminD-Health Professional/

23. Wagner CL, Greer FR, American Academy of Pediatrics Section on Breastfeeding, American Academy of Pediatrics Committee on Nutrition Prevention of rickets and vitamin D deficiency in infants, children, and adolescents. *Pediatrics.* 2008;122(5):1142–1152.

24. Institute of Medicine Ross AC, Taylor CL, Yaktine AL, Valle HBD. *Dietary reference intakes for calcium and vitamin D.* In: *Overview of Vitamin D.* National Academies Press (United States); 2011. https://www.ncbi.nlm.nih.gov/books/NBK56061/.

25. Simon AE, Ahrens KA. Adherence to vitamin D intake guidelines in the United States. *Pediatrics.* 2020;145(6): e20193574.

26. Sosa Henríquez M, Gómez de Tejada Romero M. Calcium and vitamin D supplementation in the management of osteoporosis. What is the advisable dose of vitamin D? *Rev Osteoporos Metab Min.* 2021;13(2):77–83.

27. United States Food and Drug Administration, Center for Food Safety and Applied Nutrition. *The New Nutrition Facts Label.* FDA; 2022. https://www.fda.gov/food/nutrition-education-resources-materials/new-nutrition-facts-label

28. Ames BN, Grant WB, Willett WC. Does the high prevalence of vitamin D deficiency in African Americans contribute to health disparities? *Nutrients.* 2021;13(2):499.

29. Religi A, Backes C, Chatelan A, et al. Estimation of exposure durations for vitamin D production and sunburn risk in Switzerland. *J Expo Sci Env Epidemiol.* 2019;29(6):742–752.

30. Marcos-Pérez D, Sánchez-Flores M, Proietti S, et al. Low vitamin D levels and frailty status in older adults: a systematic review and *meta*-analysis. *Nutrients.* 2020;12(8):2286.

31. Chalcraft JR, Cardinal LM, Wechsler PJ, et al. Vitamin D synthesis following a single bout of sun exposure in older and younger men and women. *Nutrients.* 2020;12(8):2237.

32. United States Food and Drug Administration, Center for Food Safety and Applied Nutrition. *Vitamin D for Milk and Milk Alternatives.* FDA; 2020. https://www.fda.gov/food/food-additives-petitions/vitamin-d-milk-and-milk-alternatives

33. United States Food and Drug Administration. *Food Additives Permitted for Direct Addition to Food for Human Consumption; Vitamin D3.* Federal Register; 2023. https://www.federalregister.gov/documents/2023/01/05/2022-28428/food-additives-permitted-for-direct-addition-to-food-for-human-consumption-vitamin-d3

34. Raisi-Estabragh Z, Martineau AR, Curtis EM, et al. Vitamin D and coronavirus disease 2019 (COVID-19): rapid evidence review. *Aging Clin Exp Res.* 2021;33(7):2031–2041.

35. Melo van Lent D, Egert S, Wolfsgruber S, et al. Low serum vitamin D status is associated with incident Alzheimer's dementia in the oldest old. *Nutrients.* 2022;15(1):61.

36. Kahwati LC, Weber RP, Pan H, et al. Vitamin D, calcium, or combined supplementation for the primary prevention of fractures in community-dwelling adults: an evidence review for the United States Preventive Services Task Force. *Agency Healthc Res Qual.* 2018 http://www.ncbi.nlm.nih.gov/books/NBK525398/.

37. Bolland MJ, Grey A, Avenell A. Effects of vitamin D supplementation on musculoskeletal health: a systematic review, *meta*-analysis, and trial sequential analysis. *Lancet Diabetes Endocrinol.* 2018;6(11):847–858.

38. Haffner D, Leifheit-Nestler M, Grund A, Schnabel D. Rickets guidance: part I—diagnostic workup. *Pediatr Nephrol.* 2022;37(9):2013–2036.

39. Thacher TD, Fischer PR, Tebben PJ, et al. Increasing incidence of nutritional rickets: a population-based study in Olmsted county, Minnesota. *Mayo Clin Proc.* 2013;88(2):176–183.

40. Creo AL, Thacher TD, Pettifor JM, Strand MA, Fischer PR. Nutritional rickets around the world: an update. *Paediatr Int Child Health.* 2017;37(2):84–98.

41. Singleton RJ, Day GM, Thomas TK, et al. Impact of a prenatal vitamin D supplementation program on vitamin D deficiency, rickets and early childhood caries in an Alaska Native population. *Nutrients.* 2022;14(19):3935.

42. Gjørup H, Beck-Nielsen SS, Haubek D. Craniofacial and dental characteristics of patients with vitamin-D-dependent rickets type 1A compared to controls and patients with X-linked hypophosphatemia. *Clin Oral Investig.* 2018;22(2):745–755.

43. Purvis RJ, Mackay GS, Cockburn F, et al. Enamel hypoplasia of the teeth associated with neonatal tetany: a manifestation of maternal vitamin D deficiency. *Lancet.* 1973;302(7833):811–814.

44. Carvalho Silva C, Mendes R, Manso Mda C, Gavinha S, Melo P. Prenatal or childhood serum levels of vitamin D and dental caries in paediatric patients: a systematic review. *Oral Health Prev Dent.* 2020;18(1):653–667.

45. Machado V, Lobo S, Proença L, Mendes JJ, Botelho J. Vitamin D and periodontitis: a systematic review and *meta*-analysis. *Nutrients.* 2020;12(8):2177.

46. Jagelavičienė E, Vaitkevičienė I, Šilingaitė D, Šinkūnaitė E, Daugėlaitė G. The relationship between vitamin D and periodontal pathology. *Medicina.* 2018;54(3):45.

47. Uday S, Högler W. Nutritional rickets & osteomalacia: a practical approach to management. *Indian J Med Res.* 2020;152(4):356–367.

48. Çakur B, Sümbüllü MA, Dağistan S, Durna D. The importance of cone beam CT in the radiological detection of osteomalacia. *Dentomaxillofac Radiol.* 2012;41(1):84–88.

49. O'Connor EA, Evans CV, Ivlev I, et al. Vitamin and mineral supplements for the primary prevention of cardiovascular disease and cancer: updated evidence report and systematic review for the United States Preventive Services Task Force. *JAMA.* 2022;327(23):2334–2347.

50. Zhang Y, Darssan D, Pascoe EM, Johnson DW, Pi H, Dong J. Vitamin D status and mortality risk among patients on dialysis: a systematic review and *meta*-analysis of observational studies. *Nephrol Dial Transpl.* 2018;33(10):1742–1751.

51. Office of Dietary Supplements. *Vitamin E: Fact Sheet for Health Professionals.* 2021. https://ods.od.nih.gov/factsheets/VitaminE-HealthProfessional/

52. Booth SL, Golly I, Sacheck JM, et al. Effect of vitamin E supplementation on vitamin K status in adults with normal coagulation status. *Am J Clin Nutr.* 2004;80(1):143–148.

53. Institute of Medicine. *Dietary Reference Intakes for Vitamin C, Vitamin E, Selenium, and Carotenoids.* National Academies Press; 2000. https://doi.org/10.17226/9810.

54. Reboul E. Vitamin E bioavailability: mechanisms of intestinal absorption in the spotlight. *Antioxidants.* 2017;6(4). https://doi.org/10.3390/antiox6040095.

55. Abner EL, Schmitt FA, Mendiondo MS, Marcum JL, Kryscio RJ. Vitamin E and all-cause mortality: a *meta*-analysis. *Curr Aging Sci.* 2011;4(2):158–170.

56. Miller ER, Pastor-Barriuso R, Dalal D, Riemersma RA, Appel LJ, Guallar E. *Meta*-analysis: high-dosage vitamin E supplementation may increase all-cause mortality. *Ann Intern Med.* 2005;142(1):37–46.

57. Assunção DGF, Silva LTPda, Camargo JDde AS, Cobucci RN, Ribeiro KDda S. Vitamin E levels in preterm and full-term infants: a systematic review. *Nutrients.* 2022;14(11):2257.

58. Sherf-Dagan S, Buch A, Ben-Porat T, Sakran N, Sinai T. Vitamin E status among bariatric surgery patients: a systematic review. *Surg Obes Relat Dis.* 2021;17(4):816–830.

59. Okebukola PO, Kansra S, Barrett J. Vitamin E supplementation in people with cystic fibrosis. *Cochrane Database Syst Rev.* 2020;9(9): CD009422.

60. Fabisiak N, Fabisiak A, Watala C, Fichna J. Fat-soluble vitamin deficiencies and inflammatory bowel disease: systematic review and meta-analysis. *J Clin Gastroenterol*. 2017;51(10):878–889.

61. Farina N, Llewellyn D, Isaac MGEKN, Tabet N. Vitamin E for Alzheimer's dementia and mild cognitive impairment. *Cochrane Database Syst Rev*. 2017;4(4): CD002854.

62. Violi F, Nocella C, Loffredo L, Carnevale R, Pignatelli P. Interventional study with vitamin E in cardiovascular disease and meta-analysis. *Free Radic Biol Med*. 2022;178:26–41.

63. Evans JR, Lawrenson JG. Antioxidant vitamin and mineral supplements for preventing age-related macular degeneration. *Cochrane Database Syst Rev*. 2017;7(7): CD000253.

64. Behfarnia P, Dadmehr M, Hosseini SN, Mirghaderi SA. The effect of Vitamin E supplementation on treatment of chronic periodontitis. *Dent Res J*. 2021;18:62.

65. Shadisvaaran S, Chin KY, Shahida MS, Ima-Nirwana S, Leong XF. Effect of vitamin E on periodontitis: evidence and proposed mechanisms of action. *J Oral Biosci*. 2021;63(2):97–103.

66. Office of Dietary Supplements. *Vitamin K: Fact Sheet for Health Professionals*. 2021. https://ods.od.nih.gov/factsheets/vitaminK-HealthProfessional/

67. Mladěnka P, Macáková K, Kujovská Krčmová L, et al. Vitamin K – sources, physiological role, kinetics, deficiency, detection, therapeutic use, and toxicity. *Nutr Rev*. 2021;80(4):677–698.

68. Hand I, Noble L, Abrams SA. Vitamin K and the newborn infant. *Pediatrics*. 2022;149(3): e2021056036.

69. Jagannath VA, Fedorowicz Z, Thaker V, Chang AB. Vitamin K supplementation for cystic fibrosis. *Cochrane Database Syst Rev*. 2015;1 CD008482.

70. Sherf-Dagan S, Goldenshluger A, Azran C, Sakran N, Sinai T, Ben-Porat T. Vitamin K-what is known regarding bariatric surgery patients: a systematic review. *Surg Obes Relat Dis*. 2019;15(8):1402–1413.

71. Office of Dietary Supplements. *Vitamin C: Fact Sheet for Health Professionals*. 2021. https://ods.od.nih.gov/factsheets/VitaminC-HealthProfessional/

72. Doseděl M, Jirkovský E, Macáková K, et al. Vitamin C-sources, physiological role, kinetics, deficiency, use, toxicity, and determination. *Nutrients*. 2021;13(2):615.

73. Rowe S, Carr AC. Global vitamin C status and prevalence of deficiency: a cause for concern? *Nutrients*. 2020;12(7):2008.

74. Carr AC, Rowe S. Factors affecting vitamin C status and prevalence of deficiency: a global health perspective. *Nutrients*. 2020;12(7):1963.

75. Tada A, Miura H. The relationship between vitamin C and periodontal diseases: a systematic review. *Int J Env Res Public Health*. 2019;16(14):2472.

76. Fageeh HN, Fageeh HI, Prabhu A, Bhandi S, Khan S, Patil S. Efficacy of vitamin C supplementation as an adjunct in the nonsurgical management of periodontitis: a systematic review. *Syst Rev*. 2021;10(1).5

77. Dodington DW, Fritz PC, Sullivan PJ, Ward WE. Higher intakes of fruits and vegetables, β-carotene, vitamin C, α-tocopherol, EPA,

and DHA are positively associated with periodontal healing after nonsurgical periodontal therapy in nonsmokers but not in smokers. *J Nutr*. 2015;145(11):2512–2519.

78. Deirawan H, Fakhoury JW, Zarka M, Bluth MH, Moossavi M. Revisiting the pathobiology of scurvy: a review of the literature in the context of a challenging case. *Int J Dermatol*. 2020;59(12):1450–1457.

79. Hemilä H, Chalker E. Vitamin C for preventing and treating the common cold. *Cochrane Database Syst Rev*. 2013;2013(1): CD000980.

80. Léger D. Scurvy. *Can Fam Physician*. 2008;54(10):1403–1406.

81. Maxfield L, Crane JS. *Vitamin C deficiency*. In: *StatPearls*. StatPearls Publishing; 2022. http://www.ncbi.nlm.nih.gov/books/NBK493187/.

82. Lee SK, Kader AA. Preharvest and postharvest factors influencing vitamin C content of horticultural crops. *Postharvest Biol Technol*. 2000;20(3):207–220.

83. Aune D, Keum N, Giovannucci E, et al. Dietary intake and blood concentrations of antioxidants and the risk of cardiovascular disease, total cancer, and all-cause mortality: a systematic review and dose-response meta-analysis of prospective studies. *Am J Clin Nutr*. 2018;108(5):1069–1091.

84. Rienks J, Barbaresko J, Nöthlings U. Association of polyphenol biomarkers with cardiovascular disease and mortality risk: a systematic review and meta-analysis of observational studies. *Nutrients*. 2017;9(4):415.

85. Rienks J, Barbaresko J, Oluwagbemigun K, Schmid M, Nöthlings U. Polyphenol exposure and risk of type 2 diabetes: dose-response meta-analyses and systematic review of prospective cohort studies. *Am J Clin Nutr*. 2018;108(1):49–61.

86. Rienks J, Barbaresko J, Nöthlings U. Association of isoflavone biomarkers with risk of chronic disease and mortality: a systematic review and meta-analysis of observational studies. *Nutr Rev*. 2017;75(8):616–641.

87. Inchingolo AD, Inchingolo AM, Malcangi G, et al. Effects of resveratrol, curcumin and quercetin supplementation on bone metabolism—a systematic review. *Nutrients*. 2022;14(17):3519.

88. Kris-Etherton PM, Lichtenstein AH, Howard BV, Steinberg D, Witztum JL. Nutrition Committee of the American Heart Association Council on Nutrition, Physical Activity, and Metabolism. Antioxidant vitamin supplements and cardiovascular disease. *Circulation*. 2004;110(5):637–641.

89. Shah S, Shiekh Y, Lawrence JA, et al. A systematic review of effects of vitamin E on the cardiovascular system. *Cureus*. 2021;13(6): e15616.

▶ Evolve Resources

Please visit http://evolve.elsevier.com/Mallonee/nutritional for additional practice and study support tools.

9

Minerals Essential for Calcified Structures

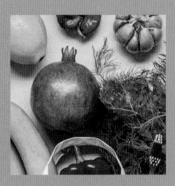

STUDENT LEARNING OUTCOMES

On completion of this chapter, the student will be able to achieve the following learning outcomes:

1. Discuss the following related to bone mineralization and growth, formation of teeth, and the mineral elements of the body:
   - List the minerals found in collagen, bones, and teeth. Describe their main physiologic roles and sources.
   - List the three calcified tissues of which teeth are composed.
   - List and discuss major minerals and trace elements of the body.
2. For calcium, phosphorus, magnesium, and fluoride:
   - Describe the physiologic roles of each mineral involved in calcified structures.

- Discuss the RDA (or AI), Tolerable Upper Intake level, and estimated average requirement for each mineral.
- Discuss the importance of calcium and phosphorus balance in the body, and name common sources of the minerals (calcium, phosphorus, magnesium, and fluoride).
- Discuss clinical conditions associated with excess and deficiency of these minerals.
- Customize nutrition recommendations for these minerals to meet patient's needs of these minerals.
- Discuss the role of water fluoridation in the prevention of dental caries.

KEY TERMS

Alveolar bone
Amorphous
Apatite
Bioavailability
Compressional forces
Fluorapatite
Fluorosis

Hydroxyapatite
Hypercalcemia
Hypercalciuria
Hypocalcemia
Mineralization
Osteoclasts
Osteoids

Osteoporosis
Periodontal disease
Phytochemicals
Remodeling
Rickets
Tensional forces
Tetany

⚙ TEST YOUR NQ

1. **T/F** Meats are good sources of phosphorus.
2. **T/F** The only nutrients essential for strong healthy bones are calcium and phosphorus.
3. **T/F** Tooth loss may be an oral sign of osteoporosis.
4. **T/F** Systemic fluoride causes changes in tooth morphology that increase caries resistance.
5. **T/F** To obtain adequate calcium, a teenager needs to drink 2 cups of milk a day.

6. **T/F** Water fluoridation is economically inefficient because very little water is actually consumed.
7. **T/F** All females should take calcium supplements to prevent osteoporosis.
8. **T/F** Calcium absorption is increased when a sugar is present.
9. **T/F** Caffeine intake may decrease calcium loss.
10. **T/F** All bottled waters contain fluoride.

Bone Mineralization and Growth

Calcified structures in the body, which include bones and teeth, are composed of a matrix of organic and inorganic substances. Dentin, cementum, and bone originate with a protein matrix, or collagen deposition. Collagen is present throughout the periodontium as the primary connective tissue fiber in the gingiva and major organic constituent of alveolar bone. Collagen is continuously remodeled (resorption and reformation of bone) throughout growth and development. Defective collagen synthesis affects formation of bones and teeth.

The organic matrix of bone is 90% to 95% collagen fibers, which are secreted by osteoblasts. Collagen formation requires the presence of a variety of substances, including protein; vitamin C; and minerals including iron, copper, and zinc. When collagen is formed, apatite, a calcium phosphate complex, automatically crystallizes adjacent to the collagen fibers.

In bones that have not undergone calcification, osteoids are formed rapidly. Most of them develop into the finished product, hydroxyapatite crystals (inorganic component of bones and teeth). The chemical formula for hydroxyapatite crystals is $Ca_{10}(PO_4)_6(OH)_2$.

Immediately after collagen formation, mineralization begins. Mineralization is the deposition of inorganic elements (minerals) on an organic matrix (mainly composed of protein in combination with some polysaccharides and lipids). In addition to calcium and phosphorus, numerous other minerals, especially magnesium, sodium, potassium, and carbonate ions, are incorporated into the mineral matrix.

Adequate nutritional components are necessary during collagen formation and mineral deposition phases to prevent structural imperfections. The crystalline mineral matrix provides compressive and tensile strength. The combination of collagen and crystalline mineral matrix forms a material resembling reinforced concrete.

The skeleton is constantly growing, changing, and remodeling itself. A small portion of total bone calcium remains in a shapeless or amorphous form. This calcium is a reserve source that can be rapidly used when serum calcium levels decrease. Osteoblasts deposit fresh calcium salts where new stresses have developed, and where osteoclasts (connected with absorption of bone) are removing calcium deposits. Bone absorption by osteoclasts is controlled by parathyroid hormone (PTH). The rate of osteoblast and osteoclast activity is normally in equilibrium, except during periods of growth. In older adults, bone resorption may exceed mineralization, causing osteoporosis.

This dynamic state accommodates changing demands of the body. Bone strength is adjusted in proportion to the degree of stress on the bone. Continual physical stress stimulates calcification and osteoblastic deposition of bone.

Formation of Teeth

Teeth are composed of three calcified tissues: enamel, dentin, and cementum. Enamel and dentin are primarily comprised of hydroxyapatite crystals similar to those in bone. Approximately 30% of dentin, 50% of cementum, and 35% of alveolar bone is organic material, principally collagen; only 4% of the enamel is organic material. Dentin lacks the osteoblasts and osteoclasts found in bone; enamel and dentin do not contain blood vessels or nerves. As with bone, the mineral crystallization structure makes teeth extremely resistant to compressional forces; collagen fibers make teeth tough and resistant to tensional forces. Actions in which pressure attempts to diminish a structure's volume are referred to as compressional forces; tensional forces are actions in which pressure stretches or strains the structure.

After a tooth erupts, no more enamel is formed, but mineral exchanges occur slowly in response to the oral environment. Changes in mineral composition of enamel occur by exchange of minerals in saliva, rather than from the pulp cavity. Minerals—such as fluoride, sodium, zinc, and strontium—can replace calcium ions. Carbonate can be substituted for phosphate; carbonate and fluoride can be substituted for hydroxyl ions. These changes may alter the solubility of apatite. Despite changes that occur in enamel composition, enamel maintains most of its original mineral components throughout life.

The crystalline structure of enamel is one of the most insoluble and resistant proteins known. This special protein matrix, in combination with a crystalline structure of inorganic salts, makes enamel harder than dentin. In fact, it is the hardest structure in the human body. It is comparable to quartz in terms of hardness. Enamel is more resistant to acids, enzymes, and other corrosive agents than dentin.

Dentin, the main tissue of teeth, contains the same constituents as bone, but its structure is denser than bone. It is a hard, yellowish substance. Its principal components are hydroxyapatite crystals embedded in a strong meshwork of collagen fibers. Odontoblasts line the inner surface of dentin and provide nourishment for the dentin.

Cementum, which covers the dentin in the root area, is another bonelike substance, but because it contains fewer minerals, it is softer than bone. Just like dentin, it is also a hard, yellowish substance that contains many collagen fibers. The outer layer of cementum is lined with cementoblasts, capable of producing cementum throughout the life of the tooth. Compressional forces cause the cementum to become thicker and stronger. Cementum exhibits more typical characteristics of bone than enamel and dentin. Minerals are absorbed and deposited at rates similar to that of alveolar bone.

Development of normal, healthy teeth is affected by metabolic factors, such as PTH secretion, and the availability of calcium, phosphate, vitamin D, protein, and many other nutrients. If these factors are deficient, calcification of teeth may be defective and abnormal throughout life.

Introduction to Minerals

Minerals are inorganic elements with many physiologic functions. Numerous inorganic elements in the body account for only about 5% of total body weight, or 7.5 lb for a 150-lb person.[1] Minerals are subdivided into those required in larger amounts (major minerals) and those required in smaller amounts (micronutrients, also called trace elements) (Box 9.1). Despite the smaller amounts required, trace elements are just as important as major minerals.

Calcium

Physiologic Roles

At least 99% of the body's calcium is found in the skeleton and teeth. Calcium is indispensable for skeletal function, which requires adequate dietary calcium to achieve full accretion of bone mass prescribed by genetic potential. Calcium (and phosphorus) in the bone, but not in the enamel of teeth, functions as a "savings account" for maintaining serum calcium levels. Only 1% of the body's calcium is found in blood, but as such, it controls body functions such as blood clotting, transmission of nerve impulses, muscle contraction and relaxation, membrane permeability, and activation of certain enzymes.[2] Research indicates that calcium intake is important not only for bone health but also for reducing the risk of many other disorders, from hypertension to obesity to certain cancers.[2]

• BOX 9.1   Mineral Elements in the Body

Major Minerals (>100 mg/day)

Calcium (Ca)[a]
Phosphorus (P)[a]
Sodium (Na)[a]
Potassium (K)
Magnesium (Mg)[a]
Chlorine (Cl)[a]
Sulfur (S)

Trace Elements (<100 mg/day)

Iron (Fe)[a]
Copper (Cu)[a]
Zinc (Zn)[a]
Manganese (Mn)[a]
Iodine (I)[a]
Molybdenum (Mo)[a]
Fluorine (F)[a]
Selenium (Se)[a]
Chromium (Cr)
Cobalt (Co)

Ultratrace Elements (No Recommended Dietary Allowances)

Boron (B)[a]
Arsenic (As)
Nickel (Ni)[a]
Silicon (Si)
Tin (Sn)
Vanadium (V)[a]
Cadmium (Cd)
Lead (Pb)
Bromide (Br)
Lithium (Li)
Aluminum (Al)

[a]Tolerable Upper Intake Levels have been established.

Saliva is supersaturated with calcium and phosphorus; saliva is a source of calcium to mineralize an immature or demineralized enamel surface and reduce caries risk.[3] Calcium and phosphate in saliva provide a buffering action to inhibit demineralization of enamel (and dentin) by plaque biofilm.[3]

Requirements

The National Academy of Medicine (NAM, formerly the Institute of Medicine) has established a recommended dietary allowance (RDA) and an estimated average requirement for calcium. The RDA is 1000 mg/day for ages 19 to 50 years.[4] During growth periods, primarily from 9 to 18 years of age, the requirement is higher (1300 mg/day) because peak bone mass appears to be related to calcium intake during periods of increased bone mineralization (Table 9.1).[4] Peak bone mass occurs between 18 and 20 years of age for females and 20 to 24 years of age for males.[5] Typical calcium intake from food sources and supplements of teens between ages 12 and 19 years was 1212 mg/day for males and females which was slightly below the RDA for calcium.[6]

Females are less likely than males to exceed their RDA. The estimated mean calcium intake for females aged 60 to 69 years during the 2017–2020 National Health and Nutrition Examination Survey was 825 mg/day compared with 1045 mg/day for males in the same age category. The lowest intake was for those aged 70 and over with 771 mg/day for females and 933 for mg/day for males. Fortunately, intake for both groups when including a calcium supplement is 1456 mg/day for males and 1474 mg/day for females.[6] This points to the need to gather history on supplement use as well as dietary intake when assessing nutritional status.

Americans usually consume an average of 842 mg/day for females and 1056 mg of calcium per day for males from food sources.[6] Inadequate calcium intake can be attributed to (1) uninformed choices or not selecting adequate sources of calcium on a

TABLE 9.1	Adequate Intake for Calcium			
Life Stage Group	EAR (mg/day)	RDA (mg/day)	AI (mg/day)	UL (mg/day)
Infants (birth–6 months)			200	1000
Infants (7–12 months)			260	1500
Children (1–3 years)	500	700		2500
Children (4–8 years)	800	1000		2500
Adolescents (9–13 years)	1100	1300		3000
Adolescents (14–18 years)	1100	1300		3000
Adults (19–30 years)	800	1000		2500
Adults (31–50 years)	800	1000		2500
Adults (51–70 years)	800	1200		2000
Males	800	1000		2000
Females	1000	1200		2000
>70 years	1000	1200		2000
Pregnancy and lactation	Same as for their age group			

AI, Adequate intake; *EAR,* estimated average requirement; *RDA,* recommended dietary allowance; *UL,* tolerable upper intake level.
Data from Institute of Medicine, Food and Nutrition Board. *Dietary Reference Intakes for Calcium and Vitamin D.* National Academy Press; 2011.

daily basis; (2) the mistaken beliefs that adults do not need milk or that milk contributes too many calories to the diet; (3) economic hardships, plus a lack of knowledge regarding inexpensive sources of calcium-rich foods; (4) self-diagnosed lactose intolerance or allergies to dairy products; (5) access to and consumption of soda and other beverages; and (6) dislike of calcium-rich foods.

Generally, inadequate calcium intake affects bone mass more than tooth structure. Inadequate calcium and vitamin D intake during tooth formation and maturation may result in hypomineralization of developing teeth. After tooth formation, dietary calcium does not affect caries rate.

Calcium Balance

Despite variations in calcium intake, serum calcium is relatively constant. If the serum calcium level declines, bones are used as calcium reserves. Skeletal calcium turns over (transfers from in and out of bone) daily to promote bone homeostasis and maintain a constant serum calcium concentration. When calcium withdrawal from bones exceeds deposits, calcium imbalance occurs. Decreased bone density caused by insufficient calcium is a slow process.

Calcium-Phosphorus Balance

Serum levels of calcium and phosphorus are inversely related. If the calcium level increases, phosphorus levels decrease and vice versa. This relationship acts as a protective mechanism to prevent high combined concentrations, which can lead to calcification of soft tissue and stone formation or contraction of the heart muscle.

Absorption and Excretion

Calcium balance, achieved when intake equals excretion, does not solely depend on adequate calcium intake. Several hormones—including PTH, calcitonin, vitamin D—help to regulate calcium absorption.[7,8] Calcium homeostasis also involves estrogens, thyroxine, and corticoid steroids.[8] Under normal conditions, about 25% of the calcium consumed is absorbed.[4] Maximum calcium absorption occurs when it is consumed in small to moderate amounts and ingested several times throughout the day.[4] In other words, individuals should consume 30% of the daily value or 300 mg per serving three to four times a day to maximize absorption.

Absorption occurs primarily in the small intestine. It is affected by many factors, as shown in Fig. 9.1.[9] Calcium absorption from various dairy products is similar, whereas calcium present in many dark-green leafy vegetables is not readily absorbed. During periods of increased need—especially during growth, pregnancy, and lactation—calcium absorption increases.[8]

Calcium absorption decreases with age, probably because of lower hormone levels and diminished function of organs such as kidneys.[8] The rate of absorption is the lowest in postmenopausal females because of diminished estrogen levels.

Although several plant foods contain large amounts of calcium, absorption is poor. Oxalates (oxalic acid) in vegetables and phytates (phytic acid) from wheat bran, bind with calcium in these foods to reduce absorption, but they do not interfere with calcium absorption from other foods.[8] Dark-green leafy vegetables (e.g., kale, turnip greens) contain minimal amounts of oxalic acid, and calcium from these vegetables is readily absorbed. Excessive dietary fiber (more than 35 g/day) also interferes with calcium absorption.[8]

Typically in the United States, the effect of intake of a high-protein diet, on calcium absorption and secretion is inconsistent with some research stating that it has no effect on bone density while other studies finding excess excretion of calcium.[8] However, the usual intake of protein and phosphorus does not cause calcium

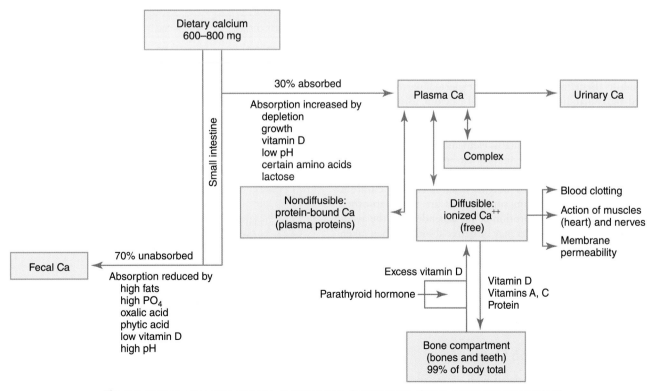

• **Fig. 9.1** Calcium absorption and use. (Adapted from Schlenker ED, Gilbert J. Williams' *Essentials of Nutrition and Diet Therapy*. 11th ed. Elsevier; 2015.)

loss when intake is adequate, whereas a diet low in protein and phosphorus may have adverse effects on calcium balance with inadequate calcium intake.

Generally, weight loss causes bone mineral loss and this is particularly true for individuals post-bariatric surgery.[8,10] Stimulation of PTH results in the possible loss of bone mass to restore the levels to normal. PTH works concurrently with vitamin D to prevent calcium from being excreted and stimulates calcium release from bone when serum levels of calcium are low. Increasing synthesis of vitamin D by PTH also results in increased calcium absorption.

Sources

Milk and other dairy products supply the greatest amount of available calcium (Table 9.2). Not only are they preferred sources of calcium because of their high calcium content, but lactose and other nutrients in dairy products enhance calcium absorption to between 30 and 45%.[9] Milk also provides other essential nutrients. Box 9.2 lists portion sizes for various foods that provide approximately 300 mg of calcium.

Since 1999, food manufacturers have been fortifying products such as fruit juices, fruit-flavored drinks, breakfast cereals, and breads with calcium. Numerous calcium-fortified foods introduced to the market have been well-received. Food products containing natural or fortified calcium must use certain terminology on packaging, as shown in Table 9.3.

An increasing percentage of the US population purchases supplements containing calcium. The US Preventive Services Task Force found inconclusive evidence to support the use of a calcium supplement in males and premenopausal females, however, this recommendation is currently undergoing review.[11] In addition, research is not consistent about whether excessive calcium intake may increase the risk of cardiovascular disease (CVD) with the most recent systematic review and *meta*-analysis suggesting no effect.[2,12] In individuals with inadequate intake from food, calcium supplements combined with vitamin D may result in small but significant reductions in bone loss.[2] This strong trend toward the use of calcium supplements is especially evident among older adults. Benefits may be less than expected, partly because of limited bioavailability of supplemental calcium. **Bioavailability** refers to the amount of a nutrient available physiologically, and it is based on its absorption rate.

A calcium supplement contains elemental calcium along with other substances, such as carbonate or citrate. The amount of elemental calcium varies among supplements. For example, calcium carbonate is 40% calcium by weight, whereas calcium citrate is 21% calcium. Some calcium supplements are better absorbed when taken with food, absorption being dependent on the availability of gastric acids. Others may be better absorbed when taken on an empty stomach. Calcium-citrate-malate, calcium lactate, calcium gluconate, and calcium sulfate are other forms of calcium in supplements or fortified foods. Choosing a supplement that has the US Pharmacopeia (USP) designation means that the quantity in the supplement is more likely to be consistent with the label.

Hyper States and Hypo States

Clinical conditions are associated with excess and deficiency of calcium. Hypercalcemia (too much calcium) and hypocalcemia (too little calcium) are critical metabolic conditions that can lead

TABLE 9.2	Calcium and Phosphorus Content of Selected Foods		
Food	Portion	Calcium (mg)	Phosphorus (mg)
Coconut milk, fortified	1 cup	459	0
Almond milk, vanilla	1 cup	422	73
Orange juice, calcium fortified	1 cup	414	221
Yogurt, nonfat plain	6 oz	388	267
Milk (2%)	1 cup	307	251
Buttermilk, low-fat	1 cup	284	368
Swiss cheese	1 oz	249	161
Parmesan cheese	1 oz	248	178
Soy milk, calcium fortified	1 cup	237	161
Rice milk	1 cup	228	137
Pizza, cheese (large)	1 piece	224	257
Cheddar cheese	1 oz	198	128
American cheese	1 slice	192	118
Kale, cooked	½ cup	177	38
Cottage cheese	1 cup	174	334
Ice cream, vanilla	1 cup	173	142
Tofu, raw, firm	½ cup	138	114
Hamburger bun	1	121	80
Turnip greens, cooked	½ cup	125	28
Spinach, cooked	½ cup	71	43
Okra, cooked	½ cup	70	52
Black beans, canned	½ cup	46	142
Oatmeal, instant	1 cup	29	156
Broccoli, cooked	½ cup	27	54
Ground beef, cooked	3 oz	23	162
Spinach, raw	1 cup	17	10
Salmon, grilled	3 oz	7	183
Cola	12 oz	4	33

Data from United States Department of Agriculture (USDA), Agricultural Research Service. *What's in the Foods You Eat Search Tool.* 2019–2020. https://www.ars.usda.gov/northeast-area/beltsville-md-bhnrc/beltsville-human-nutrition-research-center/food-surveys-research-group/docs/whats-in-the-foods-you-eat-search-tool/.

to loss of consciousness, fatal respiratory failure, or cardiac arrest. These problems are seldom caused directly by calcium intake from food sources.

Calcium Excess

Hypercalcemia, or excessive levels of calcium in the blood, is rarely the result of dietary intake. Hypercalcemia can result in renal insufficiency, gastrointestinal symptoms (e.g., nausea and vomiting),

• BOX 9.2 **Calcium Equivalents¹**

The following foods contain approximately 300 mg of calcium:
1 cup milk
1 cup soy milk or coconut milk, fortified
1 cup almond milk
1 cup orange juice, fortified
1½ oz cheddar cheese
1½ oz mozzarella cheese
1½ oz American cheese
1½ cup tofu
1 cup yogurt
2 cups ice cream
1½ servings cheese pizza

¹RDA for calcium is 1000 mg for individuals 19 to 50 years old.
Data from United States Department of Agriculture (USDA), Agricultural Research Service.
What's in the Foods Your Eat Search Tool. 2019–2020. https://www.ars.usda.gov/northeast-area/beltsville-md-bhnrc/beltsville-human-nutrition-research-center/food-surveys-research-group/docs/whats-in-the-foods-you-eat-search-tool/.

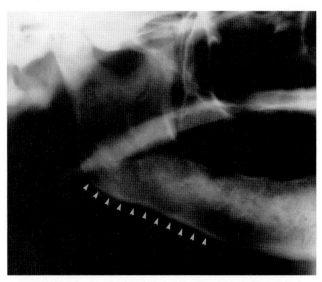

• **Fig. 9.2** Radiographic appearance of osteoporosis affecting bone of the maxillofacial complex. This portion of a panoramic radiograph depicts thinning of the gonial and interior cortices of an edentulous mandible (*arrows*). A slight increase in the general size of marrow spaces is also apparent. (Courtesy B. W. Benson, DDS, MS, Associate Professor, Department of Diagnostic Sciences, Texas A&M University College of Dentistry, Dallas, TX.)

TABLE 9.3	**Food Labeling for Calcium**

DV of Calcium in a Food	FDA-Authorized Labeling Terms
10% DV of calcium	Calcium enriched Calcium fortified More calcium
10%–19% DV of calcium	Contains calcium Provides calcium Good source of calcium
≥20% DV of calcium	High in calcium Rich in calcium Excellent source of calcium

DV, Daily value; *FDA*, US Food and Drug Administration.

bone pain, pathologic fractures, fatigue, polyuria, constipation, or hypercalciuria (high levels of calcium in the urine).[2,13] Overdoses of cholecalciferol or excessive amounts of vitamin D preparations can also cause hypercalcemia.[14] Hyperparathyroidism, certain types of bone disease, vitamin D poisoning, sarcoidosis, cancer, and prolonged excessive intake of milk may also cause adult hypercalcemia.[13]

Although findings are inconsistent, some research suggests excessive calcium intake is associated with prostate cancer and risk of death from CVD.[2,15–17] It also may inhibit absorption of other minerals like iron and zinc. Calcium carbonate supplements can interfere with absorption of levothyroxine.[2] Supplements may also interact with some antibiotics (e.g., ciprofloxacin) and HIV medications reducing absorption so the medications should be taken 2 hours before taking supplements.[2]

Calcium Deficiency

Hypocalcemia, or deficient levels of serum calcium, is typically due to vitamin D or magnesium deficiency, hypoparathyroidism,

critically ill patients, and certain medications (e.g., proton pump inhibitors [PPIs] and bisphosphonates).[2,18] In critically ill patients, hypocalcemia is often associated with poor outcomes.[18,19] Symptoms include muscle cramps that may progress to tetany, a neuromuscular disorder of uncontrollable cramps and tremors involving the muscles of the face, hands, feet, and eventually abnormal heart rhythm.[20]

Rickets, discussed in Chapter 8 in connection with vitamin D deficiency, results in porous, soft bones. Rickets develops during childhood as a result of inadequate amounts of calcium being deposited in the bone. Calcium intake may be adequate, but absorption is poor because of inadequate vitamin D.

Osteoporosis is referred to as a "pediatric disease with geriatric consequences" because adequate calcium and vitamin D intake in childhood and adolescence during growth and development is critical to building peak bone mass.[21] Osteoporosis is characterized by decreased bone mass, mineral density, and/or changes in the structure or strength of bone leading to increased risk for fracture.[22] Numerous factors, including genetics, age, sex (females have higher risk), decreased estrogen, body mass index (BMI) <18.5, smoking, previous history of major fractures, inadequate calcium or vitamin D intake, and lack of weight-bearing activity are implicated.[21,23] Calcium intake has a protective effect on bone density in females reporting a high lifetime calcium intake, but not in females who increased intake after menopause. Building bone during the formative years is the best insurance against osteoporosis.

An oral sign of osteoporosis may be loss of attachment associated with periodontal disease, but the research findings have been inconsistent (Fig. 9.2).[24,25] However, calcium intake should be encouraged to aid in maintaining alveolar bone.[26]

Osteoporosis usually goes undetected, however, until pain or spontaneous fracture occurs. Osteoporosis is discussed further in *Health Application 9.*

DENTAL CONSIDERATIONS

- Physical inactivity results in lower bone mass.[27,28] Weight-bearing physical activity is important at every age to maintain bone mass.
- Inadequate calcium can lead to incomplete calcification of the tooth, abnormalities of the teeth and bones, periodontal disease, and early tooth loss.
- Achlorhydria (the absence of hydrochloric acid in the stomach) with the use of PPIs for gastroesophageal reflux may interfere with calcium absorption and may increase the risk for bone fracture long term. Recommendations are to increase dietary sources of calcium and/or use calcium citrate supplements.[29]
- Individuals with hyperparathyroidism are at increased risk of periodontal disease and tooth loss.[30]
- Patients who have had bariatric surgery for obesity may be at risk for clinical attachment loss although the research is inconsistent.[31,32]
- Interventions for limiting or preventing further bone loss include encouraging exercise and foods rich in vitamin D and calcium.
- Patients who smoke cigarettes are at risk of osteoporosis.[33]
- Suggest alternatives for increasing calcium intake for patients with lactose intolerance (see Chapter 4, *Health Application 4*).
- Calcium supplements may alter absorption of certain medications, including glucocorticoids, cellulose sodium phosphate (Calcibind), etidronate (Didronel), phenytoin (Dilantin), levothyroxine (Synthroid),[34] bisphosphonates, and tetracycline. Supplements should be taken 1 to 4 hours before or after the medication.
- Poor patient compliance may be expected if several tablets are necessary, the supplement is too expensive, or gastrointestinal problems (e.g., gas, bloating, diarrhea) occur.

NUTRITIONAL DIRECTIONS

- Adequate daily calcium, phosphorus, and vitamin D intake is important to support bone formation and maintenance. Try to consume adequate amount of the nutrients from food sources daily. If calcium supplements are necessary, absorption can be enhanced by taking it with some form of sugar; lactose, dextrose, and sucrose.
- Evaluate calcium supplements for their solubility, which affects absorption. For calcium to be absorbed from a supplement, the tablet must first dissolve. To measure how well a calcium tablet dissolves in the body, drop a tablet in a cup of vinegar (pH 2.8) to produce an environment similar to of gastric acid (pH 1.5–3.0) in the stomach. Stir occasionally. At least two-thirds of a high-quality tablet dissolves within 30 minutes.
- Calcium supplements are available in tablets, gel capsules, liquids, gummies, and chewables.
- Compare the amount of elemental calcium provided (actual amount of calcium in the supplement) and cost per tablet. Refer patients who are appropriate candidates for calcium supplementation to a health care provider or RDN.
- Higher calcium intake in females, particularly from food sources, results in lower levels of estrogen production which has positive effects on bone health.[35] Estrogen enhances calcium absorption and enables more efficient use of calcium.
- Moderate alcohol intake enhances bone density mass as a result of less bone remodeling.[33]
- Weight-bearing exercise has a positive effect on calcium deposition in bone during childhood and adolescence.[21] Weight-bearing exercise and resistance training prevent, and in some cases reverse, bone loss in adults.[21]
- When daily calcium intake appears to be low, encourage increased consumption of food sources of calcium such as dairy products. If the patient is unable to consume dairy products, explore other calcium-fortified food sources.

- Green leafy sources of calcium that are low in oxalic acid include kale, arugula, turnip greens, broccoli, and Brussel sprouts. Oxalates inhibit the absorption of calcium. This is particularly helpful information for vegans or those not consuming dairy products.
- Do not take calcium supplements within 1 to 2 hours of eating large amounts of fiber, especially foods containing large amounts of phytates and oxalates.
- In postmenopausal females, calcium and vitamin D from food sources increase bone mineral density (BMD).[36] In addition, calcium and vitamin D helps to reduce the risk of fractures when coupled with an approved osteoporosis-related therapy, such as bisphosphonate.

Phosphorus

Physiologic Roles

Phosphorus is the second most abundant mineral in the body, with approximately 85% in the skeleton and teeth.[37] Its presence in all body cells is necessary for almost every aspect of metabolism, including (1) transfer and release of energy stored as adenosine triphosphate; (2) composition of phospholipids, DNA, and RNA; and (3) metabolism of fats, carbohydrates, and proteins. Phosphorus also helps regulate the acid-base balance in the body.

Requirements

The RDA of phosphorus for adults older than 18 years of age is 700 mg.[38] Because phosphorus is more readily available than calcium in the US food supply, intake is approximately 1.5 times higher than calcium.[6] Although harmful effects from excessive amounts of phosphorus have not been reported, the NAM established a tolerable upper intake level (UL) to reflect normal serum levels (Table 9.4).[38] Note that pregnant and lactating females consume the same amount of phosphorus as nonpregnant females of the same age.

Absorption and Excretion

Approximately 40% to 70% of dietary phosphorus is absorbed in the jejunum.[37] Its absorption can be inhibited by the same dietary factors affecting calcium absorption: phytate, excessive fat, iron, aluminum, and calcium intake. The kidneys excrete excessive amounts of phosphorus to maintain optimal body levels.

Sources

Phosphorus is abundant in foods, which is the reason why deficiencies have not been observed. A diet adequate in calcium and protein contains enough phosphorus because all three minerals are present in the same foods (see Table 9.2). In addition to milk products, meats are a good source of phosphorus. Dietary restriction of phosphorus is extremely difficult because of its wide use as a food additive in baked goods, cheese, processed meats, and soft drinks.

Hyper States and Hypo States

Both excesses and inadequacies of phosphorus can lead to medical complications, including impaired bone health.

TABLE 9.4	National Academy of Medicine Recommendations for Phosphorus			
Life Stage[a]	EAR (mg/day)	RDA (mg/day)	AI (mg/day)	UL (mg/day)
Birth–6 months	—	—	100	ND
7–12 months	—	—	275	ND
1–3 years	380	460	—	3000
4–8 years	405	500	—	3000
9–18 years	1055	1250	—	4000
19–70 years	580	700	—	4000
>70 years	580	700	—	3000
Pregnancy				
≤18 years	1055	1250	—	3500
19–50 years	580	700	—	3500
Lactation				
≤18 years	1055	1250	—	4000
19–50 years	580	700	—	4000

[a]All groups except pregnancy and lactation include males and females.
AI, Adequate intake; *EAR*, estimated average requirement; *RDA*, recommended dietary allowance; *UL*, tolerable upper intake level.
Data from Institute of Medicine (IOM), Food and Nutrition Board. *Dietary Reference Intakes For Calcium, Phosphorus, Magnesium, Vitamin D, and Fluoride.* National Academy Press; 1997.

Phosphorus Excess

Excessive phosphorus seldom has effects in healthy individuals. Inconsistent research suggests that high intake may be associated with negative effects on cardiovascular, kidney, and bone heath.[39,40]

In conditions like hypoparathyroidism or renal insufficiency, hyperphosphatemia (serum level > 2.6 mg/dL) may occur. Excessive amounts of phosphorus bind with calcium, resulting in tetany and convulsions.

Phosphorus Deficiency

Hypophosphatemia (phosphorus deficiency) is rare in the United States and may be associated with medical conditions such as hyperparathyroidism.[37] The principal clinical symptom of hypophosphatemia is muscle weakness, anemia, skeletal effects (e.g., bone pain), risk of infection, confusion, and paresthesias.[37]

Those at risk for inadequate phosphorus status include preterm infants, genetic disorders, and severe malnutrition.[37] During tooth development, a phosphorus deficiency can result in incomplete calcification of teeth, failure of dentin formation, and increased caries risk.[41]

NUTRITIONAL DIRECTIONS

- Encourage dietary patterns with adequate intake of meat, fish, dairy, vegetables, fruits, and whole grains which are good sources of phosphorus.[43]
- Evidence for intake of phosphorus alone as a factor in lower blood pressure is lacking, however, dietary patterns consistent with the Dietary Guidelines rich in potassium, magnesium, calcium, and phosphorus may be a component of managing hypertension.[44]

Magnesium

Physiologic Roles

Bones contain almost 50% to 60% of the body's magnesium.[45] It is the third most prevalent mineral in teeth, with dentin containing about two times more than enamel. Magnesium has an important function in maintaining calcium homeostasis and preventing skeletal abnormalities. Magnesium is involved in more than 300 enzymatic reactions, including protein synthesis, muscle and nerve function, DNA/RNA synthesis, blood pressure regulations, insulin activity, and glucose use.[45] Its role in enzymes is fundamental to energy (adenosine triphosphate) production. Magnesium balance is largely controlled by the kidney through urinary excretion.

Requirements

The RDA for magnesium ranges from 240 mg/day for 9 to 13-year-old children to 320 mg/day for females and 420 mg/day

DENTAL CONSIDERATIONS

- A phosphorus deficiency (hypophosphatemia) is more likely to develop in individuals with malnutrition due to alcohol and substance use disorder; malabsorption conditions (e.g., celiac disease); older adults with chronic inadequate dietary intake; kidney failure/hemodialysis; and anorexia nervosa.[42] Referral to the health care provider or RDN may be needed.
- Low phosphate intake during tooth development may lead to an increased caries risk.

TABLE 9.5 **National Academy of Medicine Recommendations for Magnesium**

Life Stage[a]	EAR (mg/day) Male	EAR (mg/day) Female	RDA (mg/day) Male	RDA (mg/day) Female	AI (mg/day) Male	AI (mg/day) Female	UL (mg/day)
Birth–6 months	—	—	—	—	30	30	ND
7–12 months	—	—	—	—	75	75	ND
1–3 years	65	65	80	80			65
4–8 years	110	110	130	130			110
9–13 years	200	200	240	240			350
14–18 years	340	300	410	360			350
19–30 years	330	255	400	310			350
>30 years	350	265	420	320			350
Pregnancy							
≤18 years		335		400			350
19–30 years		290		350			350
31–50 years		300		360			350
Lactation							
≤18 years		300		360			350
19–30 years		255		310			350
31–50 years		265		320			350

[a]All groups except pregnancy and lactation include males and females.

AI, Adequate intake; *EAR*, estimated average requirement; *RDA*, recommended dietary allowance; *UL*, tolerable upper intake level.

Data from Institute of Medicine (IOM), Food and Nutrition Board. *Dietary Reference Intakes For Calcium, Phosphorus, Magnesium, Vitamin D, and Fluoride*. National Academy Press; 1997.

for males (Table 9.5).[38] The most current NHANES data suggests that intake may be below the RDA with an average intake 270 mg/day for females to 339 mg/day for males aged 19 years and over.[6]

Although it is impossible to get too much magnesium from food alone, excessive amounts can be obtained from supplements. The UL is provided only for supplements, laxatives, and *not* food sources of magnesium.[45]

Sources

Magnesium is widely distributed in plants and animal foods; however, whole-grain products, nuts, beans, and fortified foods are some of the best sources of magnesium (Table 9.6).[45] Magnesium (Mg) is a part of the chlorophyll molecule (Fig. 9.3); therefore, green leafy vegetables are also good sources of magnesium. In addition, bananas and chocolate are the sources of magnesium. Although whole grains are good sources of magnesium, enrichment of refined grain products does not replace magnesium lost during processing. Varying amounts of magnesium can be found in tap, mineral, and bottled waters. Non-food sources of magnesium include laxatives and antacids.

Hyper States and Hypo States

Magnesium Excess

There is no evidence of harmful effects related to overconsumption of magnesium from food sources. Because kidneys regulate plasma magnesium levels, toxicity has been associated with kidney failure or impaired renal function. A high dose of magnesium acts like a laxative (e.g., milk of magnesia) and may cause diarrhea, nausea, and/or abdominal cramping.[45]

Magnesium Deficiency

In certain diseases or under stressful conditions, deficiencies may occur. Magnesium in bone is not available to replace serum magnesium deficits. A deficiency may result from numerous disease states, including gastrointestinal conditions (e.g., celiac disease, Crohn's disease) with diarrhea, Type 2 diabetes mellitus, older adults, and alcohol use disorder.[45] Magnesium deficiency symptoms include fatigue, anorexia, nausea, neuromuscular dysfunction, personality changes, disorientation, muscle spasms, seizures, tremors, and cardiac arrhythmias.[45]

Dietary deficiencies of magnesium may affect teeth and their supporting structures. Magnesium is required for the enzymes that activate vitamin D.[46] Changes in ameloblasts and odontoblasts

TABLE 9.6 Magnesium Content of Selected Foods

Food	Portion	Magnesium (mg)
Spinach, cooked	½ cup	98
Sesame seeds	1 oz	97
Hummus	½ cup	85
Potato, baked	1 medium	71
Cashew nuts	1 oz	71
Navy beans, cooked	½ cup	68
Peanut butter	2 tbsp	54
Soy milk, vanilla	1 cup	51
Pinto beans, cooked	½ cup	50
Edamame, cooked	½ cup	50
Black beans, canned	½ cup	46
Dark chocolate	1 oz	43
Brown rice, cooked	½ cup	38
Sunflower seeds	1 oz	36
Banana	1 medium	35
Bread, multigrain	1 slice	28
Broccoli, cooked	½ cup	17
Mini-wheats cereal	1 cup	16

Data from United States Department of Agriculture (USDA), Agricultural Research Service. *What's in the Foods Your Eat Search Tool.* 2019–2020. https://www.ars.usda.gov/northeast-area/beltsville-md-bhnrc/beltsville-human-nutrition-research-center/food-surveys-research-group/docs/whats-in-the-foods-you-eat-search-tool/.

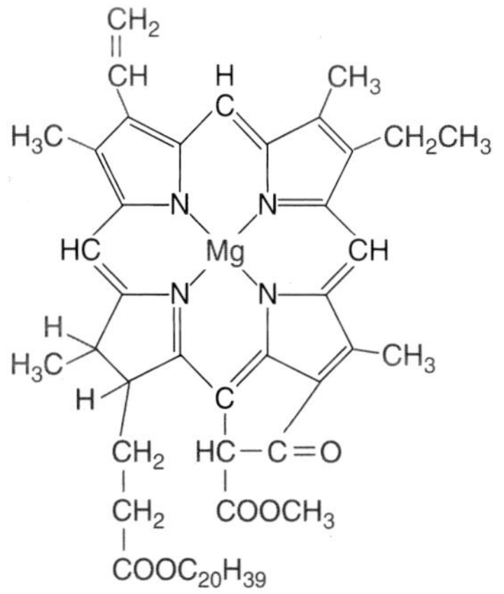

• **Fig. 9.3** Structure of chlorophyll. All chlorophyll molecules are essentially alike; they differ only in details of the side chains. Magnesium is basic to all chlorophyll molecules.

result in hypoplasia of the enamel and dentin during development. Magnesium also seems to have a role in the remineralization process to prevent progression to caries.[46] Serum magnesium levels are also associated with less attachment loss as well as less tooth loss.[46]

DENTAL HYGIENE CONSIDERATIONS

- Decreased food intake, impaired magnesium absorption, or the use of certain diuretics may contribute to hypomagnesemia, or a below-normal blood serum concentration of magnesium. Encourage the patient to follow a healthy eating pattern as defined by the *Dietary Guidelines*.
- Supplements containing magnesium can decrease the absorption of oral bisphosphonates[47] and interfere with the effectiveness of certain antibiotics. Encourage the patient to seek assistance from a pharmacist.

NUTRITIONAL DIRECTIONS

- Diets high in unrefined grains and vegetables provide more magnesium than diets that include a lot of refined foods, meats, and milk products.
- Magnesium plays a major role in blood pressure regulation; both foods rich in magnesium and supplements have been effective at lowering blood pressure.[44,48]

Fluoride

Physiologic Roles

In a strict nutritional sense, fluoride is not a nutrient essential for health. Fluoride present in low concentrations in soft tissues does not have any known metabolic function. However, because of its benefits to dental and bone health, fluoride is considered a desirable element for humans. Varying amounts of fluoride in food and/or beverages remaining in the oral cavity after ingestion will be absorbed through the mucosa or become part of plaque biofilm and saliva.

Fluoride is also advantageous to dental health because of its systemic effects before tooth eruption and topical effects after tooth eruption (Fig. 9.4). The caries-preventing properties of systemic and topical fluoride are cumulative.

Fluoride ions can replace hydroxyl ions in the hydroxyapatite crystal lattice. This fluoridated hydroxyapatite, or **fluorapatite**, is less soluble and makes the tooth more resistant to acid demineralization. Additionally, it enhances remineralization when the tooth is exposed to the caries process (Fig. 9.5). Calcium and phosphate are present in saliva and plaque at higher concentrations than fluoride. When small pits develop in the enamel, fluoride is believed to promote deposition of calcium phosphate to remineralize the enamel surface.

Primary teeth benefit from the presence of fluoride during tooth development beginning at 6 months of age. Fluoride is present in the inner part of the enamel and dentin at lower concentrations; this occurs mainly during the amelogenesis/odontogenesis stage. Enhanced concentration in the surface enamel occurs during the maturation stage of tooth development. Fluoride can be readily incorporated into the apatite crystal from topically available fluoride during the maturation stage, but this reversible process is superficial rather than fluoride being distributed throughout the enamel thickness.

The presence of fluoride in saliva interferes with the demineralization process, resulting in a less cariogenic environment. Topically available fluoride reduces dental caries by inhibiting demineralization, promoting remineralization, and interfering with formation and function of acidogenic bacteria.[49] Higher concentrations of fluoride inhibit *Streptococcus mutans, Streptococcus*

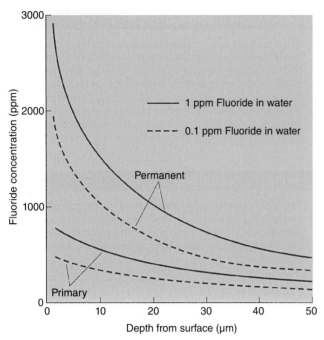

• **Fig. 9.4** Concentration gradients of fluoride in outer enamel from permanent and deciduous teeth, from areas with 1 part per million (ppm) and 0.1 ppm of fluoride in the drinking water. (From Gron P. Inorganic chemical and structural aspects of oral mineralized tissues. In: Shaw JH, ed. *Textbook of Oral Biology.* Saunders; 1978:484–507.)

sobrinus, and *Lactobacillus* in plaque biofilm, and accelerate remineralization during early stages of enamel caries development.

Maximum protection by fluoride against caries occurs during the first 6 to 10 years of life, but adults and children continue to benefit from the presence of fluoride. Systemic fluoride uptake by calcified tissues is high from infancy until age 16 years, when mineralization of unerupted permanent teeth occurs. Compared with healthy enamel, demineralized enamel retains more fluoride.

Fluoride stimulates osteoblast growth and increases new mineral deposition in cancellous bone, improves bone integrity, and decreases bone resorption and bone solubility. Concurrent adequate intake of calcium, vitamin D, and fluoride is essential.

Requirements

Because of the risk of toxicity, adequate intake of fluoride has been established at 3 mg/day for all females and 4 mg/day for males (Table 9.7). Average intake in the United States in Canadian and US studies found that the intake in adults was 0.3 to 1.0 mg/day in areas with nonfluoridated water and 1.4 to 3.4 mg/day in areas of water with fluoridation.[38] The UL for healthy individuals age 9 years and older is 10 mg/day, including food, beverages, supplements, rinses, and toothpaste.

Absorption and Excretion

Most fluoride is absorbed in the stomach, with small amounts also absorbed in the intestine. The rate and degree of absorption

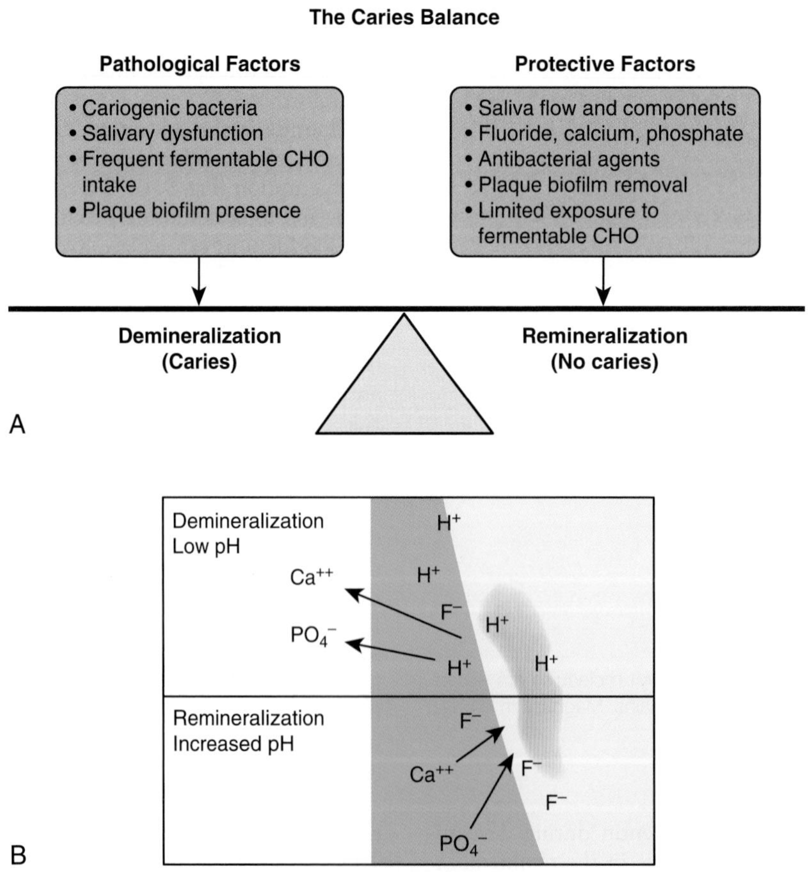

The Caries Balance

Pathological Factors	Protective Factors
• Cariogenic bacteria • Salivary dysfunction • Frequent fermentable CHO intake • Plaque biofilm presence	• Saliva flow and components • Fluoride, calcium, phosphate • Antibacterial agents • Plaque biofilm removal • Limited exposure to fermentable CHO

Demineralization (Caries)   **Remineralization (No caries)**

A

Demineralization Low pH H^+
Ca^{++} H^+
    F^- H^+
PO_4^-
    H^+ H^+

Remineralization Increased pH F^-
Ca^{++} F^-
    F^-
PO_4^-

B

• **Fig. 9.5** (A) The action of fluoride in the demineralization-remineralization process. (B) Fluoride ions replace hydroxyl ions. Fluoride promotes the deposition of calcium and phosphate to remineralize the enamel.

TABLE 9.7	National Academy of Medicine Recommendations for Fluoride		
	AI (mg/day)		
Life Stage Group	**Male**	**Female**	**UL**
Birth–6 months	0.01	0.01	0.7
7–12 months	0.5	0.5	0.9
1–3 years	0.7	0.7	1.3
4–8 years	1	1	2.2
9–13 years	2	2	10
14–18 years	3	3	10
>18 years	4	3	10
Pregnancy and Lactation			
≤50 years	—	3	10

AI, Adequate intake; *UL*, tolerable upper intake level.
Data from Institute of Medicine (IOM), Food and Nutrition Board. *Dietary Reference Intakes for Calcium, Phosphorus, Magnesium, Vitamin D, and Fluoride.* National Academy Press; 1997.

depend on the solubility of the fluoride and amount ingested at a particular time. Absorption of orally ingested fluoride is estimated to be 50% to 80%, depending on physiologic need.[50] Incorporation of fluoride into bones and enamel is proportional to total intake and need. Children retain a larger percentage of fluoride in developing bones and teeth, whereas adults retain less in calcified structures. Protein-bound fluoride in foods is not as well absorbed.

Fluoride is primarily filtered by the kidneys and excreted in the urine.[51] Aluminum (aluminum-containing antacids), soy (soy-based foods), and calcium bind with fluoride and decrease absorption.

Sources

Water

The Centers for Disease Control and Prevention (CDC) recognizes water fluoridation as one of the 10 most important public health measures of the 20th century.[52] Fluoride is available through community water supplies, food, beverages, dentifrices, and other fluoridated dental products. Fluoridation of community water contributes to fluoride intake and is a practical, cost-effective means of achieving significant decrease in the prevalence of dental caries. Approximately 80% of fluoride consumed is provided from tap and bottled water and water-based beverages, especially teas. To ensure that everyone receives adequate amounts of fluoride, the US Department of Health and Human Services, Public Health Service recommendation for community water fluoridation is 0.7 parts per million (ppm) of fluoride (equivalent to 1 mg/L).[53] Scientists do not all agree on the maximum acceptable fluoride level and the Environmental Protection Agency (EPA) continues to monitor emerging evidence to determine appropriate guidelines for water fluoridation.[54] Home water purification and filtration systems can reduce the fluoride content of tap water.

Approximately 72.8% of the US population has access to optimally fluoridated drinking water; the goal, as stated by *Healthy People 2030*, targets 77.1% of the population.[55] Water fluoridation is particularly beneficial for children and teens in economically disadvantaged communities who have less access to oral health care and alternative fluoride resources. Children who do not regularly receive dental care or have no dental insurance are at high risk for dental caries.

Many households and businesses are using bottled water, water treatment systems, or water filters for various reasons, including taste preference and convenience. Bottled water may be chosen as a healthy alternative to soft drinks and alcoholic beverages. The US Food and Drug Administration requires that naturally occurring fluoride not exceeding 1.4 to 2.4 mg/L depending on the average temperature at the location where the water is sold.[56] If fluoride is added to the water, it may not exceed 0.7 mg/L.[56] Fluoride amounts in bottled water may or may not be listed on the label. Bottled water containing 0.6 to 1.0 mg/L of fluoride may state on the packaging, "Drinking fluoridated water may reduce the risk of [dental caries or tooth decay]."[57]

In some areas of the United States, the water supply naturally contains much higher levels of fluoride than the recommended amounts. Naturally occurring fluoride is found in soils and bedrock, which will dissolve into ground water. The EPA allows a maximum level of 4 mg/L.[54] This level could possibly cause adverse health effects.

Food

Food is not a major source of fluoride for adults. All foods contain some fluoride, but the amounts provided in vegetables, meats, cereals, and fruits are insignificant (less than 0.5 mg/100 g; Table 9.8).[38] Marine fish may contain 0.1 to 0.17 mg of fluoride per 100 g.[38] Brewed tea provides approximately 1 to 6 ppm of fluoride per cup, depending on the amount of tea, brewing time, and amount of fluoride in the water, but herbal tea has negligible fluoride levels.[38] Carbonated beverages can be a significant source of fluoride if the water used in the bottling process is fluoridated. Foods prepared in fluoridated water will also be a source.

Because of varied levels of fluoride in the water supply, the amount of fluoride in infant formulas was reduced in 1979 with ranges of 0.1 to 0.3 mg of fluoride per liter.[38] Components in soy bind fluoride; soy-based formulas usually contain some fluoride.

Topical

Topical applications of fluoride include gels, foams, varnishes, dentifrices, prophylactic paste (polishing paste), and mouth rinses. These high-concentration fluoride sources prevent demineralization when oral pH decreases. When used in combination with other fluoride sources, a decline in prevalence or severity of dental caries occurs.

Hyper States and Hypo States

Fluoride Excess

Mottling of tooth enamel results from overexposure (approximately three to four times the amount necessary to prevent caries) during tooth formation. Ameloblasts are extremely sensitive to excessive fluoride ingestion. Dental fluorosis (hypomineralization of enamel) is directly related to fluoride exposure during

TABLE 9.8	Fluoride Content of Selected Foods	

Food	Fluoride (µg/100 g)
Black tea, brewed	322
Instant tea	335
Raisins	234
Crab, canned	210
Wine, white	202
Shrimp, canned	201
Coffee, brewed	91
Grape juice	72
Oysters, cooked	63
Cola	57
Potatoes, boiled	50
Carrots, cooked	47
Rice, white, cooked	41
Cheese, American, processed	35
Tomato sauce	35
Cottage cheese	32

Data from United States Department of Agriculture (USDA), Agricultural Research Service. *USDA National Fluoride Database of Selected Beverages and Foods, Release 2.* 2005. https://www.ars.usda.gov/ARSUserFiles/80400535/Data/Fluoride/F02.pdf.

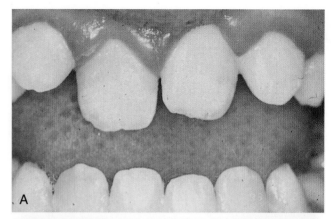
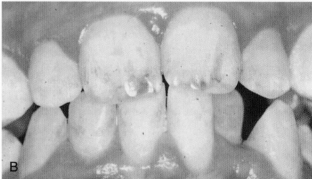
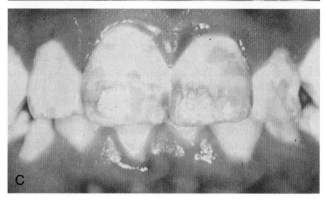

• **Fig. 9.6** (A) Mild fluorosis: white opaque areas in the enamel over less than 50% of the tooth. (B) Moderate fluorosis: all enamel surfaces of the teeth are affected; a brown stain is frequently present. (C) Severe fluorosis: hypoplasia affecting the general shape of the tooth; widespread brown stains, corroded-like appearance of teeth. (Courtesy Alton McWhorter, DDS, MS, Associate Professor, Department of Pediatric Dentistry, Texas A&M University College of Dentistry, Dallas, TX.)

tooth development and cannot occur after tooth development is complete. Fluorosed enamel contains a total protein content similar to normal enamel, but it contains a relatively high proportion of immature matrix proteins. Mild to moderate enamel fluorosis on early forming enamel surfaces was strongly associated with the use of infant formula before 1979. Frequent brushing with fluoridated toothpaste was encouraged, and fluoride supplements were used.

When drinking water contains more than recommended levels of fluoride, dental fluorosis may occur and varies from very mild cases characterized by whitish opaque flecks to white or brown staining (Fig. 9.6A), to severe dental fluorosis with secondary, extrinsic, brownish discoloration and varying degrees of enamel pitting (Fig. 9.6C). Mild to moderate fluorosis is primarily cosmetic.

Excessive fluoride intake for adults can result in adverse effects on bone health with negative impact on bone quality due to abnormal mineralization and altered collagen.[50,58] Some research suggests neurotoxicity of fluoride during early development that may affect cognitive function, however, the evidence is weak at this time so more research is needed.[50,59,60]

Fluoride Inadequacy

Lack of exposure to adequate fluoride levels may result in increased risk for dental caries.[61,62] The protective effect against caries is greatest during tooth formation. The American Dental Association and the American Academy of Pediatrics recommend exposure of the teeth to fluoride until calcification of all teeth is completed (about age 16 years).[63,64] Dosages for fluoride supplements for children are presented in Table 14.2. Various conditions warrant topical fluoride treatment in adults, such as hypersensitivity, exposed root surfaces, white spot lesions, xerostomia, use of smokeless tobacco, and radiation therapy.

Continued use of fluoridated water by adults is beneficial in maintaining the integrity of teeth. Posteruption, systemic fluoride is present in saliva and plaque, creating an environment that inhibits demineralization and enhances remineralization of tooth surfaces.

Safety

The addition of fluoride in the US water supply continues to be opposed by a small but vocal and aggressive minority of people. Antifluoridation groups have attempted to link water fluoridation to cancer, acquired immunodeficiency syndrome, Alzheimer's disease, mental illness, lowered IQ in children, CVD, fertility, and Down syndrome, but strong scientific evidence to support these allegations has not been provided. Regardless, a handful of communities in the United States have banned the addition of fluoride to their water.

Fluoridation is one of the most thoroughly researched health issues in recent history. No negative trends have been identified that could be attributed to the introduction or duration of fluoride in drinking water. In contrast, almost all professional health organizations have concluded the results of numerous long-term community trials of adding fluoride to public water supplies at optimal levels verify the effectiveness, safety, and cost-benefit of this public health measure in reducing the prevalence of dental caries. Water fluoridation is the most cost-effective method of preventing dental caries, providing the greatest benefit to individuals who can least afford preventive and restorative dentistry.

DENTAL HYGIENE CONSIDERATIONS

- Educate patients about the purpose and value of fluoridation for oral health.
- Go to the CDC website, My Water's Fluoride (https://nccd.cdc.gov/DOH_MWF/), or contact the state or local health department to determine the fluoride content of the water system in the area. Encourage patients to send samples of well water or home water treatment systems to their state health department to determine fluoride content.
- If the water source is a well, the local or state health department should be contacted about water sample testing.[64]
- Request the content of fluoride in bottled water from the manufacturer.
- Long-term use of infant formulas, particularly powdered formulas reconstituted with fluoridated water, can be a factor for mild fluorosis.
- Carefully estimate the total amount of fluoride the patient consumes daily in foods and water. Because fluoride is available from multiple sources, the possibility of toxic levels should be considered when recommending fluoride supplements or providing treatment, especially for children. Consider the number of carbonated beverages consumed and consumption of all beverages using fluoridated water. The fluoride content is not listed on the label, making it difficult to approximate the amount of fluoride being consumed.
- Educate patients about the caries process. Encourage patients to practice optimal oral hygiene. Plaque biofilm is the primary factor in caries formation. Appropriate oral hygiene when using topical fluorides at home also increases their effectiveness.
- Recommend fluoride supplements only when the fluoride level of the home water supply is known to be deficient.

- Fluoride supplements can be in liquid or tablet form. Tablet forms that dissolve slowly in the mouth also provide a topical effect.[64]
- An adequate fluoride intake is beneficial during development of teeth. Encourage fluoride-fortified foods, water, or supplements for breastfed infants and fluoridated water for children and adolescents, if applicable.
- Growth of cariogenic bacteria is reduced by the presence of fluoride. Suggest using dentifrices or mouthwashes with fluoride for oral self-care for individuals older than 3 years.
- Caution parents of children between 2 and 6 years of age to (1) use only small (pea size) amounts of fluoridated dentifrices, (2) minimize swallowing toothpaste, (3) avoid using fluoride mouth rinse, (4) keep fluoride products out of the reach of children, and (5) use a nonfluoridated toothpaste for children age 2 years and younger. Fluoride levels in children's toothpastes often equal the levels in adult fluoridated toothpastes.
- If fluoride and calcium supplements are given concurrently, absorption of both is decreased.
- For individuals living in an area where the fluoride content of water is naturally 2 to 4 ppm, recommend drinking bottled water without fluoride or using commercially available filters that can reduce the fluoride to safer levels.
- There is no risk of fluorosis after enamel has developed.
- Dental professionals need to be alert and active in their communities and prepared to present factual information to governing bodies should antifluoride advocates attempt to block addition or removal of fluoride from the community water supply.

NUTRITIONAL DIRECTIONS

- A 2.2-mg amount of sodium fluoride contains 1 mg of fluoride ion.
- To provide maximum benefits, systemic fluoride is important before tooth eruption, when development of unerupted permanent teeth is occurring.
- Fluoride supplementation is recommended for patients 6 months to 16 years old with less than 0.6 ppm of fluoride in their water source (home, childcare settings, school, or bottled) if there is no other significant source of fluoride.
- Fluoride supplements are not recommended during pregnancy.
- If a child receives suboptimal levels of fluoride, an increase in dental caries may occur. Exposure to multiple sources of fluoride increases the risk of excess fluoride, causing fluorosis.

- Fluoride supplements are inappropriate for individuals living in areas where the fluoride content of drinking water is optimal.
- Topical availability of fluoride at low concentrations on a daily basis after tooth eruption is important to deter development of dental caries.
- If caries risk is high, professionally applied and self-applied home fluoride therapies may be an integral component of dental hygiene care.
- When bottled water is being used, obtain the fluoride content from the distributor or the label.
- Aluminum antacids decrease fluoride absorption.
- High levels of calcium can interfere with the absorption of fluoride.

◆ HEALTH APPLICATION 9

Osteoporosis

Osteoporosis is a serious, common, and costly disease, increasing in prevalence in males and females. This condition is partly genetically determined. Globally the prevalence of osteoporosis is 19.7% and prevalence of low bone mass (osteopenia) is 40.4%.[23] The global prevalence of osteoporosis in females is more than twice that of men (24.8 vs. 10.6%).[23]

Osteoporotic bone is characterized as porous with reduced mineralization and density. Fig. 9.7 shows the enlargement of cancellous bone combined with a reduced and weakened trabecular bone. Osteoporotic bones are fragile and fracture easily.

Osteoporosis is more likely to develop in individuals with at least some of the risk factors listed in Box 9.3. The incidence of osteoporosis is greatest in White non-Hispanic, Asian non-Hispanic, and Hispanic females.[65] A female's risk of osteoporosis starts around menopause (age 50 years or older). Females can lose bone mass at an annual rate of approximately 2% during the 2 to 3 years before and 3 to 4 years after menopause for a total loss of bone density of 10% to 12%.[66,67] Those with low body weight may have higher rates of bone loss.[66] Bone loss in males increases after age 65 years. Risk of death during the year after a hip fracture is 8% to 36% and males are at twice the risk of dying when compared to females.[68] For individuals at risk for osteoporosis, an objective of treatment is to slow or stop disease progression before irreversible structural changes have occurred. The Bone Health and Osteoporosis Foundation recommends steps for preventing osteoporosis[69]:

1. Get the daily recommended amounts of calcium and vitamin D. Dietary modifications for patients at risk of developing osteoporosis should include at least two portions of dairy products daily (to provide 75% of RDAs). Serum vitamin D levels should be monitored and those below recommended levels may be prescribed vitamin D supplements.
2. Engage in regular weight-bearing and muscle-strengthening exercises.
3. Avoid tobacco use and excessive alcohol intake.
4. Talk to a health care provider about bone health and supplement use.
5. Take steps to prevent falling, such as regular vision and hearing exams, investigate neurologic problems, and improve safety concerns at home.
6. Have a BMD test and take medication when appropriate. Specialized tests to assess BMD should be conducted on females aged 65 years or older, males 70 years and older, those older than 50 years with risk factors for osteoporosis, and all individuals who have got their bone broken after age 50 years.

The bone health of the oral cavity (alveolar bone, maxilla, and mandible) can be affected by osteoporosis.[70] When identifying periodontal issues, such as tooth mobility, resorption of alveolar bone, temporomandibular disorders, and clinical attachment loss, a relationship to osteoporosis should

be considered.[70] Advise patients with osteoporosis about the importance of regular oral hygiene care to reduce the risk of these dental issues and also explain development of periodontitis may be more rapid and severe. Postmenopausal females treated with estrogen for osteoporosis have been found to have significantly greater attachment gains after periodontal treatment.[71]

Glucocorticoids often used in autoimmune conditions (e.g., rheumatoid arthritis), post organ transplant, asthma, chronic obstructive pulmonary disease, and inflammatory bowel disease may lead to steroid-induced osteoporosis.[72] Glucocorticoids reduce calcium absorption and increase breakdown of bone while decreasing new bone formation.[72] Patients taking these medications should be encouraged to consume adequate amounts of calcium and vitamin D, engage in weight-bearing activity, stop tobacco use, and limit alcohol intake.

To date, osteoporosis cannot be cured, but medications can help prevent or deter bone loss. Medications used to slow bone loss include estrogen-related therapy, bisphosphonates (alendronate, ibandronate, risedronate, and zoledronic acid), calcitonin, RANK-ligand inhibitor (denosumab), sclerostin inhibitor (romosozumab) and parathyroid analogs.[69] A significant dental consideration for the use of bisphosphonates, particularly following intravenous bisphosphonate or denosumab treatment for patients with cancer, is the risk for the development of osteonecrosis of the jaw.[73,74] Commonly used medications for other conditions have a documented effect on bone mineralization. Thiazide diuretics, principally used for blood pressure control, positively affect bone mineralization and decrease the risk for fracture.[75]

An adequate calcium intake is important at all stages of life, with a daily minimum intake of 1000 mg for all healthy adults and 1200 mg for females older than 51 years. Adequate exposure to sunlight and vitamin D intake are also important to maintain bone health. The action of these two nutrients is complementary; calcium supports bone formation and repair, and vitamin D helps with calcium absorption. Other nutritional considerations include adequate intake of magnesium,[76] B vitamins, and vitamin K, which may reduce fracture risk by improving BMD. Several studies have reported a positive association between the use of phytochemicals (plant chemicals) and preventing bone loss.[77,78] Phytochemicals are found in soy products (isoflavones), green tea (flavanols), and berries (anthocyanins) and have a protective effect on prevention of bone loss.[78] In addition, dietary patterns high in fiber may be protective against bone loss.[79] The overall take away message for the dental hygienist is to support the patient in following a dietary pattern consistent with those recommended by the *Dietary Guidelines*. A health care provider or RDN can further tailor the osteoporosis regimen to meet the patient's needs.

• BOX 9.3 Risk Factors for Osteoporosis

Certain people are more likely to develop osteoporosis than others. Factors that increase the likelihood of developing osteoporosis and broken bones are called "risk factors." These risk factors include non-modifiable and modifiable risk factors along with secondary cause for osteoporosis as follows:

- Non-modifiable risk factors:
  - Being female (two times higher risk)
  - Older age
  - Family history of osteoporosis or broken bones
  - History of broken bones
  - Certain races/ethnicities such as White or Asian
  - Being small and thin (low BMI <18.5)
  - Socioeconomic status and lower level of education (less than a college degree)
- Modifiable risk factors:
  - Low sex hormones (estrogen in females; testosterone in males)
  - Inadequate calcium, vitamin D, and vitamin K intake
  - Excessive intake of protein, sodium, and caffeine
  - Inactive lifestyle

- Smoking
- Excessive alcohol (three or more drinks/day)
- Secondary causes of osteoporosis
  - Chronic use of certain medications such as glucocorticosteroids, anticonvulsants
  - Disordered eating (e.g., anorexia nervosa, bulimia, athletic amenorrhea)
  - Inflammatory diseases (e.g., rheumatoid arthritis)
  - Gastrointestinal conditions leading to malabsorption (e.g., ulcerative colitis, cystic fibrosis)
  - Hyperparathyroidism
  - Chronic liver disease
  - Diabetes mellitus

Data from Pouresmaeili F, Kamalidehghan B, Kamarehei M, Goh YM. A comprehensive overview on osteoporosis and its risk factors. *Ther Clin Risk Manage.* 2018;14:2029–2049; Xiao PL, Cui AY, Hsu CJ, Peng R, Jiang N, Xu XH, Ma YG, Liu D, Lu HD. Global, regional prevalence, and risk factors of osteoporosis according to the World Health Organization diagnostic criteria: a systematic review and *meta*-analysis. *Osteoporos Int.* 2022;33(10):2137–2153.

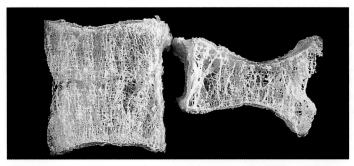

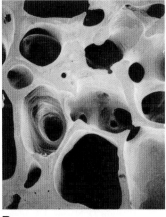

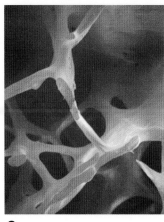

A

B   C

• **Fig. 9.7** Osteoporosis. (A) Compare the normal vertebral body (*left*) with the osteoporotic specimen (*right*). Note that the osteoporotic vertebral body has been shortened by compression fractures. (B) Microscopic normal bone. (C) Microscopic osteoporotic bone. Note the loss of trabecular bone and appearance of enlarged pores caused by osteoporosis. (Modified from Patton KT, Thibodeau GA. *Anatomy and Physiology*. 9th ed. Elsevier; 2016.)

◆ CASE APPLICATION FOR THE DENTAL HYGIENIST

During Annie's routine dental examination, her mother asked the dental hygienist whether she should start (Annie, age 5 years) on a fluoride supplement. Annie's examination revealed a caries-free mouth. She reports brushing her teeth twice a day.

Nutritional Assessment
- Food consumption pattern
- Frequency of carbohydrate intake
- Fluoride content of water consumed; average amount of water/water-based beverages consumed
- Type and amount of toothpaste and mouth rinses used

Nutritional Diagnosis
Health-seeking behaviors related to inadequate knowledge about fluoride supplementation.

Nutritional Goals
The patient will practice good oral self-care with supevision from mother and receive adequate fluoride to prevent dental caries.

Nutritional Implementation
Intervention: Explain the benefits of fluoride.
Rationale: Fluoride is advantageous to dental health because of its systemic effect before tooth eruption and its topical effects after tooth eruption. The caries-preventive properties of systemic and topical fluoride are additive.

Intervention: Discuss the toxic effects of fluoride.
Rationale: Dental fluorosis is directly related to the level of fluoride exposure during tooth development. It can also have adverse effects on bone structure.
Intervention: Assess current fluoride consumption from (1) food, (2) water supply, (3) carbonated beverages, and (4) fluoridated dentifrices and mouth rinses.
Rationale: (1) All foods contain some fluoride, but the amounts provided in vegetables, meats, cereals, and fruits are insignificant unless large amounts of seafood, tea, or deboned poultry are consumed; (2) water is usually the main source of fluoride, but some municipal water supplies and bottled waters may contain negligible amounts of fluoride; and (3) fluoride is added to 90% of all dentifrices in the United States. Because younger children swallow most of the toothpaste used, they should be provided with a dentifrice without fluoride.
Intervention: Show Annie and her mother how much toothpaste to use, and discuss the importance of not swallowing it.
Rationale: Because fluoride in toothpaste can be readily absorbed, toothpaste should not be swallowed to prevent the harmful effects of systemically available fluoride.
Intervention: Encourage the patient and her mother to consume a well-balanced diet with limited amounts of fermentable carbohydrates at snack time.
Rationale: Not only is fluoride important, but also other nutrients are essential for dental health. Snacks, especially carbohydrate-containing foods, increase the risk for dental caries.

◆ CASE APPLICATION FOR THE DENTAL HYGIENIST–CONT'D

Intervention: Suggest fluoride supplements only if fluoride intake seems to be low.

Rationale: In many cases, total fluoride exposure seems to be higher than necessary to prevent tooth decay. No more than the amount of fluoride necessary to provide the desired effect should be used.

Intervention: Recommend parental supervision and assistance for Annie's toothbrushing and flossing.

Rationale: Monitoring the child's brushing technique and assisting with flossing will ensure that effective biofilm removal occurs once a day.

Evaluation

If the patient and her mother can demonstrate the toothbrushing procedure, the patient says that she will brush her teeth after every meal and will try to eat the foods that her mother provides, and dental caries continues to be minimal, dental hygiene care was effective.

◆ Student Readiness

1. A patient claims that she dislikes milk. How would you advise her to obtain the calcium she needs?
2. What are the main physiologic roles of calcium, phosphorus, magnesium, and fluoride?
3. How do minerals differ from vitamins?
4. How would you respond to a patient who states that milk is only for babies?
5. Discuss three dietary factors that affect calcium absorption.
6. Determine the level of fluoride in your community's drinking water.
7. If an adult patient (weight about 75 kg) is drinking only bottled water that does not contain fluoride, and the patient dislikes fish and tea, how much topical fluoride would be necessary to furnish the recommendation for fluoride?
8. List five types of over-the-counter calcium supplements available. Evaluate these items for primary sources of calcium and elemental calcium per unit consumed. Find how many tablets or units would have to be consumed daily to receive 1000 mg of elemental calcium.
9. Discuss how to communicate with a patient who is opposed to community water fluoridation.
10. Why would you advise patients to obtain their mineral requirement from food sources rather than mineral supplements (unless ordered by the health care provider)?

◆ CASE STUDY

Mrs. J. M., a 69-year-old female with osteoporosis, fell and fractured her hip 6 months ago. She reports taking calcium supplements occasionally, when she can afford them. She does not like milk and has been unable to walk much since her fall.

1. What additional questions would you ask to clarify the situation?
2. What nutritional advice could you give her about her osteoporosis?
3. What is her RDA for calcium?
4. What foods could you suggest she consume to increase calcium intake?
5. When should she take her calcium supplement to maximize its absorption?
6. What oral changes might you expect to find in your assessment?
7. What effect would increased vitamin D intake have on her condition?

References

1. Haftek M, Abdayem R, Guyonnet-Debersac P. Skin minerals: key roles of inorganic elements in skin physiological functions. *Int J Mol Sci.* 2022;23(11):6267.
2. Office of Dietary Supplements. *Calcium: Fact Sheet for Health Professionals.* 2022. https://ods.od.nih.gov/factsheets/Calcium-HealthProfessional/
3. Farooq I, Bugshan A. The role of salivary contents and modern technologies in the remineralization of dental enamel: a narrative review. *F1000Res.* 2020;9:171.
4. Institute of Medicine. *Dietary Reference Intakes for Calcium and Vitamin D.* National Academies Press; 2011.
5. Xue S, Kemal O, Lu M, Lix LM, Leslie WD, Yang S. Age at attainment of peak bone mineral density and its associated factors: The National Health and Nutrition Examination Survey 2005–2014. *Bone.* 2020;131:115163.
6. Agricultural Research Service, USDA. *What We Eat in America, NHANES 2017–2020.* Food Surveys Research Group; 2022. https://www.ars.usda.gov/ARSUserFiles/80400530/pdf/1720/Table_1_NIN_GEN_1720.pdf
7. Matikainen N, Pekkarinen T, Ryhänen EM, Schalin-Jäntti C. Physiology of calcium homeostasis: an overview. *Endocrinol Metab Clin North Am.* 2021;50(4):575–590.
8. Wawrzyniak N, Suliburska J. Nutritional and health factors affecting the bioavailability of calcium: a narrative review. *Nutr Rev.* 2021;79(12):1307–1320.
9. Shkembi B, Huppertz T. Calcium absorption from food products: food matrix effects. *Nutrients.* 2022;14(1):180.
10. Jaruvongvanich V, Vantanasiri K, Upala S, Ungprasert P. Changes in bone mineral density and bone metabolism after sleeve gastrectomy: a systematic review and *meta*-analysis. *Surg Obes Relat Dis.* 2019;15(8):1252–1260.
11. United States Preventive Services Task Force, Grossman DC, Curry SJ, et al. Vitamin D, calcium, or combined supplementation for the primary prevention of fractures in community-dwelling adults: United States Preventive Services Task Force Recommendation Statement. *JAMA.* 2018;319(15):1592.
12. Jenkins DJA, Spence JD, Giovannucci EL, et al. Supplemental vitamins and minerals for cardiovascular disease prevention and treatment. *J Am Coll Cardiology.* 2021;77(4):423–436.
13. Sadiq NM, Naganathan S, Badireddy M. *Hypercalcemia.* In: *StatPearls.* StatPearls Publishing; 2023. http://www.ncbi.nlm.nih.gov/books/NBK430714/.
14. Ataide FL, Carvalho Bastos LM, Vicente Matias MF, Skare TL, Freire de Carvalho J. Safety and effectiveness of vitamin D megadose: a systematic review. *Clin Nutr ESPEN.* 2021;46:115–120.
15. Rahmati S, Azami M, Delpisheh A, Hafezi Ahmadi MR, Sayehmiri K. Total calcium (dietary and supplementary) intake and prostate

cancer: a systematic review and *meta*-analysis. *Asian Pac J Cancer Prev.* 2018;19(6):1449–1456.

16. Myung SK, Ju W, Cho B, et al. Efficacy of vitamin and antioxidant supplements in prevention of cardiovascular disease: systematic review and *meta*-analysis of randomised controlled trials. *BMJ.* 2013;346:f10.

17. Li K, Wang XF, Li DY, et al. The good, the bad, and the ugly of calcium supplementation: a review of calcium intake on human health. *Clin Interv Aging.* 2018;13:2443–2452.

18. Martha JW, Wibowo A, Pranata R. Hypocalcemia is associated with severe COVID-19: a systematic review and *meta*-analysis. *Diabetes Metab Syndr.* 2021;15(1):337–342.

19. Vasudeva M, Mathew JK, Groombridge C, et al. Hypocalcemia in trauma patients: a systematic review. *J Trauma Acute Care Surg.* 2021;90(2):396–402.

20. Lewis JL. *Hypocalcemia (low level of calcium in the blood).* In: *Merck Manuals Consumer Version.* Merck & Co., Inc; 2022. https://www.merckmanuals.com/home/hormonal-and-metabolic-disorders/electrolyte-balance/hypocalcemia-low-level-of-calcium-in-the-blood.

21. Weaver CM, Gordon CM, Janz KF, et al. The National Osteoporosis Foundation's position statement on peak bone mass development and lifestyle factors: a systematic review and implementation recommendations. *Osteoporos Int.* 2016;27(4):1281–1386.

22. National Institute of Health, National Institute of Arthritis and Musculoskeletal and Skin Diseases. *Osteoporosis.* 2022. https://www.niams.nih.gov/health-topics/osteoporosis

23. Xiao Pl, Cui Ay, Hsu Cj, et al. Global, regional prevalence, and risk factors of osteoporosis according to the World Health Organization diagnostic criteria: a systematic review and *meta*-analysis. *Osteoporos Int.* 2022;33(10):2137–2153.

24. Jepsen S, Caton JG, Albandar JM, et al. Periodontal manifestations of systemic diseases and developmental and acquired conditions: consensus report of workgroup 3 of the 2017 World Workshop on the Classification of Periodontal and Peri-Implant Diseases and Conditions. *J Periodontol.* 2018;89(Suppl 1):S237–S248.

25. Penoni DC, Fidalgo TKS, Torres SR, et al. Bone density and clinical periodontal attachment in postmenopausal women: a systematic review and *meta*-analysis. *J Dent Res.* 2017;96(3):261–269.

26. Varela-López A, Giampieri F, Bullón P, Battino M, Quiles JL. A systematic review on the implication of minerals in the onset, severity and treatment of periodontal disease. *Molecules.* 2016;21(9):1183.

27. Koedijk JB, van Rijswijk J, Oranje WA, et al. Sedentary behaviour and bone health in children, adolescents and young adults: a systematic review. *Osteoporos Int.* 2017;28(9):2507–2519.

28. McMichan L, Dick M, Skelton DA, et al. Sedentary behaviour and bone health in older adults: a systematic review. *Osteoporos Int.* 2021;32(8):1487–1497.

29. Eusebi LH, Rabitti S, Artesiani ML, et al. Proton pump inhibitors: risks of long-term use. *J Gastroenterol Hepatol.* 2017;32(7):1295–1302.

30. Lexomboon D, Tägt M, Nilsson IL, Buhlin K, Häbel H, Sandborgh-Englund G. Effects of primary hyperparathyroidism on oral health. A longitudinal register-based study. *Oral Dis.* 2023;29(7):2954–2961.

31. Ferraz AX, Gonçalves FM, Ferreira-Neto PD, et al. Impact of bariatric surgery on oral health: a systematic review and *meta*-analysis. *Clin Oral Investig.* 2023;27(5):1869–1884.

32. Dos Santos MCM, Pellizzer EP, SoutoMaior JR, et al. Clinical periodontal conditions in individuals after bariatric surgery: a systematic review and *meta*-analysis. *Surg Obes Relat Dis.* 2019;15(10):1850–1859.

33. Yuan S, Michaëlsson K, Wan Z, Larsson SC. Associations of smoking and alcohol and coffee intake with fracture and bone mineral density: a mendelian randomization study. *Calcif Tissue Int.* 2019;105(6):582–588.

34. Wiesner A, Gajewska D, Paśko P. Levothyroxine interactions with food and dietary supplements-a systematic review. *Pharm (Basel).* 2021;14(3):206.

35. Napoli N, Thompson J, Civitelli R, Armamento-Villareal RC. Effects of dietary calcium compared with calcium supplements on estrogen metabolism and bone mineral density. *Am J Clin Nutr.* 2007;85(5):1428–1433.

36. Liu C, Kuang X, Li K, Guo X, Deng Q, Li D. Effects of combined calcium and vitamin D supplementation on osteoporosis in postmenopausal women: a systematic review and *meta*-analysis of randomized controlled trials. *Food Funct.* 2020;11(12):10817–10827.

37. Office of Dietary Supplement. *Phosphorus: Fact Sheet for Health Professionals.* 2021. https://ods.od.nih.gov/factsheets/Phosphorus-HealthProfessional/

38. Institute of Medicine. *Dietary Reference Intakes for Calcium, Phosphorus, Magnesium, Vitamin D, and Fluoride.* National Academies Press; 1997. http://www.ncbi.nlm.nih.gov/books/NBK109825/.

39. Vorland CJ, Stremke ER, Moorthi RN, Hill Gallant KM. Effects of excessive dietary phosphorus intake on bone health. *Curr Osteoporos Rep.* 2017;15(5):473–482.

40. Nishi T, Shuto E, Ogawa M, et al. Excessive dietary phosphorus intake impairs endothelial function in young healthy men: a time- and dose-dependent study. *J Med Invest.* 2015;62(3–4):167–172.

41. Foster BL, Tompkins KA, Rutherford RB, et al. Phosphate: Known and potential roles during development and regeneration of teeth and supporting structures. *Birth Defects Res C Embryo Today.* 2008;84(4):281–314.

42. da Silva JSV, Seres DS, Sabino K, et al. ASPEN consensus recommendations for refeeding syndrome. *Nutr Clin Pract.* 2020;35(2):178–195.

43. United States Department of Agriculture, United States Department of Health and Human Services. *Dietary Guidelines for Americans.* 9th ed. 2020. dietaryguidelines.gov.

44. Mahmood S, Shah KU, Khan TM, et al. Non-pharmacological management of hypertension: in the light of current research. *Ir J Med Sci.* 2019;188(2):437–452.

45. Office of Dietary Supplements. *Magnesium: Fact Sheet for Health Professionals.* 2022. https://ods.od.nih.gov/factsheets/Magnesium-HealthProfessional/

46. Uwitonze AM, Rahman S, Ojeh N, et al. Oral manifestations of magnesium and vitamin D inadequacy. *J Steroid Biochem Mol Biol.* 2020;200 105636.

47. Wiesner A, Szuta M, Galanty A, Paśko P. Optimal dosing regimen of osteoporosis drugs in relation to food intake as the key for the enhancement of the treatment effectiveness—a concise literature review. *Foods.* 2021;10(4):720.

48. Asbaghi O, Hosseini R, Boozari B, Ghaedi E, Kashkooli S, Moradi S. The effects of magnesium supplementation on blood pressure and obesity measure among type 2 diabetes patient: a systematic review and *meta*-analysis of randomized controlled trials. *Biol Trace Elem Res.* 2021;199(2):413–424.

49. Zhang J, Sardana D, Li KY, Leung KCM, Lo ECM. Topical fluoride to prevent root caries: systematic review with network *meta*-analysis. *J Dent Res.* 2020;99(5):506–513.

50. Office of Dietary Supplements. *Fluoride: Fact Sheet for Health Professionals.* 2022. https://ods.od.nih.gov/factsheets/Fluoride-HealthProfessional/

51. Idowu OS, Azevedo LB, Valentine RA, et al. The use of urinary fluoride excretion to facilitate monitoring fluoride intake: a systematic scoping review. *PLoS One.* 2019;14(9):e0222260.

52. Centers for Disease Control and Prevention Ten great public health achievements – United States, 1900–1999. *MMWR Morb Mortal Wkly Rep.* 1999;48(12):241–243.

53. Centers for Disease Control and Prevention, Division of Oral Health. *Public Health Service (PHS) Recommendation: Community Water Fluoridation.* 2020. https://www.cdc.gov/fluoridation/faqs/public-service-recommendations.html

54. Environmental Protection Agency, Office of Water. *Six-Year Review 3 – Health Effects Assessment for Existing Chemical and Radionuclide National Primary Drinking Water Regulations – Summary Report.* EPA;

2015. https://www.epa.gov/dwsixyearreview/support-documents-epas-third-review-existing-drinking-water-standards

55. Centers for Disease Control and Prevention, Division of Oral Health, National Center for Chronic Disease Prevention and Health Promotion (United States). *Healthy People 2030: OH-11 Objective.* 2020. https://health.gov/healthypeople/objectives-and-data/browse-objectives/health-policy

56. Food and Drug Administration. *CFR – Code of Federal Regulations Title 21 Section 165.110 Bottled Water.* 2023. https://www.accessdata.fda.gov/scripts/cdrh/cfdocs/cfcfr/cfrsearch.cfm?fr=165.110

57. United States Food and Drug Administration. *Health Claim Notification for Fluoridated Water and Reduced Risk of Dental Caries.* FDA; 2022. https://www.fda.gov/food/food-labeling-nutrition/health-claim-notification-fluoridated-water-and-reduced-risk-dental-caries

58. Godebo TR, Jeuland M, Tekle-Haimanot R, et al. Bone quality in fluoride-exposed populations: a novel application of the ultrasonic method. *Bone Rep.* 2020;12 100235.

59. Miranda GHN, Alvarenga MOP, Ferreira MKM, et al. A systematic review and *meta*-analysis of the association between fluoride exposure and neurological disorders. *Sci Rep.* 2021;11(1):22659.

60. Veneri F, Vinceti M, Generali L, et al. Fluoride exposure and cognitive neurodevelopment: systematic review and dose-response *meta*-analysis. *Env Res.* 2023;221:115239.

61. Takahashi R, Ota E, Hoshi K, et al. Fluoride supplementation (with tablets, drops, lozenges or chewing gum) in pregnant women for preventing dental caries in the primary teeth of their children. *Cochrane Database Syst Rev.* 2017;10(10): CD011850.

62. Iheozor-Ejiofor Z, Worthington HV, Walsh T, et al. Water fluoridation for the prevention of dental caries. *Cochrane Database Syst Rev.* 2015;2015(6): CD010856.

63. Clark MB, Keels MA, Slayton RL, et al. Fluoride use in caries prevention in the primary care setting. *Pediatrics.* 2020;146(6): e2020034637.

64. American Dental Association. *Fluoride: Topical and Systemic Supplements.* 2021. https://www.ada.org/resources/research/science-and-research-institute/oral-health-topics/fluoride-topical-and-systemic-supplements

65. Sarafrazi N, Wambogo EA, Shpherd JA. Osteoporosis or low bone mass in older adults: United States, 2017–2018. *MMWR Morb Mortal Wkly Rep.* 2021;405:1–8.

66. Finkelstein JS, Brockwell SE, Mehta V, et al. Bone mineral density changes during the menopause transition in a multiethnic cohort of women. *J Clin Endocrinol Metab.* 2008;93(3):861–868.

67. North American Menopause Society Management of osteoporosis in postmenopausal women: the 2021 position statement of The North American Menopause Society. *Menopause.* 2021;28(9):973.

68. Abrahamsen B, van Staa T, Ariely R, Olson M, Cooper C. Excess mortality following hip fracture: a systematic epidemiological review. *Osteoporos Int.* 2009;20(10):1633–1650.

69. LeBoff MS, Greenspan SL, Insogna KL, et al. The clinician's guide to prevention and treatment of osteoporosis. *Osteoporos Int.* 2022;33(10):2049–2102.

70. Yu B, Wang CY. Osteoporosis and periodontal diseases - An update on their association and mechanistic links. *Periodontol 2000.* 2022;89(1):99–113.

71. Cekici A, Baser U, Isik G, Akhan SE, Issever H, Onan U. Periodontal treatment outcomes in post menopausal women receiving hormone replacement therapy. *J Istanb Univ Fac Dent.* 2015;49(3):39–44.

72. Leder B., Martinez R., Harris S., Topiwala S. *Glucocorticoid-Induced Osteoporosis.* Endocrine Society; 2022. https://www.endocrine.org/patient-engagement/endocrine-library/glucocorticoid-induced-osteoporosis

73. Martins LHI, Ferreira DC, Silva MT, Motta RHL, Franquez RT, Bergamaschi Cde C. Frequency of osteonecrosis in bisphosphonate users submitted to dental procedures: a systematic review. *Oral Dis.* 2023;29(1):75–99.

74. Limones A, Sáez-Alcaide LM, Díaz-Parreño SA, Helm A, Bornstein MM, Molinero-Mourelle P. Medication-related osteonecrosis of the jaws (MRONJ) in cancer patients treated with denosumab vs. zoledronic acid: a systematic review and *meta*-analysis. *Med Oral Patol Oral Cir Bucal.* 2020;25(3):e326–e336.

75. Desbiens LC, Khelifi N, Wang YP, et al. Thiazide diuretics and fracture risk: a systematic review and *meta*-analysis of randomized clinical trials. *JBMR Plus.* 2022;6(11):e10683.

76. Groenendijk I, van Delft M, Versloot P, van Loon LJC, de Groot LCPGM. Impact of magnesium on bone health in older adults: a systematic review and *meta*-analysis. *Bone.* 2022;154:116233.

77. Inchingolo AD, Inchingolo AM, Malcangi G, et al. Effects of resveratrol, curcumin and quercetin supplementation on bone metabolism—a systematic review. *Nutrients.* 2022;14(17):3519.

78. Bellavia D, Dimarco E, Costa V, et al. Flavonoids in bone erosive diseases: perspectives in osteoporosis treatment. *Trends Endocrinol Metab.* 2021;32(2):76–94.

79. Dai Z, Zhang Y, Lu N, Felson DT, Kiel DP, Sahni S. Association between dietary fiber intake and bone loss in the Framingham Offspring Study. *J Bone Min Res.* 2018;33(2):241–249.

▶ Evolve Resources

Please visit http://evolve.elsevier.com/Mallonee/nutritional for additional practice and study support tools.

10

Microminerals and Ultratrace Minerals in Calcified Structures

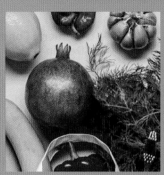

STUDENT LEARNING OUTCOMES

On completion of this chapter, the student will be able to achieve the following learning outcomes:

1. For copper, selenium, chromium, manganese, and molybdenum:
   - Describe the physiologic roles of each micromineral involved in oral health and calcified structures.
   - Discuss the RDA (or AI), Tolerable Upper Intake level (UL), and estimated average requirement (EAR) for each mineral.
   - Name common sources of microminerals and explain their importance.

   - Discuss clinical conditions associated with excess and deficiency of microminerals.
   - Customize nutrition recommendations for these microminerals to meet patient needs.
   - Counsel a patient on nutrition recommendations to meet the patient's needs for these microminerals.
2. List and explain the role of ultratrace elements present in the body.

KEY TERMS

Enteral feedings
Kayser-Fleischer ring

Keshan disease
Neurotransmitters

Stannous
Total parenteral nutrition (TPN)

◆ TEST YOUR NQ

1. **T/F** The National Academy of Medicine (formerly the Institute of Medicine) has established tolerable upper intake levels (ULs) for copper, manganese, chromium, and molybdenum.
2. **T/F** Lead levels in dental enamel can be used to determine environmental exposure to lead.
3. **T/F** Copper is important in the formation of collagen.
4. **T/F** Aluminum toxicity causes Alzheimer's disease.

5. **T/F** Selenium functions as an antioxidant.
6. **T/F** Refined foods are good sources of trace minerals.
7. **T/F** The function of many trace minerals present in enamel and dentin is unknown.
8. **T/F** Sugar is a good source of chromium.
9. **T/F** Selenium supplements are a good way to increase longevity.

Very small amounts of several minerals are essential for optimal growth and development. Many of these microminerals (Table 10.1) are found in enamel and dentin. The role of minerals may not be obvious as you clinically assess patients; nevertheless, patients with inadequate amounts may exhibit deficiency symptoms.

Tolerable upper intake levels (ULs) have not been established for several of these nutrients because of the lack of data. The requirement for these nutrients should be obtained from food sources because even small amounts may be toxic. Available evidence suggests that ultratrace minerals—especially arsenic, boron, nickel, and silicon—may be physiologically essential. Because no human deficiencies have been determined, their importance

in humans can only be inferred from results of animal studies. Human requirements have not been quantified. If they are required, the amounts needed are easily met by naturally occurring sources in food, water, and air. Other elements present in calcified structures, such as cadmium, lead, and tin, have no known function and may be contaminants.

Copper

Physiologic Roles

Copper is the third largest micromineral found in the human body, following iron and zinc. Copper is a cofactor for many enzymes that

TABLE 10.1 **Micromineral Concentrations in Human Enamel and Dentin**

	Enamel[a] (ppm)	Dentin[a] (ppm)
Aluminum	1.5–700	10–100
Boron	0.5–39	1–10
Cadmium	0.3–10	
Chromium	< 0.1–100	1–100
Copper	0.1–130	0.2–100
Iron	0.8–200	90–1000
Lead	1.3–100	10–100
Lithium	0.23–3.40	
Manganese	0.8–20	0.6–1000
Molybdenum	0.7–39	1–10
Nickel	10–100	10–100
Selenium	0.1–10	10–100
Strontium	26–1000	90–1000
Sulfur	130–530	
Tin	0.03–0.9	
Vanadium	0.01–0.03	1–10
Zinc	60–1800	

[a]µg/g dry weight.
ppm, parts per million.
Adapted from Gron P. Inorganic chemical and structural aspects of oral mineralized tissues. In: Shaw JH, ed. *Textbook of Oral Biology*. Saunders; 1978:484–507.

TABLE 10.2 **National Academy of Medicine Recommendations for Copper**

Life Stage	EAR (µg/day) Male	EAR (µg/day) Female	RDA (µg/day) Male	RDA (µg/day) Female	AI (µg/day)
Birth–6 months	–	–	–	–	200
7–12 months	–	–	–	–	220
1–3 years	260	260	340	340	
4–8 years	340	340	440	440	
9–13 years	540	540	700	700	
14–18 years	685	685	890	890	
>18 years	700	700	900	900	
Pregnancy					
14–18 years		785		1000	
19–50 years		800		1000	
Lactation					
14–18 years		985		1300	
19–50 years		1000		1300	

AI, Adequate intake; *EAR*, estimated average requirement; *RDA*, recommended dietary allowance.
Data from Institute of Medicine (IOM), Food and Nutrition Board. *Dietary Reference Intakes for Vitamin A, Vitamin K, Arsenic, Boron, Chromium, Copper, Iodine, Iron, Manganese, Molybdenum, Nickel, Silicon, Vanadium, and Zinc*. National Academy Press; 2001.

function in oxidative reactions, energy production, iron metabolism, production of neurotransmitters (including norepinephrine and dopamine), connective tissue synthesis.[1] Its function as a catalyst is important in the maturation of collagen from a precollagenous stage by catalyzing cross-linking of collagen to enhance flexibility and strength of connective tissue. Other roles include regulation of gene expression, brain development, and immune function.[1]

Copper is readily incorporated into tooth enamel.[2] The literature is inconsistent in regard to whether copper is associated with caries, however, it is suggested that copper reduces and inhibits demineralization.[2,3] Copper also inhibits bacterial growth and may have a cariostatic effect.[2]

Requirements

The National Academy of Medicine (formerly the Institute of Medicine) established the recommended dietary allowance (RDA) for copper as 900 µg/day for adults.[4] The UL has been set at 10 g/day for adults (Table 10.2). The average intake from National Health and Nutrition Examination Survey (NHANES) 2017–2020 in the United States among adults was 1.2 mg.[5]

Absorption and Excretion

Approximately one-third of dietary copper is absorbed, occurring primarily in the small intestine.[1] Absorption is enhanced by a low pH and is diminished by large amounts of calcium and zinc. Copper is stored mostly in the skeleton and muscle and is excreted through bile in feces.

Sources

Copper is widely distributed in foods. The richest sources include shellfish, oysters, crabs, liver, nuts, sesame and sunflower seeds, soy products, legumes, whole grains, and cocoa.

Hyper States and Hypo States

Toxicity

Copper toxicity is seldom encountered. Copper taken orally is an emetic; 10 mg of oral copper can produce nausea. Serum copper levels are elevated in patients with rheumatoid arthritis, myocardial infarction, conditions requiring administration of estrogen, and pregnancy.

Wilson disease is a special metabolic disorder in which abnormally high amounts of copper accumulate in the liver, kidney, brain, and cornea.[1] The liver releases less copper into the bile due to a genetic abnormality, resulting in a build-up which causes neurologic and liver damage that can result in liver cirrhosis.[1] Copper concentrates in the cornea, causing a characteristic brown, gold, or green ring called the Kayser-Fleischer ring (Fig. 10.1).[6]

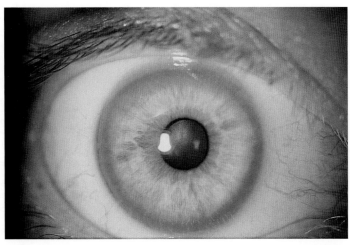

• **Fig. 10.1** Cornea in Wilson disease. Copper deposits in the corneal periphery produce the characteristic Kayser-Fleischer ring. This is a complete or incomplete brown-to-green ring near the cornea, best seen in early stages of the disease. (From Swartz MH. *Textbook of Physical Diagnosis: History and Examination.* 7th ed. Elsevier; 2014.)

Deficiency

Copper deficiency is uncommon. Copper deficiency results in osteoporosis and other bone defects; connective tissue disorders; decreased hair and skin pigmentation; hypercholesteremia; and increased risk of infection. Most of these effects may result from inadequate copper to act as a cofactor for enzymes involved in many metabolic processes in the body.

Groups at risk for inadequate copper include those with celiac disease due to malabsorption; Menkes disease, and those taking large doses of zinc supplements.[1] Zinc interferes with copper absorption and should be avoided.

DENTAL CONSIDERATIONS

- Anemia that cannot be corrected with iron supplements may be caused by copper deficiency.
- High doses of zinc supplements decrease copper absorption, possibly leading to anemia-related fatigue.

NUTRITIONAL DIRECTIONS

- Generally, diet composition has little effect on copper bioavailability.
- Infants fed formula with high iron levels may interfere with copper absorption.

Selenium

Physiologic Roles

Selenium functions mainly as a cofactor for many enzymes and as an antioxidant.[7] These selenoproteins are involved with cardiovascular, thyroid, and reproductive function and are involved in DNA synthesis.[7,8] It also has an impact on bone mineral density and contributes to the maintenance of normal immune function.[9,10] Selenium works hand in hand with vitamin E as an antioxidant; a deficiency of either nutrient increases the requirement for the other.

Selenium is present in tooth enamel and dentin.[11] It is probably incorporated into the enamel during amelogenesis. Large amounts during tooth formation may be detrimental to the mineralization process.

Requirements

The RDA establishes the adult requirement at 55 μg. The UL is 400 μg/day for adults (Table 10.3).[12] Typical intake in the United States for adults averages 94 μg daily for females and 132 μg for males.[5]

Sources

Animal products—especially seafood, kidney, liver, and other meats—are rich in selenium. Selenium intake correlates closely with caloric and protein consumption. Selenium in dairy products and eggs is more readily absorbed than selenium from other foods. Whole-grain products, nuts, and mushrooms are also good sources.

Hyper States and Hypo States

Toxicity

Toxicity and deficiency symptoms have occurred in animals from irregular distribution of selenium in soil, but these are rarely seen in humans. Routine ingestion of 2 to 3 mg of selenium can cause toxic symptoms, including nausea and vomiting, neurological symptoms, acute respiratory distress, myocardial infarction, facial flushing, skin rashes, hair and nail loss or brittleness, mottled teeth, tremors, lightheadedness, and kidney failure.[8]

While research from the 1950s and 1960s suggests an association between high levels of selenium and caries, more recent research suggests that caries activity in children is not affected by selenium in saliva.[13] However, topically selenium in sealants has been shown to have antibacterial properties.[14]

Deficiency

In parts of China, an endemic cardiomyopathy called Keshan disease is associated with severe selenium deficiency.[7] Oral selenium

| TABLE 10.3 | National Academy of Medicine Recommendations for Selenium |

Life Stage	EAR (µg/day)	RDA (µg/day)	AI (µg/day)
0–6 months			15
7–12 months			20
1–3 years	17	20	
4–8 years	23	30	
9–13 years	35	40	
>13 years	45	55	
Pregnancy			
≤14–50 years	49	60	
Lactation			
≤14–50 years	59	70	

AI, Adequate intake; *EAR*, estimated average requirement; *RDA*, recommended dietary allowance.
Data from Institute of Medicine (IOM), Food and Nutrition Board. *Dietary Reference Intakes For Vitamin C, Vitamin E, Selenium, and Carotenoids.* National Academy Press; 2000.

| TABLE 10.4 | National Academy of Medicine Recommendations for Chromium |

Life Stage Group	AI (µg/day)	
	Male	Female
Birth–6 months	0.2	0.2
7–12 months	2.2	2.2
1–3 years	11	11
4–8 years	15	15
9–13 years	25	21
14–18 years	35	24
19–50 years	35	25
>50 years	30	20
Pregnancy		
14–18 years		29
19–50 years		30
Lactation		
14–18 years		44
19–50 years		45

AI, Adequate intake.
Data from Institute of Medicine (IOM), Food and Nutrition Board. *Dietary Reference Intakes for Vitamin A, Vitamin K, Arsenic, Boron, Chromium, Copper, Iodine, Iron, Manganese, Molybdenum, Nickel, Silicon, Vanadium, and Zinc.* National Academy Press; 2001.

prophylaxis is extremely effective in reducing Keshan disease but not in eradicating it.

Deficiency in the United States and Canada is rare. However, groups at risk of a deficiency of selenium include those living in selenium-deficient areas, patients undergoing kidney dialysis, and those living with human immunodeficiency virus.[8]

Some research suggests that individuals with low selenium levels may have greater progression of periodontal disease and it may impact the wound healing process, but more research is needed.[15,16]

DENTAL CONSIDERATIONS

- Stay current with the literature about association of low selenium levels and progression of periodontal disease, and its effect on caries risk.
- Selenium is essential for health, but its excess can also be toxic.

NUTRITIONAL DIRECTIONS

- Because of increased risk of toxicity, selenium supplements should not be taken by patients unless recommended by a health care provider.
- Gastrointestinal disorders, such as Crohn's disease, can impair selenium absorption.

Chromium

Physiologic Roles

Chromium is an odorless and tasteless metallic element. Chromium is involved in carbohydrate, protein, and lipid metabolism through potentiating the action of insulin.[17] Chromium

is present in primary and permanent teeth, but the function is unknown as the content seems to be similar in carious and noncarious teeth.[18,19] There is ongoing debate about whether chromium is an essential nutrient and in 2014 the European Food and Safety Authority Panel on Dietetic Products found inadequate evidence to support making recommendations.[20]

Requirements

The adequate intake (AI) of a healthy adult has been estimated as 20 to 35 µg/day. No UL has been set (Table 10.4).[4] The 2001 National Academy of Medicine reports the average chromium content in well-balanced diets as 13.4 µg/1000 cal. Chromium is poorly absorbed; whether intestinal absorption compensates for increased demand is unclear.

Sources

Chromium is found in meats, whole-grain cereals, wheat germ, nuts, mushrooms, green beans, broccoli, brewer's yeast, beer, wine, and tap water. The refining process depletes chromium from grains and cereal.

Because chromium is naturally occurring in the environment, the United States Environmental Protection Agency (EPA) requires drinking water be monitored for harmful levels of chromium. The current EPA standard for chromium in public water systems is not to exceed 100 parts per billion (ppb) or 0.1 mg/L.[21]

Hyper States and Hypo States

Chromium Excess

Chromium toxicity has been caused by the use of chromium supplements resulting in renal failure, dermatitis, liver dysfunction, and weight loss.[17] Industrial exposure may result in liver damage and lung cancer.

Chromium Deficiency

Chromium deficiencies are rare in healthy individuals.

DENTAL CONSIDERATIONS

- Assess patients employed in industrial settings or artists using supplies with high chromium content for chromium toxicity.
- Chromium supplements may cause serious renal and liver impairment when taken in excess.

NUTRITIONAL DIRECTION

- Do not take chromium supplements unless instructed by a health care provider. Currently, the evidence is unclear as to whether supplemental chromium can help with insulin resistance, metabolic syndrome, polycystic ovary syndrome, dyslipidemia, or weight/fat loss.[17]

Manganese

Physiologic Roles

Manganese is cofactor for many enzyme systems involved in amino acid, cholesterol, and carbohydrate metabolism; optimal bone matrix development; immune function; and the antioxidant process to reduce cell damage.[22] It is absorbed in the small intestine, transported to the liver, and excreted through bile into the feces.

Requirements

As shown in Table 10.5, an adequate intake is 1.8 to 2.3 mg/day for adults.[4] The absorption of iron and manganese is inversely proportional, so a large amount of one reduces absorption of the other.[22] The UL has been established as 11 mg/day for adults. Little is known about the average intake since data was gathered in 1991, and at that time, the estimated dietary intake in the United States was 2.64 to 2.81 mg/day for males and 2.14 to 2.23 mg/day for females suggesting that most people had an adequate intake.[23]

Sources

Foods high in manganese include whole-grain cereals, legumes, nuts, tea, leafy greens, and infant formula. The bioavailability of manganese from meats, milk, and eggs makes these important sources despite their smaller quantities.

Hyper States and Hypo States

Manganese Excess

Dietary intake of manganese has not been shown to result in toxicity. However, industrial or occupational exposure is a concern in occupations such as welding and mining. Symptoms of toxic

TABLE 10.5	National Academy of Medicine Recommendations for Manganese	
	AI (mg/day)	
Life Stage Group	Male	Female
Birth–6 months	0.003	0.003
7–12 months	0.6	0.6
1–3 years	1.2	1.2
4–8 years	1.5	1.5
9–13 years	1.9	1.6
14–18 years	2.2	1.6
>18 years	2.3	1.8
Pregnancy		
14–50 years		2
Lactation		
14–50 years		2.6

AI, Adequate intake.
Data from Institute of Medicine (IOM), Food and Nutrition Board. *Dietary Reference Intakes for Vitamin A, Vitamin K, Arsenic, Boron, Chromium, Copper, Iodine, Iron, Manganese, Molybdenum, Nickel, Silicon, Vanadium, and Zinc.* National Academy Press; 2001.

exposure include ataxia, headache, fatigue, anxiety, hallucinations, lower cognitive scores, psychosis, and a syndrome similar to Parkinson disease (marked by memory loss, tremors, and rigid body posture).[24]

Like chromium, manganese is naturally present in the environment and from other sources like air pollution and agricultural fungicides. There is ongoing research about how low levels of excess manganese may impact health in the long term.

Manganese Deficiency

Manganese deficiencies have never been reported in individuals consuming a normal diet.[22] There is limited evidence about the symptoms of manganese deficiency, but it may include bone demineralization, growth retardation, loss of hair pigmentation, decreased serum cholesterol, impaired glucose tolerance, and dysregulation of lipid and carbohydrate metabolism.[22]

DENTAL CONSIDERATIONS

- Inhaling manganese dust can cause neurodegenerative symptoms similar to Parkinson disease in patients whose occupations expose them to increased inhalation of manganese (i.e., factory workers, welders, or manganese miners).

NUTRITIONAL DIRECTIONS

- An iron-rich diet may reduce absorption of manganese as they compete for the same proteins that help with absorption.[25]
- Manganese should not be confused with magnesium.

Molybdenum

Physiologic Roles

Molybdenum functions as a cofactor for enzymes related to amino acid metabolism and those involved in metabolizing drugs and toxins.[26]

Requirements

The RDA for molybdenum is 45 µg/day for adults.[4] The UL is set at 2000 µg/day for adults (Table 10.6).

Sources

Legumes, whole-grain cereals, and nuts are the best sources; milk, liver, and many vegetables are poor sources.

Hyper States and Hypo States

Except for deficiency reported during administration of total parenteral nutrition (TPN), molybdenum deficiency has not been documented in the United States.

DENTAL CONSIDERATIONS

- Molybdenum is present in small amounts in both permanent and primary teeth, but does not seem to have an association with caries.[18]

NUTRITIONAL DIRECTIONS

- Legumes (e.g., lentils, beans, peas), nuts, and whole grains are good sources of molybdenum.

Ultratrace Elements

Many ultratrace elements have been studied for their potential influence on dental caries. Results of research investigations are complicated by many factors. Nevertheless, some studies suggest some ultratrace elements tend to be present in higher amounts in carious enamel.[13,18,19] Further research is warranted to determine the mechanism of their effects.

More attention has been given to ultratrace elements as contaminants in the environment and foods. Some are considered to have no harmful effects and are used therapeutically, such as aluminum in antacids.

Boron

Boron is not considered an essential nutrient for humans, but may have an effect on metabolism of calcium, phosphorus, magnesium, or vitamin D, and may be needed to maintain membrane structure.[27] It may be involved in modulating the inflammatory response and in antioxidant activities.[28] Boron is present in the highest concentration in teeth, bones, and the gastrointestinal tract.[29]

The National Academy of Science has not identified a dietary reference intake for boron. The median dietary intake in adults

TABLE 10.6 National Academy of Medicine Recommendations for Molybdenum

Life Stage	EAR (µg/day) Male	EAR (µg/day) Female	RDA (µg/day) Male	RDA (µg/day) Female	AI (µg/day)
Birth–6 months	–	–	–	–	2
7–12 months	–	–	–	–	3
1–3 years	13	13	17	17	
4–8 years	17	17	22	22	
9–13 years	26	26	34	34	
14–18 years	33	33	43	43	
>18 years	34	34	45	45	
Pregnancy					
14–50 years		40		50	
Lactation					
14–18 years		35		50	
19–50 years		36		50	

AI, Adequate intake; *EAR*, estimated average requirement; *RDA*, recommended dietary allowance.
Data from Institute of Medicine (IOM), Food and Nutrition Board. *Dietary Reference Intakes for Vitamin A, Vitamin K, Arsenic, Boron, Chromium, Copper, Iodine, Iron, Manganese, Molybdenum, Nickel, Silicon, Vanadium, and Zinc.* National Academy Press; 2001.

ranges from 0.87 to 1.35 mg/day. Despite no RDA or AI for boron, the upper intake levels have been identified by the United States, Canada, the World Health Organization, and the European Food Safety Authority which ranges from 11.2 to 28 mg/day for adults.[4,29]

Boron is principally present in foods of plant origin, especially fruits, vegetables, nuts, legumes, and wine. Boron is also considered a contaminant in water, air, and soil. The Environmental Protection Agency monitors boron in water and the Occupational Safety and Health Administration monitors the air quality in workplaces where individuals might be exposed to boron.

Boron toxicity includes gastrointestinal symptoms (e.g., vomiting, nausea, diarrhea), dermatitis/rash/flushing, convulsions, headache, kidney damage, and can cause death.[27]

Low boron levels appear to affect urinary calcium and magnesium excretion as well as vitamin D levels resulting in the increase of calcitonin and osteocalcin which potentially results in negative changes in bone mineral density.[27] However, more research is needed to determine if boron supplementation enhances bone health.

Nickel

The physiologic role of nickel is still unclear. It may be a cofactor of certain metalloenzymes involved in functions like iron absorption, energy metabolism as well as the metabolism of vitamin B_{12} and folic acid.

Although an RDA or Adequate Intake has not been established by the National Academy of Science, an Upper Limit for intake is set at 1.0 mg/day for adults.[4]

Food sources of nickel include dried beans and peas, grains, nuts, crustaceans, cocoa, and chocolate.[30] However, it also comes from cookware and may be a contaminant in the environment.[30]

Toxicity is a concern due to variable exposure to environmental contamination by nickel. Chronic exposure may result in sensitivity and systemic contact dermatitis. Excess has adverse effects on the liver, kidneys, bones, inhibition of DNA/RNA repair, and potentially iron homeostasis.[30]

Nickel deficiency results in suboptimal growth in animals. Inadequate nickel alters trace-element composition of bone and impairs iron use.

Silicon

The role for silicon in human nutrition and health has not been identified.[4] Animal research suggests that silicon plays a role in connective tissue and bone formation, and maintenance.[31] Silicon is present in tooth enamel in larger amounts in primary than in permanent teeth, but its function, if any, is unknown.[18]

Plant-based foods like whole grains and root vegetables are sources of silicon with the majority of silicon coming from beverages like beer, coffee, and water.[4] Average intake in adults is 14–21 mg/day.[4]

Deficiencies in animal studies result in depressed collagen in bone and long bone abnormalities, resulting in malformed joints and defective bone growth.[4]

Tin

Tin is a heavy metal widely distributed in the environment with no known function in human nutrition.[32,33] The primary source of tin is from canned foods and beverages. Foods packed in tin cans that are coated with lacquer, contain very little tin, but acidic foods such as pineapple and orange juice and tomato sauce, packed in cans that are not coated with lacquer, contain significant amounts of tin. Other sources of tin include stannous (chemical term for tin) chloride, approved for use as a food additive, and fluoride, the active ingredient in some self-applied dentifrices and mouth rinses.

Higher intake of tin is associated with age (higher in children and those over age 60 years), lower socioeconomic status, and race/ethnicity.[33] Exposure to tin can cause acute gastrointestinal distress, liver, and kidney problems.

Aluminum

Aluminum probably is not an essential nutrient. Aluminum is found primarily in bone, but is also present in dental enamel.[18]

Aluminum may come from environmental and occupational exposure as well as in food, cosmetics (e.g., antiperspirant), and medications (e.g., vaccines, dialysis fluids).[34] Food packaging, aluminum foil, baking sheets, and cooking utensils can also be sources of aluminum.[34] Under normal conditions, very little aluminum is absorbed[34]; the kidneys excrete about the same amount as is absorbed.

Aluminum is neurotoxic and it is present in the brains of those with Alzheimer's disease, it has not been shown that it causes Alzheimer's disease. It has also been suggested that using aluminum containing antiperspirant increases the risk of breast cancer, but the evidence does not support this association.[34]

Lead

Lead is a heavy metal that is a contaminant in water obtained primarily from corroding lead pipes. It is not an essential nutrient for human nutrition.[35] As a result of implementation of aggressive public health measures to remove lead from paint and gasoline, blood lead levels in children have decreased markedly since the late 1970s.[36]

Lead impacts neurodevelopment of children and may be involved in neurodegenerative disease in adults. Lead is more readily absorbed from the gastrointestinal tract during infancy and early childhood than in adulthood, meaning children are more susceptible to lead exposure. Children also develop more rapidly and experience more neurodevelopmental effects from lead exposure.[37] Longer duration and/or higher concentrations of lead exposure is associated with lower IQ and cognitive function in children.[38,39] In adults who were exposed to lead during childhood, there is ongoing research to identify possible adverse effects.

Lead is present in the enamel of primary and permanent teeth.[18] The amount of lead in deciduous teeth can be used as an index of lead exposure. Evidence about an association between lead and increased caries risk is inconsistent and more research is needed.[18,40]

Lithium

Although there is no evidence for lithium being an essential nutrient in human nutrition, it is found in calcified structures including bone and dentin.[41] When this substitution is made in apatite of bone and teeth, the structure and solubility properties are altered.[41] However, the effect on dentin apatite morphology is unknown.

Vanadium

Studies on the essentiality of vanadium have been inconsistent in their findings.[4] Most research has not found that vanadium deficiency consistently impairs any biologic function in animals. However, research suggests that vanadium is involved in carbohydrate, lipid, and cholesterol metabolism as well as mineralization of bones, teeth, and thyroid and red blood cell metabolism.[18,42]

Shellfish, mushrooms, grains and grain products, wine, beer, and parsley contain small amounts of vanadium.[4] While there have been no adverse effects from food sources of vanadium, supplements and intake from contaminated water may be a concern. Adverse effects may include abdominal cramps, diarrhea, anemia, and possible kidney toxicity.[4] Based on possible toxicity, the UL was set at 1.8 mg/day for adults.[4]

Vanadium seems to be present in higher amounts in the saliva of individuals with chronic periodontitis which may be the result of alveolar bone breakdown, but this needs more research.[16] Vanadium may have a mild cariostatic effect.[18]

Mercury

Mercury is a contaminant often found in the food (e.g., seafood) and water supply either naturally in the environment, industrial pollution, and occupational exposure (e.g., dental personnel exposure to mercury and gold mining).[43] Adverse effects of mercury include neurologic and reproductive changes in adults along with negative effects on physical and cognitive development in infants and children.[44] High blood levels of mercury has also been associated with lower bone mineral density and may put individuals at risk of osteopenia and osteoporosis.[45]

The US Food and Drug Administration (FDA) monitors the presence of contaminants in food, issuing warnings as needed.[46]

Females of childbearing age, pregnant and nursing females, and young children should choose seafood low in methyl mercury and higher in omega-3 fatty acids (EPA and DHA) which includes: salmon, trout, oysters, anchovies, sardines, and Pacific and Atlantic mackerel.[47]

DENTAL CONSIDERATIONS

- Boron deficiency signs may be related to abnormalities in vitamin D, calcium, phosphorus, or magnesium levels.
- Aluminum is a cariostatic agent, especially in combination with fluoride.
- Seafood is a good source of important nutrients, including omega-3 fats that promote neurodevelopment. The American Heart Association and the *Dietary Guidelines* recommend at least two servings of fish each week.

- Encourage fish and shellfish with lower mercury levels, such as salmon, clams, sardines, crab, tilapia, scallops, shrimp, catfish, perch, whitefish, and cod. Large, older fish higher on the food chain—such as shark, swordfish, king mackerel, orange roughly, tuna, and tilefish, contain higher levels of mercury (see Fig. 13.4). For example, a scallop may have a mercury concentration of 0.003 ppm while tilefish may have 1.123 ppm.

NUTRITIONAL DIRECTIONS

- A diet low in boron increases calcium excretion; thus patients with osteoporosis should be encouraged to consume recommended amounts of fresh fruits and vegetables.
- Acidic foods and foods with high nitrate content, such as tomatoes, can accumulate very high levels of tin if left in unlacquered, opened cans in the refrigerator for more than 3 days. Once opened, these foods should be stored in glass or plastic containers.
- Consumption of a variety of foods and fluids helps people obtain trace minerals and avoid excessive amounts.

- Unrefined foods generally provide more trace minerals than highly refined foods.
- Supplements of these trace elements are not encouraged.
- Some bone meal and oyster shell used for calcium supplementation may contain dangerous amounts of lead.
- Patients who use well water can contact the local health department or water system for information on contaminants or they may have the water tested for contaminants.

◆ HEALTH APPLICATION 10

Alzheimer's Disease

Globally 55 million people have dementia and the World Health Organization has declared it a public health priority.[48] Identified more than 100 years ago, Alzheimer's disease (AD) is the most common type of dementia in individuals, comprising 60% to 70% of dementia cases.[48] An estimated 6.2 million (or 1 in 9) individuals 65 years and older in the United States are living with Alzheimer's disease.[49] These numbers will be refined in future years, as it will become more feasible for the biomarkers of AD, to test and identify those in the preclinical stages of the disease. Alzheimer's disease is the sixth leading cause of death and a leading cause of disability and morbidity.[49] Direct and indirect health care costs together exceed $355 billion and this does not include the value of family caregivers, and their health and economic burden.[49]

AD is a brain disease in which changes begin 20 years or more before the diagnosis of AD can be made.[49] AD is a continuum with three phases including preclinical AD, mild cognitive impairment (MCI), and dementia (mild-moderate-severe) due to AD.[49] The length of each phase can vary greatly based on factors such as age and sex.[49]

Lifetime risk for AD at age 45 is 20% or 1 in 5 for females, and the risk for males being 10% or 1 in 10.[49] This difference is in part because females live longer and older age is a significant risk factor for AD.[49] There are also racial and ethnic differences with older Black Americans (18%) having the highest risk followed by Hispanic (14%) and White (10%) Americans.[49] Genetics is another significant risk factor for the development of AD in old age. First degree family members with AD is also a risk factor. Individuals with Down syndrome are at increased risk with about 30% of those in their 50s and half of those in their 60s having AD.[49]

However, there may be modifiable risk factors which include controlling diabetes, hypertension, and high cholesterol along with tobacco cessation and maintaining a healthy weight.[49] Prevention of traumatic brain injury can also reduce risk for AD. In addition, to modifiable risk factors associated with chronic disease, being socially and mentally active may support brain health.[49]

A key element of disease management is early diagnosis to initiate therapy. Some causes of dementia can be treated, and some of the symptoms can possibly be reversed. A series of evaluations are used to make a clinical diagnosis of Alzheimer's disease, including medical and behavioral assessments. Often, reports from family members and friends provide valuable information regarding mental status of the individual. The National Institute of Aging and Alzheimer's Association has developed "warning signs" for detection of Alzheimer's disease (Box 10.1).[50]

Risk reduction is a focus for prevention and management of progression of dementia to AD and includes: nutrition; physical activity; hearing; sleep; cognitive training and stimulation; social engagement and education; and avoidance of certain medications (Box 10.2).[51,52] A recent study suggests that in the preclinical stage of AD, periodontal treatment may reduce AD-related brain atrophy, however, more research is needed.[53]

The FDA has approved medications for AD falling into three categories: (1) slow the disease progression, (2) to improve cognitive symptoms, and (3) to manage noncognitive symptoms.[54] Behavioral and psychiatric symptoms include physical or verbal outbursts, restlessness, hallucinations, sleep disturbances, and delusions. Research is ongoing for effective treatment for AD.

Alternative therapies such as traditional Chinese medicine (TCM), Ayurveda, and traditional Native American medicine have been used for

◆ HEALTH APPLICATION 10—CONT'D

centuries in many cultures to address disease, however, scientific research on use and effects, is in its infancy. Patients see marketing for supplements that enhance memory on a daily basis, but the research to confirm the claims is lacking. Consumers also need to be reminded that dietary supplements including vitamins, minerals, and herbal supplements are not approved by the FDA for safety or effectiveness.[55] Only adverse events are reported and monitored by the FDA and some instances have resulted in supplements being removed from the market. The FDA specifically warns consumers about unproven claims about AD treatments.[56]

There is no single diet, food, vitamin, or supplement "proven" to prevent or treat dementia or AD at this time.[57] However, there is ongoing research in this area. Food patterns like the Mediterranean diet recommended by the *Dietary Guidelines* may be of benefit and is an overall healthy eating plan and appropriate for all adults.[47,52] Individuals vitamins and minerals have also been investigated,[58,59] but separating nutrients from food sources to explore effect on AD is difficult which is why the focus should be on healthy eating patterns.

Alzheimer's disease has significant effects on nutrition and hydration status. Those with AD have significant risk for dehydration as they may forget to drink, or they may not be able to communicate their thirst to a caregiver.[60] The relationship between hydration and AD is bi-directional. Dehydration also impairs cognitive performance and is associated with developing dementia like AD.[60,61]

Malnutrition puts individuals at risk for AD and malnutrition is often present in those with AD.[62] Initially, individuals with Alzheimer's disease

may have problems with food purchasing and meal preparation and a meal delivery service like Meals on Wheels may be a helpful option for healthy meals. Appetite and food intake fluctuate with mood swings and increasing confusion. Forgetting when they last ate, the patients may skip some meals, eat twice, or forget about food cooking on the stove creating a safety issue. Malnutrition is also associated with progression of AD, therefore it is important to find ways to assist the patient with consuming an adequate diet.[63] Of equal importance is a healthy dietary pattern as poor quality patterns are associated with AD progression.[63]

Ways to encourage intake at meals is by creating a routine, serving favorite foods, ensuring a calm environment, and avoid rushing the individual. Healthy snacks and smaller meals may be more appropriate for those without a good appetite. Nutrition supplements such as protein shakes may be needed to ensure adequate nutrition intake. Finger foods allow self-feeding when the individual has challenges with using eating utensils. Foods should be cut up and offered in bite-size pieces. Serving foods one at a time may help decrease confusion. A larger meal at midday, when cognitive abilities are at their peak, is recommended.

During the final stage, which is characterized by severe intellectual impairment, food may not be recognized and may be refused. The individual also may forget how to swallow. Enteral feedings (the provision of nutrients through a tube placed in the nose, stomach, or small intestine) may be indicated to maintain nutritional status as a result of severely impaired cognition.

• BOX 10.1   Warning Signs of Alzheimer's Disease

- Memory loss that disrupts daily life
- Challenges in problem solving
- Difficulty performing familiar tasks or taking longer for normal daily tasks
- Confusion with time or place
- Problems with speaking or writing new words
- Misplacing things or losing the ability to retrace steps
- Forgetting new information learned or repeating questions

- Poor judgment
- Withdrawal from social activities they previous enjoyed
- Changes in mood or personality
- Increased anxiety or aggressive behavior

Data from National Institute on Aging. *Symptoms and Diagnosis of Alzheimer's Disease: What Are the Signs of Alzheimer's Disease?* National Institute on Aging; 2022. https://www.nia.nih.gov/health/what-are-signs-alzheimers-disease

---

• BOX 10.2   Maintain Your Brain

- Stay physically active. Physical exercise is essential for maintaining good blood flow to the brain as well as to encourage new brain cells. It also can significantly reduce the risk of heart disease, stroke, and diabetes, and thereby delay or slow age-related cognitive decline and dementia.
- Manage blood pressure to prevent cardiovascular and cerebrovascular disease to reduce risk of stroke leading to cognitive decline and dementia.
- Stay mentally active. Mentally stimulating activities or cognitive training to enhance problem solving, memory, and speed of processing.
- While the evidence for diet in delaying or preventing cognitive decline is inconsistent, research suggests adopting eating patterns recommended by the Dietary Guidelines such as the Mediterranean diet or combination of the Mediterranean and DASH (Dietary Approaches to Stop Hypertension) eating patterns may reduce the risk of Alzheimer's disease and slow the cognitive decline. This combination diet is referred to as the MIND (Mediterranean–DASH Intervention for Neurodegenerative Delay) diet.

- Hearing should be assessed and managed as hearing loss is significantly associated with dementia. Rather than asking if someone has hearing loss, ask if they have difficulty hearing in their everyday life.
- Adequate sleep. Anyone suspected of having sleep apnea should be referred to the doctor for treatment.
- Remain socially active. Social activity not only makes physical and mental activity more enjoyable, it can reduce stress levels, which helps maintain healthy connections among brain cells.

Data from National Academies of Sciences, Engineering, and Medicine. *Preventing Cognitive Decline and Dementia: A Way Forward.* The National Academies Press; 2017; van den Brink AC, Brouwer-Brolsma EM, Berendsen AAM, van de Rest O. The Mediterranean Dietary Approaches to Stop Hypertension (DASH), and Mediterranean-DASH Intervention for Neurodegenerative Delay (MIND) diets are associated with less cognitive decline and a lower risk of Alzheimer's disease—a review. *Adv Nutr.* 2019;10(6):1040–1065; Ismail Z, Black SE, Camicioli R, et al. Recommendations of the 5th Canadian Consensus Conference on the diagnosis and treatment of dementia. Alzheimer Demen. 2020;16(8):1182–1195.

◆ CASE APPLICATION FOR THE DENTAL HYGIENIST

A young female executive confides in you that she always feels tired and sometimes finds it difficult to get through the day. When you bring up the subject of nutrition, she tells you that she read a book about the importance of minerals and began taking supplements approximately 1 year ago. These self-prescribed supplements included selenium and zinc. She also takes vitamin C supplement daily. She is concerned about her lack of energy, which she relates to her poor eating habits. Meals are frequently missed or eaten at her desk.

Nutritional Assessment

- Assess readiness to change health behavior
- Knowledge level regarding food consumption guidelines, such as the *MyPlate* and the *Dietary Guidelines*
- Desire for improving nutritional and general health
- Cultural or religious influences
- Knowledge of the physiological roles of vitamins and minerals
- Recognition of the interactive effects of vitamins and minerals, especially when taken in excess of RDAs

Nutritional Diagnosis

Health-seeking behaviors related to inadequate knowledge of optimal nutrition, healthy eating habits, and the deleterious effects associated with consumption of excess vitamins and minerals.

Nutritional Goals

The patient will use the *Dietary Guidelines* and *MyPlate* to focus on healthy eating patterns and dietary intake of nutrient-dense foods rather than individual trace minerals. The patient will recognize the health risks associated with improper supplementation and will decrease reliance on supplements.

Nutritional Implementation

Intervention: Review the *Dietary Guidelines* and discuss how these guidelines support healthy eating patterns for disease prevention.
Rationale: Healthy eating patterns can improve energy reserves and overall nutritional status.
Intervention: Encourage consumption of a variety of foods from each of the five main food groups.

Rationale: A healthy eating pattern is composed of a variety of foods that together supply all the essential nutrients needed for good health.
Intervention: Review serving sizes and emphasize more servings of nutrient-dense foods. Encourage a meal timetable that is planned according to her daily schedule.
Rationale: Eating an inadequate number of calories from foods containing limited nutrients can contribute to fatigue and poor nutrition. Advance planning and a schedule of mealtimes throughout the day help to supply an adequate number of calories when appropriate serving sizes of nutritious food are selected.
Intervention: Describe the body's metabolic need for vitamins and minerals. Inform the patient that a healthy eating pattern can supply all the nutrients needed without supplementation.
Rationale: Vitamins and minerals are required for normal metabolic and physiologic functions. When supplements are taken in excess of the RDAs, some nutrients can be harmful.
Intervention: Describe how zinc supplements interact with copper absorption and relate to fatigue. Inform the patient that large amounts of vitamin C in excess of the RDAs may decrease the availability of copper in the blood. List the toxic effects of selenium.
Rationale: Because most minerals are supplied by a varied diet, supplementation can result in toxic levels and harmful nutrient interactions.
Intervention: Advise the patient to see her health care provider if fatigue persists or worsens.
Rationale: Poor eating patterns may act as a contributing factor to fatigue when the actual cause may be related to a systemic disease or condition.

Evaluation

The patient will improve eating patterns by planning meals and snacks each day. Meal planning will accommodate the patient's work schedule. The patient will use *MyPlate* and the *Dietary Guidelines* to improve the nutritional quality and quantity of her diet. The patient can state the symptoms associated with large quantities of zinc, selenium, and vitamin C, and will stop taking supplements. Persistent or worsening symptoms of fatigue will prompt the patient to seek the advice of a health care provider.

◆ Student Readiness

1. List all nutrient interactions indicated in this chapter that decrease the absorption or alter the metabolism of another nutrient. Why would a dental hygienist advise a patient to obtain mineral requirements from food sources rather than mineral supplements (unless ordered by a health care provider)?
2. Which trace minerals incorporated into enamel are beneficial? Which of them weaken the teeth or make them more susceptible to decay?
3. Which trace mineral is involved in insulin metabolism?
4. If a patient is concerned about obtaining adequate amounts of trace minerals, what are some suggestions that a dental hygienist can give?
5. Name some trace minerals (or ultratrace minerals) that may be useful as well as toxic to patients.

References

1. Office of Dietary Supplements, National Institutes of Health. *Copper: Fact Sheets for Health Professionals.* 2022. https://ods.od.nih.gov/factsheets/Copper-HealthProfessional/

2. Klimuszko E, Orywal K, Sierpinska T, Sidun J, Golebiewska M. The evaluation of zinc and copper content in tooth enamel without any pathological changes – an in vitro study. *Int J Nanomedicine.* 2018;13:1257–1264.

3. Brookes SJ, Shore RC, Robinson C, Wood SR, Kirkham J. Copper ions inhibit the demineralisation of human enamel. *Arch Oral Biol.* 2003;48(1):25–30.

4. Institute of Medicine, Panel on Micronutrients. *Dietary Reference Intakes for Vitamin A, Vitamin K, Arsenic, Boron, Chromium, Copper, Iodine, Iron, Manganese, Molybdenum, Nickel, Silicon, Vanadium, and Zinc.* National Academies Press; 2001. https://www.ncbi.nlm.nih.gov/books/NBK222322/.

5. Agricultural Research Service, USDA. *What We Eat in America, NHANES 2017–2020.* Food Surveys Research Group; 2022. https://www.ars.usda.gov/ARSUserFiles/80400530/pdf/1720/Table_1_NIN_GEN_1720.pdf

6. National Institute of Diabetes and Digestive and Kidney. *Symptoms & Causes of Wilson disease.* 2018. https://www.niddk.nih.gov/health-information/liver-disease/wilson-disease/symptoms-causes

7. Kieliszek M. Selenium–fascinating microelement, properties, and sources in food. *Molecules.* 2019;24(7):1298.

8. Office of Dietary Supplements. *Selenium: Fact Sheet for Health Professionals.* 2021. https://ods.od.nih.gov/factsheets/Selenium-HealthProfessional/

9. Xue G, Liu R. Association between dietary selenium intake and bone mineral density in the United States general population. *Ann Transl Med.* 2022;10(16):869.

10. Niu R, Yang Q, Dong Y, Hou Y, Liu G. Selenium metabolism and regulation of immune cells in immune-associated diseases. *J Cell Physiol.* 2022;237(9):3449–3464. https://doi.org/10.1002/jcp.30824.

11. Saghiri MA, Vakhnovetsky J, Vakhnovetsky A, Morgano SM. Functional role of inorganic trace elements in dentin apatite tissue—part III: Se, F, Ag, and B. *J Trace Elem Med Biol.* 2022;72:126990.

12. Institute of Medicine, Panel on Micronutrients. *Dietary Reference Intakes for Vitamin C, Vitamin E, Selenium, and Carotenoids.* National Academies Press; 2000. https://nap.nationalacademies.org/catalog/9810/dietary-reference-intakes-for-vitamin-c-vitamin-e-selenium-and-carotenoids.

13. Sekhri P, Sandhu M, Sachdev V, Chopra R. Estimation of trace elements in mixed saliva of caries free and caries active children. *J Clin Pediatr Dent.* 2018;42(2):135–139.

14. AlShahrani SS, AlAbbas MS, Garcia IM, et al. The antibacterial effects of resin-based dental sealants: a systematic review of in vitro studies. *Materials.* 2021;14(2):413.

15. Gaur S, Agnihotri R. Trace mineral micronutrients and chronic periodontitis-a review. *Biol Trace Elem Res.* 2017;176(2):225–238.

16. Inonu E, Hakki SS, Kayis SA, Nielsen FH. The association between some macro and trace elements in saliva and periodontal status. *Biol Trace Elem Res.* 2020;197(1):35–42.

17. Office of Dietary Supplements. *Chromium—Fact Sheet for Health Professionals.* 2022. https://ods.od.nih.gov/factsheets/Chromium-HealthProfessional/

18. Shashikiran ND, Subba Reddy VV, Hiremath MC. Estimation of trace elements in sound and carious enamel of primary and permanent teeth by atomic absorption spectrophotometry: an in vitro study. *Indian J Dent Res.* 2007;18(4):157–162.

19. Gierat-Kucharzewska B, Braziewicz J, Majewska U, Gódz S, Karasinski A. Concentration of selected elements in the roots and crowns of both primary and permanent teeth with caries disease. *Biol Trace Elem Res.* 2003;96(1–3):159–167.

20. EFSA Panel on Dietetic Products, Nutrition and Allergies (NDA). Scientific opinion on dietary reference values for chromium. *EFSA J.* 2014;12(10):3845.

21. United States Environmental Protection Agency. *Chromium in Drinking Water.* 2023. https://www.epa.gov/sdwa/chromium-drinking-water

22. Office of Dietary Supplements. *Manganese: Fact Sheet for Health Professionals.* 2021. https://ods.od.nih.gov/factsheets/manganese-HealthProfessional/

23. Pennington JA, Young BE. Total diet study nutritional elements, 1982–1989. *J Am Diet Assoc.* 1991;91(2):179–183.

24. Martin KV, Edmondson D, Cecil KM, et al. Manganese exposure and neurologic outcomes in adult populations. *Neurol Clin.* 2020;38(4):913–936.

25. Linus Pauling Institute. *Manganese.* Linus Pauling Institute; 2021. https://lpi.oregonstate.edu/mic/minerals/manganese

26. Office of Dietary Supplements. *Molybdenum: Fact Sheet for Health Professionals.* 2021. https://ods.od.nih.gov/factsheets/Molybdenum-HealthProfessional/

27. Office of Dietary Supplements. *Boron: Fact Sheet for Health Professionals.* 2022. https://ods.od.nih.gov/factsheets/Boron-HealthProfessional/

28. Nielsen FH, Eckhert CD. Boron. *Adv Nutr.* 2020;11(2):461–462.

29. Mitruţ I, Scorei IR, Manolea HO, et al. Boron-containing compounds in dentistry: a narrative review. *Rom J Morphol Embryol.* 2022;63(3):477–483.

30. Cubadda F, Iacoponi F, Ferraris F, et al. Dietary exposure of the Italian population to nickel: The National Total Diet Study. *Food Chem Toxicol.* 2020;146:111813.

31. Rondanelli M, Faliva MA, Peroni G, et al. Silicon: a neglected micronutrient essential for bone health. *Exp Biol Med.* 2021;246(13):1500–1511.

32. Agency for Toxic Substances and Disease Registry. *Tin and Compounds: ToxFAQsTM.* Toxic Substances Portal; 2014. https://wwwn.cdc.gov/TSP/ToxFAQs/ToxFAQsDetails.aspx?faqid=542&toxid=98

33. Lehmler HJ, Gadogbe M, Liu B, Bao W. Environmental tin exposure in a nationally representative sample of United States adults and children: the National Health and Nutrition Examination Survey 2011–2014. *Environ Pollut.* 2018;240:599–606.

34. Klotz K, Weistenhöfer W, Neff F, Hartwig A, van Thriel C, Drexler H. The health effects of aluminum exposure. *Dtsch Arztebl Int.* 2017;114(39):653–659.

35. Environmental Protection Agency. *Basic Information About Lead in Drinking Water.* 2023. https://www.epa.gov/ground-water-and-drinking-water/basic-information-about-lead-drinking-water

36. Brown TA. *Confirmatory Factor Analysis for Applied Research.* The Guilford Press; 2006.

37. Levallois P, Barn P, Valcke M, Gauvin D, Kosatsky T. Public health consequences of lead in drinking water. *Curr Environ Health Rep.* 2018;5(2):255–262.

38. Heidari S, Mostafaei S, Razazian N, Rajati M, Saeedi A, Rajati F. Correlation between lead exposure and cognitive function in 12-year-old children: a systematic review and *meta*-analysis. *Environ Sci Pollut Res Int.* 2021;28(32):43064–43073.

39. Heidari S, Mostafaei S, Razazian N, Rajati M, Saeedi A, Rajati F. The effect of lead exposure on IQ test scores in children under 12 years: a systematic review and *meta*-analysis of case-control studies. *Syst Rev.* 2022;11(1):106.

40. Wu Y, Jansen EC, Peterson KE, et al. The associations between lead exposure at multiple sensitive life periods and dental caries risks in permanent teeth. *Sci Total Environ.* 2019;654:1048–1055.

41. Saghiri MA, Vakhnovetsky J, Vakhnovetsky A. Functional role of inorganic trace elements in dentin apatite—Part II: Copper, manganese, silicon, and lithium. *J Trace Elem Med Biol.* 2022;72:126995.

42. Scibior A, Pietrzyk Ł, Plewa Z, Skiba A. Vanadium: risks and possible benefits in the light of a comprehensive overview of its pharmacotoxicological mechanisms and multi-applications with a summary of further research trends. *J Trace Elem Med Biol.* 2020;61:126508.

43. Aaseth J, Hilt B, Bjørklund G. Mercury exposure and health impacts in dental personnel. *Environ Res.* 2018;164:65–69.

44. Saavedra S, Fernández-Recamales Á, Sayago A, Cervera-Barajas A, González-Domínguez R, Gonzalez-Sanz JD. Impact of dietary mercury intake during pregnancy on the health of neonates and children: a systematic review. *Nutr Rev.* 2022;80(2):317–328.

45. Tang Y, Yi Q, Wang S, Xia Y, Geng B. Normal concentration range of blood mercury and bone mineral density: a cross-sectional study of National Health and Nutrition Examination Survey (NHANES) 2005–2010. *Environ Sci Pollut Res Int.* 2022;29(5):7743–7757.

46. Food and Drug Administration, Center for Food Safety and Applied Nutrition. *Mercury in Food and Dietary Supplements.* FDA; 2023. https://www.fda.gov/food/environmental-contaminants-food/mercury-food-and-dietary-supplements

47. United States Department of Agriculture, United States Department of Health and Human Services. *Dietary Guidelines for Americans.* 9th ed. 2020. dietaryguidelines.gov

48. World Health Organization. *Dementia.* 2021. https://www.who.int/news-room/fact-sheets/detail/dementia

49. Alzheimer's Association, Gaugler J, James B, Johnson T, Reimer J, Weuve J. 2021 Alzheimer's disease facts and figures. *Alzheimers Dement.* 2021;17(3):327–406.

50. National Institute on Aging. *Symptoms and Diagnosis of Alzheimer's Disease: What Are the Signs of Alzheimer's Disease?* National Institute on Aging; 2022. https://www.nia.nih.gov/health/what-are-signs-alzheimers-disease

51. Ismail Z, Black SE, Camicioli R, et al. Recommendations of the 5th Canadian Consensus Conference on the diagnosis and treatment of dementia. *Alzheimer Demen.* 2020;16(8):1182–1195.

52. van den Brink AC, Brouwer-Brolsma EM, Berendsen AAM, van de Rest O. The Mediterranean, dietary approaches to stop hypertension (DASH), and Mediterranean-DASH intervention for

neurodegenerative delay (MIND) diets are associated with less cognitive decline and a lower risk of Alzheimer's disease—a review. *Adv Nutr.* 2019;10(6):1040–1065.

53. Schwahn C, Frenzel S, Holtfreter B, et al. Effect of periodontal treatment on preclinical Alzheimer's disease—results of a trial emulation approach. *Alzheimer Demen.* 2022;18(1):127–141.

54. Alzheimer's Association. Medications for memory, cognition and dementia-related behaviors. In: *Alzheimer's Disease and Dementia*; 2023. https://alz.org/alzheimers-dementia/treatments/medications-for-memory

55. Food and Drug Administration. *FDA 101: Dietary Supplements.* FDA; 2022. https://www.fda.gov/consumers/consumer-updates/fda-101-dietary-supplements

56. Food and Drug Administration. *Watch Out for False Promises About So-Called Alzheimer's Cures.* FDA; 2021. https://www.fda.gov/consumers/consumer-updates/watch-out-false-promises-about-so-called-alzheimers-cures

57. Alzheimer's Association. Alternative treatments. In: *Alzheimer's Disease and Dementia*; 2023. https://alz.org/alzheimers-dementia/treatments/alternative-treatments

58. Palimariciuc M, Balmus IM, Gireadă B, et al. The quest for neurodegenerative disease treatment-focusing on Alzheimer's disease personalised diets. *Curr Issues Mol Biol.* 2023;45(2):1519–1535.

59. Shah H, Dehghani F, Ramezan M, et al. Revisiting the role of vitamins and minerals in Alzheimer's disease. *Antioxidants.* 2023;12(2):415.

60. Lauriola M, Mangiacotti A, D'Onofrio G, et al. Neurocognitive disorders and dehydration in older patients: clinical experience supports the hydromolecular hypothesis of dementia. *Nutrients.* 2018;10(5):562.

61. Wittbrodt MT, Millard-Stafford M. Dehydration impairs cognitive performance: a *meta*-analysis. *Med Sci Sports Exercise.* 2018;50(11):2360.

62. Loeffler DA. Modifiable, non-modifiable, and clinical factors associated with progression of Alzheimer's disease. *J Alzheimers Dis.* 2021;80(1):1–27.

63. Doorduijn AS, de van der Schueren MAE, van de Rest O, et al. Nutritional status is associated with clinical progression in Alzheimer's disease: the NUDAD project. *J Am Med Dir Assoc.* 2023;24(5):638–644.

▶ Evolve Resources

Please visit http://evolve.elsevier.com/Mallonee/nutritional for additional practice and study support tools.

11

Vitamins Required for Oral Soft Tissues and Salivary Glands

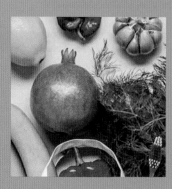

STUDENT LEARNING OBJECTIVES

On completion of this chapter, the student will be able to achieve the following learning objectives:

1. Describe the physiology of soft tissues.
2. Discuss the following related to thiamin (vitamin B_1):
   - Describe the physiologic roles of thiamin, as well as list the Recommended Dietary Allowance (RDA) and sources of thiamin.
   - Identify dental considerations and nutritional directions for hypo states related to thiamin.
3. Discuss the following related to riboflavin (vitamin B_2):
   - Describe the physiologic roles of riboflavin, as well as list the Recommended Dietary Allowance (RDA) and sources of riboflavin.
   - Identify dental considerations and nutritional directions for hypo states related to riboflavin.
4. Discuss the following related to niacin (vitamin B_3), pantothenic acid (vitamin B_5), and vitamin B_6 (Pyridoxine):
   - Describe the physiologic roles of each vitamin, as well as list the Recommended Dietary Allowance (RDA) and sources of each.

- Identify dental considerations and nutritional directions for hyper and hypo states related to each vitamin.
5. Discuss the following related to folate/folic acid, vitamin B_{12} (Cobalamin), and biotin (vitamin B_7):
   - Describe the physiologic roles of each vitamin, as well as list the Recommended Dietary Allowance (RDA) and sources of each.
   - Explain to a patient who is vegan why vitamin B_{12} is important.
   - Identify dental considerations and nutritional directions for hyper and hypo states related to each vitamin.
6. Discuss the importance of vitamins C, A, and E in oral soft tissues and salivary glands.

KEY TERMS

Achlorhydria
Antigenic
Ariboflavinosis
Ataxia
Avidin
Beriberi
Bradycardia
Candida
Cheilosis
Cholinergic
Circumvallate lingual papillae
Epithelialization
Filiform papillae
Foliate papillae

Fungating
Fungiform papillae
Glossitis
Glossopyrosis
Hypotonic
Intrinsic factor
Keratinized epithelium
Megaloblastic anemia
Myelin
Neoplasia
Neural tube defects
Nystagmus
Parasympathetic autonomic nerves
Pellagra

Periodontal disease
Pernicious anemia
Pyogenic
R-binder
Sensory neuropathy
Signs
Squamous metaplasia
Stomatitis
Sympathetic autonomic nerves
Symptoms
Tachycardia
Thiaminase

✦ TEST YOUR NQ

1. **T/F** Milk is a good source of riboflavin.
2. **T/F** Vitamin B_6 is the sunshine vitamin.
3. **T/F** Beriberi is caused by niacin deficiency.
4. **T/F** Vegans may be prone to vitamin B_{12} deficiency.
5. **T/F** Complaints of flushing and intestinal disturbances are symptoms of thiamin toxicity.
6. **T/F** A smooth purplish red or magenta tongue may be observed in patients with vitamin B_6 deficiency.
7. **T/F** Enriched breads and cereals are good sources of thiamin.
8. **T/F** Carrots are a good source of folate.
9. **T/F** Thiamin requirement is determined by one's energy requirement.
10. **T/F** The first signs of a nutritional deficiency often occur in the oral cavity.

Physiology of Soft Tissues

The oral cavity can reflect systemic disease before other signs (noticeable to the clinician) and symptoms (perceived by the patient) become evident; the condition of the oral cavity may also cause systemic problems by affecting the patient's nutrient intake. The oral cavity is the site of a wide variety of systemic disease manifestations for several reasons: (1) it has a rapid cellular turnover rate, (2) it is under constant assault by microorganisms, and (3) it is a trauma-intense environment.

The systemic circulation provides nutrients and removes metabolic waste products from underlying structures and the salivary glands via the blood supply. Fig. 11.1 shows healthy gingiva; changes in color, size, shape, texture, and functional integrity of the oral tissues often reflect systemic nutritional disorders. Signs and symptoms in soft oral tissues can be caused by deficiencies of many of the B-complex vitamins, vitamins A, C and E. (Box 11.1). Nutritional deficiencies result in similar oral signs and symptoms, such as pain, erythema, atrophy of tissues, and infection. Pyogenic (producing pus) and fungating (skin lesions with ulcerations, necrosis, and foul smell) microorganisms cause local infections in cracked epithelial surfaces. Approximately 90% of saliva is produced and secreted by three paired sets of major salivary glands: the parotid, submandibular, and sublingual glands (Fig. 11.2). Additionally, the lips and inner lining of the cheeks are equipped with hundreds of minor salivary glands.

Saliva keeps surfaces of the oral cavity healthy and lubricated and is necessary to maintain functional integrity of taste buds. Solid substances first must be dissolved in saliva to be tasted. Healthy adults produce approximately 1 to 1.5 L/day of saliva. Sympathetic autonomic nerves stimulate the body in times of stress and crisis; sympathetic impulses influence salivary composition. Parasympathetic autonomic nerves balance or slow down impulses from sympathetic nerves; parasympathetic stimulation increases the amount of saliva secreted.

Compared with plasma, saliva is hypotonic, with its main constituent being water. Hypotonic solutions have a lower solute concentration than plasma. Saliva contains more than 20 proteins and glycoproteins along with many electrolytes, including sodium, potassium, calcium, chloride, bicarbonate, inorganic phosphate, magnesium, sulfate, iodide, and fluoride. Saliva functions as a buffer to maintain the oral pH. Buffering substances resist changing the pH of the solution. The pH of unstimulated saliva is approximately 6.1, but this can rise to 7.8 at high flow rates. Antimicrobial properties of saliva provide protective benefits.

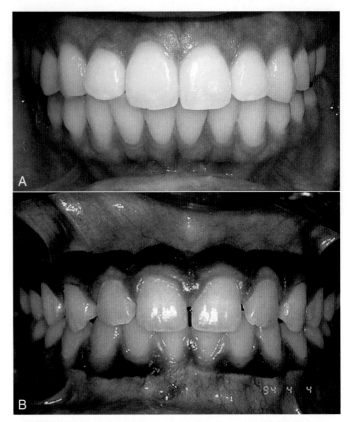

• **Fig. 11.1** Healthy gingiva. (A) Light-skinned individual. (B) Physiologic pigmentation in gingiva of dark-skinned individual. (From Perry DA, Essex G. *Periodontology for the Dental Hygienist*. 4th ed. Elsevier Saunders; 2014.)

• BOX 11.1	Vitamins Required for Healthy Oral Soft Tissues

Water-Soluble Vitamins

B Vitamins
    Thiamin
    Riboflavin
    Niacin
    Pantothenic acid
    Pyridoxine
    Biotin
    Folate
    Cobalamin
Vitamin C

Fat-Soluble Vitamins

Vitamin A
Vitamin E

The oral cavity is lined with nonkeratinized mucosa except for the hard palate, dorsum of the tongue, and gingiva surrounding the teeth, which are covered with a keratinized epithelium (a protein, the main component of the epidermis and horny tissues). The oral cavity may contain antigenic (capable of inducing an immune response with specific antibodies) substances; the oral mucosa separates a potentially adverse environment from underlying connective tissue.

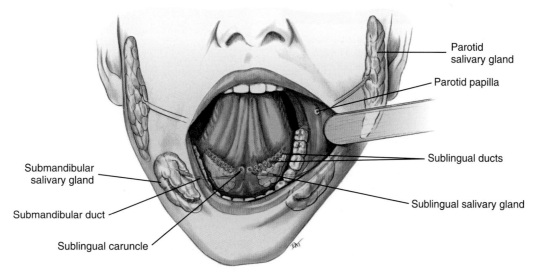

• **Fig. 11.2** The major salivary glands and associated structures. (From Fehrenbach MJ, Herring SW. *Illustrated Anatomy of the Head and Neck*. 4th ed. Elsevier Saunders; 2012.)

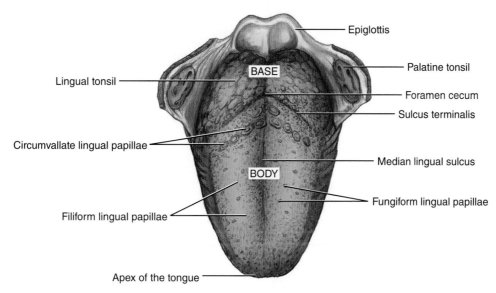

• **Fig. 11.3** Papillae on the tongue with its landmarks noted. (Reproduced with permission from Fehrenbach MJ, Herring SW. *Illustrated Anatomy of the Head and Neck*. 4th ed. Philadelphia, PA: Elsevier Saunders; 2012.)

Mucosal cells have a very rapid turnover rate, resulting in complete turnover in 3 to 5 days. Rapid generation of new cells in the oral epithelia provides replacement tissue for trauma resulting from friction of the teeth and mastication. Additionally, hundreds of cells in the filiform papillae and fungiform papillae are in constant transition, from their anabolism until their catabolism (Fig. 11.3). Filiform papillae are smooth, threadlike structures on the dorsum surface of the tongue, whereas fungiform papillae are red, mushroom-shaped structures scattered throughout the filiform papillae. There are greater numbers of fungiform papillae at the tip of the tongue.

Taste buds are located on the foliate papillae (vertical grooves located on the lateral borders of the tongue), circumvallate lingual papillae (large, mushroom-shaped distinct structures forming a V) on the dorsal surface, and the fungiform papillae of the tongue. Atrophy of fungiform and foliate papillae leads to the loss of taste buds and changes in taste acuity.

Many filiform papillae cover the anterior two-thirds of the tongue. If the filiform papillae become denuded or atrophied, the tongue appears red and pebbled, giving it a strawberry-like appearance. Fungiform papillae are bright red because of a rich vascular supply. Keratinized cells normally cover the fungiform papillae on the tongue surface. Chronic severe nutrient deficiencies result in the loss of fungiform papillae and a smooth red tongue.

🦷 DENTAL CONSIDERATIONS

- Because of rapid turnover rate of oral tissues, the first signs of nutritional deficiency are frequently evident in the oral cavity. The epithelium of the tongue is usually the first to be affected, followed by areas around the lips. Assess patients for oral signs of nutritional deficiencies.
- The tongue may become edematous as a result of disease or nutritional deficiency.

🔷 DENTAL CONSIDERATIONS—CONT'D

- Angular cheilitis or cheilosis (cracks around the corners of the mouth; Fig. 11.5) and glossitis (inflammation of the tongue; Figs. 11.4 and 11.6) are commonly associated with deficiencies of several B-complex vitamins.
- Saliva aids in the ability to speak properly, and taste and swallow foods.
- The composition of saliva affects taste and can be a determining factor in food choices.
- Xerostomia may result in increased incidence of caries, stomatitis (inflammation of oral mucosa), gingival inflammation, and greater susceptibility to oral infections.
- Saliva may be used to diagnose some local and systemic diseases and heavy-metal toxicity, such as mercury toxicity.
- Salivary secretion is controlled primarily by cholinergic (nerves stimulated by acetylcholine) parasympathetic (autonomic) nerves; patients taking anticholinergic medications (which usually contain atropine) exhibit decreased salivary flow. These medications may be prescribed for bradycardia (low heart rate), diarrhea, peptic ulcers, and occasionally asthma.

🔷 NUTRITIONAL DIRECTIONS

- Saliva helps maintain integrity of the teeth, tongue, and mucous membranes of the oral and oropharyngeal areas.
- Nutritional abnormalities affect oral soft tissues in a variety of ways (e.g., angular cheilitis and glossitis).
- The RDA is higher than the average need for an individual. If the amount consumed is slightly under the listed RDA, most individuals will still be healthy. However, the lower the requirement of a vitamin or mineral, the greater the risk of a deficiency.

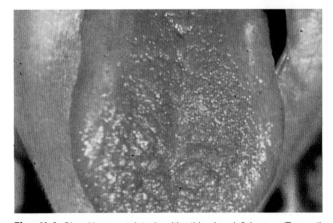

• **Fig. 11.4** Glossitis associated with thiamin deficiency. (From the American Dental Association Council on Dental Therapeutics. *Oral Manifestations of Metabolic and Deficiency Changes.*)

Thiamin (Vitamin B₁)

Physiologic Roles

Thiamin functions as a coenzyme in metabolism of energy nutrients via the TCA cycle (or Krebs or citric acid cycle) to produce energy. This role makes it crucial for normal functioning of the brain, nerves, muscles, and heart. However, the main effects of thiamin deficiency are disturbances of carbohydrate metabolism,

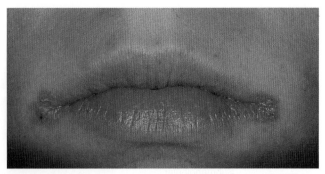

• **Fig. 11.5** Angular cheilitis. (Reproduced with permission from Ibsen OAC, Phelan JA. *Oral Pathology for the Dental Hygienist*. 6th ed, St. Louis, MO: Elsevier Saunders; 2014.)

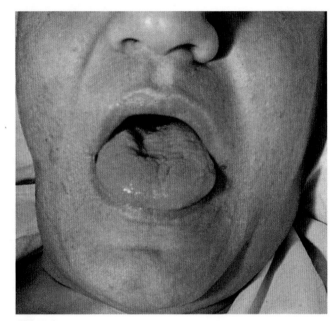

• **Fig. 11.6** Glossitis associated with severe riboflavin deficiency. (From McLaren DS. *A Colour Atlas and Text of Diet-Related Disorders*. 2nd ed. Mosby-Year Book; 1992.)

which is impossible without thiamin. Thiamin is a component necessary for the synthesis of niacin, and it also helps regulate appetite. It is a constituent of enzymes that degrade sucrose to organic acids that can ultimately dissolve tooth enamel.

Requirements

Thiamin is involved in using carbohydrates for energy; the requirement is based on total calorie need. The Recommended Dietary Allowance (RDA) for males (≥14 years old) is 1.2 mg/day and for females (≥19 years old) is 1.1 mg/day (Table 11.1). Participation in rigorous physical activity uses more energy, which requires more thiamin. Also, requirements are increased by pregnancy and lactation, hemodialysis or peritoneal dialysis, fever, hyperthyroidism, cardiac conditions, bariatric surgery, alcohol use disorder, and the use of loop diuretics. No known adverse effects are evident from excessive thiamin intake, including supplements. Although a Tolerable Upper Intake Level (UL) is not established for thiamin, care should be taken when consumption routinely exceeds the RDA.

TABLE 11.1   National Academy of Medicine Recommendations for Thiamin

Life Stage	EAR (mg/day) Male	EAR (mg/day) Female	RDA (mg/day) Male	RDA (mg/day) Female	AI (mg/day)
0–6 months					0.2
7–12 months					0.3
1–3 years	0.4	0.4	0.5	0.5	
4–8 years	0.5	0.5	0.6	0.6	
9–13 years	0.7	0.7	0.9	0.9	
14–18 years	1	1	1.2	1	
≥19 years	1	0.9	1.2	1.1	
Pregnancy					
14–50 years		1.2		1.4	
Lactation					
14–50 years		1.2		1.4	

AI, Adequate intake, *EAR*, estimated average requirement; *RDA*, recommended dietary allowance.
Data from Institute of Medicine (IOM), Food and Nutrition Board. *Dietary Reference Intakes for Thiamin, Riboflavin, Niacin, Vitamin B₆, Folate, Vitamin B₁₂, Pantothenic Acid, Biotin, and Choline.* National Academy Press; 1998.

TABLE 11.2   Thiamin Content of Selected Foods

Food	Portion	Thiamin (mg)
Lean pork chop, broiled	4 oz	0.78
Black beans, boiled	½ cup	0.4
English muffin, plain, enriched	1	0.3
Macaroni, whole wheat, cooked	1 cup	0.2
Peas acorn squash, cubed, baked	½ cup	0.2
White rice, enriched, cooked	1 cup	0.1
Sweet potato, baked	1 cup	0.1
Bread, whole wheat	1 slice	0.1
Sunflower seeds, toasted	1 oz	0.1

Data from National Institutes of Health. Office of Dietary Supplements. *Thiamin Fact Sheet for Health Professionals.* https://ods.od.nih.gov/factsheets/Thiamin-HealthProfessional/U.S; Department of Agriculture (USDA), Agricultural Research Service. *Food Data Central 2019.* https://fdc.nal.usda.gov/fdc-app.html#/food-details/168251/nutrients.

Sources

Thiamin is widely distributed in foods, and intake of a variety of foods, including enriched grains or whole grains, can ensure adequate amounts (Table 11.2). The most common sources of thiamin are enriched breads, cereals, and pasta. Enriched grains may contain almost twice as much thiamin as whole grains. In the protein group, pork is an exceptionally good source. Other good sources include nuts and legumes. Following the recommendations of the *MyPlate* website and the *Dietary Guidelines*, which both emphasize eating a variety of foods, ensures adequate intake.

Hypo States

Thiamin is required for metabolism of carbohydrates, proteins, and fats; insufficient intake adversely affects most organ systems. Primary dietary deficiency usually occurs in developing countries where polished rice is the staple diet. In developed countries, thiamin deficiency is secondary to alcoholism, ingestion of raw fish containing microbial thiaminase (an enzyme that inactivates thiamin), chronic febrile states, and total parenteral nutrition (TPN). Cooking deactivates thiaminase.

Thiamin is often called the "morale vitamin" because short-term deficiency may cause depression, irritability, weight loss and anorexia, fatigue, and inability to concentrate.[1] The brain and central nervous system, almost entirely dependent on glucose for energy, are seriously impaired when thiamin is unavailable.

Severe thiamin deficiency results in beriberi, which causes extensive damage to the nervous and cardiovascular systems. There are two major types of beriberi: wet beriberi which affects the cardiovascular system and dry beriberi which affects the central nervous system. The classic chronic form of beriberi manifests with impairment of sensory and motor function without involvement of the central nervous system. Symptoms of dry beriberi include muscular wasting, and diminished reflexes. Symptoms of wet beriberi include edema, deep muscle pain in the calves, peripheral paralysis, tachycardia (rapid heartbeat), and an enlarged heart that may result in congestive heart failure.

A thiamin deficiency in infancy may result in less calcified and smaller percentage of inorganic material in enamel.[2] Whether or not a thiamin deficiency is evident in oral tissues is controversial. Some clinicians have associated a flabby, red, and edematous tongue with thiamin deficiency (see Fig. 11.4). The fungiform papillae become enlarged and hyperemic or swollen in appearance due to excess blood.

Wernicke-Korsakoff syndrome is another thiamin deficiency disease, typically associated with alcoholism, which is characterized by mental confusion, nystagmus (involuntary rapid movement of the eyeball), and ataxia (a gait disorder characterized by uncoordinated muscle movements). These symptoms occur most frequently in malnourished alcoholics. Alcohol intake increases thiamin requirement, yet total nutrient intake is usually poor in alcoholics. Early diagnosis is essential to initiate thiamin therapy early in the course of the disease to prevent permanent damage and death.

DENTAL CONSIDERATIONS

- A careful medical, social, and dietary history—including a clinical assessment of the oral cavity, alcohol consumption, and activity level—helps identify early stages of thiamin deficiency.
- Risk of alcohol abuse or dependence is based on how much and how often an individual drinks. Moderation is considered 2 drinks or less a day for males and 1 drink or less a day for females. Heavy drinking is defined as more than 4 drinks per day or more than 14 drinks per week for males and more than 3 drinks per day or more than 7 drinks per week for females; 5 or more drinks per occasion is considered excessive for any adult.[3]
- Vitamin deficiencies seldom occur in isolation. If a deficiency is suspected, symptoms of other vitamin B deficiencies may also be present.

DENTAL CONSIDERATIONS—CONT'D

- Because thiamin is essential for carbohydrate metabolism, a thiamin deficiency is closely linked to abnormalities of brain function. For patients who are confused or have altered thought processes, referral to a primary care provider or an RDN may be indicated to further assess health status and nutrient intake.
- Carbohydrate loading or a very-high-carbohydrate diet and high physical activity slightly increase the thiamin requirement.
- Thiamin deficiency has been reported in patients after gastrectomy and bariatric surgery (gastric bypass) related to decreased absorption.

NUTRITIONAL DIRECTIONS

- Certain products such as tea, coffee, raw fish, and shelf fish contain an active enzyme, thiaminase, which destroys thiamin.[4]
- Baking soda added to cooking water to enhance the color of vegetables can destroy thiamin.[5]
- Overcooking and high temperatures destroy thiamin. [6]
- Antacids reduce use of thiamin[7]
- Some diuretics can increase thiamin excretion.[7]

Riboflavin (Vitamin B_2)

Physiologic Roles

Riboflavin functions as a coenzyme in metabolism of carbohydrate, protein, and fat to release cellular energy. Closely related to the metabolism of protein, all conditions requiring increases in protein (e.g., growth spurts or burns) lead to additional riboflavin requirements. Riboflavin is also essential for healthy eyes and skin and maintenance of mucous membranes. Along with thiamin, riboflavin is necessary for synthesis of niacin.

Requirements

As shown in Table 11.3, the National Academy of Medicine (formerly the Institute of Medicine) recommends an intake of 1.3 mg/day for males (14 years old and older) and 1.1 mg/day for females (19 years old and older). This level is influenced by individual energy requirements. Additionally, when nitrogen balance is positive, more riboflavin is retained. No UL has been established.

Sources

Although milk and milk products are excellent sources of riboflavin, most dietary intake is furnished by fortified breads and cereals in the grain group Meat, poultry, and fish are also good sources (Table 11.4).

Hypo States

Primary riboflavin deficiency is uncommon but is encountered in patients with multiple nutrient deficiencies as a result of poor nutrient absorption or use. Because riboflavin is essential in vitamin B_6 and niacin functions, riboflavin deficiency leads to symptoms related to secondary deficiency of these nutrients.

TABLE 11.3 National Academy of Medicine Recommendations for Riboflavin

Life Stage	EAR (mg/day) Male	EAR (mg/day) Female	RDA (mg/day) Male	RDA (mg/day) Female	AI (mg/day)
0–6 months					0.3
7–12 months					0.4
1–3 years	0.4	0.4	0.5	0.5	
4–8 years	0.5	0.5	0.6	0.6	
9–13 years	0.8	0.8	0.9	0.9	
14–18 years	1.1	0.9	1.3	1	
≥19 years	1.1	0.9	1.3	1.1	
Pregnancy					
14–50 years		1.2		1.4	
Lactation					
14–50 years		1.3		1.6	

AI, Adequate intake, *EAR*, estimated average requirement; *RDA*, recommended dietary allowance.

Data from Institute of Medicine (IOM), Food and Nutrition Board. *Dietary Reference Intakes for Thiamin, Riboflavin, Niacin, Vitamin B₆, Folate, Vitamin B₁₂, Pantothenic Acid, Biotin, and Choline.* National Academy Press; 1998.

TABLE 11.4 Riboflavin Content of Selected Foods

Food	Portion	Riboflavin (mg)
Beef liver, pan fried	3 oz	2.9
Oats, instant, fortified, cooked with water	1 cup	1.1
Milk, 2 % milkfat	1 cup	0.5
Yogurt, low-fat, 1% milkfat, plain	8 oz	0.37
Cottage cheese, low-fat	1 cup	0.37
Trail mix, regular, with chocolate chips, unsalted nuts and seeds	1 cup	0.33
Egg, whole, scrambled	1 large	0.2
Rotisserie chicken, breast meat only	3 oz	0.2
Bagel, enriched	1 medium, 3½–4 inches diameter	0.2
Quinoa, cooked	1 cup	0.2
Salmon, pink, canned	3 oz	0.2
Spinach, raw	1 cup	0.1

Data from National Institutes of Health. Office of Dietary Supplements. *Riboflavin Fact Sheet for Health Professionals.* https://ods.od.nih.gov/factsheets/Riboflavin-HealthProfessional/; U.S. Department of Agriculture (USDA), Agricultural Research Service. National Agricultural Library. *USDA National Nutrient Database for Standard Reference Legacy.* 2018. https://www.nal.usda.gov/sites/default/files/page-files/riboflavin.pdf.

Symptoms associated with riboflavin deficiency, or ariboflavinosis, include angular cheilitis (see Fig. 11.5), glossitis (see Fig. 11.6), dermatitis, and anemia with pale oral mucosa. Along with angular cheilosis, the lips may become extremely red and smooth. Fungiform papillae become swollen and slightly flattened and mushroom shaped during early stages of riboflavin deficiency; the tongue has a pebbly or granular appearance. Severe chronic deficiencies lead to progressive papillary atrophy and patchy, irregular denudation of the tongue. The tongue may become purplish red or magenta in color because of vascular proliferation and decreased circulation. In more advanced cases, the entire tongue may become atrophic and smooth (see Fig. 11.6). These symptoms, especially glossitis and dermatitis, may be secondary to vitamin B_6 deficiency.

DENTAL CONSIDERATIONS

- Hyperthyroidism, fevers, the added stress of injuries or surgery, excessive alcohol consumption, and malabsorption syndromes increase riboflavin requirements. Assess patients with these conditions for signs of deficiency: cheilitis, papillary atrophy, glossitis, and dermatitis.
- Congenital facial developmental abnormalities such as cleft lip and palate deformities may occur if the mother is deficient in riboflavin at the time of conception.
- Bilateral cheilosis may not be due to riboflavin deficiency; consider improperly constructed dentures, fungal (candidiasis) or yeast infection, and aging that may contribute to cheilosis.
- Some antibiotics may increase excretion of riboflavin; thus monitor for a deficiency in patients on long-term therapy.

NUTRITIONAL DIRECTIONS

- Enriched products provide more riboflavin than their whole-grain counterparts.
- Lighted display cases have the potential to cause decomposition of riboflavin when milk is marketed in translucent plastic containers.
- A mixed diet that contains 2 cups of low-fat milk and 4 to 6 oz of meat protein daily ensures adequate riboflavin intake.
- Vegans and those who consume minimal or no dairy products (e.g., patients who are lactose intolerant) are at risk of developing riboflavin deficiency.
- Riboflavin is not known to be toxic, but there is no benefit from high doses.
- A riboflavin deficiency typically does not occur in isolation but rather is a result of a variety of vitamin B–complex deficiencies.

Niacin (Vitamin B₃)

Physiologic Roles

The term *niacin* is loosely used to refer to two compounds, nicotinic acid and nicotinamide. Both compounds are used by the body. Niacin is crucial as a coenzyme in energy (adenosine triphosphate) production. It functions with riboflavin in glucose production and metabolism and is involved in lipid and protein metabolism. Niacin also functions in enzymes involved in microbial degradation of sucrose to produce organic acids.

Requirements

The body obtains niacin not only directly from food but also indirectly from conversion of an amino acid, tryptophan, and from synthesis by intestinal microorganisms. RDAs are given in terms of niacin equivalents, which include dietary sources of niacin plus its precursor, tryptophan. Approximately 1 mg of niacin may be formed from 60 mg of dietary tryptophan. Niacin requirements are related to caloric intake. The RDA niacin equivalents for adults are 14 to 16 mg daily (Table 11.5). The UL for adults is 35 mg daily. Naturally occurring niacin in foods has not been shown to cause adverse effects.

Sources

Niacin is widely distributed in plant and animal foods. Good sources include meats, fortified cereals, legumes, seeds, and nuts (Table 11.6). The majority of niacin in the United States diet is obtained from meat and milk. Tryptophan is found mainly in milk and meats. The RDA for niacin equivalents is easily met by consuming foods high in niacin and foods containing tryptophan.

Hyper States and Hypo States

Effects of excessive nicotinamide, the water-soluble active form of niacin from supplements has been observed, but not from food or beverage sources. The use of 50 mg of niacin taken daily can function as a vasodilator, producing flushing of the skin, itching, tachycardia, nausea and vomiting, and severe liver damage. Extended-release niacin is associated with few gastrointestinal symptoms without increasing liver damage. Because the body is able to store some niacin, larger doses associated with supplements may lead to serious problems, including abnormal liver function and gout. Supplemental doses of nicotinic acid (1–3 g/day) prescribed by a physician are a treatment option for reducing low-density lipoprotein cholesterol and triglycerides, while increasing high-density lipoprotein cholesterol. (Nicotinamide does not function in this role.) Larger supplemental doses of niacin should be closely monitored by a health care provider.

Niacin deficiency is usually associated with a maize (corn) diet because corn products contain all the essential amino acids except tryptophan. This diet increases the body's requirements for tryptophan and niacin. A deficiency is also seen in alcohol use disorder, malnutrition, and poverty, but is unlikely in individuals who consume adequate protein. Niacin deficiency results in degeneration of the skin, gastrointestinal tract, and nervous system, a condition known as pellagra. Symptoms of pellagra have been referred to as "the 4 Ds"—dermatitis, diarrhea, depression or dementia, and death. The term *pellagra* is derived from the Latin word for animal hide; the skin may become rough and resemble goose flesh. The most striking and characteristic sign of pellagra is a reddish skin rash—especially on the face, hands, or feet—which is always bilaterally symmetrical (i.e., appears on both sides of the body at the same time; Fig. 11.7A). It flares up when skin is exposed to strong sunlight. Neurologic symptoms include depression, apathy, headache, fatigue, and loss of memory. If untreated, it may lead to death.

Deficiency also affects mucous membranes: (1) painful stomatitis causes diminished food intake, and (2) lesions in the gastrointestinal tract result in diarrhea and less vitamin absorption.

TABLE 11.5   Institute of Medicine Recommendations for Niacin

Life Stage	EAR (mg/day)[a] Male	EAR (mg/day)[a] Female	RDA (mg/day) Male	RDA (mg/day) Female	AI (mg/day)[b]	UL (mg/day)
0–6 months					2	ND[c]
7–12 months					4	ND[c]
1–3 years	5	5	6	6		10
4–8 years	6	6	8	8		15
9–13 years	9	9	12	12		20
14–18 years	12	11	16	14		30
≥19 years	12	11	16	14		35
Pregnancy						
14–18 years		14		18		30
≥19 years		14		18		35
Lactation						
14–18 years		13		17		30
≥19 years		13		17		35

[a]Niacin equivalents.

[b]Preformed niacin.

[c]ND—not determinable because of lack of data of adverse effects in this age group and concern with regard to lack of ability to handle excess amounts. Source of intake should be from food and formula to prevent high levels of intake.

AI, Adequate intake; *EAR*, estimated average requirement; *RDA*, recommended dietary allowance; *UL*, tolerable upper intake level.

Data from Institute of Medicine (IOM), Food and Nutrition Board: *Dietary Reference Intakes for Thiamin, Riboflavin, Niacin, Vitamin B$_6$, Folate, Vitamin B$_{12}$, Pantothenic Acid, Biotin, and Choline.* National Academy Press; 1998.

TABLE 11.6   Niacin Content of Selected Foods

Food	Portion	Niacin (mg)
Beef liver, pan fried	3 oz	14.9
Chicken breast, skinless, grilled	3 oz	10.3
Turkey breast, skinless, roasted	3 oz	10.0
Salmon, sockeye cooked	3 oz	8.6
Tuna, light, canned in water	3 oz	8.6
Rice, brown, cooked	1 cup	5.2
Potato, white, baked	1 med	2.3
Rice, enriched white, cooked	1 cup	2.3
Sunflower seeds, dry roasted	1 oz	2.0
Lentils, boiled with or without salt	½ cup	1.06
Cashews, dry roasted	1 oz	0.4
Milk, 1% milkfat	1 cup	0.2

Data from National Institutes of Health. Office of Dietary Supplements. *Niacin Fact Sheet for Health Professionals.* https://ods.od.nih.gov/factsheets/Niacin-HealthProfessional/; U.S. Department of Agriculture (USDA), Agricultural Research Service. National Agricultural Library. *USDA National Nutrient Database for Standard Reference Legacy.* 2018. https://www.nal.usda.gov/sites/default/files/page-files/niacin.pdf.

Pellagrous glossitis begins with swelling of the papillae at the tip and lateral borders of the tongue. The tongue becomes painful, scarlet, and edematous (Fig. 11.7B). Atrophic changes involve loss of filiform and fungiform papillae, and the tongue becomes smooth and shiny. The mucosa is also reddened. Fissures occur in the epithelium and along the sides of the tongue; these become infected rapidly. The gingiva may become inflamed, resembling ulcerative gingivitis. Corners of the lips are initially pale; fanlike fissuring occurs that radiates into the perioral epithelium and may leave permanent scars.

🦷 DENTAL CONSIDERATIONS

- Assess patients—especially those consuming excessive amounts of alcohol, who are malnourished, or those with a heavy dependence on corn or maize—for oral signs of niacin deficiency. Symptoms to watch for include complaints of a nonspecific burning sensation throughout the oral cavity; a smooth, shiny, bright-red tongue swollen at the tip and lateral margins; stomatitis; and red and inflamed marginal and attached gingiva. Refer to a physician for further consult if indicated.
- Prolonged treatment with isoniazid for tuberculosis may lead to niacin deficiency. Niacin supplements may be prescribed by the health care provider to prevent deficiency.

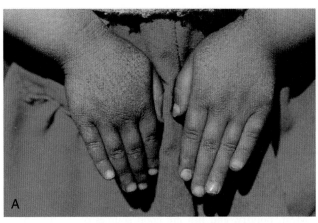
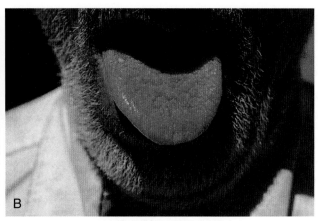

• **Fig. 11.7** (A) Symmetrical chapping of the dorsum of the hands. This is a common site for the skin changes of pellagra to occur. A careful history and full examination permit the diagnosis to be made. (B) Scarlet tongue. The tongue in pellagra is frequently scarlet in appearance and extremely painful. However, this may occur in many nonnutritional conditions; other signs, especially those on the skin, have to be present to make the clinical diagnosis. Fissuring of the tongue alone is not significant. (From McLaren DS. *A Colour Atlas and Text of Diet-Related Disorders*. 2nd ed. Mosby-Year Book; 1992.)

NUTRITIONAL DIRECTIONS

- Patients should understand that a frequent side effect of a therapeutic dose of nicotinic acid is flushing (i.e., feeling warm; redness; itching or tingling of the face, neck, arms or upper chest). A therapeutic dose should only be prescribed by a physician or comparably licensed health care provider and any side effects should be discussed with them.
- Nicotinic acid, nicotinamide, and niacinamide are correct terms for the water-soluble active form of niacin and should not be confused with nicotine.

Pantothenic Acid (Vitamin B5)

Physiologic Roles

Pantothenic acid is similar to other B vitamins in its metabolic roles. Pantothenic acid plays a key role in carbohydrate, fat, and protein metabolism. Additionally, it is important in synthesis and degradation of triglycerides, phospholipids, and sterols and in formation of certain hormones and nerve-regulating substances.

Requirements

The Estimated Average Requirement (EAR), RDA, or UL has not been determined for pantothenic acid for any age group. The Adequate Intake (AI) for adults is 5 mg/day (Table 11.7).

Sources

Pantothenic acid is synthesized by most microorganisms and plants. It is particularly abundant in animal foods and whole-grain cereals (Table 11.8). Bacteria in the digestive tract also produce pantothenic acid.

Hypo States

Naturally occurring dietary deficiency of pantothenic acid is very rare. A deficiency results in dysfunctional lipid synthesis and

TABLE 11.7	National Academy of Medicine Recommendations for Pantothenic Acid	
Life Stage	**AI (mg/day)**	
0–6 months	1.7	
7–12 months	1.8	
1–3 years	2	
4–8 years	3	
9–13 years	4	
14–18 years	5	
≥19 years	5	
Pregnancy		
14–50 years	6	
Lactation		
14–50 years	7	

AI, Adequate intake.
Data from Institute of Medicine (IOM), Food and Nutrition Board. *Dietary Reference Intakes for Thiamin, Riboflavin, Niacin, Vitamin B6, Folate, Vitamin B12, Pantothenic Acid, Biotin, and Choline*. National Academy Press; 1998.

energy production. Symptoms include burning sensations in the feet, depression, fatigue, insomnia, and weakness.

DENTAL CONSIDERATIONS

- Pantothenic acid deficiency rarely occurs alone but may occur along with other B-vitamin deficiencies.
- Pantothenic acid may help in wound healing; thus encourage patients undergoing oral or periodontal surgery to eat a well-balanced diet comprised of nutrient-dense foods.

TABLE 11.8   **Pantothenic Acid Content of Selected Foods**

Food	Portion	Pantothenic Acid (mg)
Corn, sweet, yellow, canned	1 cup	1.4
Beef liver, cooked	3 oz	8.3
Sunflower seeds	½ cup	4.8
Tuna, fresh, bluefin, cooked	3 oz	1.2
Chicken, skinless, cooked	3 oz	1.3
Pork loin chop, broiled	3 oz	1.0
Avocado, raw	1/2	1.0
Portobello mushroom, grilled	½ cup	0.76
Egg, hard boiled	1 large	0.7
Milk 2% milkfat	1 cup	0.9
Salmon, cooked	3 oz	0.7
Ground beef, 85% lean, broiled	3 oz	0.60
Rice, white, long grain, regular, unenriched, cooked with salt	1 cup	0.6
Broccoli, boiled	1/2 cup	0.5
Mixed nuts, lightly salted	1 oz	0.3

Data from National Institutes of Health. Office of Dietary Supplements. *Pantothenic Acid Fact Sheet for Health Professionals.* https://ods.od.nih.gov/factsheets/PantothenicAcid-HealthProfessional/U.S; Department of Agriculture (USDA), Agricultural Research Service. National Agricultural Library. *USDA National Nutrient Database for Standard Reference Legacy.* 2018. https://www.nal.usda.gov/sites/default/files/page-files/pantothenic_acid.pdf.

⬤ NUTRITIONAL DIRECTIONS

- Pantothenic acid is naturally present in meat, poultry, fish, some fruits, vegetables and added to other foods such as enriched cereals and grains.
- Diets including fresh meats, vegetables, and whole-grain foods that are unprocessed contain more pantothenic acid than refined, canned and frozen food.

Pyridoxine (Vitamin B_6)

Vitamin B_6 is the term commonly used for a group of three compounds: pyridoxine, pyridoxal, and pyridoxamine. All three forms can be used by the body in their role as coenzymes.

Physiologic Roles

Several essential roles for vitamin B_6 have been identified. In addition to (1) its role as a coenzyme in protein metabolism, vitamin B_6 plays a part in (2) conversion of tryptophan to niacin, (3) hemoglobin synthesis, (4) synthesis of unsaturated fatty acids from essential fatty acids, (5) energy production from glycogen, (6) production of antibodies and immune cells, and (7) proper functioning of the nervous system, including synthesis of neurotransmitters.

Requirements

The current RDA for vitamin B_6 ranges from 1.1 to 1.7 mg daily for adults (Table 11.9). The requirement for vitamin B_6 increases with protein intake because of its major role in amino acid metabolism. Limited amounts of vitamin B_6 are produced by microorganisms in the digestive tract. The UL has been determined to be 100 mg/day for adults. Teenagers, females of childbearing age, smokers, non–Hispanic African American males, and individuals who are underweight are frequently deficient in vitamin B_6.

Sources

Meat, poultry, and fish are good sources of vitamin B_6. Other good sources include some fruits, nuts, fortified cereals, whole-grain products, and vegetables (Table 11.10). Vitamin B_6 from animal sources has greater bioavailability than that provided by plants. Pyridoxine in some plants (potatoes, spinach, beans, and other legumes) is frequently bound to proteins, resulting in low bioavailability. Canning, roasting, boiling, or stewing meat and various food-processing techniques can reduce pyridoxine content of food, as the vitamin is leached into the liquid.

Absorption and Excretion

Absorption of vitamin B_6 differs from other B-complex vitamins. All three forms of the vitamin are converted to an absorbable form by an intestinal enzyme. Body stores are small and repletion is gradual.

Hyper States and Hypo States

Science and media suggest possible benefits of supplemental amounts of vitamin B_6 in cardiovascular disease (CVD), sickness during pregnancy, premenstrual syndrome, and neuropathies.[8,9] Due to low levels of evidence, supplemental amounts beyond the UL are not currently recommended. Acute pyridoxine toxicity is uncommon; however, routine supplementation with megadoses has documented side effects, including ataxia and severe sensory neuropathy (impairment of the ability to feel) and, in some instances, bone pain and muscle weakness. In most cases, complete recovery occurs with discontinuation of megadose supplementation.

Deficiency rarely occurs alone; vitamin B_6 deficiency is most commonly observed along with deficiency of several other B vitamins. Individuals with poor-quality diets in addition to overall low nutrient intake (e.g., alcohol use disorder and older adults) may experience a deficiency. Clinical signs include central nervous system abnormalities or convulsions, dermatitis with cheilosis, glossitis, impaired immune responses, and anemia. Pyridoxine deficiency–induced glossitis is denoted by pain, edema, and papillary changes. Initially, the tongue has a scalded sensation, followed by reddening and hypertrophy of filiform papillae at the tip, margins, and dorsum (Fig. 11.8).

Stores of vitamin B_6 in a mother's body are critical to the well-being of her newborn infant. Oral contraceptive agents (OCAs) taken before conception may reduce maternal vitamin B_6 levels during pregnancy and in breast milk. An increase in dietary intake of vitamin B_6 may be recommended for females taking OCAs, especially if a pregnancy is planned in the near future.

TABLE 11.9	National Academy of Medicine Recommendations for Pyridoxine(Vitamin B$_6$)

	EAR (mg/day)		RDA (mg/day)			
Life Stage	Male	Female	Male	Female	AI (mg/day)	UL (mg/day)^a
0–6 months					0.1	ND^b
7–12 months					0.3	ND^b
1–3 years	0.4	0.4	0.5	0.5		30
4–8 years	0.5	0.5	0.6	0.6		40
9–13 years	0.8	0.8	1	1		60
14–18 years	1.1	1	1.3	1.2		80
19–50 years	1.1	0.9	1.3	1.3		100
≥51 years	1.4	1.3	1.7	1.5		100
Pregnancy						
14–18 years		1.6		1.9		80
≥19 years		1.6		1.9		100
Lactation						
14–18 years		1.7		2		80
≥19 years		1.7		2		100

^{a}Vitamin B$_6$ as pyridoxine.
^{b}ND—not determinable because of lack of data of adverse effects in this age group and concern with regard to lack of ability to handle excess amounts. Source of intake should be from food and formula to prevent high levels of intake.
AI, Adequate intake, *EAR*, estimated average requirement; *RDA*, recommended dietary allowance; *UL*, tolerable upper intake level.
Data from Institute of Medicine (IOM), Food and Nutrition Board. *Dietary Reference Intakes for Thiamin, Riboflavin, Niacin, Vitamin B$_6$, Folate, Vitamin B$_{12}$, Pantothenic Acid, Biotin, and Choline.* National Academy Press; 1998.

⬡ DENTAL CONSIDERATIONS

- Patients may present with pain of the tongue, which precedes redness and swelling of the tip of the tongue. Eventually, atrophy of papillae results in a smooth, purplish tongue. Angular cheilitis, oral ulcers, and stomatitis also may be noted.
- Encourage foods high in vitamin B$_6$, and monitor for deficiency signs and symptoms, especially in females of childbearing age, excessive alcohol intake, and older adults. Referral to a primary care provider or a registered dietitian may be indicated.
- Use of drugs affecting vitamin B$_6$ metabolism warrants supplementation to avoid secondary vitamin B$_6$ deficiency. These drugs include isoniazid and cycloserine (for tuberculosis), penicillamine (for Wilson disease, lead poisoning, kidney stones, and arthritis), and theophylline (for asthma).

⬡ NUTRITIONAL DIRECTIONS

- Vitamin B$_6$ supplements should not be taken unless prescribed by a health care provider.
- If supplements are needed, signs and symptoms improve within 1 week.
- Adequate daily intake of nutrient-dense food sources of pyridoxine is important.
- Vitamin B$_6$ is removed during grain processing and not replaced during enrichment; whole-grain breads and cereals are better sources.

Folate/Folic Acid (Vitamin B$_9$)

The generic term *folate* encompasses several compounds that have nutritional properties similar to those of folic acid. Several different metabolically active forms have been identified. The terms *folate*, *folic acid*, and *folacin* are used interchangeably. Folate is the natural form found in foods, whereas folic acid is a synthetic form used in vitamin supplements and food fortification. The body converts folic acid to folate.

Physiologic Roles

Folate functions as a coenzyme for approximately 20 enzymes. As such, the methylenetetrahydrofolate reductase (MTHFR) enzyme is involved in synthesis of RNA and DNA. MTHFR is important for numerous chemical reactions involving folate and is required for the process of converting the amino acid homocysteine to methionine, which is used to make proteins and other important compounds. It functions in conjunction with vitamins B$_{12}$ and C in maintaining normal levels of mature red blood cells (RBCs). Folate has an important role in proper formation of the neural tube during the first month of fetal development.

Requirements

As shown in Table 11.11, the RDA is 400 µg for adults. Folate can be expressed as dietary folate equivalents, which are equivalent to

TABLE 11.10   Pyridoxine (Vitamin B₆) Content of Selected Foods

Food	Portion	Pyridoxine (mg)
Beef liver, pan fried	3 oz	0.90
Turkey, ground, fat free patty, broiled	4 oz	0.77
Cream of wheat, instant, prepared with water	1 cup	0.75
Pork loin, roasted	4 oz	0.65
Salmon, sockeye, cooked	3 oz	0.60
Sunflower seeds	½ cup	0.54
Chicken breast, roasted	3 oz	0.50
Banana	1 med	0.43
Potato, white, baked	1 med	0.36
Tuna, white, canned in water	3 oz	0.18
Nuts, mixed, dry roasted	1 oz	0.10
Rice, white, long grain, regular, raw, unenriched	½ cup	0.15
Tomato soup, canned, condensed reduced sodium	½ cup	0.10

Data from National Institutes of Health. Office of Dietary Supplements. *Pyridoxine Fact Sheet for Health Professionals.* https://ods.od.nih.gov/factsheets/VitaminB6-HealthProfessional/; U.S. Department of Agriculture (USDA), Agricultural Research Service. National Agricultural Library. *USDA National Nutrient Database for Standard Reference Legacy.* 2018. https://www.nal.usda.gov/sites/default/files/page-files/Vitamin%20B-6.pdf.

1 μg of folate. Requirements for folate are increased during periods of growth and development, such as adolescence, pregnancy, and lactation, because of its role in DNA synthesis. The National Academy of Medicine (formerly the Institute of Medicine) established a UL for the synthetic forms of folic acid available in dietary supplements and fortified foods, but the UL does not pertain to folate from food because a high intake from food sources has not been reported to cause adverse effects.

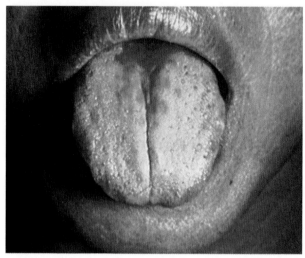

• **Fig. 11.8** Fungiform papillary hypertrophy. The condition can be seen and felt as a tongue blade is drawn lightly over the anterior two-thirds of the tongue. The tongue may have a berrylike appearance. (Courtesy Dr. H. H. Sandstead. From McLaren DS. *A Colour Atlas and Text of Diet-Related Disorders.* 2nd ed. Mosby-Year Book; 1992.)

TABLE 11.11   National Academy of Medicine Recommendations for Folate[a]

Life Stage	EAR (μg/day) Male	Female	RDA (μg/day) Male	Female	AI (μg/day)	UL (μg/day)[b]
0–6 months					65	ND[c]
7–12 months					80	ND[c]
1–3 years	120	120	150	150		300
4–8 years	160	160	200	200		400
9–13 years	250	250	300	300		600
14–18 years	330	330	400	400		800
≥19 years	320	320	400	400		1000
Pregnancy						
14–18 years		520		600		800
≥19 years		520		600		1000
Lactation						
14–18 years		450		500		800
≥19 years		450		500		1000

[a]Dietary folate equivalents.

[b]Folate from fortified foods or supplements.

[c]ND—not determinable because of lack of data of adverse effects in this age group and concern with regard to lack of ability to handle excess amounts. Source of intake should be from food and formula to prevent high levels of intake.

AI, Adequate intake; *EAR,* estimated average requirement; *RDA,* recommended dietary allowance; *UL,* tolerable upper intake level.

Data from Institute of Medicine (IOM), Food and Nutrition Board. *Dietary Reference Intakes for Thiamin, Riboflavin, Niacin, Vitamin B₆, Folate, Vitamin B₁₂, Pantothenic Acid, Biotin, and Choline.* National Academy Press; 1998.

Sources

Rich sources of folate include liver, green leafy vegetables, fortified cereals and grain products, legumes, and citrus fruits. Spinach, beef liver, asparagus, and brussel sprouts are foods with the highest folate levels (Table 11.12).

In 1996 the US Food and Drug Administration (FDA) mandated the addition of specific amounts of folic acid to all enriched cereals and grain products. Since then, folate intake and serum folate levels have been monitored because of potential risks of some individuals consuming excessive amounts.

Absorption and Excretion

Dietary folate must undergo changes to be absorbed. The intestinal enzyme that accomplishes this requires a slightly acidic pH and is activated by the presence of zinc. Folic acid from supplements and fortified foods is absorbed almost twice as well as that from naturally occurring folate in foods. Individuals needing larger amounts, especially females who may become pregnant, may need a supplement in addition to fortified folate-rich foods.

Hyper States and Hypo States

A high folic acid intake may be harmful for some people. Prolonged intake of excessive folic acid can cause kidney damage and mask symptoms of vitamin B_{12} deficiency, resulting in neurologic and cognitive symptoms. Although a decreased risk of cognitive decline has been suggested in older adults taking folic acid supplements, evidence-based research indicates only a causal relationship between high folic acid intake and risk of developing dementia.[10,11] Therefore, additional studies need to be conducted.

Abundant intake of folate-rich foods may protect against some common cancers, particularly colorectal cancer. Meta-analysis of scientific studies found no significant effect of folic acid supplementation on incidence of cancer of the large intestine, prostate, lung, breast, or any other specific site.[12,13] The UL of 1000 µg/day for adults is applicable to supplements and fortified foods, not to naturally occurring folate in food.

Folate deficiency, the most common vitamin deficiency among the B-complex vitamins, usually occurs with other nutrient deficiencies. Folate inadequacy may occur secondary to excessive alcohol consumption, malabsorptive disorders, pregnancy and lactation, kidney disease, inadequate dietary intake, or taking medications that interfere with folate absorption or metabolism (Box 11.2). Folate deficiencies are also associated with a mutation in the MTHFE gene. Variations in the MTHFR gene are common in many populations worldwide. While individuals with neural tube defects have this genetic variation, many people with a gene variation in MTHFR do not have neural tube defects, nor do their children.

Folate deficiency can produce soreness and shallow ulcerations on the tongue and oral mucosa as well as swelling of the tongue. Glossitis is usually present in individuals with folic acid deficiency. The tongue becomes fiery red and papillae are absent (Fig. 11.9). Folic acid deficiency impairs immune responses and resistance of the oral mucosa to penetration by pathogenic organisms such as *Candida*.

TABLE 11.12	Folate Content of Selected Foods	
Food	Portion	Folate (DFE; µg)
Total, whole-grain cereal	1 cup	901
Spaghetti, enriched, cooked	1 cup	185
Liver, beef, braised	3 oz	215
Bagel, enriched	3½–4 inches	171
Asparagus, cooked	4 spears	89
Spinach, cooked	½ cup	131
Navy beans	½ cup	127
Black eyed, peas cooked	½ cup	105
Turnip greens, cooked	½ cup	85
Broccoli, cooked	½ cup	84
Brussel sprouts, boiled	½ cup	78
Potato, white, baked	1 med	66
Romaine lettuce	1 cup	64
Trail mix, tropical	1 cup	59
Bread, pita, enriched	1 small	48
Orange	1 med	48
Orange juice	1 cup	47
Egg, hard-boiled	1 large	22
Peanuts, dry roasted	1 oz	41
Grapefruit	1 med	26
Banana	1 med	24
Tomato	1 med	18
Brown rice, cooked	1 cup	18
Bread, whole wheat	1 slice	13

DFE, Dietary folate equivalent.
Data from National Institutes of Health. Office of Dietary Supplements. *Folate Fact Sheet for Health Professionals.* https://ods.od.nih.gov/factsheets/Folate-HealthProfessional/; U.S. Department of Agriculture (USDA), Agricultural Research Service. https://fdc.nal.usda.gov/; National Agricultural Library. *USDA National Nutrient Database for Standard Reference Legacy.* 2018. https://www.nal.usda.gov/sites/default/files/page-files/folate.pdf

• BOX 11.2　Drugs That May Impact Folate Status

Anticonvulsants
Antiepileptic medications
Oral contraceptives
Analgesics
Metformin (antihyperglycemic)
Sulfasalazine (antiinflammatory, antiarthritic)
H_2-receptor blockers (decreased gastric acid secretion)
Antacids
Triamterene (diuretic)
Methotrexate (antiarthritic, antineoplastic)
Alcohol

From National Institutes of Health Office of Dietary Supplements. *Folate. Fact Sheet for Health Professionals.* https://ods.od.nih.gov/factsheets/Folate-HealthProfessional/.

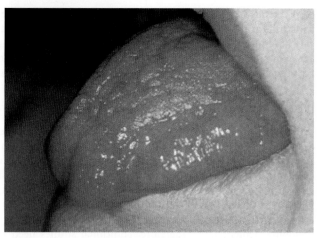

• **Fig. 11.9** Folic acid deficiency. Fiery red tongue completely devoid of papillae. (Courtesy Dr. W. R. Tyldesley. McLaren DS. *A Colour Atlas and Text of Diet-Related Disorders*. 2nd ed. Mosby-Year Book; 1992.)

Deficiency symptoms first appear in rapidly dividing cells, such as in the gastrointestinal tract, RBCs, and white blood cells. RBCs do not develop normally; they become pale and extremely large (megaloblastic) but cannot transport oxygen to cells, a condition known as megaloblastic anemia.

Folic acid deficiency during pregnancy, which may be caused by MTHFR variation, is associated with an increased risk of spina bifida and other neural tube defects (birth defects of the skull, brain, and spinal cord); cleft palate and lip; low birth weight; and premature birth. More than 300,000 infants are born each year with neural tube defects worldwide. The prevalence has decreased by about 35% since folic acid fortification was mandated. As a result of folic acid fortification, approximately 1300 babies are born without a neural tube defect.[14,15]

⬡ DENTAL CONSIDERATIONS

- Evaluate oral status for folate deficiency. Observe for swelling and pallor or reddening of the tip of the tongue (depending on the degree of anemia) with atrophy of filiform papillae, reddening of the fungiform papillae at the tip and lateral border, and formation of small ulcers. Posterior progression eventually leads to complete atrophy of the filiform papillae and formation of bright red spots (fungiform papillae). Angular cheilitis (see Fig. 11.5) and painful ulcerations of the buccal mucosa and palatal and gingival epithelia may also occur.
- Folic acid supplementation may improve resistance to periodontal inflammation in patients deficient in folate. Supplementation should be provided in consult with medical provider.
- A low serum folate level is associated with periodontal disease. Encourage patients to consume adequate intakes of folate-rich foods, along with maintaining meticulous oral hygiene.
- Folate is one of the most common nutrient deficiencies after bariatric surgery.[16] Encourage patients who have had this procedure to adhere to bariatric nutrition guidelines and supplements as recommended by their health care providers.
- Increased gingival inflammation has been associated with OCAs; encourage females taking OCAs to increase their consumption of folate-rich foods.
- Folate absorption is lower when folate is given to individuals taking anticonvulsants and OCAs. Methotrexate (drug used for chemotherapy and arthritis) interferes with the conversion of folate to the active form used by cells. Large doses of folic acid could reduce the therapeutic efficacy of the drug and should be taken under the supervision of the health care provider.

⬡ NUTRITIONAL DIRECTIONS

- Folate may be called folic acid or folacin. Folate is natural form found in foods. Folic acid is the form found in fortified foods and vitamin supplements. Folacin is the term that can be used for both naturally occurring folate and folic acid.
- Folate is easily destroyed by food processing and cooking; raw vegetables provide more folate than those that are canned or overly cooked.
- Adequate folic acid is important in the periconceptual period (400 µg/day before conception and 600 µg/day for pregnant females). The critical time for neural tube formation is the first month of pregnancy and cleft palates and/or lips develop in weeks 7 to 11.
- There is also an association between adequate intake of foods fortified with folic acid and a reduction of congenital heart defects at birth.[17]

Cobalamin (Vitamin B$_{12}$)

Cobalamin or vitamin B$_{12}$, is a complex group of compounds that contains cobalt. Cobalt is a trace mineral that serves an essential component in the structure and formation of vitamin B$_{12}$. It is the only vitamin that contains a mineral.

Physiologic Roles

Vitamin B$_{12}$ functions as a coenzyme in conjunction with folate metabolism in DNA synthesis. It also functions in metabolism of certain amino acids, fatty acids, carbohydrates, and folate. Vitamin B$_{12}$ is essential in formation and regeneration of RBCs, myelin synthesis, and cognitive function. Myelin is the lipid substance that insulates nerve fibers and affects transmission of nerve impulses. It is essential for a normal functioning nervous system.

Requirements

The RDA for adults is 2.4 µg daily (Table 11.13). A high vitamin B$_{12}$ intake results in accumulation in the liver with increasing age, but this may be desirable because serum vitamin B$_{12}$ levels decline

TABLE 11.13	National Academy of Medicine Recommendations for Cobalamin (Vitamin B$_{12}$)				
	EAR (µg/day)		RDA (µg/day)		
Life Stage	Male	Female	Male	Female	AI (µg/day)
0–6 months					0.4
7–12 months					0.5
1–3 years	0.7	0.7	0.9	0.9	
4–8 years	1	1	1.2	1.2	
9–13 years	1.5	1.5	1.8	1.8	
≥14 years	2	2	2.4	2.4	
Pregnancy					
14–50 years		2.2		2.6	
Lactation					
14–50 years		2.4		2.8	

AI, Adequate intake, *EAR*, estimated average requirement; *RDA*, recommended dietary allowance. Data from Institute of Medicine (IOM), Food and Nutrition Board. *Dietary Reference Intakes for Thiamin, Riboflavin, Niacin, Vitamin B$_6$, Folate, Vitamin B$_{12}$, Pantothenic Acid, Biotin, and Choline*. National Academy Press; 1998.

in elderly individuals due to lower absorption rates. No UL has been established, but caution against excessive intake is warranted.

Sources

Microorganisms (bacteria, fungi, and algae) can synthesize vitamin B_{12}. Vitamin B_{12} is not found in plants unless they are fortified or contaminated by microorganisms. Fortified soymilk and sea vegetables (e.g., dulse, kelp, alaria, laver, sea lettuce) are vegan sources. The primary sources of vitamin B_{12} are meat and animal products (Table 11.14). Gastrointestinal flora produce small amounts of absorbable vitamin B_{12}.

Absorption and Excretion

Vitamin B_{12} from food is released from its protein bond by hydrochloric acid and enzymes in the stomach and intestine. Free vitamin B_{12} combines with salivary R-binder (protein produced by

TABLE 11.14	Cobalamin (Vitamin B_{12}) Content of Selected Foods	
Food	Portion	Vitamin B_{12} (µg)
Beef liver, braised	3 oz	70.7
Salmon, Atlantic cooked	3 oz	2.6
Beef, ground (90/10), broiled	3 oz	2.2
Yogurt, low-fat, plain	6 oz	0.95
Skim milk	1 cup	1.1
Lean pork chop, broiled	3 oz	0.7
Cottage cheese, low fat, 2%	½ cup	0.53
Chicken breast, roasted	2 slices	0.4
Egg, hard-boiled	1 large	0.5

Data from National Institutes of Health. Office of Dietary Supplements. *Vitamin B12 Fact Sheet for Health Professionals.* https://ods.od.nih.gov/factsheets/VitaminB12-HealthProfessional/#en20; U.S. Department of Agriculture (USDA). *Agricultural Research Service.* Food Data Central. https://fdc.nal.usda.gov/; National Agricultural Library. *USDA National Nutrient Database for Standard Reference Legacy.* 2018. https://www.nal.usda.gov/sites/default/files/page-files/Vitamin%20B-12.pdf

the salivary glands) in the stomach. In the small intestine, trypsin (pancreatic enzyme) removes the R-binder, and vitamin B_{12} combines with intrinsic factor, a glycoprotein secreted by the parietal cells in the stomach. Absorption of vitamin B_{12} occurs at specific receptor sites in the ileum and is possible only if it is bound to intrinsic factor. The vitamin is recycled from bile and other intestinal secretions. Excessive amounts are bound to a protein and stored for 3 to 4 years in the liver or are excreted.

Hyper States and Hypo States

Excessive intake of folic acid from supplements delays the diagnosis of, or exacerbates the effects of, vitamin B_{12} deficiency by correcting the anemia but not the cognitive impairment. Injections of vitamin B_{12} are popular treatments for a deficiency related to malabsorption because this delivery bypasses potential barriers to absorption. Oral administration of vitamin B_{12} is not as effective as intramuscular administration in correcting the deficiency since the vitamin may not be absorbed. Although vegan populations are at increased risk, vitamin B_{12} deficiency is rarely caused by insufficient dietary sources. Lack of intrinsic factor, R-binder, or an enzyme needed for absorption of vitamin B_{12}, is the primary cause of deficiency. Pernicious anemia, which is characterized by abnormally large RBCs, glossitis, gastrointestinal disturbances, weakness, and neurologic manifestations, occurs frequently in older patients relative to achlorhydria (decreased hydrochloric acid production in the stomach) and decreased synthesis of intrinsic factor by the parietal cells. Rapid neuropsychiatric decline occurs with severe vitamin B_{12} deficiency; however, supplementation with vitamin B_{12} may not improve cognitive ability. More research is needed.[18]

Cobalamin malabsorption is caused by inability to release vitamin B_{12} from food so that it cannot be taken up by intrinsic factor for absorption. Patients develop a lemon-yellow tint of the skin and eyes as a result of concurrent anemia and jaundice from inability to produce RBCs; a smooth, beefy red tongue; and neurologic disorders. Deficiency symptoms develop very slowly.

Initial oral symptoms of vitamin B_{12} deficiency include glossopyrosis (unexplained pain of the tongue), followed by swelling and pallor with eventual disappearance of the filiform and fungiform papillae. The tongue may be completely smooth, shiny, and deeply reddened with a loss or distortion of taste (Fig. 11.10). Bright red, diffuse, excruciating lesions may occur in the buccal

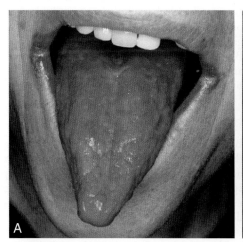
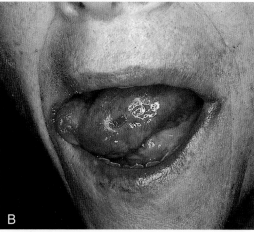

• **Fig. 11.10** Pernicious anemia. (A) Angular cheilitis and depapillation of the tongue in a patient with pernicious anemia. (B) The mucosa becomes atrophic in pernicious anemia and is easily ulcerated. Note ulcer on left lateral aspect of tongue. (From Ibsen OAC, Peters SC. Phelan JA. *Oral Pathology for the Dental Hygienist: With General Pathology Introductions.* 8th ed. Elsevier Saunders; 2023.)

and pharyngeal mucosa and undersurface of the tongue. An oral examination may reveal stomatitis or a pale or yellowish mucosa, xerostomia, cheilosis, hemorrhagic gingiva, and bone loss.

Neurologic symptoms, such as numbness or tingling, occur as a consequence of demyelination of the nerves. Deficiency symptoms are rapidly corrected with vitamin B_{12} supplements or intramuscular injections. The crystalline form of vitamin B_{12} found in supplements does not require gastric acid or enzymes for initial digestion, and large oral doses (containing more than 200 times the RDA) can reverse biochemical signs of vitamin B_{12} deficiency in older adults.[19]

Children with vitamin B_{12} deficiency (e.g., vegans) may have growth challenges. Other symptoms include anorexia (loss of appetite), altered taste sensation, abdominal pain, and general weakness. A vitamin B_{12} deficiency is also associated with poor cognitive performance.[20]

DENTAL CONSIDERATIONS

- Assess for oral signs of deficiency; signs and symptoms of vitamin B_{12} deficiency are similar to those of folic acid deficiency except that burning tongue pain precedes physical signs of vitamin B_{12} deficiency.
- Patients with xerostomia may have poor absorption of vitamin B_{12}.
- Patients older than age 50 years are encouraged to choose fortified sources of vitamin B_{12} or a dietary supplement to meet their needs because the synthetic form is better absorbed than naturally occurring vitamin B_{12} in foods.
- Concomitant ingestion of ascorbic acid via foods or supplements can reduce bioavailability of vitamin B_{12} and result in deficiency. It is recommended to take vitamin C supplements 2 or more hours after taking a vitamin B_{12} supplement. Refer them to their health care provider and/or RDN for guidance.
- Due to changes in digestive physiology after gastric bypass surgery, vitamin B_{12} may need to be administered by injection or sublingual supplement form.
- Vitamin B_{12} deficiency is associated with metformin (an antihyperglycemic medication) therapy in patients with diabetes. Patients with diabetes taking metformin may need a supplement. Levels of vitamin B_{12} should be monitored by the health care professional and/or RDN in those patients at increased risk of a deficiency. [21-23]
- Histamine receptor antagonists (H_2 blockers; ranitidine [Zantac EFFERdose], famotidine [Pepcid], and cimetidine [Tagamet]) do not affect vitamin B_{12} status, but prolonged use of proton-pump inhibitors (esomeprazole [Nexium], lansoprazole [Prevacid], omeprazole [Prilosec OTC], pantoprazole [Protonix], and rabeprazole [AcipHex]) by older adults negatively affects vitamin B_{12} status. Oral supplementation with recommended amounts of vitamin B_{12} does not prevent this decline.[23] Encourage patients taking these medications to consult their health care provider and/or RDN.

NUTRITIONAL DIRECTIONS

- Because vitamin B_{12} is found only in animal products, vegans (strict vegetarians) require vitamin B_{12}–fortified foods or a daily supplement.
- One cup of fortified cereal will provide the daily requirement for vitamin B_{12}. The synthetic form of the vitamin is easily absorbed by individuals who have limited stomach acid.

Biotin (Vitamin B_7)

Physiologic Roles

Biotin functions as a coenzyme in metabolism of carbohydrates, proteins, and fats. It has an important biochemical role in every living cell in maintaining metabolic homeostasis. Biotin also plays

TABLE 11.15	National Academy of Medicine Recommendations for Biotin
Life Stage	AI (µg/day)
0–6 months	5
7–12 months	6
1–3 years	8
4–8 years	12
9–13 years	20
14–18 years	25
>18 years	30
Pregnancy	
14–50 years	30
Lactation	
14–50 years	35

AI, Adequate intake.
Data from Institute of Medicine (IOM), Food and Nutrition Board. *Dietary Reference Intakes for Thiamin, Riboflavin, Niacin, Vitamin B₆, Folate, Vitamin B₁₂, Pantothenic Acid, Biotin, and Choline.* National Academy Press; 1998.

an important role in regulating gene transcription (synthesis of DNA and RNA) and metabolically functions closely with folic acid, pantothenic acid, and vitamin B_{12}.

Requirements

Because of insufficient data, only an adequate intake for biotin has been established for all age groups (Table 11.15). Intakes of 10 to 200 µg/day are considered safe and adequate. No UL has been established for biotin.

Sources

Although biotin is widely distributed in foods, its availability is low compared with that of other water-soluble vitamins. Rich sources of biotin include egg yolk, liver, and cereals. The microflora in the gastrointestinal tract probably provides part of the body's needs. Biotin is included in many dietary supplements, infant formulas, and baby foods. Food composition tables usually do not report biotin content of food.

Hypo States

Biotin deficiency can be produced by the ingestion of avidin, the protein found in raw egg whites. Avidin is denatured by heat; cooked egg white does not present a problem. Six raw egg whites per day over several months can produce anorexia, nausea, vomiting, glossitis, pallor, depression, and dry scaly dermatitis.[24]

Oral signs of biotin deficiency are pallor of the tongue and patchy atrophy of the lingual papillae. Although the pattern resembles geographic tongue, it is confined to the lateral margins or is generalized to the entire dorsum.

🔹 DENTAL CONSIDERATIONS

- Assess patients for signs of deficiency: glossitis, pallor of the mucosal tissue, and papillary atrophy.
- Antibiotics reduce the production of biotin by intestinal bacteria along with some antiseizure, antipsychotic, and antidepressant drugs.

🔹 NUTRITIONAL DIRECTIONS

- Drinking or eating large amounts of raw egg whites over a long period may lead to biotin deficiency.
- Eggs should be cooked to decrease avidin's binding capacity and to minimize the danger of *Salmonella* poisoning.
- A balanced diet that includes a variety of foods contains adequate amounts of biotin.

Other Vitamins

Most nutrients perform more than one physiologic function. Although one nutrient may appear to be more important in calcified structures and of lesser importance in oral soft tissues, its roles actually are equally important. The following nutrients have been discussed in previous chapters, but they have important functions in soft oral tissues that the dental hygienist should not overlook.

Vitamin C

Vitamin C is involved in improving the host defense mechanism by ensuring optimal activity of white blood cells. It has an important role in protecting soft oral tissues from infections caused by bacterial toxins and antigens and protecting tooth enamel from plaque microorganisms.

The role of vitamin C in collagen formation is well-known. Vitamin C deficiency causes weakened collagen, leading to gingivitis and poor wound healing (see Chapter 8).

Vitamin A

Vitamin A, necessary for maintaining the integrity of epithelial tissues, is a significant factor in the development and maintenance of salivary glands. Large amounts of vitamin A may inhibit keratinization of epithelial cells. Vitamin A increases synthesis of cellular proteins that stimulate growth and influence metabolism.

Vitamin A deficiency produces squamous metaplasia (change in cell structure in the oral cavity) with keratin production in the duct cells of salivary glands. This results in decreased salivary secretion and xerostomia. Oral and oropharyngeal cancers have been associated with vitamin A deficiency in humans.

Vitamin E

As discussed in Chapter 8, cell membranes contain polyunsaturated fatty acids that are susceptible to peroxidation. Vitamin E plays a major role as an antioxidant to neutralize free radicals, especially in membranes that contain a large proportion of unsaturated fatty acids. It not only prevents inflammation of the periodontium but also promotes integrity of cell membranes of the mucosa.

🔹 DENTAL CONSIDERATIONS

- One of the first signs of vitamin C deficiency is increased susceptibility to infections. During later stages, the gingiva becomes reddened and swollen, and bleeds easily with an increased risk of candidiasis and petechiae. Also, the collagenous structure is weakened and wound healing becomes slow.
- When a deficiency exists, vitamin C supplementation decreases permeability of the sulcular epithelium and increases collagen synthesis.
- Parotid gland enlargement is associated with deficiencies of vitamins A and C and protein malnutrition.
- Vitamin A deficiency may result in reduced epithelialization (natural healing), impaired wound healing and tissue regeneration, and increased risk of candidiasis.

🔹 NUTRITIONAL DIRECTIONS

- Foods rich in antioxidants (vitamins E and carotene) may suppress chemically induced neoplasia (abnormal growth of tissue) in the mouth, esophagus, and stomach. However, a meta-analysis indicated an increased risk of mortality related to supplementation of these nutrients. Encourage individuals with these neoplasias to choose nutrient-dense foods that are rich in vitamin E and beta-carotenes.
- Vitamin C functions in maintaining periodontal health. A varied and adequate diet including at least one vitamin C–rich food (see Table 8.10) daily provides adequate amounts.

◆ HEALTH APPLICATION 11

Vitamin and Mineral Supplements

Approximately one-half of the US population consumes vitamin and mineral dietary supplements. One-third of them use a multivitamin-multimineral (MVM) supplement on a daily basis. Approximately 65% of adults aged 62 to 85 years used dietary supplements in 2003 to 2006.[25,26] Supplement sales increased by 14.5% in 2020 and grew by 7.5% in 2021. An estimated $60 billion was spent on dietary supplements in 2021.[27–29] Less than 25% of supplements were recommended by a health care provider. Supplements are not regulated by the Food and Drug Administration (FDA), making them subject to misrepresentation and misuse by consumers.[25] The five most

popular products are fish oil/omega-3 fatty acid supplements, multivitamins, vitamin D, calcium, and vitamin C.[30] Most adults are taking dietary supplements to optimize their health and well-being (e.g., enhance cognition and physical performance, increase energy); prevent chronic diseases, cancer in particular; and as nutritional "insurance" to cover lifestyle choices.[30] People who take dietary supplements generally are consuming more nutrient-dense foods, resulting in higher nutrient intakes than those who do not take a supplement.[31] Use of dietary supplement is reported to increase with age and is higher among females than males.[25]

Continued

◆ **HEALTH APPLICATION 11—CONT'D**

Vitamin and Mineral Supplements

Rates of vitamin–mineral deficiencies involve less than 10% of the general population. The nutrients and their rates of deficiency are vitamin B_6 (10%); iron (9.5%); vitamin D (8.1%); vitamin C (6%); vitamin B_{12} (2%); and vitamins A and E, and folate (<1%).[32,33] MVM supplements usually contain 100% of the recommended intake for 10 vitamins and 10 minerals except for calcium (100% Reference Daily Intake for calcium makes the pill too large). There is no standard or regulation governing which vitamins and minerals or how much are included in an MVM supplement.

Vitamin and mineral supplements are drugs, but they are not subject to the same regulations as standard drugs. The *Dietary Supplement Health and Education Act* (DSHEA) of 1994 defines dietary supplements (or dietary ingredients) as vitamins, minerals, amino acids, sports nutrition and weight loss supplements, homeopathic medicines, herbs and botanicals (see Health Application 15), and other products such as enzymes, organ tissues, and metabolites to supplement dietary intake. In other words, a dietary supplement is any product not meant for use as a conventional food or as a sole item of a meal or diet. The DSHEA restricted the FDA's ability to regulate products marketed as "dietary supplements." This act allows supplement manufacturers to market products without proving purity, strength, or effectiveness of supplements to the FDA. Manufacturers are responsible for ensuring that products are safe before they put them on the market. Once a product is marketed, the FDA is responsible for showing that a dietary supplement is "unsafe" before taking action to restrict the product's use or removal from the marketplace. Manufacturers of dietary supplements must record, investigate, then forward to the FDA any reports they are aware of; however, a great majority of the adverse events (Box 11.3) that occur annually remain unreported. In summary, the FDA does not review dietary supplement products for safety and effectiveness before they are marketed. Therefore, it is essential for consumers and health care providers to report about such adverse effects to the FDA.

In 2007 the FDA implemented good manufacturing practices to ensure that supplements are produced in a quality manner, do not contain contaminants or impurities, and are labeled truthfully. The new mandate was intended to ensure that products are free of contamination and impurities. The FDA has determined that many dietary supplements contain undeclared active pharmaceutical ingredients. Of particular concern are supplements contaminated with prescription medications, controlled substances, experimental compounds, or drugs rejected by the FDA because of safety concerns. Some products on the market contain ingredients used for patients with diabetes, high cholesterol, dementia, or insomnia. Most of the products containing potentially hazardous ingredients are those promising sexual enhancement, optimal athletic performance, and weight loss.

Because there are no uniform manufacturing rules for these products, MVM supplements may not contain what the bottle claims, could be contaminated with something from the manufacturing plant, or may have tainted ingredients. ConsumerLab.com, often called the "watchdog" of the supplement industry, is a private organization that provides independent evaluations of dietary products. In a recent evaluation, almost 30% of multivitamins tested contained significantly more or less of an ingredient than

claimed, were over or close to the Tolerable Upper Intake Level (ULs), or did not dissolve fast enough for maximum absorption.[34]

Manufacturers can legally make three types of claims for a dietary supplement: health claims, structure/function claims, and nutrient content claims. Claims can describe the link between a food substance and disease or a health-related condition; intended benefits of using the product; or the amount of a nutrient or dietary substance present. The label on a product sold as a dietary supplement and promoted as a treatment, prevention, or cure for a specific disease or condition would not be allowed. Manufacturers must notify the FDA if they want to make a claim on the product and must include evidence of the product's effectiveness and safety.

If the FDA finds that supplements do not contain ingredients claimed, the agency can consider the products adulterated or misbranded. In minor cases, the FDA may ask the manufacturer to remove an ingredient or revise its label. In more serious cases, it could seize the product, file a lawsuit, or seek criminal charges.

The United States Pharmacopeia (USP), the National Sanitation Foundation International (NSF), and ConsumerLab.com (CL) are nonprofit groups that verify whether companies offer contamination-free products and use good manufacturing practices. The presence of a USP, NSF, or CL symbol on the label helps to ensure quality of a product because the symbols mean that the product has been tested to disintegrate and dissolve in the gastrointestinal tract, contains uniform quality (potency and purity), and contains ingredients as listed on the packaging. These organizations require an expiration date on the packaging. The symbols do not indicate that the supplement is safe for everyone or has any benefits. Not every brand has the seals; some manufacturers may not submit their products for testing.

In most instances, evidence does not indicate a need for most MVM supplements, but use of supplementation is endorsed when there is a demonstrated vitamin or mineral deficiency based on laboratory tests. Some nutrients are more likely to be inadequate during particular phases of life, as follows:

- Iron and folic acid—for adolescent girls and females during childbearing years, especially during pregnancy (see Chapter 13)
- Vitamin B_{12}—for people who are older than age 50 years (see Chapter 15)
- Vitamin D—for older adults, people with heavily pigmented skin, and people exposed to inadequate ultraviolet-B radiation (see Chapter 8)

Additionally, during specific circumstances, typical nutritional needs or eating patterns change; thus health care professionals should assess and determine whether a nutrient supplement is appropriate. Low-calorie food intake patterns (<1200 kcal daily) are typically inadequate in vitamins and minerals. Supplements may be used to prevent, treat, or manage disease or other conditions. This would include supplementation with calcium and vitamin D for osteoporosis and electrolyte replacement to treat acute diarrhea. Individuals who limit the variety of foods in their diet may need an MVM supplement, especially if whole food groups are omitted. Examples include vegans (inadequate amounts of calcium, iron, zinc, and vitamins D and B_{12}); people who eliminate all dairy foods (lack of calcium and vitamin D); and patients who severely restrict food choices because of allergies and food

---

• BOX 11.3   Adverse Events Related to Dietary Supplements to Report to the US Food and Drug Administration

- Itching, rash, hives, throat/lip/tongue swelling, wheezing
- Low blood pressure, fainting, chest pain, shortness of breath, palpitations, irregular heart beat
- Severe, persistent nausea, vomiting, diarrhea, or abdominal pain
- Difficulty urinating, decreased urination, dark urine
- Fatigue, appetite loss, yellowing skin/eyes

- Severe joint/muscle pain
- Slurred speech, one-sided weakness of face, arm, leg, vision
- Abnormal bleeding from nose or gingiva
- Blood in urine, stool, vomit, or sputum
- Marked mood, cognitive, or behavioral changes, thoughts of suicide
- Visit to emergency department or hospitalization

From U.S. Food and Drug Administration. *Dietary Supplements—How to Report a Problem.* https://www.fda.gov/food/dietary-supplements/how-report-problem-dietary-supplements, https://www.fda.gov/Food/DietarySupplements/ReportAdverseEvent/default.htm.

Vitamin and Mineral Supplements

intolerances, such as celiac disease (malabsorption and elimination of grain-based foods). In general, unless a health care provider specifically indicates a need for more than 100% of the RDA of a particular nutrient, supplementation is probably not wise.

Patients may be taking amino acid and folic acid supplements, unconventional items, or herbal products described as "natural." These supplements may be deemed safe and desirable, but may adversely affect an existing medical condition or interact with other supplements or prescribed medications. Heroin, cocaine, and tobacco also can be considered "natural" plant-based substances but lead to obvious health issues and are unsafe.

Megadoses of vitamins with intakes of 20 to 600 times the RDAs are sometimes advocated. Megadosage is defined as a dosage that is more than 10 times the RDA. A megadose of a vitamin is actually a misnomer because, at these levels, the vitamin is functioning as a drug rather than a nutrient. This practice is dangerous and should be supervised by a health care provider to ensure that toxicities do not occur. A well-established principle of pharmacologic therapy is that all substances are potentially toxic at large enough doses. Taking more than the National Academy of Medicine's UL means that risks likely outweigh benefits.

The body processes essential nutrients from food differently than pill form, probably because substances in foods interact with each other in a way that may affect nutrient absorption and utilization. High-dose dietary supplements may not only fail to prevent chronic disease but may actually do harm. For example, kidney stones may occur with high doses (500 mg/day) of vitamin C.[35]

Patients become their own diagnosticians by self-prescribing MVMs or single supplements without consulting their health care provider. The potencies of these self-prescribed supplements vary widely, containing from insignificant amounts to more than 5000% of the Dietary Reference Intake. Consumers use dietary supplements to achieve their self-care goals. Dietary supplements are, in their opinion, an easy means to ensure good health; treat and prevent serious illnesses, colds, and flu; increase mental acuity; and alleviate depression. These individuals may delay seeking medical attention for various health problems. Dietary supplements are not intended to treat disease. Many patients consider vitamins safe to take in any amount. However, each year, thousands of supplement toxicities occur, especially in children.

Public health nutrition would be best served by insisting on a scientifically sound basis for dietary supplementation. Many research and observational studies have shown little or no evidence of protection regarding associations of MVM use for incidence of cardiovascular disease or cancer.[36]

Despite consensus of public opinion, healthy patients do not need dietary supplements if they consume a diet well-balanced with a variety of nutrient-dense foods 80% of the time. Vitamin and mineral supplements are not recommended as a preventive measure in a well-nourished population. Foods are the best source of nutrients. US Poison Control Center has received a significant increase in the rate of calls regarding dietary supplement exposures since 2000. In 2021 increase in serious exposure of supplements were among the top 10 reasons for contacting a US Poison Control Center. Dietary supplements/herbals/homeopathic therapies were among the top five most common exposures in children 5 years or less.[37–39]

The long-term impact of supplementation is unknown. Supplements do not replace or improve the benefits of eating fruits and vegetables, and they may cause unwanted health consequences. In most situations, money is better spent on fresh fruits and vegetables. Obtaining nutrients from dietary sources rather than supplements reduces risk for nutrient deficiencies, excesses, and potential interactions with other drugs or medical conditions. A vast body of observational and epidemiologic studies has associated an increased dietary intake of antioxidants from fruits and vegetables with reduced risks of a range of diseases, including cancer.[40]

Conservative, evidence-based information is often hard to balance against dramatic claims for health in a pill. Whereas the scientific community has reached a consensus about the overall lack of scientific evidence for healthy Americans needing a supplement, several cautions, shown in Box 11.4, are offered for decision-making.

For patients who choose to self-prescribe supplements, low levels of nutrients that do not exceed the RDA are recommended. Amounts greater than 100% of the RDA should be limited to treatment of specific circumstances under medical supervision. Store brands of vitamins are often identical to name brands; expensive supplements are no better than less costly supplements. Daily MVM supplements are most effective when taken with a meal. It takes longer for a full stomach to empty, allowing more time for the supplement to dissolve and be absorbed. Some nutrients may compete with or block the action or absorption of another nutrient; taking single supplements at different meals may be necessary to avoid potential interactions.

A medical history should include specific queries about dietary and herbal supplements because many patients typically do not inform health care professionals of their usage. Document the type of supplement, amount, potential interactions, and dental implications (Box 11.5). By asking additional questions to determine why the patient is taking the supplement, the dental

---

• BOX 11.4 Red Flags to Consider about Supplements

- Beware of claims to cure, mitigate, treat or prevent disease; if it sounds too good to be true, it is usually not true. Do not assume that all supplements are safe.
- Beware of testimonials and endorsements, especially from celebrities. Even the most sincere, all-meaning success stories offered by friends and relatives without financial incentives cannot establish a product's safety or efficacy.
- Beware of the idea that if a little is good, more is better. Intake of vitamins and minerals should not exceed the established Tolerable Upper Intake Level.
- Beware of enticing terms such as all-natural, antioxidant-rich, clinically proven, antiaging, and other vague but seductive claims that a product will promote heart health, prostate health, sexual prowess, energy, weight loss, fat loss, muscle power, and the like.

- Beware of interactions between supplements and medication. Always inform all health care providers, including pharmacists, about supplements taken, and ask specifically about potential interactions with prescription and over-the-counter medications.
- Beware of products that do not contain the amounts indicated on the label (more than or less than). In general, products that have been approved by the United States Pharmacopeia or National Sanitation Foundation International are the safest.
- Beware of undocumented testimonials by patients or doctors.
- Beware of products marketed through the Internet. Whereas US Food and Drug Administration oversight is seen by many as overly obtrusive, other countries have no regulations for manufacturing dietary supplements. Most of the recalled supplements are produced in other countries.

Adapted from U.S. Food and Drug Administration. *FDA 101: Dietary Supplements.* https://www.fda.gov/consumers/consumer-updates/fda-101-dietary-supplements; U.S. Food and Drug Administration. *Health Fraud Database.* https://www.fda.gov/consumers/health-fraud-scams/health-fraud-product-database; U.S. Food and Drug Administration. *Health Fraud Scams.* https://www.fda.gov/consumers/health-fraud-scams.

Continued

◆ **HEALTH APPLICATION 11—CONT'D**

Vitamin and Mineral Supplements

• BOX 11.5 **"ABCD" Approach to Asking Patients about Use of Dietary Supplements**

Ask

- What do you take: what form, what brand, what dose, and what else?
- How long have you been taking it, how much do you take, and how often?
- Why do you take it, why was it recommended, and by whom?
- Does it do what you thought it would?

Be

- Wary of any single nutrient used (e.g., vitamin C, E, or B_{12}) not recommended by a health care provider or RDN, and of doses exceeding the National Academy of Sciences, National Academy of Medicine, Food and Nutrition Board Dietary Reference Intakes.
- Sure to look up supplements used in a reliable resource.

Communicate

- Any concerns or risks about safety, drug-nutrient interactions, toxicity to the patient.

Document

- Supplements used, risks of concern, communication with patient, interaction.

Do

- Not get into the supplement business; when in doubt or wanting to refer a patient, contact the credentialed nutrition professional, an RDN.

RDN, registered dietitian nutritionist.
From Touger-Decker R. Vitamin and mineral supplements: what is the dentist to do? *J Am Dent Assoc.* 2007;138(9):1222–1226.

---

hygienist can discuss the benefits of a balanced diet, fluids, exercise, and tobacco (nicotine) cessation (see Chapter 19, *Health Application 19*). More important, a careful investigation of peer-reviewed literature and use of scientifically based, current, quality research with valid clinical trials, a systematic review, or meta-analysis would provide dental hygienists with accurate information to help assess a patient's intake and provide advice.

All health professionals are responsible for reporting any damaging effects or illness resulting from nutritional supplements to the FDA (https://www.safetyreporting.hhs.gov/) and submitting complaints to the Federal Trade Commission regarding misleading advertising (Reportfraud.ftc.gov). Dental hygienists must consider whether their academic training and scope of practice qualifies them to provide advice regarding dietary supplement usage. Promoting healthy eating patterns and lifestyles according to national guidelines is appropriate advice to provide to patients. A complete nutritional assessment of the patient needs to be conducted by a professional with expertise to validate the use of a supplement.

◆ **CASE APPLICATION FOR THE DENTAL HYGIENIST**

A young mother of a 3-year-old says she has heard that she should be taking folate supplements because she is considering discontinuing her birth control pills. She is concerned about the effects of the birth control pills on her nutritional status and their effect on a fetus should she become pregnant.

Nutritional Assessment

- Types of foods consumed
- Knowledge base of foods rich in folate
- Current use of any dietary supplements
- Motivation to change eating habits
- Knowledge of physiologic values and absorption of folate

Nutritional Diagnosis

Health-seeking behavior related to nutritional status and effects on fetus.

Nutritional Goals

The patient will consume foods rich in folate and ask her health care provider about the need to take a multivitamin supplement or a folate supplement.

Nutritional Implementation

Intervention: Evaluate the oral area for symptoms of folate or other nutrient deficiencies.
Rationale: This will help determine whether she may be currently deficient and determine the need to consult her health care provider.

Intervention: Referral to a physician and/or registered dietitian to discuss the following about folate: (1) different names used, (2) functions, (3) requirements, and (4) sources.
Rationale: This provides the patient with a sound base of knowledge about folic acid.
Intervention: Discuss symptoms of folate deficiency and harmful effects of too much folic acid.
Rationale: Although the patient needs to consume adequate amounts of folic acid to prevent neural tube defects, too much can also be harmful.
Intervention: Discuss the stability of folate during cooking and processing.
Rationale: Knowing that folate can easily be destroyed during food preparation allows the patient to make decisions based on her eating habits and to determine whether her diet provides adequate amounts of folate.
Intervention: Explain that her requirement for folic acid is increased because of the birth control pills and because of the needs of the fetus and other physiologic changes occurring early during pregnancy.
Rationale: This knowledge will help her realize the importance of changing dietary patterns and maintaining the new healthful diet.

Evaluation

The patient should increase her intake of folate-rich foods (cereal and grain products that are fortified with folate, oranges, legumes, liver, green leafy vegetables). Additionally, she should consult her health care provider before she discontinues the OCA and begins taking a multivitamin. She can state why she has an increased requirement for folic acid and why it is important not to take excessive amounts.

◆ Student Readiness

1. Name the two water-soluble vitamins most involved in the metabolism of fats, proteins, and carbohydrates to form energy (adenosine triphosphate) through the citric acid or Krebs cycle.
2. Match the conditions associated with the appropriate vitamin deficiency:

Thiamin	Ariboflavinosis
Riboflavin	Scurvy
Niacin	Pellagra
Vitamin B_{12}	Megaloblastic anemia
Ascorbic acid	Beriberi
	Pernicious anemia
	Wernicke-Korsakoff syndrome
	Neutral tube defects

3. Why is it important that water-soluble vitamins be consumed daily?
4. Define "megadose." What are the disadvantages of taking vitamin megadoses?
5. Name three foods that are good sources of each of the following nutrients: thiamin, riboflavin, vitamin B_{12}, and folate.
6. What would you teach a vegan about vitamin B_{12}?
7. Discuss why signs and symptoms of deficiencies of water-soluble vitamins appear periorally. List signs and symptoms of deficiencies you should be alert for and list vitamins that might be implicated.
8. What recommendations could you offer to a patient to ensure the availability of folate? Why is folate so important before and during pregnancy?

◆ CASE STUDY

A 32-year-old male presents with the following symptoms: swollen tongue with reddening at the tip, small oral ulcerations, and gingival hyperplasia. The patient is being treated with long-term anticonvulsant medication.

1. Is a dietary assessment indicated? Explain your answer.
2. What are possible effects of the patient's medication on his nutritional and oral status?
3. If a deficiency exists, which vitamins/minerals are most likely lacking? Why?
4. Which types of foods and food preparation methods should be suggested? Why?
5. What advice should you give regarding oral care?

References

1. Institute of Medicine. *Food and Nutrition Board. Dietary Reference Intakes: Thiamin, Riboflavin, Niacin, Vitamin B6, Folate, Vitamin B12, Pantothenic Acid, Biotin, and Choline.* Washington, DC: National Academy Press; 1998.
2. Moskovitz M, Dotan M, Zilberman U. The influence of infantile thiamine deficiency on primary dentition. *Clin Oral Investig.* 2017;21(4):1309–1313.
3. National Institute of Health. National Institute on Alcohol Abuse and Alcoholism. *Alcohol's Effects on Health.* https://www.niaaa.nih.gov/alcohol-health/overview-alcohol-consumption/moderate-binge-drinking
4. Wiley KD, Gupta M. Vitamin B1 (thiamine) deficiency. In: *StatPearls.* StatPearls; 2022.
5. Anding R.H., Baylor College of Medicine and Texas Childrens Hospital. *Thiamine and Riboflavin and the Highway to Health.* 2020. https://www.wondriumdaily.com/thiamine-and-riboflavin-and-the-highway-to-health
6. Harvard TH, Chan School of Public Health. Thiamin—vitamin B1. In: *The Nutrition Source.* https://www.hsph.harvard.edu/nutritionsource/vitamin-b1/.
7. National Institutes of Health. Office of Dietary Supplements. *Thiamin Fact Sheet for Health Professionals.* https://ods.od.nih.gov/factsheets/Thiamin-HealthProfessional/.
8. Retallick-Brown H, Blampied N, Rucklidge JJ. A pilot randomized treatment-controlled trial comparing vitamin B6 with broad-spectrum micronutrients for premenstrual syndrome. *J Altern Complement Med.* 2020;26(2):88–97.
9. Stach K, Stach W, Augoff K. Vitamin B6 in health and disease. *Nutrients.* 2021;13(9):3229. https://doi.org/10.3390/nu13093229.
10. Horvat P, Gardiner J, Kubinova R, et al. Serum folate, vitamin B-12 and cognitive function in middle and older age: the HAPIEE study. *Exp Gerontol.* 2016;76:33–38.
11. McCleery J, Abraham RP, Denton DA, et al. Vitamin and mineral supplementation for preventing dementia or delaying cognitive decline in people with mild cognitive impairment. *Cochrane Database Syst Rev.* 2018;11(11): CD011905.
12. Vollset SE, Clarke R, Lewington S, et al. Effects of folic acid supplementation on overall and site-specific cancer incidence during the randomised trials: meta-analyses of data on 50,000 individuals. *Lancet.* 2013;381(9871):1029–1036.
13. Moazzen S, Dolatkhah R, Tabrizi JS, et al. Folic acid intake and folate status and colorectal cancer risk: a systematic review and *meta-analysis. Clin Nutr.* 2018;37(6 Pt A):1926–1934.
14. National Center on Birth Defects and Developmental Disabilities, Centers for Disease Control and Prevention, Centers for Disease Control and Prevention. *Neural Tube Defects Prevention Around the World.* https://www.cdc.gov/grand-rounds/pp/2017/20171017-neural-tube.html.
15. CDC. Updated estimates of neural tube defects prevented by mandatory folic acid fortification—United States, 1995–2011. *MMWR Morb Mort Wkly Rep.* 2015;64(01):1–5.
16. Krzizek EC, Brix JM, Stöckl A, Parzer V, Ludvik B. Prevalence of micronutrient deficiency after bariatric surgery. *Obes Facts.* 2021;14(2):197–204.
17. Wang D, Jin L, Zhang J, Meng W, Ren A, Jin L. Maternal periconceptional folic acid supplementation and risk for fetal congenital heart defects. *J Pediatr.* 2022;240:72–78.
18. Zhang D-M, Ye J-X, Mu J-S, et al. Efficacy of vitamin B supplementation on cognition in elderly patients with cognitive-related diseases: a systematic review and *meta-analysis. J Geriat Psychiatry Neurol.* 2017;30(1):50–59.
19. Wang H, Li L, Qin LL, Song Y, Vidal-Alaball J, Liu TH. Oral vitamin B(12) versus intramuscular vitamin B(12) for vitamin B(12) deficiency. *Cochrane Database Syst Rev.* 2018(3): CD004655.
20. Moore E, Mander A, Ames D, et al. Cognitive impairment and vitamin B_{12}: a review. *Int Psychogeriatr.* 2012;24(4):541–556.
21. Aroda VR, Edelstein SL, Goldberg RB, et al. Long-term metformin use and vitamin B_{12} deficiency in the Diabetes Prevention Program Outcomes Study. *J Clin Endocrinol Metab.* 2016;101(4):1754–1761.
22. Chapman LE, Darling AL, Brown JE. Association between metformin and vitamin B_{12} deficiency in patients with type 2 diabetes: a systematic review and *meta-analysis. Diabetes Metab.* 2016;42:316–327.
23. Miller JW. Proton pump inhibitors, H2-receptor antagonists, metformin, and vitamin B-12 deficiency: clinical implications. *Adv Nutr.* 2018;9(4):511S–518S.
24. Saleem F., Soos M.P. Biotin deficiency. In: *StatPearls.* StatPearls Publishing. https://www.ncbi.nlm.nih.gov/books/NBK547751/.
25. Cowan AE, Tooze JA, Gahche JJ, et al. Trends in overall and micronutrient-containing dietary supplement use in US adults and children, NHANES 2007-2018. *J Nutr.* 2023;152(12):2789–2801.
26. National Institutes of Health. *Multivitamin/Mineral Supplements Fact Sheet for Health Professionals.* https://ods.od.nih.gov/factsheets/MVMS-HealthProfessional/.
27. Qato DM, Alexander GC, Guadamuz JS, Lindau ST. Prevalence of dietary supplement use in US children and adolescents, 2003–2014. *JAMA Pediatr.* 2018;172:780–782.

28. National Institutes of Health. Multivitamin/mineral supplements fact sheet for health professionals. Updated June 6, 2023. https://ods.od.nih.gov/factsheets/MVMS-HealthProfessional/ Accessed August 14, 2023.

29. National Products Insider. *Supplement Business Report. L Changing Channels.* Nutrition Business Journal; 2021. https://www.naturalproductsinsider.com/business-operations/supplement-business-forecast-special-report.

30. Mishra S, Stierman B, Gahche JJ, Potischman N. *Dietary supplement use among adults: United States, 2017–2018. NCHS Data Brief, No 399.* National Center for Health Statistics; 2021. https://doi.org/10.15620/cdc:101131.

31. Crawford C, Brown LL, Costello RB, Deuster PA. Select dietary supplement ingredients for preserving and protecting the immune system in healthy individuals: a systematic review. *Nutrients.* 2022;14(21):4604. https://doi.org/10.3390/nu14214604.

32. Pfeiffer CM, Sternberg MR, Schleicher RL, Haynes BM, Rybak ME, Pirkle JL. The CDC's second national report on biochemical indicators of diet and nutrition in the U.S. population is a valuable tool for researchers and policy makers. *J Nutr.* 2013;143(6):938S–947SS. https://doi.org/10.3945/jn.112.172858.

33. Centers for Disease Control and Prevention (CDC). *CDC's Second Nutrition Report: A Comprehensive Biochemical Assessment of the Nutrition Status of the U.S. Population.* 2012. http://www.cdc.gov/nutritionreport/.

34. ConsumerLab. *Multivitamin and Multimineral Supplements Review.* https://www.consumerlab.com/reviews/review_multivitamin_compare/multivitamins/.

35. Ferraro PM, Curhan GC, Gambaro G, Taylor EN. Total, dietary, and supplemental vitamin C intake and risk of incident kidney stones. *Am J Kidney Dis.* 2016;67(3):400–407. https://doi.org/10.1053/j.ajkd.2015.09.005.

36. Schwingshackl L, Boeing H, Stelmach-Mardas M, et al. Dietary supplements and risk of cause-specific death, cardiovascular disease, and cancer: a systematic review and *meta-analysis* of primary prevention trials. *Adv Nutr.* 2017;8:27–39.

37. Gummin DD, Mowry JB, Beuhler MC, et al. 2021 Annual Report of the National Poison Data System© (NPDS) from America's Poison Centers: 39th annual report. *Clin Toxicol.* 2022;60(12):1381–1643.

38. Rao N, Spiller HA, Hodges NL, et al. An increase in dietary supplement exposures reported to US Poison Control Centers. *J Med Toxicol.* 2017. https://doi.org/10.1007/s13181-017-0623-7.

39. Chen F, Du M, Blumberg JB, et al. Association among dietary supplement use, nutrient intake, and mortality among U.S. adults: a cohort study. *Ann Intern Med.* 2019;170(9):604–613.

40. Fulton SL, McKinley MC, Youg IS, et al. The effect of increasing fruit and vegetable consumption on overall diet: a systematic review and *meta-analysis. Crit Rev Food Sci Nutr.* 2016;56:802–816.

 Evolve Resources

Please visit http://evolve.elsevier.com/Mallonee/nutritional for additional practice and study support tools.

12

Fluids and Minerals Required for Oral Soft Tissues and Salivary Glands

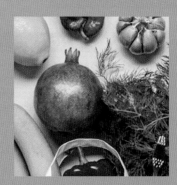

STUDENT LEARNING OUTCOMES

On completion of this chapter, the student will be able to achieve the following student learning outcomes:

1. In relation to fluids:
   - Describe the physiologic roles of fluid and list the fluid requirements for both males and females. Also, identify factors that may affect those requirements.
   - List and discuss the various sources of fluid.
   - Discuss hyper and hypo states related to fluid imbalances in the body; identify oral signs and symptoms of fluid imbalances; and discuss areas of nutritional concern with patients who have fluid imbalances.
   - Differentiate popular beverages for their benefits and/or detrimental oral health effects.
2. Explain how electrolytes affect hydration status.
3. In relation to sodium and chloride:
   - Describe the physiologic roles of sodium and chloride, and list the requirements for both males and females.
   - List and discuss the various sources of sodium and chloride, and discuss with patients how to decrease dietary sources of sodium.
   - Discuss hyper and hypo states related to sodium and chloride imbalances in the body, identify oral signs and symptoms of sodium imbalances.
   - Identify diseases and medications associated with restriction of sodium intake.
4. In relation to potassium:
   - Describe the physiologic roles of potassium, and list potassium requirements for both males and females.
   - List and discuss the various sources of potassium, and discuss with patients how to increase dietary sources of potassium.
   - Discuss hyper and hypo states related to potassium imbalances in the body, identify oral signs and symptoms of potassium imbalances, and discuss areas of nutritional concern with patients who have potassium imbalances.
5. In relation to iron:
   - Describe the physiologic roles of iron, and list the iron requirements for both males and females.
   - List and discuss the various sources of iron.
   - Discuss hyper and hypo states related to iron imbalances in the body. Identify oral signs and symptoms of iron imbalances, and discuss areas of nutritional concern with patients who have iron imbalances.
6. In relation to zinc and iodine:
   - Describe the physiologic roles of zinc and iodine, and list the zinc and iodine requirements for both males and females.
   - List and discuss the various sources of zinc and iodine, and discuss with patients how to increase dietary sources of zinc and iodine.
   - Discuss hyper and hypo states related to zinc and iodine imbalances in the body. Identify oral signs and symptoms of zinc and iodine imbalances, and discuss areas of nutritional concern with patients who have zinc and iodine imbalances.

KEY TERMS

Aldosterone	Goitrogens	Myxedema
Anions	Guarana	Nonheme iron
Antidiuretic hormone (ADH)	Heme iron	Osmoreceptors
Cations	Hemochromatosis	Peripheral edema
Cretinism	Hyperkalemia	Quercetin
Ergogenic	Hypernatremia	Renin
Erosion	Hypodipsia	Solutes
Essential hypertension	Hypokalemia	Solvent
Extracellular fluid (ECF)	Hyponatremia	Taurine
Fluid volume deficit (FVD)	Interstitial fluid	Transferrin
Fluid volume excess (FVE)	Intracellular fluid (ICF)	
Goiter	Longitudinal fissures	

⟐ TEST YOUR NQ

1. **T/F** Thirst is the primary regulator of fluid intake.
2. **T/F** Meats are made of more than half water.
3. **T/F** Water is the most abundant component in the body.
4. **T/F** Heme iron is provided by meat sources and is more readily absorbed than iron from vegetable or grain products.
5. **T/F** Normal fluid requirements are eight 8-oz cups of total water daily.
6. **T/F** The Recommended Dietary Allowance (RDA) for sodium is 5000 mg/day.
7. **T/F** Taste alteration is a symptom of zinc deficiency.
8. **T/F** Potassium is principally found in extracellular fluid.
9. **T/F** Milk is a good source of potassium.
10. **T/F** Pallor of oral mucosa is associated with iodine deficiency.

Water and several mineral elements are essential for maintenance of healthy oral tissues, including tooth enamel. Visual signs of these nutrient deficiencies in the gingiva, mucous membranes, and salivary glands are less obvious than signs observed with the B vitamin complex and vitamin C deficiencies discussed in Chapter 11. Nevertheless, water and several minerals have a significant effect on integrity of the oral cavity and, ultimately, nutritional status. Oral problems associated with hyper or hypo states of the minerals discussed in this chapter are slow to develop and may not be evident immediately. Chronically decreased salivary flow attributable to inadequate body fluids increases caries risk and may lead to rampant tooth decay and eventually loss of teeth.

Fluids

Water is the most abundant component in the body. At birth, water constitutes approximately 75% to 80% of body weight. Because such a large percentage of the infant's body weight consists of water, fluid loss is more significant in infants than in adults. Total body water decreases with age, representing 50% to 60% of an adult's body weight. Adipose tissue contains less water than muscle; a person with a large amount of fat has a lower percentage of total body water. Females' bodies, with inherently larger fat stores, contain less water than males' bodies, which have a higher percentage of lean muscle tissue.

Body fluids are distributed in compartments, separated by semipermeable membranes. Intracellular fluid (ICF), which constitutes 60% of the body's fluid weight, includes all the fluid within cells (chiefly in muscle tissue; Fig. 12.1). Extracellular fluid (ECF) consists of fluid outside the cells, including fluid in plasma and lymph and the interstitial fluid that fills the space between cells. These fluids help control movement of water and electrolytes through the body. Membranes serve as barriers by preventing movement of certain substances from one compartment to another; however, they do not completely isolate the compartments. Water is essentially unrestricted in its movement from compartment to compartment. Certain dissolved substances, or solutes, such as glucose, amino acids, and oxygen, also cross membranes freely. Cellular membranes allow maintenance of solute concentration by their selectivity.

When two compartments are separated by semipermeable membranes and movement of some solutes is restricted, osmosis occurs. Osmotic pressure within the body equalizes the solute concentration of ICFs and ECFs by shifting small amounts of water in the direction of higher concentration of solute, as shown in Chapter 3.

Physiologic Roles

Water has several important physiologic roles: (1) it acts as a solvent (fluid in which substances are dissolved), enabling chemical reactions to occur by entering into reactions, such as hydrolysis; (2) it maintains stability of all body fluids, as principal component and medium for fluids (blood and lymph), secretions (saliva and gastrointestinal fluids), and excretions (urine and perspiration); (3) it enables transport of nutrients to cells and provides a medium for excretion of waste products; (4) it acts as a lubricant between cells to permit movement without friction; and (5) it regulates body temperature by evaporating as perspiration from skin and vapor from the mouth and nose. Negative fluid balance has serious detrimental effects on many physiologic functions. A few days without water can be fatal.

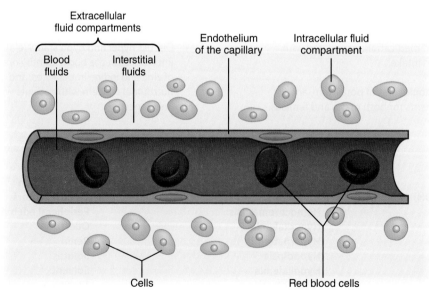

• **Fig. 12.1** Water is a key component of the fluid compartment inside (intracellular) and outside (extracellular) cells.

Requirements and Regulation

Fluid requirements are based on experimentally derived intake levels that are expected to meet nutritional needs of a healthy population. To maintain normal hydration, the National Academy of Medicine established an Adequate Intake (AI) for total fluid (beverages, water, and food). As shown in Table 12.1, males require 3.7 L/day (125 oz), and females require 2.7 L/day (91 oz). Daily fluid intake averaged 117 oz/day for males and 93 oz for females in 2009 to 2012.[1] No Tolerable Upper Intake Level (UL) is established for water, although water intoxication does occur occasionally.

Overconsumption and underconsumption of fluids can occur over short periods. However, if adequate amounts of fluids are available, consumption matches physiologic needs over an extended period. Individuals who consume a high-protein or high-fiber diet, struggle with diarrhea or vomiting, are physically active or exposed to warm or hot weather, require more fluids.

Water is lost by a variety of routes: (1) urination, (2) perspiration, (3) expiration, and (4) defecation. Urine production depends on the amount of fluid intake and type of diet eaten. However, waste products must be kept in solution; minimum urine output to eliminate waste products is 400 to 600 mL/day.

Water losses in the form of sweat can vary greatly. An increase in body temperature (fever) is accompanied by increased sweating and respiration. Strenuous exercise can greatly affect the amount of water lost through the skin. Water vapor in expired air varies with the rate of respiration. The presence of inflammation also elevates respiration rate. Approximately 100 to 200 mL of water is lost each day in feces; this dramatically increases with diarrhea.

Water losses result in stimulation of water (thirst) and decreased kidney output to maintain fluid balance. Saliva also may help maintain water balance because saliva flow is reduced in dehydration, leading to drying of the oral mucosa and sensation of thirst.

Normal fluid requirements (Fig. 12.2) can be drastically changed in different climatic environments, with various exercise levels, diet, and social activities, and with illnesses accompanied by diarrhea or vomiting. The body cannot store water, so the amount lost must be replaced.

In healthy adults, thirst is the earliest sign of the body's need for fluids but is often mistaken for hunger (Fig. 12.3). The ability to regulate water balance is not as precise in infants and older adults. Older patients often have a reduced sensation of thirst. When 2% of body water is lost, osmoreceptors are stimulated, creating a physiologic desire to ingest liquids. Osmoreceptors are neurons in the hypothalamus sensitive to changes in serum osmolality levels. Stimulation of osmoreceptors not only causes thirst but also increases the release of antidiuretic hormone (ADH) from the pituitary gland. ADH causes the body to retain fluid by decreasing urinary output (see Fig. 12.2). Conversely, ADH secretion is inhibited when fluids accumulate and excess water is eliminated.

Decreased blood pressure also stimulates release of the enzyme renin, which ultimately leads to increased release of the hormone aldosterone by the adrenal cortex. This release of aldosterone results in retention of sodium and water by the kidneys and excretion of potassium and hydrogen ions, causing blood pressure to increase.

Absorption

No digestion is necessary for water absorption; it is transported easily in both directions across the intestinal mucosa by osmosis (see Fig. 3.5). Within an hour, 1 L can be absorbed from the small intestine. Normally, almost all fluid is absorbed, with a small amount excreted in feces.

Sources

Water

Water is the only liquid nutrient essential for body hydration. During the process of metabolism, liquids and solid foods provide water. Some fruits and vegetables have a higher percentage of water than milk, and meats do contain more than half water (Table 12.2). Regardless of its source, fluids act the same physiologically. Water liberated in the process of metabolism is also available. Metabolism of fat produces approximately twice as much water as the metabolism of protein or carbohydrate; metabolism of these macronutrients supplies about 300 to 350 mL daily.

Plain tap water is the most natural source of fluids, best for quenching thirst, most economical, and healthiest. Greater than 30% of fluid intake comes from water for adults and >40% for youth (ages 2–19).[1,2] Fig. 12.4 indicates the distribution of the

TABLE 12.1	National Academy of Medicine Recommendations for Water	
	AI[a]	
Life Stage	**Male (L/day)**[b]	**Female (L/day)**[b]
0–6 months	0.7[c]	0.7[c]
7–12 months	0.8[d]	0.8[d]
1–3 years	1.3[e]	1.3[e]
4–8 years	1.7[f]	1.7[f]
9–13 years	2.4[g]	2.1[h]
14–18 years	3.3[i]	2.3[g]
>18 years	3.7[j]	2.7[k]
Pregnancy		
14–50 years		3[l]
Lactation		
14–50 years		3.8[m]

AI, Adequate intake.
[a]The AI is not equivalent to a Recommended Dietary Allowance.
[b]L = liter; 1 L = 4.2 cups.
[c]Assumed to be from human milk.
[d]Assumed to be from human milk, complementary foods, and beverages. This includes ~0.6 L (~3 cups) as total fluid, including formula or human milk, juices, and drinking water.
[e]Total water. This includes ~0.9 L (~4 cups) as total beverages, including drinking water.
[f]Total water. This includes ~1.7 L (~5 cups) as total beverages, including drinking water.
[g]Total water. This includes ~1.8 L (~8 cups) as total beverages, including drinking water.
[h]Total water. This includes ~1.6 L (~7 cups) as total beverages, including drinking water.
[i]Total water. This includes ~2.6 L (~11 cups) as total beverages, including drinking water.
[j]Total water. This includes ~3 L (~13 cups) as total beverages, including drinking water.
[k]Total water. This includes ~2.7 L (~9 cups) as total beverages, including drinking water.
[l]Total water. This includes ~3 L (~10 cups) as total beverages, including drinking water.
[m]Total water. This includes ~3.1 L (~13 cups) as total beverages, including drinking water.
Data from Institute of Medicine (IOM), Food and Nutrition Board. *Dietary Reference Intakes for Water, Potassium, Sodium, Chloride, Chloride, and Sulfate.* National Academies Press; 2005.

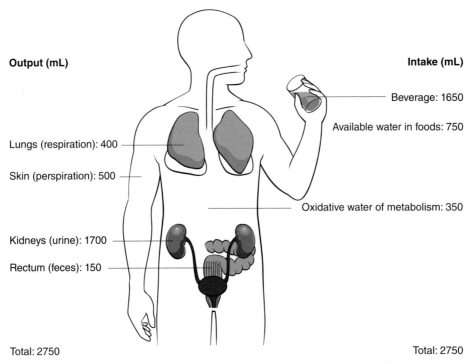

Output (mL)

Intake (mL)

Beverage: 1650

Available water in foods: 750

Lungs (respiration): 400

Skin (perspiration): 500

Oxidative water of metabolism: 350

Kidneys (urine): 1700

Rectum (feces): 150

Total: 2750

Total: 2750

• **Fig. 12.2** The role of osmoreceptors and antidiuretic hormone in fluid balance.

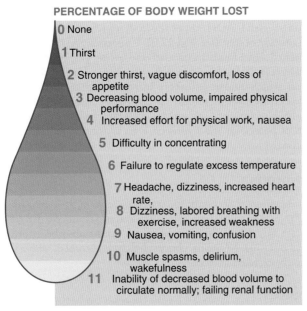

PERCENTAGE OF BODY WEIGHT LOST

0 None

1 Thirst

2 Stronger thirst, vague discomfort, loss of appetite

3 Decreasing blood volume, impaired physical performance

4 Increased effort for physical work, nausea

5 Difficulty in concentrating

6 Failure to regulate excess temperature

7 Headache, dizziness, increased heart rate,

8 Dizziness, labored breathing with exercise, increased weakness

9 Nausea, vomiting, confusion

10 Muscle spasms, delirium, wakefulness

11 Inability of decreased blood volume to circulate normally; failing renal function

• **Fig. 12.3** Percentage of body weight lost. Adverse effects of dehydration. (Reproduced with permission from Mahan LK, Raymond JL. *Krause's Food & the Nutrition Care Process*. 14th ed. St. Louis, MO: Elsevier, 2017.)

types of beverage intake for the youth. The United States has one of the safest public water supplies in the world. During the past century, many improvements in Americans' health can be attributed to improvements in drinking water, such as community fluoridation and infectious disease control. When groundwater becomes polluted, it is no longer safe to drink. Water contaminates may include naturally occurring arsenic and radon; lead from corroded pipes; fertilizer and pesticides; microbial agents, such as bacteria, viruses, parasites; medications; or waste from manufacturing processes.

The Environmental Protection Agency regulates levels of contaminants allowed in public drinking water; these amounts are provided to customers by water utility companies annually or can be obtained online for a specific area. Private well owners are responsible for ensuring that their water is safe from contaminants.

Concerns about the water supply, a desire for a more convenient form of fluid intake, may lead consumers to choose bottled water. The bottled water market continues to increase but suffered a setback as a result of environmental concerns (e.g., energy required to produce plastic nonbiodegradable plastic bottles, bisphenol A BPA content of bottles, cost of marketing, and shipping bottles of water) and the revelation that a large percentage of bottled water from well-known brands utilize groundwater (same source as the public water supply) or tap water. The letters P.W.S. on bottled water stands for "public water source." Bottled water, regulated by the US Food and Drug Administration (FDA), is available with many labels: drinking water, sparkling water, mineral water, Artesian water, alkaline water, caffeinated water, oxygenated water, and purified water (distilled, demineralized, deionized, and reverse osmosis). Bottled water also includes flavored waters and nutrient-added water beverages. Broad claims for these various waters lack research to support them.

The FDA established maximum levels for contaminants and disinfection by-products (e.g., bromate, chlorite, and so on) and disinfectants (e.g., chlorine) in bottled water. This trend has resulted in increased water intake, but numerous problems are associated with this practice. Many consumers think bottled water is healthier, but most bottled waters do not contain fluoride. Fluoride does not have to be listed on the label unless it is added.

Coffee and Tea

Coffee is the number one beverage consumed at home. For many Americans, coffee tastes good and helps "jump start" the morning. Both coffee and tea, without added sugars or creamers, contain

TABLE 12.2	Percentage of Water in Foods	
Food Item	**% Water**	
Vegetables		
Lettuce, raw	96	
Celery, raw	96	
Cabbage, raw	92	
Broccoli, boiled	91	
Spinach, boiled	91	
Fruits		
Watermelon, raw	91	
Strawberries, raw	91	
Grapefruit, raw	91	
Peach, raw	90	
Banana, raw	74	
Raisins	15	
Dairy		
Milk, nonfat	91	
Yogurt, low fat	85	
Cottage cheese, low fat	83	
Ice cream, vanilla	61	
Cheese, swiss	38	
Meat, Fish, Poultry, Eggs		
Eggs	76	
Fish, baked	72	
Chicken, roasted	67	
Beef steak, broiled	58	
Grains		
Cereals, cooked	85	
Rice, brown, boiled	70	
Pasta, cooked	62	
Bread, whole wheat	39	
Bread, white	36	
Crackers, saltines	5	

From U.S. Department of Agriculture (USDA), Agricultural Research Service. *FoodData Central, 2020. USDA National Nutrient Database for Standard Reference, Version 2.* 2020. http://fdc.nal.usda.gov.

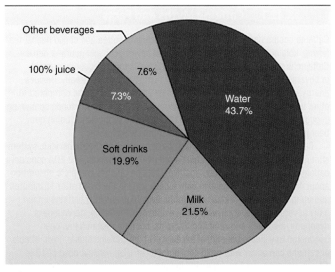

• **Fig. 12.4** Contribution of intake (grams) across beverage types, US youths (age 2–19 years). Other beverages include coffee, tea, sports and energy drinks. (NHANES 2013-2016. https://www.cdc.gov/nchs/data/factsheets/factsheet_nutrition.htm.)

compounds. These naturally present chemical compounds may be the reason numerous studies have discovered an inverse relationship between coffee consumption and chronic health conditions (Box 12.1).

Because of the addition of caffeine to many new products, it is important for the dental hygienist to recognize potential sources to educate the patient (Table 12.3). Coffee consumption has no detrimental effects on periodontal health.[3] Specifically, chlorogenic acid (a phenolic acid) may have antimicrobial qualities and can inhibit the activity and proliferation of *Porphyromonas gingivalis*.[4] More studies are needed to determine the effects of caffeine on periodontal disease.

The most common types of caffeinated teas are black, green, and oolong, while most herbal teas are decaffeinated. Antioxidants are found in both caffeinated and herbal teas. During processing, some of the antioxidants are destroyed, such as in tea powders, decaffeinated and bottle teas.

For teas containing senna, aloe, buckthorn, and other plant-derived laxatives, the FDA has issued warnings. In addition, the FDA has granted permission for unauthorized health claims for green teas and requested that other manufacturers remove health claims on their labels.

Sugar-Sweetened Beverages

Sugar-sweetened beverages (SSB) constitute up to 50% of added sugar intake in the United States and globally, with carbonated beverages being the highest contributor. The *Dietary Guidelines* recommend reducing added sugar consumption to less than 10% of total calories/day and to choose beverages with no added sugars.[5] Most notable is the observed decline in SSB consumption replaced with water.[6] SSB includes sugary carbonated beverages; noncarbonated fruit drinks; sports and energy drinks; sweetened coffees, teas, and water. The Center for Disease Control (CDC) found 26% of adults (31% in nonmetropolitan counties, 25% in metropolitan counties) and 63% youth reported consuming a SSB at least once daily.[7] According to the National Health and Nutrition Examination Survey (NHANES), a federally supported monitoring protocol coordinated by the National Center for

negligible calories, vitamins, or minerals. Both beverages contain caffeine, a compound that has received a lot of attention regarding its safety. In addition to contributing to fluid intake, both have some health benefits. In addition to caffeine, they both contain valuable polyphenols, antioxidants, and other bioactive

• BOX 12.1 Caffeine Myths and Facts*

Caffeine occurs naturally in many plants, including coffee and cacao beans, tea leaves, kola nuts (used to flavor carbonated beverages), and guarana berries. Caffeine is added to medications and foods but is most frequently present in beverages. The caffeine concentration in products varies greatly. Besides energy shots, coffee has one of the highest amounts of caffeine compared to other beverages. Coffee is highly consumed worldwide. Beside foods containing chocolate, it has been added to a multitude of food products including gum, beef jerky, waffles and maple syrup to promote wakefulness.

Caffeine is a part of the methylxanthines, a group of central nervous system stimulants, affecting the brain, spinal cord, and other nerves. The FDA considers caffeine both a drug and a food additive. Caffeine reaches complete absorption about 45 minutes after ingestion with a peak level in the blood after 15 minutes and up to 2 hours. It is metabolized in the liver. High levels of caffeine intake have adverse effects, such as anxiety, excitement, agitation, nervousness, dysphoria, insomnia and rambling thoughts, but little research has been conducted to validate benefits of excessively high caffeine intake. Toxic effects of caffeine can occur with rapid consumption of 1.2 g, while a dose of 10 to 14 g is thought to be fatal.[1] It would be atypical to consume poisonous levels of caffeine through coffees and teas, however, caffeine poisoning may occur from high dose tablets or supplements.[1]

Caffeine increases a person's metabolic rate and may be associated with increased wakefulness. Very high caffeine intake (>500 mg/day) is associated with nervousness, restlessness, anxiety, difficulty with sleeping, arrhythmia, gastrointestinal upset, tremors, and psychomotor agitation. Moderate amounts of caffeine (about 300 mg/day) do not cause these effects in most individuals.

1. Myth: Caffeine is not addictive.
   Fact: As a central nervous system stimulant, it can cause mild physical dependence, but it does not threaten physical, social, or economic health as addictive drugs do. Abruptly stopping caffeine may cause withdrawal symptoms such as headache, fatigue, anxiety, and depressed mood and concentration for a day or two.
2. Myth: Caffeine consumed within 6 hours of going to bed may cause insomnia.
   Fact: Caffeine is quickly absorbed and in most cases, the body rids of caffeine quickly. The liver metabolizes caffeine. Drinking 1 or 2 cups of coffee in the morning will not interfere with nighttime sleep for most people.
3. Myth: Caffeine enhances the risk of osteoporosis.
   Fact: Moderate amounts of caffeine do not increase risk for osteoporosis. High levels (more than 700 mg/day) do not increase risk for bone loss if adequate amounts of calcium are consumed. (The addition of 2 tbsp of milk in a cup of coffee can offset calcium loss.) However, older adults may be more sensitive to the effects of caffeine

on calcium metabolism and, to be cautious, postmenopausal females should limit caffeine intake to less than 300 mg/day.
4. Myth: Low amounts of caffeine (less than 200 mg caffeine/day) have not been found to interfere with the ability to get pregnant or cause miscarriages, birth defects, premature birth, or low birth rate.
   Fact: One cup of coffee (containing approximately 200 mg caffeine) is considered safe during pregnancy.
5. Myth: Caffeine is dehydrating.
   Fact: Caffeine acts as a mild diuretic, but fluid in caffeinated beverages offsets the effect of fluid loss and does not cause dehydration.
6. Myth: Caffeine helps individuals under the influence of alcohol to sober up.
   Fact: Caffeine has no effect in helping people under the influence of alcohol to sober up. Reaction time and judgment are still impaired.

Caffeine has some health benefits including improved alertness, concentration, and energy, and possible improvement in immune function. The International Agency for Research on Cancer (IARC), part of the World Health Organization, and the American Cancer Society determined the evidence to be inconclusive of coffee drinking causing human cancer, and it helps to reduce the risk of several forms of human cancer. Coffee consumption may reduce the risk of liver diseases, diabetes mellitus, and high blood pressure.[1,2] Evidence indicates that it is not harmful and may be beneficial in helping prevent CVD, congestive heart failure, heart arrhythmias, and stroke.[1,3,4] However, coffee has not been shown to prevent these conditions, and whether the health benefits are causal or associative findings is unknown. Researchers are unsure which elements in coffee and tea contribute to these health benefits, but they agree it is not the caffeine.

Energy drinks and soft drinks may contain sugar and/or caffeine. In general, soft drinks contain less caffeine than energy drinks per ounce. Caffeine content of many coffees, teas, soft drinks, energy drinks, and candies are listed in Table 12.3.

References

1. vanDam RM, Hu FB, Willett W. Coffee, caffeine, and health. *NEJM*. 2020;383:369–378.
2. Furman D, Chang J, Lartigue L, et al. Expression of specific inflammasome gene modules stratifies older individuals into two extreme clinical and immunological states. *Nat Med*. 2017;23:174–184.
3. Lee J, Lee JE, Kim Y. Relationship between coffee consumption and stroke risk in Korean population: the Health Examinees (HEXA) Study. *Nutr J*. 2017;16(1):7.
4. Wikoff D, Welsh BT, Henderson R, et al. Systematic review of potential adverse effects of caffeine consumption in healthy adults, pregnant women, adolescents, and children. *Food Chem Toxicol*. 2017;109:585–648.

*Adapted from Stuart A. *Caffeine Myths and Facts*. 2020 WebMD, LLC, June 12, 2021. www.webmd.com/diet/caffeine-myths-and-facts#1. Accessed March 25, 2023.

Health Statistics at the CDC, almost 30% of fluid intake for US youth (age 2–19 years) is a SSB (see Fig. 12.4). A 20-oz sugary carbonated beverage, for example, contains 15 to 18 tsp of sugar and approximately 240 calories. Although SSBs have significantly decreased among children and adults, according to the NHANES data, each group continues to consume more than the recommendation.[7,8] The declining sugary carbonated beverage consumption is being replaced with liquids such as bottled water, sports drinks, energy drinks, coffees and teas.

Approximately half of the increase in energy intake occurring over the past 20 years is attributed to sugar-sweetened beverages. Most people are unaware of how many calories or grams of added sugar are in their beverages, but these factors can be linked to dental caries, weight gain, metabolic syndrome, cardiovascular disease, and other chronic conditions.

Energy Drinks

Energy drinks are nonalcoholic fluids with a low pH value which may include ingredients such as added sugar, stimulants, electrolytes, vitamins, minerals, amino acids and herbs. Specifically, energy drinks contain ingredients such as caffeine (stimulant), guarana (a seed containing four times as much caffeine as coffee beans), and taurine (an amino acid with antioxidant properties). Guarana is one of the stimulants in the National Collegiate Athletic Association's (NCAA) 2016 banned drugs list. A concentrated version is referred to as an energy shot, found in 2 to 3 oz containers and containing the same quantity of stimulants.[9] Since the introduction in the United States in 1997, the sales of energy drinks and shots have escalated.

Energy drinks are marketed as an ergogenic (enhance physical performance, stamina, or recovery) to delay fatigue and increase

TABLE 12.3   Caffeine Content of Beverages and Chocolate

Beverage or Product	Portion or Size	Caffeine Content (mg)
Coffee		
Coffee, brewed	12 oz (small)	96
Iced coffee, brewed	12 oz	112
Latte	12 oz	130
Espresso	1 oz	64
Cappuccino	12 oz	130
Coffee, instant, reconstituted	12 oz	62
Coffee, decaffeinated, brewed	12 oz	2
Espresso, decaffeinated	1 oz	0.3
Tea		
Green tea, hot	12 oz (small)	43
Black tea, hot	12 oz	72
Oolong tea, hot	12 oz	58
Tea, bottled, ready-to-drink	12 oz	11
Black tea, hot, decaffeinated	12 oz	2
Herbal tea	12 oz	0
Soft Drinks		
Cola, regular	12 oz	34
Fruit flavored citrus, regular and diet	12 oz	56
Yellow green colored citrus	12 oz	71
Dr. Pepper type, regular	12 oz	34
Dr. Pepper type, diet	12 oz	43
Cola, diet	12 oz	43
Cola, decaffeinated	12 oz	0
Root Beer	12 oz	0
A&W Root Beer; 7 Up; Sierra Mist, regular and diet; Sprite, regular and diet	12 oz	0
Energy Drinks		
5-Hour energy	2 oz	200–207
Rockstar, regular or sugar free	8 oz	79–80
Red Bull, regular or sugar free	8.4 oz	75–80
Amp, regular or sugar free	8 oz	71–74
Full Throttle, regular or sugar free	8 oz	70–100
Chocolate Candy		
Candy, milk chocolate	1 bar (1.55 oz)	9
Candy, semi-sweet chocolate	1 bar (1.55 oz)	27
Candy, white chocolate	1 bar (1.55 oz)	0

From U.S. Department of Agriculture (USDA), Agricultural Research Service. *FoodData Central, 2020.* USDA National Nutrient Database for Standard Reference, *Version 2.* 2020. http://fdc.nal.usda.gov.

alertness. They promise to make a person feel more awake and boost attention span. This is appealing to children, adolescents, young adults, and middle-aged adults, but can have negative health outcomes. Consuming several energy drinks, especially when combined with alcohol, have been linked to serious adverse events, including cardiac arrest, myocardial infarction, atrial fibrillation, and seizures. Energy drinks may also increase risk for caffeine overdose in caffeine abstainers as well as in habitual consumers of caffeinated coffee, soft drinks, and tea. Therefore the American Academy of Pediatrics, American College of Sports Medicine, and the American Heart Association are examples of reputable health organizations that discourage intake of energy drinks.

Decaffeinated energy drinks have eliminated caffeine but are packed with B vitamins and quercetin (bioflavonoid reported to energize muscles). Energy drinks containing "natural" ingredients, such as ginkgo or guarana, are considered a dietary supplement rather than a food or medication by the FDA. Contrary to what commercial advertisements would lead one to believe, vitamins only help the body use energy from foods; extra B vitamins do not provide additional energy bursts. These vitamins and amino acids are present in larger quantities than found naturally occurring in foods and plants; their combined effect when combined with caffeine may be enhanced. Almost all Americans get adequate amounts of B vitamins in their diets, yet marketers would lead people to believe that a megadose of B vitamin will energize.

Sports Drinks

Recent emphasis on Americans increasing their physical activity appears to have sparked an interest in supplemental products by sports enthusiasts and people attempting to maintain their health. The availability of sports nutrition products is ubiquitous.

Hydration status impacts activity performance and monitoring timing and quantity of fluids is essential. Profuse sweating, electrolyte loss, and glycogen depletion may require ingestion of sports drinks. Water intake will likely be a proper rehydration choice for the majority of healthy individuals who follow adequate nutritional habits and perform physical activities lasting less than 60 to 80 minutes.[10] For most people engaged in routine physical activity, sports drinks offer little to no advantage over plain water, however, many individuals prefer the taste of a sports drink over water and will drink more.

Sports drinks and energy drinks are significantly different products, but the terms are confusing and used interchangeably by many consumers. Sports drinks (e.g., Gatorade and Powerade), popular among children and sports enthusiasts, are designed to restore fluid balance, to replace fluid and electrolytes lost in sweat during physical activity, and, ultimately, to optimize athletic performance.

Sports drinks often contain 6% to 8% carbohydrates (low pH), minerals, electrolytes, and sometimes vitamins or other nutrients, such as protein and/or amino acids. There is no advantage of consuming vitamins and/or the minerals calcium and magnesium in sports drinks; these are readily available in a well-balanced diet.

Most sports products are designed for endurance athletes who exercise at high intensity for prolonged periods. This type of athlete can benefit from a sports beverage that contains carbohydrates and electrolytes, and sometimes protein. Sports nutrition products are sometimes recommended for recreational athletes for exercising, especially in the heat and for high-intensity activities.

Scientific studies do not support claims of improved performance and recovery for many sports drinks and protein shakes, making it virtually impossible for the public to make informed choices about advertised sports products.

Dental Erosion

Many sweetened, flavored, and carbonated beverages have a pH in the acidic range (pH ≤ 4), which is associated with enamel erosion (Table 12.4).[11] Erosion is the permanent dissolution of tooth surfaces caused by the action of external (extrinsic) and internal (intrinsic) acids of non-bacterial sources. Acidic beverages would be an example of external sources, including carbonated beverages, SSBs, fruit juice, vitamin beverages, alcoholic beverages, sports and energy drinks. Frequent consumption and time of day are additional factors to consider for erosion. Damage to tooth enamel can occur in as little as 5 days of exposure to acidic beverages, especially with frequent exposure.

Calcium added to acidic beverages may lessen the erosive potential to teeth. Beverages with a low pH but containing high levels of fluoride promote some remineralization while beverages without fluoride roughen enamel surfaces.

Acids, such as phosphoric, malic or citric, are added to beverages for flavor, providing a tart, zingy, and differentiable taste to help offset the sweetness of the sugar present in beverages. Other benefits include acting as a preservative, inhibiting growth of bacteria or enhance taste which allows for a reduction of other flavoring ingredients. For example, colas will add phosphoric acid for the distinct flavor it provides, along with the ability to increase shelf life and reduce the growth of bacteria.[12]

Hyper States and Hypo States

Regulation of fluid intake and excretion by the kidneys usually maintain fluid balance in the body despite a wide range of intake (Fig. 12.5B). Imbalances may occur, however. **Fluid volume excess (FVE)** is the relatively equal gain of water and sodium in relation to their losses; **fluid volume deficit (FVD)** results from relatively equal losses of sodium and water.

🦷 DENTAL CONSIDERATIONS

- Individuals who do not ordinarily consume caffeine are not encouraged to change this habit.
- Small to moderate amounts of caffeine are not a concern for most individuals, but excessive consumption can cause disturbed sleep, headaches, irritability, and nervousness.
- If caffeine is added to a food product, it must be included in the ingredients listed on the food label. However, the amount does not have to be disclosed.
- Since primary teeth have a thinner enamel layer than permanent teeth, they are more susceptible to erosion, especially the dentin.
- Encourage patients to decrease SSBs. Recommendation: (1) substitute water, a beverage with a non-nutritive sweetener, or a beverage containing less or no added sugar. Be realistic with the recommendation. If the patient drinks multiple SSBs/day, compliance may be greater if replacing one SSB with an acceptable beverage and increasing this number as goals are met. (2) Decrease portion sizes. For example, if a patient is consuming a 20 oz SSB, suggest a 12 oz serving. (3) Encourage daily and adequate oral hygiene care.
- Although there is no conclusive evidence of effectiveness, some claim a mixture of apple cider vinegar and water every morning will reduce appetite and remove toxins. Due to the low pH value, educate the patient on dental erosion as an adverse side effect. When the patient wishes to continue use, instruct diluting the vinegar in a larger glass of water.
- Effective oral care prior to bedtime is essential to reduce the risk of erosion.

TABLE 12.4	pH of Beverages	
Beverage		**pH**
Lemon juice		2.25
Coca-cola Classic		2.37
Welch's 100% Grape Juice		2.38
Schweppes Tonic Water		2.54
Ocean Spray Cranberry Juice		2.56
Kool-Aid Mix Pink Lemonade		2.66
Rockstar Energy Drink		2.74
Powerade Lemon Lime		2.75
Crystal Light Raspberry Ice		2.77
Snapple Kiwi Strawberry		2.77
Vault		2.77
Hi-C Tropical		2.81
5-Hour Berry		2.81
Arizona Iced Tea		2.85
Crush Orange		2.87
Dr. Pepper		2.88
Lipton Green Tea with Citrus		2.93
Nestea Iced Tea with Lemon		2.94
V8 Splash Berry Blend		2.94
Vitamin Water Connect Black Cherry Lime		2.96
Gatorade Lemon Lime		2.97
Propel Berry		3.01
Dasani Strawberry		3.03
CapriSun Surfer Cooler		3.08
Full Throttle Citrus		3.09
Sobe Life Water Blackberry Grape		3.15
Mountain Dew		3.22
Red bull Shot		3.25
Red Bull Sugar Free		3.39
7UP Diet		3.48
Monster Energy		3.48
Fuze Tropical Punch		3.17
Juicy Juice Sparkling Apple		3.47
Welch's Apple Juice		3.57
AMP Energy Juice Orange		3.6
Welch's Orange Juice		3.73
Barq's Root Beer		4.11
S. Pellegrino Sparkling Mineral Water		4.96
Dasani water		5.03
Starbucks Medium Roast Coffee		5.11
Perrier Carbonated Mineral Water		5.25
Aquafina water		6.11

From Reddy A, Norris DF, Momeni SS, et al. The pH of beverages in the United States. *JADA*. 2016;147(4). https://doi.org/10.1016/j.adaj.2015.10.019.

NUTRITIONAL DIRECTIONS

- With regard to hydration and fluid intake, water is the gold standard. However, there are many acceptable fluids, such as skim milk. Although wine is acidic, it does not have the same potential for erosion as other acidic beverages do have, since it is generally not consumed as frequently.
- Habitual intake of caffeinated beverages (coffee, tea, soft drinks, and other caffeinated beverages) contributes to the daily total water intake similar to that contributed by noncaffeinated beverages.
- Consider caffeine consumption from all sources.
- Energy drinks can potentially be dangerous for individuals under 18 years, pregnant females, individuals who have a caffeine sensitivity, do not consume caffeine regularly, or are taking certain medications such as Adderall (for attention deficit disorder).
- The amount of caffeine in a product is not required on labels because it is not a nutrient.
- Beverages are important to satisfy nutritional and hydration needs and fluid preferences.
- The FDA, Health Canada, and the European Union have recommended limiting caffeine intake to 400 mg/day (4–5 cups of coffee), except for pregnant females, who should limit caffeine intake to 200 to 300 mg.
- Health Canada recommends limiting caffeine for children:
  - Ages 4 to 6 years: 45 mg, about the amount in one can of cola
  - Ages 7 to 9 years: 62 mg
  - Ages 10 to 12 years: 85 mg[13]
- Increase fluid intake and salivary production by chewing sugarless gum, preferably gum containing xylitol.
- High-protein diets, such as diets in which fruit and vegetable intake is minimal, increase fluid requirements to eliminate higher levels of urinary waste products.
- Drink fluids during exercise to replace fluid loss through perspiration. (Loss of 1 lb of body weight during exercise means at least 2 cups of water have been lost.) In most cases, water is the most appropriate choice.
- To make wise beverage choices, read labels on bottled waters to see what ingredients they contain.
- Most tap water is safe and economical.
- Make water more exciting by adding slices of lemon, lime, strawberries, cucumber, watermelon, mint leaves or add a splash of 100% juice to plain sparkling water.
- When selecting a sugar-sweetened beverage, choose a smaller size (6–8 oz).

Fluid Volume Excess

FVE mainly occurs in ECF compartments secondary to an increase in total body sodium content (Fig. 12.5C). Because water follows sodium, an excess leads to an increase in total body water. Excess fluid moves into interstitial compartments, located between cells and in body cavities such as joints, pleura, and the gastrointestinal tract, causing edema.

Congestive heart failure, chronic renal failure, chronic liver disease, and high levels of steroids may predispose an individual to FVE because of sodium retention. Conditions causing a loss of protein and reduced serum albumin levels (e.g., malnutrition and renal diseases) may contribute to FVE resulting from osmotic forces ordinarily exhibited by proteins and albumin. Common manifestations of FVE include rapid weight gain, puffy eyelids, distended neck veins, and elevated blood pressure. Peripheral edema is commonly observed in the legs and feet. Treatment involves correction of underlying problems or therapy for the specific disease; fluid or sodium (or both), may be restricted, or diuretics may be prescribed.

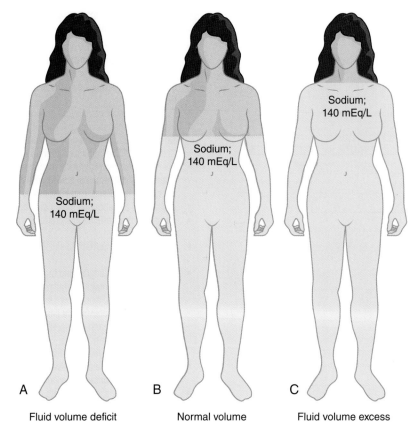

A — Fluid volume deficit

B — Normal volume

C — Fluid volume excess

• **Fig. 12.5** Fluid volume disturbances. Compared with normal body fluids (B), in fluid volume deficit (A), equal percentages of water and sodium losses occur, producing an isotonic depletion. In fluid volume excess (C), water and sodium are retained, producing an isotonic expansion. (Adapted from Davis JR, Sherer K. *Applied Nutrition and Diet Therapy for Nurses.* 2nd ed. Saunders Elsevier; 1994.)

Fluid Volume Deficit

In FVD (see Fig. 12.5A), the sodium-to-water ratio remains relatively equal; ADH and aldosterone secretions are not activated. Prolonged inadequate fluid intake can result in FVD. However, FVD is usually associated with excessive loss of fluids from the gastrointestinal tract (vomiting, diarrhea, or drainage tubes), urinary tract (diuretics, polyuria, or excessive urination), or skin (profuse sweating). Medications such as diuretics and laxatives may also increase risk of dehydration and heat-related illness in hot weather. Fever increases the need for electrolytes, increases fluid losses in dehumidified air, and causes excessive sweating.

Dehydration temporarily leads to weight loss, but more importantly, has adverse effects on cognitive function and motor control (see Fig. 12.3). Decreased food and fluid intake can result from illness, dementia, anorexia, nausea, or fatigue. Other less obvious reasons are an inability to (1) obtain water, such as with impaired movement; (2) activation of the thirst mechanism, as in **hypodipsia** (diminished thirst); or (3) swallow, as in neuromuscular problems or unconsciousness. Excessive fluid losses occasionally occur with prolonged exercise.

Common characteristics of FVD include weight loss, confusion and fatigue, sunken eyes, hypotension, and orthostatic hypotension. Classic signs are dry tongue with **longitudinal fissures** (slits or wrinkles that extend lengthwise on the tongue; Fig. 12.6), xerostomia, shrinkage of oral mucous membranes, decreased skin turgor, dry skin, and decreased urinary output. A diminished salivary flow is associated with inadequate fluid intake. Treatment involves

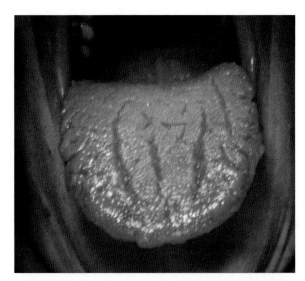

• **Fig. 12.6** Fissured tongue. (Reproduced with permission from Ibsen OAC, Phelan JA. *Oral Pathology for the Dental Hygienist.* 6th ed. St. Louis, MO: Saunders Elsevier; 2014.)

replacing lost fluid. If FVD is mild, oral fluids are likely to be sufficient; intravenous solutions are needed with significant FVD.

Electrolytes

Electrolytes are compounds or ions that dissociate in solution; they are also known as **cations** if they have a positive charge and **anions** if they have a negative charge. Cations in the body include sodium, potassium, calcium, and magnesium; anions include chloride, bicarbonate, and phosphate. The body's hydration status depends on an electrolyte balance of equal concentrations of cations to anions. Because the electrolyte concentration in plasma is so low,

DENTAL CONSIDERATIONS

- Common conversion of total water intake: 1 L = 33.8 fluid oz and 1 cup = 8 fluid oz.
- Direct measurement of the total amount of body water is impossible. Evaluation of physical signs of fluid deficit or excess is a valuable assessment to dental hygiene diagnosis and treatment.
- Assess patients for puffy eyelids or distended neck veins; inquire about recent unintentional weight changes, check blood pressure, and refer to a healthcare provider if necessary. A rapid weight loss or gain of 3% or greater of total body weight is significant.
- Observe for dry tongue with longitudinal fissures, xerostomia, or shrinkage of oral mucous membranes; adequacy of salivary flow; decreased skin turgor; and dry skin. Inquire about frequency and amount of urine output and fluid intake.
- Salivary flow measurements may be indicated for patients who present with FVD.
- Several physiologic and social factors prevalent in older patients place them at risk for dehydration (see Chapter 15). In addition, this population may drink less fluid because of dementia, immobility, or fear of incontinence.
- The oral mucosa is especially sensitive to the body's fluid volume; increases and decreases in body fluid affect the fit of a denture. FVD generates a loose-fitting prosthesis, whereas FVE may create a tight-fitting prosthesis. Patients may present with ulcerations with either fluid deficit or excess and find the prosthesis uncomfortable to wear.

NUTRITIONAL DIRECTIONS

- Rapid weight changes generally indicate loss or gain of water rather than fatty tissue; a loss or gain of 480 mL (2 cups) of fluid is equivalent to a loss or gain of 1 lb.
- Due to the larger surface area-to-body mass ratio, there is a risk for FVD in infants and children.
- Pale yellow or almost colorless urine indicates adequate hydration. Dark-yellow urine with a strong odor, advancing to painful urination, and (eventually) cessation of urine output are progressive signs of inadequate water intake and dehydration.

it is expressed as milliequivalents per liter (mEq/L). Electrolytes are important in water balance and acid-base (pH) balance.

Electrolyte distribution is different in ICF and ECF compartments. The principal cation in plasma and interstitial fluid is sodium; the principal anion is chloride. The principal cation in ICF is potassium; the principal anion is phosphate. The major difference between intravascular fluid and interstitial fluid is the large amount of protein in the former. Because sodium and potassium are the major cations, these are discussed in more detail.

Sodium

Physiologic Roles

The important physiologic roles of sodium include (1) maintaining normal ECF concentration by affecting the concentration, excretion, and absorption of potassium and chloride, and water distribution; (2) regulating acid-base balance; and (3) facilitating impulse transmission in nerve and muscle fibers. Sodium is present in calcified structures; its function in bones and teeth is unclear. It is also present in saliva. Sodium concentration in saliva determines one's recognition of salt in food.

Requirements and Regulation

Because sodium is readily available in foods, no RDA has been established. The National Academy of Medicine estimates a safe minimum intake might be 500 mg/day. This amount is increased in the face of abnormal losses. Sodium regulation involves several mechanisms. To keep the ECF concentration normal, the sodium-potassium pump is constantly moving sodium from the cell to ECF. Aldosterone released by the adrenal cortex results in sodium reabsorption or excretion by the kidneys depending on the body's need (Fig. 12.7). The kidneys can adjust sodium excretion to match sodium intake despite large variations in intake. If serum sodium is high, aldosterone is inhibited, and sodium is excreted; the opposite is true for depressed serum sodium levels.

For most individuals, the AI for sodium is 1500 mg/day (ages 9–50); and the UL is 2300 mg/day (ages 14–70+) (Table 12.5). This AI does not apply to highly active individuals, such as endurance athletes, who lose large amounts of sodium through sweat.

The vast majority of individuals in the United States and Canada have a high-sodium intake, considerably above the 2300 mg/day with an average intake of 3393 mg/day in those 20 years and older in the United States.[4] Adults with hypertension, prehypertension, diabetes, chronic kidney disease, over the age of 51 years and African Americans would benefit from reducing sodium intake to 1500 mg/day. Almost one-half of Americans have hypertension; lowering daily sodium intake could reduce blood pressure.[14] The World Health Organization recommends a maximum daily intake of 2000 mg of sodium intake for adults.[14]

Sources

Approximately 10% of the sodium consumed comes from natural content of foods and fluids regularly ingested. Sodium is a natural constituent of most foods (Table 12.6) and all food groups (except for minimal amounts from fruits); thus lowering intake requires careful choices from all food groups. Animal foods such as meat, saltwater fish, eggs, dairy products, and some vegetables (beets, carrots, celery, spinach, and other dark-green leafy vegetables) contain measurable amounts of sodium. Sandwiches are the number one source of sodium in the American diet.[4] The large quantity of bread products consumed accounts for more than twice as much sodium as snack foods such as potato chips and pretzels.[15]

Most consumers believe regular salt contains more sodium than sea salt, which has been marketed as containing "natural" nutrients and more minerals than table salt. Trace elements in sea salt are minuscule and meaningless, with no known health benefits. Far more relevant is the fact that, unlike table salt, sea salt is not fortified with iodine, which is important for thyroid health, especially during pregnancy.

Approximately 75% to 80% of the sodium consumed is added to processed foods and foods prepared in restaurants and fast-food establishments (Fig. 12.8). Processed, packaged, cured, canned, pickled, convenience, and restaurants (e.g., fast foods), as well as condiments, are significant sources of sodium (Box 12.2). "Hidden" sources include softened and bottled water, baking powder, baking soda, dentifrices (including toothpastes containing baking soda or sodium fluoride), chewing tobacco, and over-the-counter medications (e.g., antacids, cough medicines, and laxatives). As

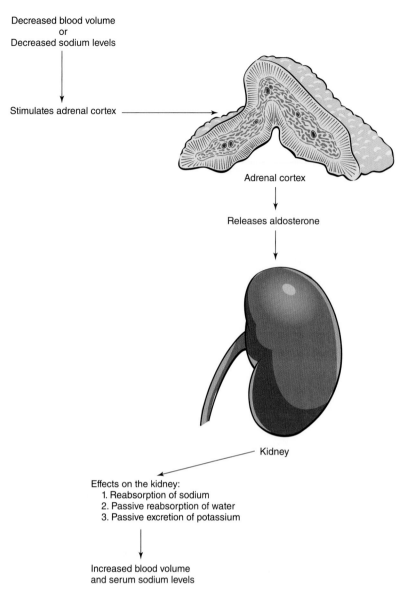

Decreased blood volume
or
Decreased sodium levels

Stimulates adrenal cortex ——————————→

Adrenal cortex

Releases aldosterone

Kidney

Effects on the kidney:
1. Reabsorption of sodium
2. Passive reabsorption of water
3. Passive excretion of potassium

Increased blood volume
and serum sodium levels

• **Fig. 12.7** Effects of aldosterone on sodium levels. (Adapted from Davis JR, Sherer K. *Applied Nutrition and Diet Therapy for Nurses*. 2nd ed. Saunders Elsevier; 1994.)

TABLE 12.5 National Academy of Medicine Recommendations for Sodium

Life Stage Group	AI[a](g/day) Male	Femaledbull	UL Male	Female	Chronic Disease Risk Reduction Intake: Reduce Intakes if Above ___g/day
0–6 months	0.11	0.11	ND	ND	ND[a]
7–12 months	0.37	0.37	ND	ND	ND[a]
1–3 years	0.8	0.8	ND	ND	1.2
4–8 years	1	1	ND	ND	1.5
9–13 years	1.2	1.2	ND	ND	1.8
14->70 years	1.5	1.5	ND	ND	2.3
Pregnancy					
14–50 years			1.5	ND	2.3
Lactation					
14–50			1.5	ND	2.3

AI, Adequate intake; *ND*, not determinable; *UL*, tolerable upper intake level.
[a]The AI is not equivalent to a Recommended Dietary Allowance.
Data from National Academies of Sciences, Engineering, and Medicine. *Dietary Reference Intakes for Sodium and Potassium*. National Academies Press; 2019.

TABLE 12.6   Where Is the Sodium?

Food Groups	Sodium (mg)
Whole and Other Grains, and Grain Products[a]	
Cooked cereal, rice, pasta, unsalted, ½ cup	0–5
Ready-to-eat cereal, 1 cup	0–360
Bread, 1 slice	110–175
Vegetables	
Fresh or frozen, cooked without salt, ½ cup	1–70
Canned or frozen with sauce, ½ cup	140–460
Tomato juice, canned, ½ cup	330
Fruit	
Fresh, frozen, canned, ½ cup	0–5
Low-Fat or Fat-Free Milk or Milk Products	
Milk, 1 cup	107
Yogurt, 1 cup	175
Natural cheeses, 1½ oz	110–450
Processed cheeses, 2 oz	600
Nuts, Seeds, and Legumes	
Peanuts, salted, ⅓ cup	120
Peanuts, unsalted, ⅓ cup	0–5
Beans, cooked from dried or frozen, without salt, ½ cup	0–5
Beans, canned, ½ cup	400
Lean Meats, Fish, and Poultry	
Fresh meat, fish, poultry, 3 oz	30–90
Tuna canned, water pack, no salt added, 3 oz	35–45
Tuna canned, water pack, 3 oz	230–350
Ham, lean, roasted, 3 oz	1020

[a]Whole grains are recommended for most grain servings.
From U.S. Department of Health and Human Services, National Institutes of Health. *Your Guide to Lowering Your Blood Pressure With Dash.* NIH Publication No. 06-4082. Revised April 2006. https://www.nhlbi.nih.gov/files/docs/public/heart/new_dash.pdf.

• BOX 12.2   Suggestions for Lowering Sodium Intake

- Avoid foods with concentrated sources of sodium and do not add salt to foods.
- Avoid adding salt to food at the table or in recipes. Flavor foods with herbs, spices, wine, lemon, lime, or vinegar (see Table 12.7 for additional ideas).
- Salt substitutes can contain sodium, potassium, and other minerals. Salt substitutes should not be used unless approved by a health care provider or RDN.
- Sodium is found naturally in most foods. Animal products such as meat, fish, poultry, milk, and eggs are naturally higher in sodium than fruits and vegetables.
- Restaurant meals should be selected carefully because of their high sodium content.
- Limit the following high-sodium processed foods:
  - *Meats*:
    - Limit: Smoked, cured, salted, or canned meats, fish, or poultry, including bacon, cold cuts, ham, frankfurters, and sausages; sardines, anchovies, and marinated herring; pickled meats or pickled eggs
    - Substitute: fresh options, such as seafood, lean meats and poultry; add cranberry sauce, applesauce as accompaniments for meat or poultry
  - *Dairy products*:
    - Limit: Processed cheese, blue cheese, buttermilk.
    - Substitute: Swiss cheese and creams cheese are relatively low in sodium; unsalted cottage cheese with herbs or fruit
  - *Vegetables*:
    - Limit: Sauerkraut, pickled vegetables prepared in brine, commercially frozen vegetable mixes with sauces
    - Substitute: fresh or frozen vegetables
  - *Breads and cereals*:
    - Limit: Breads, rolls, and crackers with salted tops
    - Substitute: baking products with sodium-free baking powder (e.g., potassium bicarbonate) and salt-free shortening; low or no sodium versions
  - *Soups*:
    - Limit: Canned soups, dried soup mixes, broth, bouillon (except salt-free)
  - *Fats*:
    - Limit: Salad dressings containing bacon bits, salt pork, dips made with instant soup mixes or processed cheese
    - Substitute: homemade salad dressings, without adding salt
  - *Beverages*:
    - Limit: Commercially softened water, cocoa mixes, club soda, sports drinks, tomato or vegetable juice
    - Substitute: unsalted tomato or vegetable juice, homemade hot cocoa
  - *Miscellaneous*:
    - Limit: Commercial pasta sauces and mixes; salted chips, popcorn, and nuts; olives; commercial stuffing; gravy mixes; seasoning salts (garlic, celery, onion), light salt, monosodium glutamate (MSG); meat tenderizer; catsup, prepared mustard, prepared horseradish, soy sauce, Worcestershire sauce, fish sauce; medications
    - Substitute: unsalted snacks

shown in Fig. 12.9, a sandwich, a staple in the American diet, may provide over 1500 mg sodium (more than 60% of the recommended *National Academy of Medicine* amount). Sodium can be replaced in foods with spices, as noted in Table 12.7, to enhance taste appeal. Recommendations for reducing sodium intake and accompanied substitutions are provided in Box 12.2.

Because people have acquired a taste for high levels of salt in their food, food products with less sodium are not as palatable; thus these products are not competitive with higher-sodium products in the market. The flavor of a food is the major determinant of food choices, overriding other factors, such as healthy choices.

Reducing sodium added to foods by food manufacturers and restaurants is fundamental to lowering sodium intake. The US government and numerous other governments are working with food manufacturers to reduce sodium content of products. The goal is to slowly, and without loss of consumers' acceptance, achieve safer levels of sodium consistent with public health recommendations. Between 2000 and 2014, sodium content decreased significantly for packaged foods overall and top food sources of sodium. Despite this reduction, 98% of households purchase foods with sodium density exceeding optimal levels.[16] Reformulation by the food industry is the most cost-effective strategy for salt reduction.

Most Sodium Comes from Processed and Restaurant Foods

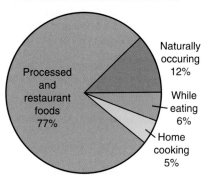

• **Fig. 12.8** Most of the sodium that Americans eat comes from packaged, processed, store-bought, and restaurant foods. Only a small amount comes from salt added during cooking or at the table. (From Centers for Disease Control and Prevention (CDC). *Salt—Sodium and Food Sources.* https://www.cdc.gov/salt/sodium-potassium-health/index.html.)

How does your sandwich stack up on sodium?

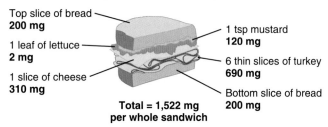

Top slice of bread **200 mg**
1 leaf of lettuce **2 mg**
1 slice of cheese **310 mg**
1 tsp mustard **120 mg**
6 thin slices of turkey **690 mg**
Bottom slice of bread **200 mg**

Total = 1,522 mg per whole sandwich

• **Fig. 12.9** How does your sandwich stack up on sodium? Total = 1522 mg per whole sandwich. (From Centers for Disease Control and Prevention (CDC). *About Sodium and Health.* https://www.cdc.gov/salt/about/.)

Hyper States and Hypo States

Serum sodium concentration is an index of water deficit or excess, not an index of total sodium levels in the body. Sodium levels in the blood are significantly higher than potassium levels because sodium is the major cation in intravascular fluid. **Hypernatremia** (elevated serum sodium level) and **hyponatremia** (low serum sodium level) are usually a result of hormonal imbalances or increased fluid loss or retention. "True" hypernatremia or hyponatremia, or imbalances caused by too much or too little sodium intake, rarely occurs in adults. If renal and hormonal mechanisms for sodium retention and excretion function efficiently, and water intake is adequate, the amount of dietary sodium causes little change in total body sodium. However, sodium fluctuations can affect plasma volume.

Because water and sodium are closely related, a change in one causes a change in the other. Hypernatremia can be associated with FVD or FVE. A very high-sodium intake can be toxic, especially if the intake is insufficient.

Water deprivation (as occurs in unconscious, debilitated individuals or infants), insensible water loss (as a result of exposure to dry heat, sweating, or hyperventilation), and watery diarrhea lead to a loss of water in excess of sodium. Infants are more prone to watery diarrhea, whereas older patients are susceptible to water deprivation. If polyuria is not balanced with increased water intake, hypernatremia may occur.

Symptoms of hypernatremia are a result of fluid moving from the ICF to the ECF in an attempt to equalize sodium and water balance. This movement of fluid causes atrophy of tissue cells.

TABLE 12.7	Herbs and Spices to Complement Foods
Food	**Herbs/Spices**
Beef	Onion, bay, chives, cloves, cumin, garlic, pepper, marjoram, rosemary, thyme, ginger, turmeric
Bread	Caraway, marjoram, oregano, poppy seed, rosemary, thyme
Carrots	Cinnamon, cloves, nutmeg, marjoram, sage
Cheese	Basil, chives, curry, dill, fennel, garlic, marjoram, oregano, parsley, sage, thyme
Fish	Dill, curry powder, paprika, fennel, tarragon, garlic, parsley, thyme
Fruit	Cinnamon, coriander, cloves, ginger, mint
Green beans	Dill, oregano, tarragon, thyme
Lamb	Garlic, marjoram, oregano, rosemary, thyme
Other vegetables	Basil, chives, dill, tarragon, marjoram, mint, parsley, pepper, thyme, turmeric
Pork	Onion, coriander, cumin, garlic, ginger, hot pepper, pepper, sage, thyme, ginger
Potatoes, rutabaga	Dill, garlic, paprika, parsley, sage, turmeric
Poultry	Garlic, ginger, oregano, rosemary, sage, tarragon
Salads	Basil, chives, French tarragon, garlic, parsley, arugula, sorrel (best if fresh or added to salad dressing, or use herbs and vinegars for extra flavor), turmeric
Soups	Bay, tarragon, marjoram, parsley, rosemary, turmeric
Winter squash/ sweet potatoes	Cloves, nutmeg, cinnamon, ginger

Cells in the central nervous system shrink, producing hallucinations, disorientation, lethargy, and possibly coma. Other signs are extreme thirst; dry, "sticky" tongue and oral mucous membranes; fever; and convulsions. A sticky tongue can be identified by slowly rolling a tongue depressor over the lateral side of the tongue; tacky filiform papillae stick to the tongue depressor.

Hyponatremia, a potentially life-threatening condition, may develop when sodium losses exceed water losses, or when fluids are retained, leading to a greater concentration of water than sodium. The resulting changes in sodium-water movement to rebalance equilibrium leads to cellular edema. Problems are especially evident in the cranium, where there is no room for expansion. Sodium deficiency may lead to a decrease in salivary flow or a decrease in sodium concentration of saliva. Water intoxication or hyponatremia can occur when individuals drink too much water (several liters a day). The blood sodium level decreases to a dangerously low level, causing headaches, blurred vision, cramps, swelling of the brain, coma, and possibly death.

Heat exhaustion in unacclimated individuals may result in a sodium deficit. Hyponatremia may also occur in individuals who drink excessive quantities of water as a part of psychiatric disorder or when excessive amounts of diuretics are given. Excessive vomiting and diarrhea, especially in infants, can also lead to a sodium deficit.

Early symptoms of hyponatremia are fatigue, nausea, headache, and abdominal cramps. Other symptoms—headache, confusion, lethargy, and coma—are the result of cellular edema. Even though there is cellular edema, peripheral edema is not present. This is because water is primarily retained within cells rather than in the interstitial compartment. Chronic hyponatremia is usually well tolerated. It may or may not be treated, depending on the precipitating cause and severity.

🦷 DENTAL CONSIDERATIONS

- The salt recognition threshold is determined by sodium concentration of saliva (i.e., the lower the level of sodium in saliva, the easier it is to detect a small amount of salt in food).
- A low salt recognition threshold is desirable for patients who should curtail salt intake for health reasons; however, in a hyponatremic patient, diminished salt consumption could contribute further to sodium depletion.
- Sodium deficiency may lead to a decreased salivary flow rate.
- Assess patients for signs and symptoms of hypernatremia (thirst; dry, sticky tongue; xerostomia) and hyponatremia.
- Patients with such conditions as hypertension, prehypertension, chronic kidney disease, or diabetes need to consume 1500 mg or less of sodium daily. Refer patients who would benefit by reducing sodium intake to 1500 mg/day to a registered dietitian nutritionist (RDN).
- Avoid adding salt to food at the table or in recipes. Encourage patients to use herbs and spices to flavor food instead of using high-sodium seasonings (see Table 12.7).
- High levels of sodium (>2 g/day) cause calcium loss in the urine.
- Identify "hidden" sources of sodium in a patient's diet. Discuss ways to reduce sodium.
- To convert milligrams of sodium to milliequivalents, divide the number by 23 (the atomic weight of sodium). For example, 1000 mg of sodium ÷ 23 = 43 mEq of sodium.
- Table salt contains sodium and chloride (40% sodium and 60% chloride): 1/4 teaspoon salt = 575 mg sodium
  1/2 teaspoon salt = 1150 mg sodium
  3/4 teaspoon salt = 1725 mg sodium
  1 teaspoon salt = 2300 mg sodium

🦷 NUTRITIONAL DIRECTIONS

- Use the Nutrition Facts label to choose foods lower in sodium.
  - Read the ingredient list to identify and avoid sources of sodium additives:
  - Disodium guanylate
  - Disodium inosinate
  - Himalayan pink salt
  - Monosodium glutamate
  - Sodium bicarbonate
  - Sodium nitrate
  - Sodium citrate
  - Sodium chloride
  - Trisodium phosphate
- Use reduced sodium or no-salt-added products. Prepare more meals at home, choosing fresh or frozen products. Limit eating at restaurants.
- Salt substitutes can contain sodium, potassium, and other minerals. Salt substitutes should not be used unless approved by a healthcare provider or RDN.
- Sodium is found naturally in most foods. Animal products such as meat, fish, poultry, milk, and eggs are naturally higher in sodium than in fruits and vegetables.
- Dietary sodium restriction is rarely the cause of hyponatremia. Sodium depletion may occur in combination with excessive losses as a result of vomiting, diarrhea, surgery, or profuse perspiration from exercise or fever.
- Sea salt, Kosher salt, and table salt, all contain similar levels of sodium.
- Foods making nutrient claims must meet certain labeling guidelines (see Box 1.4)
- Encourage the patient to make gradual changes.

Chloride

Physiologic Roles

Chlorine is the primary anion connected with sodium in ECF to help maintain ECF balance, osmotic equilibrium, and electrolyte balance. Large concentrations of chloride are present in gastric secretions, which are important for protein digestion and creating an acidic environment to inhibit bacterial growth and enhance iron, calcium, and vitamin B_{12} absorption.

Requirements and Regulation

The AI for chloride has been established by the National Academy of Medicine at 2300 mg/day (see Table 12.8). Chloride intake and losses parallel to those of sodium.

Sources

Most chloride intake is from salt (sodium chloride). Sources of chloride are the same as those for sodium, including processed foods. Water is an additional source of chloride.

Hyper States and Hypo States

Toxicity from chloride can be caused by excessive intakes of salt, dehydration, renal failure, diarrhea, and Cushing's syndrome. Conditions associated with sodium depletion, such as persistent heavy sweating, chronic diarrhea, vomiting, or chronic renal failure, may precipitate hypochloremia and an electrolyte imbalance.

Potassium

Physiologic Roles

Potassium has the following important physiologic roles: (1) maintains cellular (ICF) concentration, (2) directly affects muscle contraction (especially cardiac) and electrical conductivity of the heart, (3) facilitates transmission of nerve impulses, and (4) regulates acid-base balance. Potassium is important to maintain good muscle function for physically active individuals.

Requirements and Regulation

Potassium is a nutrient with consumption levels below the AI level. Similar to sodium, there is no RDA for potassium. As shown in Table 12.9, the AI for potassium has been established by the National Academy of Medicine at 2600 mg/day for adult females and 3400 mg/day for adult males. This is equivalent to approximately 6 to 7 servings of fruits and vegetables, however, potassium is present in all food groups. No UL has been established for healthy adults.

Fruits and vegetables are among the richest sources of potassium; low potassium intake is the result of low intakes of fruits and vegetables. High intake of meats and other animal proteins cause further depletion of this mineral. Average potassium intake of the US population is lower than recommended. Studies have reinforced an association between hypertension and sodium, potassium, and sodium to potassium ratio.[17] Low potassium consumption can cause sensitivity to salt, further increasing risk of hypertension. The sodium-potassium pump regulates potassium levels. Depending on cellular needs, potassium constantly moves

TABLE 12.8	National Academy of Medicine Recommendations for Chloride		
	AI (g/day)[a]		**UL (g/day)**
Life Stage	**Male and Female**		
0–6 months	0.18		ND
7–12 months	0.57		ND
1–3 years	1.5		2.3
4–8 years	1.9		2.9
9–13 years	2.3		3.4
14–50 years	2.3		3.6
51–70 years	2.0		3.6
>70 years	1.8		3.6
Pregnancy			
14–50 years	2.3		3.6
Lactation			
14–50 years	2.3		3.6

AI, Adequate intake; *ND,* not determinable; *UL,* tolerable upper intake level.
[a]The AI is not equivalent to a Recommended Dietary Allowance.
Data from National Academies of Sciences, Engineering, and Medicine. *Dietary Reference Intakes for Sodium and Potassium.* National Academies Press; 2019.

TABLE 12.9	National Academy of Medicine Recommendations for Potassium	
	AI[a]	
Life Stage	**Male (g/day)**	**Female (g/day)**
0–6 months	0.4	0.4
7–12 months	0.86	0.86
1–3 years	2	2
4–8 years	2.3	2.3
9–13 years	2.5	2.3
14–18 years	3	2.3
≥19 years	3.4	2.6
Pregnancy		
≤18 years		2.6
≥19 years		2.9
Lactation		
≤18 years		2.5
≥19 years		2.8

AI, Adequate intake.
[a]The AI is not equivalent to a Recommended Dietary Allowance.
Data from National Academies of Sciences, Engineering, and Medicine. *Dietary Reference Intakes for Sodium and Potassium.* National Academies Press; 2019.

either into or out of cells. Aldosterone indirectly affects serum potassium levels. If aldosterone is released, sodium is reabsorbed, but potassium is excreted. Subsequently, if aldosterone is inhibited, potassium is retained (see Fig. 12.7). Approximately 92% of ingested potassium is excreted in urine, but a small amount is lost through feces or sweat.

Sources

Potassium is naturally available from foods and fluids regularly consumed, and the average intakes are 2595 mg/day which is very close to the AI (Table 12.10). Dairy, meat, and grains contribute 31% of total dietary potassium. Fruits and vegetables contribute 20% of total dietary potassium. Milk is the number one single food source of potassium for all age groups in the United States. Processed foods usually contain less potassium than fresh products. Potassium supplements and salt substitutes are another source; salt substitutes (potassium chloride) often replace sodium with potassium.

Hyper States and Hypo States

Minor deviations in serum potassium levels can be life threatening. Abnormal levels are referred to as either hyperkalemia (elevated serum potassium level) or hypokalemia (low serum potassium level).

Hyperkalemia has three causes: (1) impaired renal excretion, (2) increased shift of potassium out of cells, and (3) increased potassium intake. Most potassium is excreted through the kidneys. Acute or chronic renal failure impairs potassium excretion, resulting in potassium being retained. Increased serum potassium levels can result from an increased dietary intake, excessive administration

of potassium supplements orally or intravenously, or excessive use of potassium-containing salt substitutes. In catabolic situations (burns, trauma, and so on), large amounts of potassium are released; a healthy kidney will increase potassium excretion.

Hyperkalemia is life threatening because cardiac arrest may occur. Elevated potassium levels are irritating to the body; symptoms include muscle weakness (the first sign), tingling and numbness in the extremities, diarrhea, bradycardia, abdominal cramps, confusion, and electrocardiographic changes. Treatment for hyperkalemia involves potassium restriction or using medications to remove potassium.

Potential consequences of chronic potassium deficiency are often unrecognized. Problems include hypertension, heart attacks, strokes, kidney stones, and a loss of bone minerals that can lead to osteoporosis. Potassium deficiency can cause individuals to feel tired, weak, and irritable while unable to pinpoint a cause.

Excessive loss or inadequate intake of potassium can result in hypokalemia. Potassium loss occurs through the gastrointestinal and renal tracts and by excessive sweating. Because potassium is contained in gastric and intestinal secretions, vomiting and diarrhea may cause hypokalemia. Some potassium is lost through sweat; excessive perspiration can lead to hypokalemia. Drugs, such as diuretics (e.g., furosemide and hydrochlorothiazide) and antibiotics (e.g., carbenicillin and amphotericin B), are major offenders. Cushing syndrome, hyperaldosteronism, an excess of insulin, hypomagnesemia, alcoholism, and alkalosis also cause hypokalemia.

Potassium is the major ICF cation; deficits can affect every body's system. Death from cardiac or respiratory arrest can occur. Clinical manifestations include anorexia muscle weakness in the legs, leg cramps, and electrocardiographic changes.

TABLE 12.10 Potassium Content of Selected Foods

Food	Portion	Potassium (mg)
Beans, mature, white, boiled	1 cup	1000
Potato, baked with skin	I med	952
Lima beans, cooked	1 cup	909
Spinach, cooked from fresh	1 cup	833
Avocado, raw, black skin	1	660
Yogurt, nonfat, plain	1 cup	625
Sweet potato with skin, baked	1 med	542
Tomato juice	1 cup	538
Beets, cooked	1 cup	518
Orange juice	1 cup	458
Tomato, fresh, chopped	1 cup	427
Banana	1 med	422
Cantaloupe	1 cup	417
Salmon, baked	3 oz	381
Milk, 1%	1 cup	366
Sirloin steak, broiled	3 oz	323
Raisins	1 small box	322
Quinoa, cooked	1 cup	291
Orange	1 med	238
Gatorade sports beverage	8 oz	37

From U.S. Department of Agriculture (USDA), Agricultural Research Service. *FoodData Central, 2020.* USDA National Nutrient Database for Standard Reference, Version 2. 2020. http://fdc.nal.usda.gov.

◆ DENTAL CONSIDERATIONS

- Be aware of factors that can cause potassium to increase or decrease. Refer the patient to the healthcare provider or RDN as needed.
- Medical conditions that can interfere with excretion of potassium include diabetes, renal failure, severe heart events, and adrenal insufficiency.
- Medications that can interfere with excretion of potassium are angiotensin-converting enzyme inhibitors, angiotensin receptor blockers, and potassium-sparing diuretics.

◆ NUTRITIONAL DIRECTIONS

- Choose at least two servings of fruit and three to four servings of vegetables daily in addition to recommended amounts of dairy to obtain adequate amounts of potassium.
- Read labels; salt substitutes may be high in potassium. Consult a healthcare provider or RDN before using potassium-containing salt substitutes.
- If a potassium-wasting diuretic has been prescribed, consume high-potassium foods or take a potassium supplement.

Iron

Physiologic Roles

Every cell contains iron; approximately 4 g (less than 1 tsp) is present in the entire body. Iron is a major component of hemoglobin, which transports oxygen from the lungs to the tissues, including both oral soft and hard tissues. It also catalyzes many oxidative reactions within cells and participates in the final steps of energy metabolism. Other roles include (1) conversion of beta-carotene to vitamin A, (2) synthesis of collagen, (3) formation of purines as part of nucleic acid, (4) removal of lipids from the blood, (5) detoxification of drugs in the liver, and (6) production of antibodies. Lactoferrin, a salivary glycoprotein, is capable of binding iron. It has an antibacterial action by competing with iron-requiring organisms in the mouth for limited amounts of available iron.

Requirements

The RDA for iron is 18 mg daily for females 19 to 50 years old, 8 mg/day for females 51 years old and older, and 8 mg/day for males 19 years old and older (Table 12.11). The RDA is higher for premenopausal females than for males or postmenopausal females because of blood loss during menstruation. During the reproductive phase of a female's life, iron loss is at least twice that of a male or of a postmenopausal female. Although premenopausal females need more iron and the average intake is 11.7 to 12.3 mg/day well below the RDA, they tend to consume less than males whose average 15.9 mg/day well above the RDA. Iron requirements also increase during times of impaired absorption (e.g., diarrhea), periods of rapid growth, and heavy physical activity because of the increased need for oxygen transport and energy production.

The RDA is based on the approximation that 10% of dietary iron is absorbed. The demand for iron replenishment is constant because cells are continually being replaced; the life of a red blood cell is 120 days. When a cell dies, iron is recycled, released and transported to various storage sites to be used again. A UL for iron was established at 45 mg/day for adults.

Absorption and Excretion

Similar to calcium, iron is poorly absorbed. Most of the iron in food is in the oxidized form of ferric iron (Fe^{3+}). Gastric acid in the stomach helps promote iron absorption. By binding to the serum protein transferrin, iron is continuously transported through the body because transferrin functions to recycle iron.

Absorption of heme iron parallels the body's need; absorption of nonheme iron depends on intraluminal and meal composition and physiologic need. Heme iron is provided by meat sources containing hemoglobin from red blood cells and myoglobin from muscle cells. The RDA is based on consumption of at least 75% of iron intake from heme sources. Nonheme iron is present in eggs, milk, and plants. Acidic conditions enhance iron absorption, but calcium and manganese interfere with its absorption. Fig. 12.10 lists factors affecting iron absorption. Combinations of food can enhance iron absorption; a meal of roast beef (rich in iron) with potatoes (rich in vitamin C) increases iron absorption.

TABLE 12.11	National Academy of Medicine Recommendations for Iron						
	EAR (mg/day)		RDA (mg/day)		AI (mg/day)[a]		UL (mg/day)
Life Stage	Male	Female	Male	Female	Male	Female	
0–6 months					0.27	0.27	
7–12 months	6.9	6.9	11	11			40
1–3 years	3	3	7	7			40
4–8 years	4.1	4.1	10	10			40
9–13 years	5.9	5.7	8	8			40
14–18 years	7.7	7.9	11	15			45
19–50 years	6	8.1	8	18			45
≥51 years	6		8	8			45
Pregnancy							
14–18 years		23		27			45
19–50 years		22		27			45
Lactation							
14–18 years		7		10			45
19–50 years		6.5		9			45

AI, Adequate intake; *EAR,* estimated average requirement; *RDA,* recommended dietary allowance; *UL,* tolerable upper intake level.

[a]For healthy human milk–fed infants, the AI is the mean intake. The AI is not equivalent to an RDA.

Data from Institute of Medicine (IOM), Food and Nutrition Board. *Dietary Reference Intakes For Vitamin A, Vitamin K, Arsenic, Boron, Chromium, Copper, Iodine, Iron, Manganese, Molybdenum, Nickel, Silicon, Vanadium, and Zinc.* National Academy Press; 2001.

Sources

Iron is probably the most difficult mineral to obtain in adequate amounts in the American diet. Although liver is often considered the best source of iron, meats (especially beef), egg yolk, dark-green vegetables, and enriched breads and cereals all contribute significant amounts (Table 12.12). Iron supplements come in two forms; the ferrous form (i.e., ferrous sulfate or ferrous gluconate) is easier on the gut and absorbed better than the ferric form. Gastrointestinal side effects can include nausea, heartburn, diarrhea or constipation. Even though iron can be considered toxic because of the body's inability to excrete excess amounts, supplementation is a safe and effective treatment to replenish iron stores for iron-deficiency anemia. In circumstances where supplemental iron is not effective, such as malabsorption due to celiac disease or hemodialysis, intravenous therapy may be indicated.

Hyper States and Hypo States

The body cannot easily eliminate excess iron; this may explain why iron absorption rates are poor. The body seldom overcomes its regulation of intestinal absorption. Iron overload may occur, however, if ingestion of iron is extremely elevated. Hemochromatosis is a hereditary disorder in which iron is absorbed at a high rate despite elevated iron stores in the liver. Accumulation of iron throughout the body may develop with excessive iron intake or multiple

blood transfusions. Initially, it is difficult to diagnose because of its resemblance to other conditions in which fatigue and general weakness are symptoms. Elevated iron stores have been associated with increased risk of cardiovascular disease (CVD) and liver disease. Iron supplements should not be taken indiscriminately and without a comprehensive laboratory workup.

Inadequate dietary iron intake, and chronic and acute inflammatory conditions are individually associated with iron-deficiency anemia. As the leading nutrient deficiency in both developed and developing countries, iron-deficiency anemia continues to be a global health issue. Anemia has been linked to unfavorable outcomes of pregnancy resulting in a high risk of preterm delivery and subsequent low birth weight and possibly poor neonatal health. A deficiency can lead to various symptoms, such as microcytic anemia, fatigue, faulty digestion, blue sclerae, pale conjunctivae, and tachycardia. Iron-deficiency anemia may be caused by inadequate dietary intake; accelerated demand or losses; and inadequate absorption secondary to diarrhea, decreased acid secretions, or antacid therapy. Iron deficiency is frequently the result of postnatal feeding practices and has a serious impact on growth, and mental and psychomotor development in infants and children.

The most prominent oral signs of iron deficiency include pallor of the lips and oral mucosa, angular cheilitis, atrophy of filiform papillae, and glossitis (see Figs. 17.1 and 17.2). Oral candidiasis and a reduced resistance to infection are frequently associated with iron deficiency.

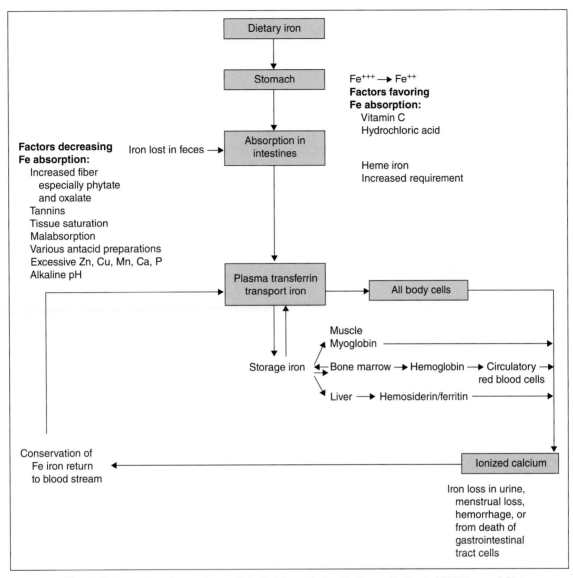

• **Fig. 12.10** Iron absorption and use. (Adapted from Davis JR, Sherer K. *Applied Nutrition and Diet Therapy for Nurses*. 2nd ed. Saunders Elsevier; 1994.)

DENTAL CONSIDERATIONS

- Despite the prevalence of iron-deficiency anemia, supplements are not recommended without laboratory testing to indicate a deficiency. Referral to the healthcare provider or RDN may be necessary.
- The most prominent sign of iron deficiency in the oral cavity is pallor and swelling of the tongue. The patient also may complain of soreness and a "burning" tongue. Atrophic changes progress from a patchy denudation of papillae to a smooth, reddened tongue.
- Hemochromatosis is common in alcohol use disorder, usually in males, who may drink more than 1 L of red wine daily. Do not recommend iron-rich and iron-fortified foods to patients with this condition.
- Iron-containing supplements are one of the leading causes of poisoning deaths in children younger than 6 years old in the United States. Encourage storing iron supplements in a place inaccessible to children.

- Patients at risk of iron deficiency include patients with renal failure, individuals experiencing periods of rapid growth (e.g., pregnant females, infants, toddlers, and teenage girls), and vegans. Referral to the healthcare provider or RDN may be necessary.
- Encourage good oral hygiene practices when iron supplements are taken to prevent extrinsic staining of teeth. Liquid forms of iron can be taken through a straw. More frequent recall appointments may be indicated.
- Because older adults may have a reduced production of gastric acid, this can interfere with iron absorption, increasing the risk of an iron deficiency. Referral to the healthcare provider or RDN may be necessary.

TABLE 12.12	Iron Content of Selected Foods		
Food	**Portion**	**Iron (mg)**
Total cereal	1 cup	24.0[a]
Wheat chex cereal	1 cup	19.3[a]
Oatmeal, instant, fortified, prepared with water	1 cup	13.6[a]
Raisin bran cereal	1 cup	10.8[a]
Chicken liver, braised	3 oz	9.8[b]
Oysters, steamed	3 ox	6.9[b]
Lentils, boiled	1 cup	6.6[a]
Spinach, boiled	1 cup	6.4[a]
Beef liver, fried	3 oz	5.2[b]
Lima beans, boiled	1 cup	4.2[a]
Pinto beans, boiled	1 cup	3.6[a]
Beef, ground, 90% lean, broiled	3 oz	2.3[b]
Beef, chuck roast, lean only, cooked	3 oz	2.0[b]
Potato, baked, with skin	1 medium	1.8[a]
Turkey, dark meat, roasted	3 oz	1.1[b]
Wine, red	1 glass	0.8[a]
Raisins, seedless	1 small box	0.8[a]
Avocado, black skin	1	0.8[a]
Turkey, light meat, roasted	3 oz	0.6[b]

[a]Nonheme iron.
[b]Heme iron.
From U.S. Department of Agriculture (USDA), Agricultural Research Service. *FoodData Central, 2020.* USDA National Nutrient Database for Standard Reference, Version 2. 2020. http://fdc.nal.usda.gov.

⚙ NUTRITIONAL DIRECTIONS

- A food rich in vitamin C with supplements or meals increases iron absorption, especially nonheme iron. Take iron with orange juice, tomato juice, or vitamin C–enriched juices, such as apple juice.
- If nonheme-containing grains or vegetables are consumed with small amounts of heme iron, absorption of the nonheme iron doubles.
- Because iron provided in a vegan diet is the nonheme form, iron absorption is lower than for individuals consuming animal foods.
- Polyphenols (not caffeine) in tea and coffee decrease iron absorption. No decrease in iron absorption occurs when tea or coffee is consumed 1 hour before or 2 hours after a meal.
- Vitamin A deficiency can cause iron deficiency because vitamin A helps to transport iron from the storage sites.
- Iron supplements are best absorbed on an empty stomach, but often may lead to gastrointestinal symptoms. When such side effects occur, the patient often takes iron supplements with food and in divided doses to reduce symptoms associated with these supplements.
- A common treatment of hemochromatosis or iron overload is to donate blood regularly.
- For maximum absorption, avoid taking an iron supplement with a large calcium supplement (>800 mg).

Zinc

Physiologic Roles

Zinc is a component in more than 300 enzymes that perform a variety of functions affecting cell growth and replication; sexual maturation, fertility, and reproduction; night vision; immune defenses; and taste, smell, and appetite. It is ubiquitous in the body—in organs, tissues, bones, fluids, and cells. Zinc is required for DNA, RNA, and protein synthesis. In this role, zinc is essential for bone growth and mineral metabolism. Zinc-containing enzymes are important in collagen synthesis and bone resorption and remodeling. Zinc might well be recognized as the most important essential trace mineral for humans.

Requirements

The National Academy of Medicine recommends a daily intake of 11 mg for males and 8 mg for females (Table 12.13). The RDA is based on the traditional American diet in which most people consume meat. Average intake for adult males is 12.6 mg/day and for females it is 9.1 mg/day. Vegans absorb less zinc so the RDA may be about one and a half times that of individuals consuming animal products, although no recommended intake has been identified. The UL for zinc is 40 mg/day.

Absorption and Excretion

Bioavailability of zinc varies widely; approximately 25% to 40% of dietary zinc is absorbed. Absorption depends on several factors, including body size; total dietary zinc; and the presence of other potentially interfering substances, such as calcium, fiber, and phosphate salts. Higher-quality protein improves zinc absorption. Many substances in plant products (e.g., fiber and phytate) interfere with zinc absorption. Zinc is lost in the feces; abnormal losses from diarrhea increase zinc requirements.

Sources

Protein-rich foods are good sources of zinc. Lamb, beef, crustaceans (especially oysters), eggs, and peanuts contain significant amounts of zinc (Table 12.14).

Hyper States and Hypo States

Consumption of high levels of zinc normally causes vomiting and diarrhea, epigastric pain, lethargy, and fatigue and can result in renal damage, pancreatitis, and death. Supplementation is recommended only under medical supervision.

Individuals at particular risk of zinc deficiency include those whose zinc requirements are high (e.g., during periods of rapid growth and during pregnancy and lactation), those with alcohol use disorder, vegans, those suffering from anorexia nervosa and individuals with severe malabsorption (ulcerative colitis, chronic diarrhea), sickle cell disease, or other chronic health problems.

Oral manifestations of zinc deficiency include changes in the epithelium of the tongue, such as thickening of epithelium; increased cell numbers; impaired keratinization of epithelial cells; increased susceptibility to periodontal disease; impaired wound healing and flattened filiform papillae. Zinc deficiency is associated with loss of taste and smell acuity, poor appetite, hallucinations,

TABLE 12.13   National Academy of Medicine Recommendations for Zinc

Life Stage	EAR (mg/day)		RDA (mg/day)		AI (mg/day)[a]		UL (mg/day)
	Male	Female	Male	Female	Male	Female	
0–6 months					2	2	4
7–12 months	2.5	2.5	3	3			5
1–3 years	2.5	2.5	3	3			7
4–8 years	4	4	5	5			12
9–13 years	7	7	8	8			23
14–18 years	8.5	7.5	11	9			34
≥19 years	9.4	6.8	11	8			40
Pregnancy							
14–18 years		10		12			34
19–50 years		9.5		11			40
Lactation							
14–18 years		10.9		13			34
19–50 years		10.4		12			40

AI, Adequate intake; *EAR*, estimated average requirement; *RDA*, recommended dietary allowance; *UL*, tolerable upper intake level.

[a]The AI is not equivalent to an RDA.

Data from Institute of Medicine (IOM), Food and Nutrition Board. *Dietary Reference Intakes for Vitamin A, Vitamin K, Arsenic, Boron, Chromium, Copper, Iodine, Iron, Manganese, Molybdenum, Nickel, Silicon, Vanadium, and Zinc.* National Academy Press; 2001.

TABLE 12.14   Zinc Content of Selected Foods

Food	Portion	Zinc (mg)
Oysters, steamed	3 oz	66
Total cereal	1 cup	20.0
Baked beans, canned, plain, or vegetarian	1 cup	5.8
Beef, chuck roast, lean, roasted	3 oz	3.8
Lobster, steamed	3 oz	3.4
Beef, hamburger, 90% lean, broiled	3 oz	5.4
Crab, broiled	3 oz	4
Yogurt, plain, low fat	8 oz	2.0
Kidney beans, cooked	1 cup	1.9
Peas, green, cooked	1 cup	1.9
Cashews	1 oz	1.5
Cheese, Swiss	1 oz	1.2
Oatmeal, instant, plain prepared with water	1 cup	1.2
Milk, skim	1 cup	1.0
Peanuts, roasted	1 oz	0.9
Chicken breast, skinless, grilled	3 oz	0.8
Peanut butter	1 tbsp	0.4
Flounder or sole, cooked	3 oz	0.3
Kale, cooked	1 cup	0.3
Red wine	5 oz	0.2

From U.S. Department of Agriculture (USDA), Agricultural Research Service. *FoodData Central, 2020.* USDA National Nutrient Database for Standard Reference, Version 2. 2020. http://fdc.nal.usda.gov.

and depression. Zinc deficiency can result in congenital defects, such as skeletal abnormalities, especially cleft palate and lip. Even when adequate amounts of zinc are provided for an extended time, abnormalities in mineral metabolism are not completely reversed. When zinc deficiency is diagnosed, supplementation is needed.

🦷 DENTAL CONSIDERATIONS

- Patients with abnormalities of taste because of zinc deficiency may respond to supplementation, but additional zinc is ineffective in reversing abnormal taste acuity associated with other conditions.
- Supplementation in zinc-depleted patients is beneficial for wound healing, but unnecessary for healthy individuals.
- Zinc supplementation interferes with use of iron and copper and adversely affects high-density lipoprotein levels. Do not advocate for indiscriminate use of zinc.
- Zinc lozenges and zinc supplements are marketed to treat cold symptoms. It is unclear if zinc reduces the onset or duration of a cold, especially if zinc status is adequate. However, notable side effects of treating cold symptoms with zinc are bad taste and nausea. Currently, zinc formulations are not standardized and the best dosage is unknown.

🍎 NUTRITIONAL DIRECTIONS

- Small amounts of animal protein can significantly improve bioavailability of zinc from a legume-based meal.
- Fruits and vegetables are low in zinc, whereas peanuts and peanut butter have higher amounts.
- Meat, fish, and poultry are the preferred sources of zinc because of its bioavailability from plant foods.
- If a well-balanced diet is consumed, zinc supplements are rarely needed and may be harmful.
- Large amounts of iron can decrease zinc absorption from food. Iron supplements between meals allow greater zinc absorption from foods.
- Due to the impact of phytates on zinc absorption, the Nutrition Societies of Germany, Austria, and Switzerland have revised the reference values of zinc. The intake is recorded based on the intake of phytates (low, moderate, and high).[18]

Iodine

Physiologic Role

Iodine is required for production of thyroxine, a hormone secreted by the thyroid gland. Thyroxine regulates the basal metabolic rate; an altered metabolic rate affects other nutrient requirements. Thyroid hormones are essential for normal brain development.

Requirements

The adult RDA for iodine is 150 μg/day. Because iodine is related to the metabolic rate, needs are increased during periods of accelerated growth, especially during pregnancy and lactation. As shown in Table 12.15, the RDA for pregnant and lactating females is higher because of critical needs of the fetus and infant during this period. The UL for iodine is 1100 μg/day.

Currently, iodine intake of the average American adult is adequate. However, iodine levels for pregnant and breastfeeding females are less than desirable—between 21% and 44% of third-trimester pregnant females in the United States may have inadequate levels of iodine.[19]

Sources

A major source of iodine is seafood (especially cod, shrimp, and tuna) and plants grown near the ocean. Other natural sources include seaweed, dairy products, grain products, and eggs. Breast milk contains iodine and hence it is added to infant formulas. The iodine content of meat and animal products depends on iodine content of foods consumed by animals; iodine content of fruits and vegetables is affected by the iodine content of soil and fertilizer and by irrigation practices. The iodine content of foods is not reflected on package labeling and is not available in the US Department of Agriculture's Nutrient Database.

The best safeguard for acquiring an AI is the use of iodized salt. Until the 1920s, endemic iodine deficiency disorders were prevalent in the Great Lakes, Appalachian, and Northwestern regions of the United States. Iodized salt virtually eliminated endemic goiter and remains the mainstay of eradicating iodine deficiency in the United States and worldwide. Iodine in salt will remain stable for many months if kept dry, preferably in a cool place away from light.

Hyper States and Hypo States

Very high levels of iodine may cause adverse effects in some individuals. Excessive amounts of iodine can result in enlargement of the thyroid gland similar to the condition produced by deficiency. Thyroiditis, hypothyroidism, hyperthyroidism, goiter (enlargement of the thyroid gland), and sensitivity reactions have occurred in relation to excessive iodine intake through foods, dietary supplements, topical medications, and iodinated contrast media.

Iodine deficiency is a major public health problem internationally, especially for pregnant females. It is considered the most common cause of preventable intellectual impairment. With insufficient iodine intake, the thyroid cannot produce adequate amounts of thyroxine. The pituitary gland continues to secrete thyroid-stimulating hormone, resulting in further hypertrophy and engorgement of the thyroid gland. Goiter is usually associated with iodine deficiency but may be caused by excessively high intake of goitrogens contained in cabbage, cauliflower, brussels sprouts, broccoli, kale, raw turnips, and rutabagas.

An iodine deficiency may cause profound metabolic and emotional disturbances ranging from a mild deceleration of catabolic functions, with sensitivity to cold, dry skin, and mildly elevated blood lipids, to mild depression of mental functions. Endemic goiter occurs where the soil or water is low in iodine content (Fig. 12.11).

Goiter is the main disorder resulting from low iodine intake. Other iodine-deficiency disorders include stillbirths, spontaneous abortions (i.e., miscarriages), and congenital anomalies; endemic cretinism, usually characterized by impaired mental development and deaf mutism related to fetal iodine deficiency; and impaired mental function. Children born to mothers with severe iodine deficiency have delayed eruption of primary and secondary teeth and an enlarged tongue. Craniofacial growth and development are altered; malocclusion is common.

TABLE 12.15	National Academy of Medicine Recommendations for Iodine						
	EAR (µg/day)		RDA (µg/day)		AI (µg/day)[a]		
Life Stage	Male	Female	Male	Female	Male	Female	UL (µg/day)
0–6 months					110	110	ND
7–12 months					130	130	ND
1–3 years	65	65	90	90			200
4–8 years	65	65	90	90			300
9–13 years	73	73	120	120			600
14–18 years	95	95	150	150			900
≥19 years	95	95	150	150			1100
Pregnancy							
≥14 years		160		220			900
Lactation							
≥14 years		209		290			900

AI, Adequate intake; *EAR*, estimated average requirement; *ND*, not determinable; *RDA*, recommended dietary allowance; *UL*, tolerable upper intake level.

[a]For healthy human milk–fed infants, the AI is the mean intake. *The AI is not equivalent to an RDA.*

Data from Institute of Medicine (IOM), Food and Nutrition Board. *Dietary Reference Intakes for Vitamin A, Vitamin K, Arsenic, Boron, Chromium, Copper, Iodine, Iron, Manganese, Molybdenum, Nickel, Silicon, Vanadium, and Zinc.* National Academy Press; 2001.

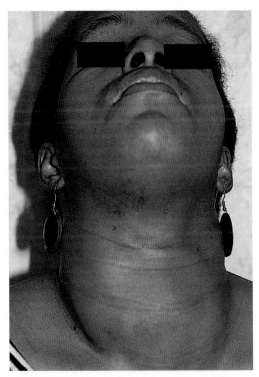

• **Fig. 12.11** Goiter resulting from iodine deficiency. (Reproduced with permission from Swartz M. *Textbook of Physical Diagnosis: History and Examination.* 6th ed. St. Louis, MO: Saunders Elsevier; 2009.)

A deficiency of iodine remains the most frequent cause worldwide, second only to starvation, of preventable mental retardation in children. Even a mild deficiency during pregnancy is related to mild and subclinical intellectual and psychomotor deficits in neonates, infants, and children. Severe iodine deficiency usually leads to infertility and increased risks for miscarriage or congenital anomalies. Further information regarding iodine deficiency in pregnancy is provided in Chapter 13.

● DENTAL CONSIDERATIONS

- During the oral examination, assess patients for possible thyroid problems.
- Enlargement of the thyroid gland can indicate hyperthyroidism or hypothyroidism. Refer these patients to a healthcare provider.
- For females who are pregnant, or breastfeeding, stress the importance of taking a prenatal multivitamin that contains iodine.
- Severe hypothyroidism is termed myxedema; hyperthyroidism is also called Graves' disease.

● NUTRITIONAL DIRECTIONS

- Sea salt has been advocated by health food promoters, but its iodine content is negligible. Purchase salt that is fortified with iodine, as indicated on the label.
- Individuals consuming large amounts of seaweed, a rich source of iodine, may be at risk for iodine toxicity.

◆ **HEALTH APPLICATION 12**

Hypertension

Hypertension is defined as a persistent elevation of systolic blood pressure greater than 120 mm Hg and diastolic pressure greater than 80 mm Hg (Table 12.16). Nearly half (46%)[20] of American adults have hypertension and 28% had prehypertension,[21] warranting some form of change in lifestyle and treatment. The prevalence of hypertension is higher in the following population groups: 60 years and older; individuals of African-American descent, Asians, and Hispanic Americans; a family history; a sedentary lifestyle; consume a large amount of alcohol; have dyslipidemia and/or diabetes; and are obese. According to NHANES estimates, 80% to 85% are aware of having hypertension; 71% to 81% of individuals with hypertension receive treatment; and 50% to 55% have control with their blood pressure.[21]

For every increment of blood pressure above normal levels, there is a commensurate increase in risk of cardiovascular complications, stroke, peripheral vascular disease, and renal insufficiency. Hypertension may result in myocardial infarction, cerebrovascular accident, or heart failure. Uncontrolled hypertension can affect blood vessels in the eyes, kidneys, and nervous system. Hypertension cannot be cured, but it can be controlled. One of the goals of *Healthy People 2030* is to reduce the proportion of adults with hypertension to 27.7%.[22]

Etiology

Several important causal factors for hypertension have been identified, including excess body weight, excess sodium intake, minimal physical activity, inadequate intake of fruits and vegetables and potassium, and excess alcohol intake. Body fat deposited in the trunk increases risk of developing essential hypertension independent of the overall level of obesity, whereas peripherally deposited fat does not. Essential hypertension is elevated blood pressure of unknown cause.

A weight loss of 10% can be as effective at reducing blood pressure as pharmacologic treatment in many cases. Despite the fact that sodium restriction alone does not always result in lower blood pressure for all patients with hypertension, sodium reduction is effective in lowering mean blood pressure in salt-sensitive adults. There is no precise method of identifying salt sensitivity. Sodium restriction enhances effectiveness of diuretics and other pharmacologic treatments. Box 12.2 provides suggestions to reduce sodium intake. Generally, when sodium must be restricted, hidden sources of sodium should be considered: (1) sodium bicarbonate and other sodium products used as leavening agents; (2) sodium benzoate, used as a preservative in margarine and relishes; (3) sodium citrate and monosodium glutamate, used to enhance flavors in gelatin desserts, beverages, and meats; (4) sodium bicarbonate or sodium fluoride added to dentifrices or used in place of commercial dentifrices and mouth rinses; (5) some medications, particularly when taken regularly and frequently, such as antacids, laxatives, and cough medicines; and (6) chewing tobacco.

High-potassium dietary intake has a protective effect against hypertension, has no adverse effect on blood lipids, and is associated with a lower risk of stroke.[24] Potassium increases urinary sodium excretion. A customary high sodium-to-low potassium ratio consumed when most foods are highly processed may be detrimental to normal blood pressure regulation. Increasing dietary potassium intake from nonprocessed foods is a factor in reducing blood pressure and development of CVD. Overall, a diet rich in nutrients can lead to a decrease in CVD and fewer strokes. For example, the National High Blood Pressure Education Program recommends the Dietary Approaches to Stop Hypertension (DASH) diet for preventing and managing hypertension by combining a flexible and individualized meal plan with lifestyle modifications. DASH promotes an overall healthy eating pattern rich in fruits, vegetables, low-fat dairy, whole grains, nuts, fish, and poultry, rather than focusing on calorie restriction or eliminating specific nutrients. In addition, the DASH diet reduces or limits saturated fat, total fat, cholesterol, red meats, and sweets. Therefore this meal plan will be rich in fiber, potassium, magnesium and calcium.

Drug therapy is effective, but for prehypertensive and treated hypertensive individuals, lifestyle changes are also important. Dietary modifications reduce blood pressure for many individuals with mild to moderate hypertension. Health-promoting lifestyle modifications (e.g., weight loss, smoking cessation, increase in physical activity) are recommended to prevent the progressive increase in blood pressure and CVD. Looking at the overall dietary pattern instead of one single nutrient is the key for assessing risk. Notable for the dental hygienist is that individuals with insufficient masticatory function, poor oral hygiene, and oral inflammation and periodontal disease[25] may be associated with hypertension; patients with these problems may need to be referred to a healthcare professional. The dental hygienist can also help by monitoring blood pressure, and educating and supporting the patient's efforts with lifestyle modifications to reduce blood pressure values. One tool to help support the patient is the AHA's How to Manage Blood Pressure—Life's Simple 7 (Fig. 12.12), which contains valuable information the dental hygienist can use for patient education.

TABLE 12.16	2017 High Blood Pressure (BP) Clinical Practice Guideline: Executive Summary Categories of BP in Adults[a]		
BP Category	**Systolic Pressure (mm Hg)**		**Diastolic Pressure (mm Hg)**
Normal	<120	and	<80
Elevated	120–129	and	<80
Hypertension			
Stage 1	130–139	or	80–89
Stage 2	≥140	or	≥90

[a]Individuals with systolic blood pressure and diastolic blood pressure in two categories should be designated to the higher BP category.

Data from Whelton PK, Carey RM, Aronow WS, et al. ACC/AHA/AAPA/ABC/ACPM/AGS/APhA/ASH/ASPC/NMA/PCNA guideline for the prevention, detection, evaluation, and management of high blood pressure in adults: a report of the American College of Cardiology/American Heart Association Task Force on Clinical Practice Guidelines. *Hypertension.* 2018:71(6);e13–e115. https://www.ahajournals.org/doi/pdf/10.1161/HYP.0000000000000065. Accessed August 28, 2020.

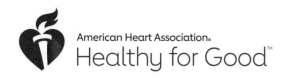

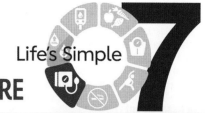

HOW TO MANAGE BLOOD PRESSURE

Life's Simple 7

① UNDERSTAND READINGS

The first step to managing blood pressure is to understand what the levels mean and what is considered normal, elevated, high blood pressure (hypertension) and hypertensive crisis. heart.org/BPlevels

Blood pressure is typically recorded as two numbers, written as a ratio like this:

117

76

Read as "117 over 76 millimeters of mercury."

Systolic
The top number, the higher of the two numbers, measures the pressure in the arteries when the heart beats (when the heart muscle contracts).

Diastolic
The bottom number, the lower of the two numbers, measures the pressure in the arteries when the heart is resting between heart beats.

BLOOD PRESSURE CATEGORY	SYSTOLIC mm Hg (top number)		DIASTOLIC mm Hg (bottom number)
Normal	Lower than 120	*and*	Lower than 80
Elevated Blood Pressure	120–129	*and*	80
High Blood Pressure (Hypertension) Stage 1	130–139	*or*	80–89
High Blood Pressure (Hypertension) Stage 2	140 or higher	*or*	90 or higher
Hypertensive Crisis (Call your doctor immediately)	Higher than 180	*and/or*	Higher than 120

② TRACK LEVELS

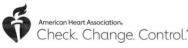

Check.   Change.   Control.

Health care providers can take blood pressure readings and provide recommendations.

Check. Change. Control. helps you track your progress in reducing blood pressure.

Track online at ccctracker.com/AHA

LEARN MORE AT HEART.ORG/MYLIFECHECK AND HEART.ORG/HBP

© Copyright 2019 American Heart Association, Inc., a 501(c)(3) not-for-profit. All rights reserved. Unauthorized use prohibited. Citations available upon request.5/19 DS14545

③ TIPS FOR SUCCESS

EAT SMART

Eat a healthy diet of vegetables, fruits, whole grains, beans, legumes, nuts, plant-based proteins, lean animal proteins and fish. Limit sodium, saturated fats and added sugars. Limit sugary foods and drinks, fatty or processed meats, salty foods, refined carbohydrates and highly processed foods. heart.org/EatSmart

MOVE MORE

Physical activity helps control blood pressure, weight and stress levels. heart.org/MoveMore

MANAGE WEIGHT

If you're overweight, even a slight weight loss can reduce high blood pressure. heart.org/Weight

DON'T SMOKE

Every time you smoke, vape or use tobacco, the nicotine can cause a temporary increase in blood pressure. heart.org/Tobacco

SLEEP WELL

Short sleep (less than 6 hours) and poor-quality sleep are associated with high blood pressure.

• **Fig. 12.12** American Heart Association. How to Manage Blood Pressure—Life's Simple 7. 2019 (https://www.heart.org/en/healthy-living/healthy-lifestyle/my-life-check--lifes-simple-7/ls7-blood-pressure-infographic).

◆ CASE APPLICATION FOR THE DENTAL HYGIENIST

Your patient, an older gentleman, complains of a dry mouth and sore tongue. He states that he has not been thirsty and his intake of fluids has been poor for 4 days. His healthcare provider recently prescribed a diuretic for hypertension and told him to eliminate salt and add more fruits and vegetables to his diet. He complains, "nothing tastes good."

Nutritional Assessment
- Blood pressure value
- Oral mucous membranes, tongue characteristics
- Fluid likes and dislikes
- Mental changes

Nutritional Diagnosis
Fluid volume deficit related to diuretic and poor fluid or food intake.

Nutritional Goals
Patient will have good skin turgor, moist oral mucous membranes, and increase in his intake of liquids and food.

Nutritional Implementation
Intervention: Explain the need for fluid intake.
Rationale: Knowledge and involvement in self-care increase compliance.
Intervention: Encourage the patient to drink his favorite fluids, preferably water, on a regular schedule.
Rationale: The patient is more apt to drink his favorite fluid, and, in doing so, he will replace fluids lost because of the diuretic.
Intervention: Identify methods to increase salivary flow and oral lubrication.
Rationale: The patient's degree of oral comfort will improve and soft tissue will heal.
Intervention: Explain the importance of oral hygiene. How to perform oral self-care procedures.
Rationale: Less saliva allows more food debris to remain on teeth, which may increase caries risk. Because oral mucosa and gingival tissues are more

susceptible to trauma, an extra-soft bristle brush may be appropriate for plaque removal, and the patient should be cautioned against aggressive oral hygiene. Other oral physiotherapy aids may be warranted for optimal plaque biofilm removal.
Intervention: Explore challenges the patient will encounter with foods low in salt and discuss ways to enhance flavors of food without using sodium (see Box 12.2 and Tables 12.6 and 12.7). Explain that as his salt intake decreases, salt in the saliva will also decrease so that after about 3 months of moderately low intake, his preferred salt level in foods will decrease and his taste for food will gradually improve.
Rationale: Most Americans can consume up to 10 times the recommended amount of sodium. Sodium concentration in saliva determines a patient's recognition of salt in food; higher levels of sodium in saliva means higher levels of sodium are needed for it to be detected.
Intervention: A dentifrice containing stannous fluoride will be consistent with the healthcare provider's order to limit sodium intake and allow improvement with oral inflammation and control of plaque biofilm.
Rationale: Sodium bicarbonate or sodium fluoride is added to some dentifrices and mouth rinses; these would increase his sodium intake, especially if oral hygiene is practiced several times a day and the patient swallows the dentifrice or mouth rinse.
Intervention: Have the patient record his dietary intake for 1 to 3 days. Compare this record with the recommendations for reduced sodium intake.
Rationale: Suggestions can be flexible and tailored to the patient's needs. The patient can set a goal based on the information presented.

Evaluation
Desired outcomes include the patient's adequate consumption of preferred beverages each day, moist oral mucous membranes, no gingival inflammation, and no dental caries.

◆ Student Readiness

1. Define ICF and ECF. What are the principal electrolytes found in each?
2. Record your daily fluid intake. How does your intake compare with the required intake? What percentage is water? What source does your water come from (e.g., tap, bottled)?
3. Fluid is essential for survival. Discuss advantages and disadvantages of water intake versus other fluids, such as milk, soft drinks, tea, and coffee.
4. Identify all of the SSBs you (or a patient) consumed yesterday. Determine the total number of grams or teaspoons of added sugar in beverages consumed. This information can be found on a food label or looking at nutrition information for brand names. Compare this total to the recommended intake of 9 tsp/day (36 g) for male or 6 tsp/day (24 g) for female. Instructions to determine the number of teaspoons of sugar in a serving can be found in Chapter 4.
5. List five clinical observations indicating FVD. What type of medication is frequently prescribed that affects hydration status?
6. What can cause FVD or FVE?

7. What can cause hypernatremia and/or hyponatremia? Why is altering salt intake of patients with these conditions not usually the mode of treatment? Class activity: Obtain a 24-hour recall (instructions in Chapter 21) of a partner. Circle the high sodium foods/beverages. Provide the partner with lower sodium choices.
8. Discuss dental hygiene interventions for iron-deficiency anemia. Discuss factors affecting iron absorption.
9. Which two nutrients discussed in this chapter are important for collagen formation?
10. Name the electrolyte(s) or mineral(s) discussed in this chapter associated with the following symptoms:
    - Shrinkage of mucous membranes
    - Thirst
    - Oral pallor
    - Taste abnormalities
    - Lethargy
    - Enlargement of thyroid
    - Poor wound healing
    - Swollen tongue
    - Loss of appetite
11. Identify dietary guidelines that would be beneficial to the older adult in the Case Application in this chapter.

◆ CASE STUDY

A 17-year-old boy complains of a dry mouth; difficulty in swallowing food; dry, sticky tongue; and dry skin. The patient reports that he has just recovered from the flu with fever, diarrhea, and vomiting. He also informs you that he is currently undergoing training for an athletic competition and exercises 3 to 4 hours/day. A 24-hour diet recall reveals the patient's fluid intake includes 48 to 72 oz of caffeinated soft drinks without any other beverages and a high-protein intake.

1. What other information should you obtain about the patient's dietary intake?
2. Could the patient's oral symptoms be attributed to his current fluid intake?
3. Is salivary analysis indicated for this patient?
4. What suggestions could you make that would decrease his symptoms of xerostomia? List suggestions to increase his fluid intake.
5. What oral self-care practices would you recommend to relieve his oral discomfort and facilitate swallowing?

◆ CASE STUDY

A 15-year-old girl comes into the dental office reporting a history of iron-deficiency anemia. She has clinical symptoms typical of this anemia: glossitis; smooth, shiny, red tongue; and painful cracks at the corners of her mouth. Her healthcare provider has prescribed ferrous sulfate and zinc to correct this deficiency.

1. When evaluating dietary intake, what are some foods that are good sources of iron?
2. If the patient is having problems with the ferrous sulfate supplement (e.g., constipation or nausea), would it be advisable to resolve the anemia by just increasing dietary iron intake? Why or why not?
3. Why has the healthcare provider ordered zinc supplements?
4. What should you tell her about iron from plant or animal foods?
5. What can she do to help increase absorption of iron and zinc?

References

1. Rosinger A, Herrick K. Daily water intake among US men and women, 2009-2012. *NCHS Data Brief No. 242*. National Center for Health Statistics; 2016.
2. Herrick CA, Terry AL, Afful J. Beverage consumption among youth in the United States: 2013-2016. *HANES NCHS Data Brief No. 320*. NCHS; 2018. https://www.cdc.gov/nchs/products/databriefs/db320.htm.
3. Duarte PM, Reis AF. Coffee consumption has no deleterious effects on periodontal health but its benefits are uncertain. *J Evid Based Dent Pract*. 2015;15(2):77–79.
4. Tsou SH, Hu SW, Yang JJ, et al. Potential oral health care agent from coffee against virulence factor of periodontitis. *Nutrients*. 2019;11:2235. https://doi.org/10.3390/nu11092235. https://pubmed.ncbi.nlm.nih.gov/31527555/.
5. U.S. Department of Health and Human Services and U.S. Department of Agriculture. *2015–2020 Dietary Guidelines for Americans*. 8th ed. 2015. https://health.gov/our-work/food-nutrition/2015-2020-dietary-guidelines/guidelines/chapter-1/.
6. Imoisili OO, Park S, Lundeen EA, et al. Sugar-sweetened beverage consumption among adults, by residence in metropolitan and nonmetropolitan counties in 12 states and the District of Columbia, 2017. *Prev Chronic Dis*. 2020;17:190108. https://doi.org/10.5888/pcd17.190108.
7. Vieux F, Maillot M, Rehm CD, et al. Trends in tap and bottled water consumption among children and adults in the United States: analyses of NHANES 2011-16 data. *Nutr J*. 2020 https://doi.org/10.1186/s12937-020-0523-6. https://nutritionj.biomedcentral.com/articles/10.1186/s12937-020-0523-6.
8. Marriott BP, Hunt KJ, Malek AM, Newman JC. Trends in intake of energy and total sugar from sugar-sweetened beverages in the United States among children and adults, NHANES 2003-2016. *Nutrients*. 2019. https://www.mdpi.com/2072-6643/11/9/2004.
9. Bleich SN, Vercammen KA, Koma JW, Zhonghe L. Trends in beverage consumption among children and adults, 2003-2014. *Obesity*. 2018;26(2):432–441.
10. National Institutes of Health, National Center for Complementary and Integrative Health. *Energy Drinks*. 2018. https://nccih.nih.gov/health/energy-drinks.
11. Nutrition and Enhanced Sports Performance.. In: Meyer F, Timmons BW, Wilk B, Leites GT, eds. *Water: Hydration and Sports Drink*. 2nd ed. Elsevier; 2019.
12. Reddy A, Norris DF, Momeni SS, et al. The pH of beverages in the United States. *JADA*. 2016;147(4):255–263.
13. Chan AS, Tran TTK, Hsu YH, et al. A systematic review of dietary acids and habits on dental erosion in adolescents. *Int J Paediatr Dent*. 2020;00:1–21. https://doi.org/10.1111/ipd.12643.
14. Health Canada. *Health Canada Is Advising Canadians About Safe Levels of Caffeine Consumption*. 2017. https://healthycanadians.gc.ca/recall-alert-rappel-avis/hc-sc/2017/63362a-eng.php.
15. Benjamin EJ, Muntner P, Alonso A, et al. Heart disease and stroke-2019 update: a report from the American Heart Association. *Circulation*. 2019;139:56–528.
16. World Health Organization. *WHO Guideline: Sodium Intake for Adults and Children*. Geneva. https://iris.who.int/bitstream/handle/10665/77985/9789241504836_eng.pdf.
17. Centers for Disease Control and Prevention (CDC). Top 10 Sources of Sodium. June;6:2023https://www.cdc.gov/salt/food.htm.
18. Poti J, Dunford EK, Popkin BM. Sodium reduction in US households' packaged food and beverage purchases, 2000 to 2014. *JAMA Intern Med*. 2017;177(7):986–994.
19. Li M, Yan S, Li X, et al. Association between blood pressure and dietary intakes of sodium and potassium among US adults using quantile regression analysis NHANES 2007–2014. *J Hum Hypertens*. 2020;34:346–354.
20. Haase H, Ellinger S, Linseisen J, et al. Revised D-A-CH-reference values for the intake of zinc. *J Trace Elem Med Biol*. 2020;61. https://doi.org/10.1016/j.jtemb.2020.126536.
21. Lumen A, George NI. Estimation of iodine nutrition and thyroid function status in late-gestation pregnant women in the United States: development and application of a population-based pregnancy model. *Toxicol Appl Pharmacol*. 2017;314:24–38.
22. Salim V, Alonso A, Benjamin E. Heart disease and stroke statistics—2020 update: a report from the American Heart Association. *Circulation*. 2020;141:e139–e596.
23. US Department of Health and Human Services. Office of Disease Prevention and Healthy Promotion. *Progress Toward Healthy People 2030 Objectives: Heart Disease and Stroke*. https://health.gov/healthypeople/objectives-and-data/browse-objectives/heart-disease-and-stroke.
24. Whelton SP, Blumenthal RS. Insights on potassium supplementation for the treatment of hypertension from the Canadian Hypertension Education Program Guidelines (CHEP). *Circulation*. 2017;135:3–4.
25. Pietropaoli D, Del Pinto R, Ferri C, et al. Definition of hypertension-associated oral pathogens in NHANES. *J Periodontol*. 2019;90:866–876.

▶ Evolve Resources

Please visit http://evolve.elsevier.com/Mallonee/nutritional for additional practice and study support tools.

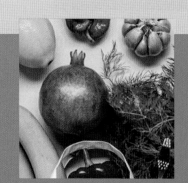

13

Nutritional Requirements Affecting Oral Health in Females

STUDENT LEARNING OBJECTIVES

On completion of this chapter, the student will be able to achieve the following learning outcomes:

1. Discuss the following related to factors affecting fetal development:
   - Explain the importance of prenatal weight and weight gain during pregnancy.
   - Advise prenatal patients who have unusual dietary patterns.
   - Discuss why good oral health is important before and during a pregnancy.
   - List foods that pregnant females should avoid to decrease the risk of foodborne illness.
2. Discuss factors affecting oral development.
3. Discuss nutritional requirements for pregnancy, including:
   - Name nutrients needed in larger amounts by pregnant females and explain why those increases are needed.
   - Identify nutrients frequently consumed in inadequate amounts by pregnant females and suggest ways to improve their intake.

   - Discuss nutrients commonly supplemented during pregnancy.
4. Discuss nutritional requirements for lactation, including:
   - Name nutrients needed in larger amounts by lactating females and explain why those increases are needed.
   - Identify nutrients frequently consumed in inadequate amounts by lactating females and suggest ways to improve their intake.
   - Discuss nutrients commonly supplemented during lactation.
5. List the nutrients affected by oral contraceptive agents (OCAs), as well as the increased risks associated with the use of OCAs.
6. Describe the many hormonal changes that occur in a female's body during menopause, as well as nutritional approaches that can be used to reduce menopausal symptoms.

KEY TERMS

Anencephaly
Atrophic gingivitis
Dysesthesia
Erythropoiesis
Gravidas
Hormone replacement therapy (HRT)

Listeriosis
Low birth weight (LBW)
Menopausal gingivostomatitis
Menopause
Nutritional insult
Perimenopause

Pica
Preeclampsia
Premature
Primigravida
Toxoplasmosis

TEST YOUR NQ

1. **T/F** All efforts should be made to satisfy a pregnant female's food cravings because cravings reflect an innate need for certain nutrients.
2. **T/F** The fetus is nourished from the mother's nutrient stores.
3. **T/F** After pregnancy, most mothers have at least one carious lesion because calcium is pulled from teeth for the developing fetus.
4. **T/F** A female should eat twice as much food when she is pregnant because she has to eat for both herself and the fetus.
5. **T/F** Weight gain depends on health and body mass before prepregnancy; most females should gain 25 to 35 lb during pregnancy.

6. **T/F** Vitamin A is the only nutrient warranting global supplementation during pregnancy.
7. **T/F** Although there are some cases of low milk production, most females can produce enough milk to support nutritional needs of the infant.
8. **T/F** Breast milk that is too thin must be nutritionally inadequate.
9. **T/F** If breast milk supply is inadequate, omit a feeding to have more milk available later.
10. **T/F** WIC is a governmental program that provides supplemental foods for females, infants, and children.

Healthy Pregnancy

Although there is no specific definition of a healthy pregnancy, the health of both mother and infant is important. A healthy baby begins with a healthy mother. In addition to continued preservation of the mother's physical health, her emotional and psychological well-being is important. Goals for the infant include being (1) full term (born between the 39th and 41st week of gestation) and (2) mature (weighing more than 6 lb). Infants with a low birth weight (**LBW**; weighing less than 5½ lb) or who are premature (gestational age less than 37 weeks, especially a gestational age of less than 32 weeks) have more long-term health and developmental problems, oral problems, and increased risk of early mortality. In 2014, approximately 34% of all infants who died, were born at less than 32 weeks' gestation. The number of infants born prematurely rose from 10.1% in 2020 to 10.5% in 2021.[1] Primary factors for a successful pregnancy are nutritional status before conception, appropriate weight gain, and adequate intake of essential nutrients during pregnancy.

The classic report published in 1970 by the National Academy of Sciences established a basis for increased nutritional requirements during pregnancy.[2] More recent workshops acknowledge that the report principally addressed undernutrition and inadequate weight gain, whereas current concern has shifted to focus on increased body weight of females in their childbearing years who are more likely to have chronic conditions such as hypertension or diabetes mellitus.[3] Many health care providers and females of childbearing age are unaware of these guidelines for weight gain. Gaining either too little or too much weight during pregnancy can lead to poor outcomes of the mother and the infant. With the exception of chromosomal issues, fetal health is determined by the mother's diet, exercise, and lifestyle choices. The quality of daily food choices is the most important and most ignored factor determining pregnancy outcomes (Fig. 13.1).

Factors Affecting Fetal Development

Preconceptional Nutritional Status

Health status is important for a female, but it is especially critical for conception. Preconceptual obesity or underweight not only hampers fertility but can also set the stage for metabolic problems during pregnancy.[4] Ideally, weight adjustments should be achieved

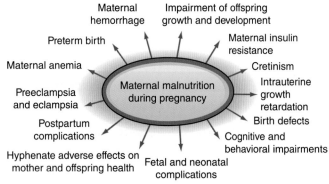

• **Fig. 13.1** Major negative effects of maternal malnutrition (both undernutrition and overnutrition) on mother and infant. (Reproduced with permission from Mahan LK, Raymond JL. *Krause's Food and the Nutrition Care Process*. 14th ed. St. Louis, MO: Elsevier; 2016.)

before pregnancy begins. Because of the detrimental influence of maternal overweight and obesity on pregnancy outcomes, the Academy of Nutrition and Dietetics (AND) recommends counseling for all females of reproductive age (especially those who are overweight or obese) about maternal and fetal risks, addressing prepregnancy obesity, excessive weight gain, and postpartum weight retention, including benefits of lifestyle changes prior to pregnancy.[5] Severe dietary restrictions are inappropriate when a female is trying to conceive even though she is attempting to lose weight in anticipation of the pregnancy. Achieving a healthy weight prior to conception can reduce weight-related complications such as high blood pressure, gestational diabetes, and the risk of preterm birth.[6] Preeclampsia is a potentially serious complication of pregnancy involving high blood pressure that often leads to premature delivery. A health care provider should be consulted to determine healthy weight goals.

Globally, nearly half of all pregnancies are unintended.[7] By the time a female has her first prenatal visit, fetal development has progressed beyond the critical period when a lack of folic acid or certain exposures may have already compromised the health and well-being of the mother and/or the fetus. In addition to eating a well-balanced diet, prenatal vitamins are encouraged in anticipation of a pregnancy. Prenatal food choices may have enduring effects on the child's lifelong food preferences and negative metabolic outcomes.[8]

In pregnancies conceived in less than 1 year after the previous pregnancy, maternal nutritional reserves may be inadequate, contributing to increased incidence of preterm births and fetal growth retardation. Risk of maternal mortality and morbidity is also higher.[9] Body parts and organs develop rapidly during the first trimester; birth defects are likely to occur if usual dietary patterns are poor or if drugs are used during this critical period. With some nutrients, such as calcium and iron, higher requirements are met by increased maternal absorption, but for others, inadequate maternal intake may deplete the mother's stores (e.g., folic acid), potentially resulting in suboptimal infant stores at birth.[10]

Unusual Dietary Patterns

Pica, or an abnormal consumption of specific food and nonfood substances—such as dirt, clay, baking soda, paint chips, stones, cloth, baby powder, starch (laundry and corn), large quantities of ice/frost, or other inedible items—remains a millennia-old nutritional enigma. Females practicing pica behaviors are usually from lower socioeconomic groups or have less than a high school education; are in poor nutritional health; may be adolescents having clinical problems; or are affected by behavioral/environmental factors, such as alcohol or substance abuse. Pica is more frequently practiced by African American females living in rural areas with a childhood and family history of pica.[11] Micronutrient deficiencies, especially iron and zinc, may result from these abnormal behaviors.[5,12] Pica may result in lead poisoning and, depending on the nonfood item, the substance consumed can cause teeth to wear down quickly.[13]

Personal beliefs about cravings and customs influencing dietary selections are cultural and regional. Familiarity with local beliefs is beneficial in assessing how these practices affect nutritional status and in advising a gravida (pregnant female) about habits potentially detrimental to both her and the fetus. Patients may be more receptive to changing their food habits when the dental hygienist provides unbiased guidance about desirable food choices and how this relates to their oral health and systemic health.

Health Care

Availability, use and access to health care services may contribute to pregnancy outcomes. Inadequate prenatal care leads to problems for both mother and fetus. Prenatal care is important to protect the embryo from the effects of chronic health problems later in life. A goal of *Healthy People 2030* is to increase the proportion of pregnant females who receive early and adequate prenatal care. Current data demonstrates that 76.4% of pregnant females receive adequate prenatal care with a goal of increasing this to 80.5%.[14]

Age

Maternal age can be a factor in the increased number of LBW infants among gravidas younger than 18 years old. Most adolescent girls do not complete linear growth and achieve gynecologic maturity until age 17 years. Nutritional requirements are quite high to meet growth needs for both the adolescent and fetus. Additionally, many adolescents have an inadequate intake of numerous crucial nutrients (see Chapter 14). Pregnancy during adolescence may have an adverse effect on postmenopausal bone density; greater calcium and vitamin D consumption during pregnancy may protect against bone loss[15]

Intake of calorie-dense foods and erratic eating may preclude adequate intake of required nutrients. Socioeconomic disadvantages of these young mothers may affect their diet as a result of the amount of food available and their uninformed selections.

More females are choosing to become pregnant at an older age. A female needs to be particularly aware of maintaining her nutritional health if a pregnancy after age 35 years is anticipated. Maternal risks involve chronic conditions, including overweight or obesity, and diabetes and hypertension. These conditions should be closely supervised by an obstetrician to lessen their impact on the fetus.

Weight Gain

Successful pregnancies depend on ideal preconceptional weight plus appropriate weight gain during gestation. Prepregnancy obesity in the United States rose from 26.1% in 2016 to 29.0% in 2019.[5,16,17] The goal for females who are overweight before pregnancy is to avoid excessive weight gain, but to consume adequate calories to allow optimal fetal growth.

Current National Academy of Medicine (NAM) recommendations take into consideration the factors for weight gain that affect pregnancy before conception and continue through the first year postpartum with regard to the health of both infant and mother.[18,19] These guidelines are based on body mass index (BMI) categories and include a relatively narrow range of recommended gain for obese females. The suggested range of weight gain accommodates differences such as age, race/ethnicity, and other factors that affect pregnancy outcomes. The guidelines are intended to be used along with good clinical judgment and a discussion between the female and her health care provider about diet and exercise. Females whose prepregnancy weight is within a normal BMI should have a total weight gain of 25 to 35 lb, or 0.8 to 1 lb/week during the second and third trimesters (Table 13.1). More research is needed to determine appropriate weight gain for adolescents. Some females are concerned about gaining too much weight during pregnancy; others, recognizing the need to eat for two, consume excessive amounts of food. Excessive weight gain during pregnancy can increase maternal risk of gestational diabetes, pregnancy-induced high blood pressure, preeclampsia, assisted deliveries, postpartum hemorrhage, and weight retention. Fetal risks include preterm delivery, increased mortality, large-for-gestational age, and congenital anomalies.[20] Physical activity, such as walking briskly for 30 minutes a day, can help avoid adding many pounds during pregnancy. Among primigravida (first-time pregnancies) females, 66% experience gestational weight gain exceeding NAM recommendations.[21] Females who gain more than the recommended amount of weight during pregnancy are more likely to retain the weight and retain the postpartum weight. Excess weight gain in pregnancy is associated with an increased incidence of having a larger baby which can complicate delivery and lead to obesity in childhood.[22] On the other hand, underweight females are at increased risk for spontaneous preterm birth and LBW, which is associated with health problems for the infant.[22]

Oral Health

A recent study demonstrates that slightly more than half of pregnant females report getting dental care during their pregnancy.[23] Of those females who experienced problems during pregnancy, less than 35% scheduled a visit to the dentist. If they have not received routine dental care either before or during pregnancy, they may be unaware of the importance of oral health care during this period. Even though a pregnant woman may not have overt dental problems, maintaining proper oral hygiene care is important. Oral hygiene practices and dental service utilization are highly related to racial, ethnic, and economic disparities.[24,25]

TABLE 13.1	Recommendation for Total and Rate of Weight Gain During Pregnancy by Prepregnancy Body Mass Index (BMI)		
Prepregnancy BMI	BMIa (kg/m²) (WHO)	Total Weight Gain Range (lb)	Rates of Weight Gainb Second and Third Trimester (Mean Range in lb/week)
Underweight	<18.5	28–40	1 (1–1.3)
Normal weight	18.5–24.9	25–35	1 (0.8–1)
Overweight	25.0–29.9	15–25	0.6 (0.5–0.7)
Obese (includes all classes)	≥30.0	11–20	0.5 (0.4–0.6)

aTo determine BMI, go to https://www.nhlbi.nih.gov/health/educational/lose_wt/BMI/bmicalc.htm or use this formula: BMI = (weight in pounds/[height in inches × height in inches]) × 703.
bCalculations assume a 0.5–2 kg (1.1–4.4 lb) weight gain in the first trimester.
From Institute of Medicine (IOM) and National Research Council (NRC). *Weight Gain During Pregnancy: Reexamining the Guidelines*. National Academies Press: 2009. http://www.nationalacademies.org/hmd/Reports/2009/Weight-Gain-During-Pregnancy-Reexamining-the-Guidelines.aspx.

Attitudes and behaviors about dental care during pregnancy may be influenced by fear of harm to the female or fetus. Routine dental care (dental prophylaxis and tooth scaling) during pregnancy is not associated with an increased risk of serious medical events, preterm deliveries, spontaneous abortions, or fetal deaths or anomalies.

Hormonal changes (estrogen and progesterone) associated with pregnancy contribute to an increased susceptibility to pregnancy gingivitis and periodontitis. Obstetricians or prenatal care providers should be aware of these changes and encourage routine prophylaxis during pregnancy.[26] Oral health education and therapeutic protocol may decrease gingivitis during pregnancy.[27] Pregnancy gingivitis (Fig. 13.2A) usually becomes evident in the second month of pregnancy. If plaque biofilm is allowed to accumulate and irritate the gingiva, gingivitis occurs and may result in large growths called "pregnancy tumors" (Fig. 13.2B). Some studies indicate that periodontal disease during pregnancy is possibly a risk factor for adverse pregnancy outcomes such as preeclampsia, premature birth, and/or LBW infant.[28,29] However, treatment of periodontal disease during pregnancy does not appear to improve perinatal outcomes.[30–33] The etiology of preterm birth and/or LBW is multifactorial, involving consumption habits and socioeconomic and health factors. Periodontal disease is more prevalent in populations at the highest risk of adverse pregnancy outcomes; whether or not periodontal disease increases the risk for adverse pregnancy outcomes, use of dental services for pregnant females needs to be encouraged.

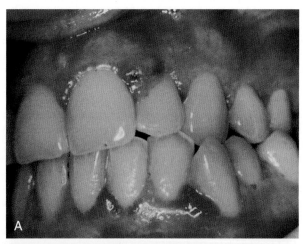

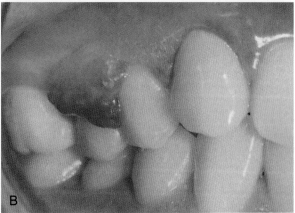

• **Fig. 13.2** (A) Moderate form of pregnancy gingivitis. (B) Pyogenic granuloma (i.e.) pregnancy tumor. (Reproduced with permission from Perry DA, Beemsterboer PL. *Periodontology for the Dental Hygienist.* 4th ed. St. Louis, MO: Saunders; 2014.)

Nausea is common during pregnancy; recurring vomiting increases oral exposure to gastric acid secretions, which may erode tooth enamel. In addition to nausea and vomiting, gastroesophageal reflux disease occurs frequently during pregnancy because of normal physiologic changes that affect the lower esophageal sphincter. Evidence shows a strong association between gastroesophageal reflux disease and dental erosion.[34] Acidity from repeated regurgitation can be treated by a sodium bicarbonate rinse to neutralize oral pH, rinse for 30 seconds, then brush and floss.[35]

Drugs and Medications

Use of tobacco, alcohol, caffeine, some medications, megadoses of nutrients, and illegal drugs can harm the fetus. Caffeine, a stimulant and a diuretic, crosses the placenta. Epidemiologic studies have shown inconsistent conclusions about the effect of caffeine intake during pregnancy on the risk of LBW or preterm birth.[36,37] However, the current recommendation is to eliminate caffeine or limit it to less than 200 mg/day.[38–40] Brewed coffee, for example, can contain 150 to 500 mg caffeine per 16-oz cup. Considering the popularity of coffee, sodas, and energy drinks, minimizing caffeine intake may be challenging for some pregnant females.

Alcohol is a folic acid antagonist and can cross the placenta. For decades, doctors and researchers have known that alcohol intake during pregnancy may cause birth defects, especially fetal alcohol syndrome (discussed in *Health Application 13*). Prenatal exposure to alcohol can harm the fetus and is the leading preventable cause of birth defects, and intellectual and neurodevelopmental disabilities. The effects of a small amount of alcohol on the fetus are not well understood.[41] Alcohol-related birth defects and developmental disabilities are completely preventable when females abstain from alcohol. During pregnancy, no amount of alcohol intake is considered safe; all forms of alcohol (beer, wine, liquor) pose similar risks.[42]

Artificial Sweeteners

Nonnutritive sweeteners, while classified as generally safe, have received little attention regarding their safety during pregnancy and the guidelines are limited. The US Food and Drug Administration (FDA) has approved aspartame, acesulfame-K, rebaudioside (Stevia), and sucralose for moderate consumption during pregnancy.[43,44] There is an evidence that nonnutritive sweeteners cross the placenta. It is a concern that exposure to these alternative sweeteners can adversely affect the metabolic health of the developing fetus. Saccharin has been shown to cross the placenta and remain in fetal tissue so the FDA does not recommend this nonnutritive sweetener as safe during pregnancy.[44,45] Pregnant females with the genetic disorder phenylketonuria should not use aspartame throughout their life span.

Food Safety

During pregnancy, females are at high risk for foodborne illness because of physiologic changes that may increase exposure of the gravida and fetus to hazardous substances. Pregnant and breastfeeding females, in particular, should heed food-handling precautions discussed in Chapter 16 in addition to other precautions discussed here.

The US FDA advises pregnant females to avoid unpasteurized (raw) milk and cheese, and juices; raw or undercooked animal foods such as seafood, meat, poultry, and eggs; and raw sprouts because of high risk of foodborne illness.[46] Certain foodborne illnesses can be especially dangerous; for example, listeriosis can cause miscarriage, premature birth, stillbirth, or acute illness in newborns.[47] Listeriosis is a disease usually caused by food contaminated with the bacterium *Listeria monocytogenes*, which principally affects infants and adults with weakened immune systems. These harmful bacteria grow slowly at refrigerated temperatures. The disease caused by *Listeria* can be transmitted to the fetus even if the mother does not show any signs of illness. Symptoms include gastrointestinal problems followed by fever and muscle aches. To reduce the risk of listeriosis, pregnant females should heat leftovers and ready-to-eat foods (e.g., deli meats, hot dogs, and luncheon meats) until steaming (165°F); and avoid unpasteurized (raw) milk, soft cheeses (Brie, feta, blue-veined, Camembert, and queso blanco, queso fresco) and homemade cheese if prepared with unpasteurized milk; smoked fish and pâtés; meat spreads from a meat counter or refrigerated section of the store; and store-prepared salads such as ham, chicken, egg, tuna, and seafood salads.[48]

Toxoplasmosis, caused by a parasite, is a leading cause of death related to foodborne illness in the United States.[49] The gravida may be symptom free because the immune system prevents the parasite from causing illness, but the infection is passed on to the fetus. In addition to observing safe food-handling precautions listed in Box 16.3, pregnant females should be especially mindful of cooking meat, poultry, and seafood to safe minimum internal temperatures; washing all cutting boards and knives with hot soapy water after use; avoiding drinking untreated water; washing hands with soap and water after touching soil, sand, cat litter, raw meat, or unwashed vegetables; and wearing gloves when gardening or handling sand, or cleaning cat litter boxes.[50]

Pregnant females are encouraged to consume at least 8–12 oz (2–3 servings) of cooked seafood weekly (especially salmon, herring, mussels, trout, sardines, and pollock, which are rich in omega-3 fatty acids).[50] White tuna, also known as albacore tuna and tuna steaks, should be limited to 6 oz.[51] Raw fish should be avoided. Evidence is unclear about the impact that mercury has on the developing brain and nervous system of a fetus or young baby.[51,52] Therefore it is recommended to use caution and limit the intake of fish and seafood by choosing those with lower mercury content. As shown in Fig. 13.3, the FDA and the Environmental Protection Agency have provided advice about the best or good choices and fish to avoid while ensuring two to three servings of fish weekly to prevent ingesting dangerous levels of mercury.[53,54] Lead, present in tap water leached from plumbing, and in dust from deteriorating lead-based paint, can negatively affect socialization and behaviors. Absorbed lead accumulates; maternal bones can release stored lead into the bloodstream.[55] Regardless of the source, lead is absorbed by fetal brain cells in place of calcium needed for thought processes.[56] This results in lifelong developmental problems, such as reduced attention span, increased impulsive behavior, and lower intelligence.[57]

Other chemicals, or pesticides in the food supply may pass through the placenta. As a prudent measure, encourage pregnant females to wash all produce thoroughly, or purchase organic fruits and vegetables most likely to contain pesticides (Box 16.4).

Factors Affecting Oral Development

Variations in the arrangement of teeth, their eruption time, and pits and fissures on enamel can be attributed to environmental and genetic factors.[58] Critical periods for various stages of tooth development occur at different times. Nutrients supplied by the mother must be available when needed for the development of preeruptive teeth and soft tissues. All primary teeth and many permanent teeth are at various stages of development at birth.

Tooth development begins by the sixth week of gestation. Calcification of deciduous teeth begins about the fourth month; development of more than 60% of the 52 deciduous and permanent teeth is initiated during gestation (Table 13.2). By the fourth month of pregnancy, the mandible is calcified.

Severe and irreversible damage results if nutritional insult (deficiency or excessive amounts of specific nutrients) or infection occurs during critical stages, especially in dentin or enamel formation (Table 13.3). After eruption, the tooth has no mechanism to repair itself. Severe nutrient deficiencies can result in oral malformations such as cleft palate, cleft lip, and shortened mandible. Less-severe nutrient deficiencies can reduce the size of the tooth, interfere with tooth formation, delay the time of tooth eruption, and increase the susceptibility of teeth to caries. Most nutrient deficiencies that occur in utero affecting developing teeth increase the child's susceptibility to dental caries.[59,60]

Dentin and enamel depend on many nutrients: vitamin C for formation of collagen matrix; and calcium, magnesium, phosphorus, and vitamin D for mineralization. An inadequate amount of any of these nutrients during tooth development results in an imperfect matrix, with subsequent imperfection of mineralization (see Table 13.3). Infants whose mothers have low levels of vitamin D during pregnancy may be at increased risk for tooth enamel defects and early childhood tooth decay.[59,61] Keratin in enamel depends on vitamin A for its synthesis. Folate deficiency, known to cause neural tube defects, can result in incomplete formation of cranial bones.

Benefits of fluoride supplements during pregnancy in preventing infant dental caries are uncertain. Although fluoride supplements are considered safe for the mother and fetus, oral fluoride supplements during pregnancy seem to have minimal benefits on the developing fetus and are not recommended.[62] Use of fluoridated products, such as toothpaste and mouth rinses, and fluoridated water are encouraged.

Nutritional Requirements for Pregnancy

Dietary Reference Intakes (DRIs) for pregnancy indicate advisable nutrient intake for optimal health of both mother and fetus. Accelerated growth and metabolism increases most nutrient requirements to some extent. Each vitamin and mineral is not separately discussed in this chapter; Table 13.4 shows the increased amounts recommended for each of the nutrients. The following mean nutrient intakes are commonly below the Recommended Dietary Allowances (RDAs) for pregnant females: fiber, vitamin D, folate, iron, and polyunsaturated fatty acids (PUFA). In addition to low intake of these nutrients, gravidas on vegan diets frequently consume inadequate amounts of vitamin B_{12} and are at increased risk of an inadequate intake of iron and vitamin D.[63] Adolescent females with childbearing potential frequently have inadequate intakes of nutrients, potentially affecting pregnancy outcomes.[64]

Energy and Calories

During pregnancy, calorie requirements increase slightly to ensure nutrient and energy needs. The estimated energy requirement does not increase during the first trimester of pregnancy, allows an additional 340 cal/day during the second, and allows an additional 452 cal during the third trimester.[18] This additional energy is needed to (1) build new tissues, including added maternal tissues and growth of the fetus and placenta; (2) support increased metabolic expenditure; and (3) enable physical movement of additional

ADVICE ABOUT EATING FISH

For Those Who Might Become or Are Pregnant or Breastfeeding and Children Ages 1 – 11 Years

 Fish‡ provide key nutrients that support a child's brain development.

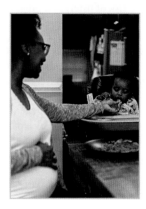

Fish are part of a healthy eating pattern and provide key nutrients during pregnancy, breastfeeding, and/or early childhood to support a **child's brain development**:

- Omega-3 (called DHA and EPA) and omega-6 fats
- Iron
- Iodine (during pregnancy)
- Choline

Choline also supports development of the **baby's spinal cord**. Fish provide iron and zinc to support **children's immune systems**. Fish are a source of other nutrients like protein, vitamin B12, vitamin D, and selenium too.

 ## Choose a variety of fish that are lower in mercury.

While it is important to limit mercury in the diets of those who are pregnant or breastfeeding and children, many types of fish are both nutritious and lower in mercury.

This chart can help you choose which fish to eat, and how often to eat them, based on their mercury levels.

What is a serving? As a guide, use the palm of your hand.

 Pregnancy and breastfeeding:
1 serving is 4 ounces

Eat 2 to 3 servings a week from the "Best Choices" list
(OR 1 serving from the "Good Choices" list).

 Childhood:
On average, a serving is about:

1 ounce at age 1 to 3
2 ounces at age 4 to 7
3 ounces at age 8 to 10
4 ounces at age 11

Eat 2 servings a week from the "Best Choices" list.

Best Choices

Anchovy	Herring	Scallop
Atlantic croaker	Lobster, American and spiny	Shad
Atlantic mackerel		Shrimp
Black sea bass	Mullet	Skate
Butterfish	Oyster	Smelt
Catfish	Pacific chub mackerel	Sole
Clam		Squid
Cod	Perch, freshwater and ocean	Tilapia
Crab	Pickerel	Trout, freshwater
Crawfish	Plaice	Tuna, canned light (includes skipjack)
Flounder	Pollock	Whitefish
Haddock	Salmon	Whiting
Hake	Sardine	

Good Choices

Bluefish	Monkfish	Tilefish (Atlantic Ocean)
Buffalofish	Rockfish	
Carp	Sablefish	Tuna, albacore/ white tuna, canned and fresh/frozen
Chilean sea bass/ Patagonian toothfish	Sheepshead	
Grouper	Snapper	Tuna, yellowfin
Halibut	Spanish mackerel	Weakfish/seatrout
Mahi mahi/dolphinfish	Striped bass (ocean)	White croaker/ Pacific croaker

Choices to Avoid HIGHEST MERCURY LEVELS

King mackerel	Shark	Tilefish (Gulf of Mexico)
Marlin	Swordfish	Tuna, bigeye
Orange roughy		

What about fish caught by family or friends? Check for fish and shellfish advisories to tell you how often you can safely eat those fish. If there is no advisory, eat only one serving and no other fish that week. Some fish caught by family and friends, such as larger carp, catfish, trout and perch, are more likely to have fish advisories due to mercury or other contaminants.

www.FDA.gov/fishadvice
www.EPA.gov/fishadvice

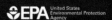

‡ This advice refers to fish and shellfish collectively as "fish" / Advice revised October 2021

• **Fig. 13.3** Advice about eating fish. From United States Environmental Protection Agency and United States Food and Drug Administration. https://www.fda.gov/media/102331/download?attachment; EPA-FDA Advice about Eating Fish and Shellfish: For Those Who Might Become Pregnant, Are Pregnant, Are Breastfeeding, and for Children. https://www.epa.gov/choose-fish-and-shellfish-wisely/epa-fda-advice-about-eating-fish-and-shellfish. Accessed April 27, 2024.

CONTINUED

ADVICE ABOUT EATING FISH
For Those Who Might Become or Are Pregnant or Breastfeeding and Children Ages 1 – 11 Years

 The ***Dietary Guidelines for Americans*** recommends eating fish as part of a healthy eating pattern.

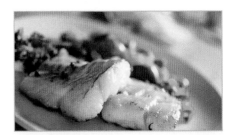

The *Dietary Guidelines for Americans* recommends:

- At least 8 ounces of seafood (less for children§) per week based on a 2,000 calorie diet.

- Those who are pregnant or breastfeeding consume between 8 and 12 ounces per week of a variety of seafood from choices that are lower in mercury.

 Eating fish can provide other health benefits too.

Fish intake during pregnancy is recommended because moderate scientific evidence shows it can help your baby's cognitive development.

Strong evidence shows that eating fish, as part of a healthy eating pattern, may have heart health benefits . Healthy eating patterns that include fish may have other benefits too. Moderate scientific evidence shows that eating patterns relatively higher in fish but also in other foods, including vegetables, fruits, legumes, whole grains, low- or non-fat dairy, lean meats and poultry, nuts, and unsaturated vegetable oils, and lower in red and processed meats, sugar-sweetened foods and beverages, and refined grains are associated with:

> A healthy eating pattern consists of choices across all food groups (vegetables, fruits, grains, dairy, and protein foods, which includes fish), eaten in recommended amounts, and within calorie needs. Healthy eating patterns include foods that provide vitamins, minerals, and other health-promoting components and have no or little added sugars, saturated fat, and sodium.

 Promotion of bone health – decreases the risk for hip fractures *

 Decreases in the risk of becoming overweight or obese *

 Decreases in the risk for colon and rectal cancers *

This advice supports the recommendations of the *Dietary Guidelines for Americans*, which reflects current science on nutrition to improve public health. The *Dietary Guidelines for Americans* focuses on dietary patterns and the effects of food and nutrient characteristics on health.

§ For some children, the amounts of fish in the *Dietary Guidelines for Americans* are higher than in this FDA/EPA advice. The *Dietary Guidelines for Americans* states that to consume those higher amounts, children should only be fed fish from the "Best Choices" list that are even lower in mercury – these fish are anchovies, Atlantic mackerel, catfish, clams, crab, crawfish, flounder, haddock, mullet, oysters, plaice, pollock, salmon, sardines, scallops, shad, shrimp, sole, squid, tilapia, trout, and whiting.

* There is moderate scientific evidence of a relationship between the eating pattern as a whole and the potential health benefit.

‡ This advice refers to fish and shellfish collectively as "fish" / Advice revised October 2021

• **Fig. 13.3 cont'd**

TABLE 13.2   Chronology of Development of the Human Dentition

Tooth	Hard Tissue Formation Begins	Amount of Enamel Formed at Birth	Enamel Completed	Eruption	Root Completed
Primary Dentition					
Maxillary					
Central incisor	4 months in utero	Five-sixths	1½ months	7½ months	1½ years
Lateral incisor	4½ months in utero	Two-thirds	2½ months	9 months	2 years
Canine	5 months in utero	One-third	9 months	18 months	3½ years
First molar	5 months in utero	Cusps united	6 months	14 months	2½ years
Second molar	6 months in utero	Cusp tips still isolated	11 months	24 months	3 years
Mandibular					
Central incisor	4½ months in utero	Three-fifths	1½ months	6 months	1½ years
Lateral incisor	1½ months in utero	Three-fifths	3 months	7 months	1½ years
Canine	5 months in utero	One-third	9 months	16 months	3¼ years
First molar	5 months in utero	Cusps united	5½ months	12 months	2¼ years
Second molar	6 months in utero	Cusp tips still isolated	10 months	20 months	3 years
Permanent Dentition					
Maxillary					
Central incisor	3–4 months	–	4–5 years	7–8 years	10 years
Lateral incisor	10–12 months	–	4–5 years	8–9 years	11 years
Canine	4–5 months	–	6–7 years	11–12 years	13–15 years
First premolar	1½–1¾ years	–	5–6 years	10–11 years	12–13 years
Second premolar	2–2¼ years	–	6–7 years	10–12 years	12–14 years
First molar	At birth	Sometimes a trace	2½–3 years	6–7 years	9–10 years
Second molar	2½–3 years	–	7–8 years	12–13 years	14–16 years
Mandibular					
Central incisor	3–4 months	–	4–5 years	6–7 years	9 years
Lateral incisor	3–4 months	–	4–5 years	7–8 years	10 years
Canine	4–5 months	–	6–7 years	9–10 years	12–14 years
First premolar	1¾–2 years	–	5–6 years	10–12 years	12–13 years
Second premolar	2–2¼ years	–	6–7 years	11–12 years	13–14 years
First molar	At birth	Sometimes a trace	2½–3 years	6–7 years	9–10 years
Second molar	2½–3 years	–	7–8 years	11–13 years	14–15 years

Adapted and slightly modified by Massler and Shour from Logan WAG, Kronfeld R. Development of the human jaws and surrounding structures from birth to the age of 15 years. *J Am Dent Assoc* 1933;20:379–428; From Touger-Decker R, Radler DR, Depaola DP. Nutrition and dental medicine. In: Ross AC, Caballero B, Cousins, RJ, et al., eds. *Modern Nutrition in Health and Disease*. 11th ed. Wolters Kluwer Health/Lippincott Williams & Wilkins; 2014:1016–1040.

weight. Appropriate weight gain reflects adequacy of energy intake and influences birth weight. When calorie intake is slightly inadequate, physiologic adaptations spare energy for fetal growth.[65]

Gestational weight gain within the recommended range produces optimal pregnancy outcomes; many females exceed the guidelines. Increasing energy intake as recommended may encourage excessive weight gain, and increases risk for adverse pregnancy outcomes.[66,67] Clearly, the key to adhering to the NAM guidelines for weight gain is to limit energy intake while increasing nutrient density and maintaining levels of physical activity.[68] Focusing on portion size may be a valuable tool to help prevent excess weight gain.[69]

TABLE 13.3	Nutrient Deficiencies and Tooth Development
Nutrient	Effect on Tissue
Protein	Delayed tooth eruption; increased caries susceptibility; dysfunctional salivary glands
Vitamin A	Disturbed keratin matrix of enamel; increased enamel hypoplasia; increased caries susceptibility; decreased epithelial tissue development; dysfunction of tooth morphogenesis
Vitamin D	Poor calcification; pitting
Calcium/phosphorus	Decreased calcium concentration; hypomineralization (hypoplastic defects)
Ascorbic acid	Disturbed collagen matrix of dentin; alterations of dental pulp
Fluoride/iron/zinc	Increased caries susceptibility
Iodine	Delayed tooth eruption
Magnesium	Hypoplasia of enamel

Compiled from information in Touger-Decker R, Radler DR, Depaola DP. Nutrition and dental medicine. In: Ross AC, Caballero B, Cousins RJ, et al., eds. *Modern Nutrition in Health and Disease.* 11th ed. Wolters Kluwer Health/Lippincott Williams & Wilkins; 2014:1016–1040; Nizel AE. Preventing dental caries: the nutritional factors. *Pediatr Clin North Am* 1977;24:144–155; Shaw JH, Sweeney EA. Oral health. In: Schneider HA, Anderson CD, Coursin DB, et al., eds. *Nutritional Support of Medical Practice.* Harper & Row; 1983:517–540.

Dieting for weight loss is not recommended during pregnancy even though studies indicate that interventions can improve some outcomes for the mother and the baby. Dietary interventions are effective to control the amount of weight gain since most females tend to gain too much weight. Avoidance of carbohydrate-rich foods—such as enriched breads and cereals—to reduce calories, either preconceptionally or during pregnancy, negatively affects folic acid intake; this situation may be detrimental to the fetus. Moreover, added sugars and excess saturated fat should be avoided in favor of nutrient-dense foods.

A gravida who is significantly underweight before conception may need additional calories during the first trimester. Because requirements for many nutrients are increased, it is more important that foods be chosen wisely, principally using nutrient-dense foods.[18]

Fat

Vitamin and mineral requirements during pregnancy increase proportionately higher than calorie needs. Saturated fats should be limited because of their minimal nutrient contribution, but PUFAs are needed to reduce serum lipids and for adequate fetal central nervous system development. Hormonal changes result in significant elevations of serum cholesterol and triglycerides during the second trimester of pregnancy.

More important during pregnancy (and lactation) is the fact that maternal intake of omega-3 fatty acids has a positive impact on maternal, infant, and child health.[70] Omega-3 fatty acids are crucial for infant's brain and visual development, especially during the latter part of gestation and early postnatal life. Requirements for omega-3 fatty acids (docosahexaenoic acid/DHA) have not been established, but some experts have recommended at least

200 to 300 mg/day of DHA during pregnancy.[71] Two servings of fatty fish per week can provide the 200 to 300 mg/day needed.[70]

Protein

Protein is the basic nutrient for growth; an additional 25 g of protein, or a total of 71 g daily, is recommended. The Dietary Guidelines Advisory Committee reported that almost half of pregnant females consume less than the recommended amount of protein.[72] Pregnant females should be advised to consume adequate levels of protein from a variety of sources to include lean meats, poultry, eggs, seafood, and plant-based proteins.[73]

Calcium and Vitamin D

Calcium and vitamin D work together in the formation of skeletal tissue and teeth. During pregnancy, hormonal and physiologic adjustments promote increased calcium absorption and retention; thus, the DRI is the same as that of nonpregnant females of the same age. This extra calcium is thought to be stored in maternal bone for fetal availability in the third trimester, when fetal bone growth is rapid.[74] If calcium intake meets the DRI, additional calcium supplementation is believed to be unnecessary.

The recommended 1000 mg/day of calcium for females older than 19 years of age can be met by three servings of milk or dairy products. Pregnant females younger than 19 years of age may need 4 cups of milk to provide the necessary 1300 mg/day. Dairy products may be incorporated into cooking, or eaten in different forms—such as cheese, ice cream, or yogurt—for variety (see Table 9.2 and Box 9.2).

Vitamin D intake during pregnancy has traditionally been associated with infant growth, bone ossification, tooth enamel formation, and neonatal calcium homeostasis, but the function of vitamin D during pregnancy is uncertain.[75] The NAM established 600 IU/day for pregnant females; current Tolerable Upper Intake Level is 4000 IU (100 µg). The American College of Obstetrics and Gynecology and the NAM currently recommend 600 IU (15 µg) daily vitamin D supplementation during pregnancy to support maternal and fetal bone metabolism.[76]

Clinical studies have established relationships between vitamin D levels and adverse pregnancy outcomes.[77,78] Vitamin D supplements improve serum levels, but the needs, safety, and effectiveness of supplementation during pregnancy remain controversial.[79] Screening for pregnant females thought to be at increased risk of vitamin D deficiency, should be considered; if justified, 1000 to 2000 IU/day of vitamin D is considered safe.[76]

B Vitamins

Several of the B-vitamin requirements are based on energy or calorie intake; usually, their intake increases automatically with the intake of additional calories. However, adequate intake of some B vitamins may be difficult to achieve without careful selection of foods or supplementation.

The RDA for folate (600 µg) during pregnancy is significantly more than that for the nonpregnant female (400 µg). The role of folate as a coenzyme is essential for nucleic acid synthesis. Folate is also required for increased red blood cell formation. Folate deficiency impairing cell growth and replication may cause fetal anomalies. Orofacial clefts and neural tube defects, such as spina bifida and anencephaly (absence of a major portion of the brain and skull), are attributed to inadequate folate intake before conception and during the first trimester. It is recommended that females take 400 µg of folic acid daily prior to conception to help prevent up to 7 in 10 (70%) of neural tube defects.[80] The US

TABLE 13.4 Vitamin and Mineral Recommended Dietary Allowances

Nutrient	Nonpregnant Females (19–30 Years Old)	Pregnant (14–18 Years Old)	PREGNANT (19–30 YEARS OLD)		Lactating (14–18 Years Old)	LACTATING (19–30 YEARS OLD)	
			Amount of Nutrient	Percent Increase[a]		Amount of Nutrient	Percent Increase[a]
Vitamin A	700 µg	750 µg RE	770 µg RE	10	1200 µg RE	1300 µg RE	71
Vitamin D	15 µg	15 µg	15 µg	0	15 µg	15 µg	0
Vitamin E	15 α–TE	15 α–TE	15 α–TE	0	19 α–TE	19 α–TE	27
Vitamin K	90 µg*	75 µg*	90 µg*	0	75 µg*	90 µg*	0
Vitamin C	75 mg	85 mg	85 mg	13	115 mg	120 mg	60
Thiamin	1.1 mg	1.4 mg	1.4 mg	27	1.4 mg	1.4 mg	27
Riboflavin	1.1 mg	1.4 mg	1.4 mg	27	1.4 mg	1.6 mg	45
Niacin	14 mg NE	18 mg NE	18 mg NE	28	17 mg NE	17 mg NE	21
Vitamin B_6	1.3 mg	1.9 mg	1.9 mg	46	2.0 mg	2 mg	54
Folate	400 µg	600 µg	600 µg	50	500 µg	500 µg	25
Vitamin B_{12}	2.4 µg	2.6 µg	2.6 µg	8	2.8 µg	2.8 µg	17
Calcium	1000 mg	1300 mg	1000 mg	0	1300 mg	1000 mg	0
Phosphorus	700 mg	1350 mg	700 mg	0	1250 mg	700 mg	0
Magnesium	310 mg	400 mg	350 mg 360 mg[b]	9	360 mg	310 mg	0
Fluoride	3 mg*	3 mg*	3 mg*	0	3 mg*	3 mg*	0
Iron	18 mg	27 mg	27 mg	50	10 mg	9 mg	[–50%]
Zinc	8 mg	12 mg	11 mg	38	13 mg	12 mg	50
Iodine	150 µg	220 µg	220 µg	47	290 µg	290 µg	93
Selenium	55 µg	60 µg	60 µg	9	70 µg	70 µg	27
Copper	900 µg	1000 µg	1000 µg	11	1300 µg	1300 µg	44

Note: This table presents Recommended Dietary Allowances in **bold type** and adequate intakes in regular type followed by an asterisk (*).
[a]Percent increase for pregnant females above nonpregnancy recommendation.
[b]Ages 31–50 years old.
Data from National Research Council. *The Guide to Nutrient Requirements*. National Academies Press; 2006; National Research Council. *Dietary Reference Intakes for Calcium and Vitamin D*. National Academies Press; 2011.

Preventive Services Task Force recently reviewed its 2009 recommendation on folic acid supplementation in females of childbearing age, examining the effectiveness of supplementation and new evidence on the benefits and harms of supplements, and reaffirmed its previous recommendation.[80]

Because of crucial effects on pregnancy, the FDA requires supplementation of all enriched grain products with specific amounts of folic acid. Since implementation of folic acid fortification in the United States in 1996, neural tube defects have decreased by 35%.[80,81] Even with folic acid fortification, nearly 25% of reproductive-age females, especially Hispanic females, fail to get enough of the B vitamin. In 2016 the FDA approved folic acid fortification of corn masa flour, allowing manufacturers to voluntarily add folic acid in amounts consistent with the levels of other enriched cereal grains.[82] The seal "Folic Acid for a Healthy Pregnancy" was developed to help females quickly and easily identify products fortified with folic acid.

Meeting the requirement for folate solely from food intake is difficult for most pregnant females. Education promoting consumption of folic acid from folate-rich foods, supplements, and foods fortified with folic acid can help prevent neural tube defects. Conscientious daily selections of raw fruits and vegetables, especially green leafy vegetables, can help ensure adequate intake. Folic acid–fortified breads and cereals also contribute significant amounts (see Tables 1.4 and 11.12). Every female of reproductive age should be encouraged to consume a daily supplement containing 400 µg folic acid; absorption from supplements is better than from natural folate in foods. The March of Dimes indicates that only 33% females take a multivitamin supplement containing folic acid.[83]

Iron

A common problem among nonpregnant females is iron-deficiency anemia; many females begin pregnancy with diminished iron stores. Increased iron during gestation is needed for producing red blood cells and the placenta, and to compensate for cord and blood loss at delivery.[84]

The fetus acts as a parasite in that fetal erythropoiesis (the formation of red blood cells) occurring at the expense of maternal iron stores. Iron-deficiency anemia is seldom seen in full-term infants. During a normal pregnancy, the fetus consumes 500–800 mg of iron from the mother.[85] Fetal accumulation of iron occurs principally in the last trimester. Premature infants, having a shortened gestation, have insufficient time to acquire adequate iron and may be born with iron-deficiency anemia; however, premature infants absorb iron very efficiently.[86]

Approximately 27 mg of iron is needed daily during pregnancy. Because the average American diet does not provide this amount within normal calorie requirements, daily supplements of 30 mg of ferrous iron are recommended to provide adequate amounts of iron during the second and third trimesters of pregnancy.[87] Initiation of supplements before gestational week 24 prevents iron deficiency. Low-dose iron supplementation during pregnancy, even if the gravida is not anemic, improves the female's iron status and seems to protect the infant from iron-deficiency anemia. Infant iron status has been associated with cognitive and neurobehavioral outcomes, indicating the importance of optimal iron status at birth.[88]

Iron supplements frequently cause nausea and constipation, and occasionally high hemoglobin levels. Iron supplements taken one to three times weekly on nonconsecutive days reduce side effects and increase acceptance and adherence while maintaining safe hemoglobin levels.[89] If iron supplements are not provided, it may take 2 years after delivery for maternal serum iron levels to return to normal.[90]

High hemoglobin levels have been associated with an increased risk of LBW and premature births; thus levels should be routinely monitored.[91]

Zinc

Zinc is crucial early in pregnancy during the formation of fetal organs, but requirements are the highest in late pregnancy for fetal growth and development. The RDA for zinc is 12 mg during pregnancy. An increase in high-protein foods, especially meats, improves zinc intake.

Iodine

Dietary iodine requirements are higher during pregnancy as a result of increased maternal thyroid hormone production and fetal iodine requirements. Iodine nutritional status is on the decline among US females of childbearing age.[92] Adherence to the Dietary Guidelines recommendation to decrease the use of salt (usually iodized), increased use of processed foods (not iodized), and increased popularity of sea salt (contains no iodine), may be affecting iodine intake. Adverse effects of iodine deficiency in pregnancy include maternal and fetal goiter; cretinism; fetal brain development and intellectual impairments; neonatal hypothyroidism; and infant mortality.[93] Iodine deficiency is a significant global public health problem.[94]

The NAM recommends a daily iodine intake of 220 μg during pregnancy. Because many females of reproductive age in the United States are marginally deficient in iodine, the American Thyroid Association, Teratology Society, and the American Academy of Pediatrics recommend a supplement containing adequate iodine during pregnancy and lactation.[95,96] The American Thyroid Association has stressed that adequate maternal iodine is necessary to ensure the health of the mother and the infant; the addition of 150 μg of potassium iodide in prenatal vitamins would be effective.[97]

Although an infrequent occurrence, congenital hypothyroidism may also result from excess prenatal intake of iodine supplements.[98] The NAM has not determined a safe upper limit for iodine during pregnancy and lactation.

Vitamin-Mineral Supplements

Keeping vitamin and nutrient levels up during pregnancy is essential for a healthy baby. In the United States, vitamin and mineral supplementation is commonly recommended during pregnancy. The specific nutrient amounts for a daily multivitamin-mineral supplement appropriate for gravidas of any age are shown in Table 13.5.

Supplementation should be based on an identified nutritional need, evidence of a benefit, and lack of harmful effects. Multivitamins seem to improve brain development and cognitive abilities with long-term benefits.[99] Nutrient-dense foods are the ideal source for providing nutrients, but supplements may be warranted during this period because many females fail to meet their prenatal nutrient requirements through diet alone. Excessive amounts of many nutrients may have detrimental effects on the fetus (Table 13.6).

The NAM subcommittee concluded that iron is the only known nutrient warranting global supplementation during pregnancy. A goal for Healthy People 2030 is to reduce iron-deficiency anemia among pregnant females. Approximately 11% of pregnant females were iron deficient in 2015–16.[100]

TABLE 13.5 Nutrient Supplementation During Pregnancy

Nutrient	Amount of Supplement Recommended
Calcium	1000 mg for ages 19 to 50; 1300 mg for ages 14–18
Vitamin A	770 μg for ages 19 to 50; 770 mg for ages 14–18
Vitamin C	50 mg (85 mg)
Vitamin D	600 IU
Vitamin B$_6$	1.9 mg
Vitamin B$_{12}$	2.6 μg
Folate	600 μg
Iron	27 mg
Iodine	220 μg
Choline	450 μg

Data from Institute of Medicine, Food and Nutrition Board. Nutrition During Pregnancy. National Academy Press; 1990; National Academies of Sciences, Engineering, and Medicine; Health and Medicine Division; Food and Nutrition Board; Harrison M, eds. In: 2, Macronutrient Requirements. Nutrition During Pregnancy and Lactation: Exploring New Evidence: Proceedings of a Workshop. National Academies Press (United States); 2020. https://www.ncbi.nlm.nih.gov/books/NBK562630/; The American College of Obstetricians and Gynecologists. Nutrition During Pregnancy. https://www.acog.org/womens-health/faqs/nutrition-during-pregnancy.

TABLE 13.6	Nutrient Supplementation Associated With Deleterious Fetal Outcomes
Nutrient	**Effects on Fetus**
Vitamin A	Pharmacologic use of vitamin A analogs has resulted in major congenital defects (malformation of cranium, face, heart, thymus, and central nervous system) and spontaneous abortion, especially during first trimester.
Vitamin D	Excessive intake of vitamin D can result in hyperabsorption of calcium, hypercalcemia, calcification of soft tissues, and mental retardation.
Vitamin E	Excessive intake of vitamin E is associated with higher incidence of spontaneous abortions.
Vitamin K	Menadione administered parenterally has been associated with hemolytic anemia, hyperbilirubinemia, and kernicterus in the newborn.
Vitamin C	Megadoses of vitamin C have been reported to cause vitamin C dependency, with the symptoms of conditional scurvy observed postpartum.
Iodine	Large amounts of iodides have resulted in infants with congenital goiter, hypothyroidism, and intellectual disability.
Zinc	Large amounts of zinc supplements during the third trimester were implicated in premature delivery and stillbirth.
Fluoride	Well water containing 12–18 parts/million (ppm) fluoride produced offspring with significant mottling of deciduous teeth.

Data from Worthington-Roberts B. Nutrition deficiencies and excesses: impact on pregnancy, part 2. *J Perinatol* 1985;5(4):12.

Dietary folate intake does not usually meet the RDA, but since folate enrichment of cereal products began in 1998, maternal folate status has improved significantly. Whole-grain products do not contain as much folate (and are not absorbed as well) as enriched grains and cereals; therefore, only one-half of the gravida's grain selections should be whole grains. A supplement containing folate may be prudent if intake is questionable. It should be initiated before conception because birth defects from inadequate folate intake may occur before the woman realizes she is pregnant. A multivitamin supplement containing folic acid is recommended for all young females 18 to 24 years old because of the number of unintentional pregnancies in that age group.[101]

Excess vitamin A (10,000 IU of vitamin A preformed from animal sources) during the first trimester can result in severe craniofacial and oral clefts and limb defects.[102] Intake of preformed vitamin A should be limited to approximately 100% of the Daily Value (5000 IU). Liver and other animal products and fortified foods and vitamin supplements listing retinyl palmitate and retinyl acetate as ingredients contain preformed vitamin A. Beta-carotene, which the body converts to vitamin A, is much less toxic. Fortified foods containing beta-carotene, and fruits and vegetables that contain natural beta-carotene should be chosen whenever possible.

Nutritional supplementation may be warranted in high-risk pregnancies, including adolescent pregnancies; multiple gestations (carrying more than one fetus); and pregnancies in females who use cigarettes, alcohol, or other drugs. Females who do not routinely consume milk, dairy products, or foods fortified with calcium and vitamin D—may benefit from taking a calcium supplement. Vitamin D supplementation may be beneficial for some females living in northern latitudes with limited exposure to sunlight; more study is needed to determine the most effective dosage. Iron supplements containing more than 30 mg of iron necessitate supplemental amounts of zinc and copper.[103]

Compliance with taking a nutrition supplement is poor; only about half of females in the United States take prenatal vitamins.[104] Many females do not take the supplement because of nausea and vomiting or previous adverse effects, whereas others indicate that the size of the pill is a factor. Patients should be encouraged to take the prescribed supplement and informed of the importance and reasons why it is needed. Compliance with the use of prenatal supplements will be more likely based on a convenient supply, affordability, and reinforcement by health care providers.

Dietary Intake and Education

Prenatal nutritional care may improve outcomes by saving lives, reducing risk of LBW, and decreasing costs of care that are the consequences of LBW. Nutrient intake warrants more attention than weight gain. Although adequate weight gain is the most reliable measurable tool for assessing the adequacy of energy intake, food choices can provide adequate calories yet may be deficient in vital nutrients. For this reason, the NAM subcommittee recommends routine assessment of dietary practices for all pregnant women in the United States to determine the need for improved diet or vitamin-mineral supplementation. Most females are highly motivated to make dietary changes during their pregnancy.

Because maternal nutrition has profound effects on infant health, the *MyPlate* website (https://www.myplate.gov/life-stages/pregnancy-and-breastfeeding) has links that provide a myriad of information for pregnant and breastfeeding mothers, including calculations for a healthy weight gain and other tips for making healthy food choices. Dental hygienists can use these tools to discuss nutritional requirements and shortages in patients' diets. *MyPlatePlan* (https://www.myplate.gov/myplate-plan) can be used to personalize a food plan based on age, height, prepregnancy weight, and physical activity level. Other topics for the gravida covered through links on the *MyPlate* website include dietary supplements, food safety, and special health needs.

Some pregnant females may have little or no nutritional knowledge. Although knowledge is the key to wise food choices, nutrition counseling is often unavailable or ignored during pregnancy. It is recommended that females receive nutritional counseling during pregnancy for optimal outcomes.[105] Interventions prior to conception, as well as during pregnancy, improve fetal development and long-term health. Low-income expectant mothers have more opportunities to receive nutritional information through established programs such as the Supplemental Nutrition Program for Women, Infants, and Children (WIC) more than affluent females receive through the private sector.

Identification of poor and desirable food habits and dietary patterns can serve as the foundation for appropriate nutrition education and intervention. Identified nutritional problems, such as pica or fad dieting, or risk factors, such as alcohol abuse, may require special attention. Most important, the gravida should understand what foods she should eat and the importance of choosing nutrient-dense foods. Breastfeeding should also be promoted during pregnancy.

🦷 DENTAL CONSIDERATIONS

Assessments

- *Physical:* Level of education, income status, culture, religion, prenatal health care, medical history (including drugs taken), dental history, oral examination, feelings about weight gain.
- *Dietary:* Health and nutritional knowledge and skills; adequacy of intake based on a well-balanced diet using a variety of foods, including enriched grain products; vegetarianism; food budget; food cravings and aversions; fad diets; beliefs about nutrition during pregnancy; pica; alcohol use; and caffeine intake.

Interventions

- Become familiar with local nutritional practices and beliefs about pregnancy; these beliefs are regional and may be affected by cultural beliefs.
- During routine dental recare for females of childbearing age, discuss the importance of maintaining oral health and dental appointments during pregnancy.
- Refer patients at risk of inadequate intakes of specific nutrients to a registered dietitian nutritionist (RDN) or health care provider.
- Emphasize consumption of a nutrient-dense diet, with three to six meals throughout the day to ensure optimal intake of nutrients. Discuss the importance of consuming two servings of low-mercury fish per week, focusing on the benefits of consumption and not just the risks by providing a broad range of fish that are low in mercury and high in omega-3 fatty acids.
- Patients who might become pregnant should have a high folate intake. If a female of childbearing age is not taking a multivitamin supplement and is following a carbohydrate-restricted diet, refer her to a health care provider or an RDN.
- Ask pregnant patients whether they are taking a prenatal supplement. If not, refer them to a health care provider.
- Pregnancy is the ideal opportunity to discuss good nutritional and oral hygiene habits needed during this period and for the newborn infant. Proper oral tissue development of the fetus depends on adequate maternal nutrition. Refer to an RDN if more in-depth nutrition counseling is needed.
- Encourage foods high in calcium. Low calcium intake may impair bone-mineral deposition, especially in females younger than 25 years of age. Consuming the recommended 1300 mg of calcium daily is particularly important for pregnant teens to meet calcium demands. The use of dietary calcium is preferred because these foods also provide other valuable nutrients—protein, riboflavin, vitamin D, and other components that enhance calcium absorption.
- Snacking is acceptable for pregnant females. Provide information on avoidance of acid attacks and resultant tooth decay by recommending appropriate oral hygiene techniques after snacking and encouraging foods such as nuts, raw vegetables, yogurt, and popcorn.
- If the mother has a strong preference for sweets, the infant's diet is also likely to be high in sugar. Review the gravida's diet for the form and frequency of sugar-containing foods, and suggest modifications or substitutions as indicated. This could create a healthier pattern for the patient and alleviate potential dental problems for the infant.
- Discuss the risk of early childhood caries with all pregnant females (see Chapter 14).
- Encourage pregnant patients to use iodized salt, and choose good dietary sources of iodine (e.g., milk and dairy products and fish). Avoid kelp supplements because of excessive levels of iodine.
- Because of potentially increased risk of preterm or LBW infants associated with pregnancy gingivitis and other periodontal issues, encourage excellent oral hygiene habits throughout the day.
- Encourage sexually active females of childbearing age who drink alcohol to use reliable methods to prevent pregnancy, plan their pregnancies, and stop drinking before becoming pregnant.
- Stress the importance of enrolling in educational breastfeeding classes that address benefits, techniques, common problems, myths, and skills training.

🦷 NUTRITIONAL DIRECTIONS

- Pregnant females should consult their health care provider before taking any drug, including nonprescription drugs and herbal products.
- Preventive oral care, including limiting frequency of fermentable carbohydrate intake and adequate oral hygiene care (brush the teeth at least two times a day, floss daily, and use an antibacterial mouthwash), is important for both mother and fetus.
- Nutrient needs must be met by deliberate preplanning and informed food choices.
- Low-fat or skim milk may be used to control weight, decrease saturated fat intake, and provide equivalent nutrients.
- Although the pregnant patient is "eating for two," energy requirements are not double.
- Moderate increases in whole grains, milk, and legumes can provide additional protein and other important nutrients.
- Calcium, vitamin D, and vitamin B$_{12}$ supplements are advisable for vegans because they exclude all animal products. Pregnant vegans should be referred to an RDN.
- Vitamin D may be a special concern for females with minimal exposure to sunlight or routine use of sunscreens. Regular exposure to sunlight and foods fortified with vitamin D (e.g., milk and cheese) are recommended.
- Powdered milk (⅓ cup) can be added to soups, cooked cereals, mashed potatoes, or casseroles if the gravida has an aversion to drinking milk.
- Adverse symptoms, such as nausea or constipation, frequently occur from iron supplementation. Rather than discontinuing the supplement, take it with meals, or consult the health care provider about possibly decreasing the dosage or taking it three to four times a week.
- Absorption of iron from supplements or foods is enhanced if taken between meals with vitamin C-rich foods, such as orange juice, while avoiding milk or tea.
- Moderately intense exercise during pregnancy (such as 30-minute brisk walks) is beneficial if medical reasons do not prevent it. Exercise enhances blood flow, which delivers nutrients to the fetus, improves mood and energy level, and increases cardiovascular fitness and endurance.

Lactation

Exclusive breastfeeding for 4 to 6 months and continuing until 12 months is the ideal method of feeding infants. Complementary foods should begin at least by 6 months. US health authorities began to promote breastfeeding about 25 years ago, a healthy practice that has been slowly gaining popularity. In 2019, approximately 62.6% of infants were initially exclusively breastfed. At 6 months, this number fell to 45.3%, and by 12 months, only 24.9% were exclusively breastfed.[106] The target for breastfeeding established in *Healthy People 2030* is 42.4% exclusively at 6 months, and 54.1% for any breastfeeding at 1 year.[107,108] Breastfeeding rates vary by race/ethnicity, participation in the WIC supplemental nutrition program, mother's age and education, and geography. Despite increases in the prevalence of infants initially being breastfed, the prevalence of breastfeeding among African American infants remains below that for Whites and Hispanics. Despite improvements in trends among Hispanic or non–Hispanic Whites, Blacks, Asian, American Indian and Alaskan Natives, breastfeeding rates for Black infants still remains the lowest.[109] Numerous breastfeeding initiatives have been launched to increase breastfeeding rates: the Baby-Friendly Hospital Initiative, *Ten Steps to Successful Breastfeeding,* launched by WHO and UNICEF and numerous initiatives by state health departments and state and local WIC agencies designed to raise awareness of the importance and benefits of breastfeeding infants.[110] In 2016, the US Preventive Services Task Force recommended providing supportive interventions during pregnancy and after birth to support breastfeeding.[111]

Despite extensive evidence for short-term and long-term health benefits from breastfeeding for both mother and baby, and practical

• BOX 13.1 Advantages of Breastfeeding

For the Mother

- Maternal hormones produced as a result of lactation facilitate contractions of the uterus and control postpartum bleeding.
- Prepregnancy weight is achieved sooner because breastfeeding burns calories.
- Breastfeeding is less expensive than formula feeding.
- Mother-infant bonding is enhanced with breastfeeding.
- Breastfeeding saves time because there are no bottles to clean, prepare, warm, or sterilize.
- Prolactin, the hormone that helps the milk "let down," relaxes the mother.
- The mother is at reduced risk of premenopausal breast and ovarian cancer.
- Breastfeeding is associated with reduced visceral adiposity, leading to lower rates of high blood pressure, reduced risk of type 2 diabetes and hyperlipidemia.

For the Infant

- Human milk is nutritionally balanced with maximum bioavailability of nutrients for infants; easy for the infant to digest.
- Breast milk contains antibodies to promote immunologic properties that help reduce infant morbidity and mortality.
- Breast milk constantly changes in composition to meet the changing needs of the infant, especially a premature infant.
- Human milk reduces the risk of food allergies and asthma and prevents or delays the occurrence of atopic dermatitis in early childhood.
- Breastfeeding promotes infant oral-motor and structural development.
- Incidence of thumb sucking and tongue thrusting is lower in breastfed infants.
- Breastfed infants are exposed to a variety of tastes through the mother's milk.
- Breast milk can help reduce the risk of many short-term and long-term health problems that may affect preterm babies.
- Breast milk promotes brain development. Longer periods of exclusive breastfeeding during an infant's first year increase some measures of a child's cognitive development.
- Prolonged breastfeeding may reduce the risk of overweight in childhood.
- Breastfeeding longer than 6 months may provide health benefits well beyond the breastfeeding period.
- Breastfeeding is associated with a reduction in the risk of sudden death syndrome (SIDS)

Adapted from Meek JY, Noble L; Section on Breastfeeding. Policy Statement: Breastfeeding and the Use of Human Milk. *Pediatrics.* 2022;150(1):e2022057988; The American College of Obstetricians and Gynecologists. *Breastfeeding Benefits. How Does Breast Feeding Benefit My Baby?* https://www.acog.org/femaless-health/faqs/Breastfeeding-Your-Baby.

work. Breastfeeding continues to meet important nutritional needs and provides protection from illness and infection beyond the first 6 months of life. Mothers are encouraged to continue breastfeeding beyond the minimum of 6 months. However, prolonged breast feeding (>2 years) may increase the risk for dental caries.[113]

Nutritional Recommendations for Breastfeeding

For most nutrients, recommendations for lactating females are similar to those for pregnant females. Energy requirements are proportional to the quantity of milk produced. Approximately 85 cal are needed for every 100 mL of milk produced, requiring approximately a 500-cal daily increase. Although this increase may not be fully adequate to cover the needs for milk production, the 2 to 4 kg of fat accumulated during pregnancy is available to supply additional calories. Return to prepregnancy weight is accelerated. The major determinant of milk production is the infant's demand for milk, not maternal energy intake. Weight loss during lactation has no apparent deleterious effects on milk production.

Carbohydrate intake from whole grains, dairy, fruits, and vegetables is important for maintaining lactose synthesis and milk volume. The amount of protein recommended is slightly higher than for pregnancy—an additional 25 g or a total of 70 g daily. Breastfeeding is positively related to mental development of the infant but may be more influenced by maternal education, social class, a nurturing environment, and intelligence of the parents than diet. Long-chain PUFAs, especially DHA, seem to play a beneficial role in children's mental development and possibly immune response; thus a prenatal omega-3 fatty acid supplement should be considered. Other nutrients needed in larger quantities during pregnancy include vitamins A, E, C, riboflavin, B_6, and B_{12}, along with the minerals copper, zinc, iodine, and selenium. Maternal vitamin B_6 status affects amounts found in breast milk, and, thus infant growth. A source of vitamin B_{12} intake, from either foods or supplements, is crucial for optimal infant nutrition. Neurologic impairments have occurred in children of breastfeeding vegan mothers who were eating no or very limited foods of animal origin, the source of vitamin B_{12}. A lactating female also requires additional fluids to replace those secreted in the milk. An additional 1000 mL/day (4 cups) of fluids is needed.

Dietary Patterns for Lactating Females

The dietary pattern of a lactating female is similar to that of a pregnant female. Consumption of 3 cups of milk or dairy products fortified with vitamin D daily provides approximately 1000 mg of calcium and 300 IU of vitamin D, which are adequate amounts for females older than 19 years. Much higher doses of vitamin D are needed to achieve adequate concentrations in exclusively breastfed infants; thus vitamin D supplementation for these infants is recommended.[114,115] Other high-calcium foods may also be used. High-protein foods may include 6 to 8 oz of meat daily, depending on the quantity of milk consumed. Adequate servings of fresh fruits, vegetables, and whole-grain products help provide the additional calories.

Low-iron stores have a deleterious effect on the mother; a prenatal vitamin is encouraged for postpartum females to provide adequate iron and folate to replenish stores. Females who have mild iron deficiency are less sensitive to their infants' cues and have more difficulty bonding with their infants. Females who are anemic are more likely to experience postpartum depression.

Many foods consumed by the mother may affect breast milk. Certain foods, especially strongly flavored foods such as raw

benefits, such as lower cost (Box 13.1), many females choose to bottle-feed. Personal and social biases (such as attitudes of family and close friends, and problems with breastfeeding in public and employment practices) are principal factors in this decision. A mother's decision to breastfeed can be positively influenced by health education and peer support; her success is greatly improved through active support from her family, friends, communities, clinicians, health care providers, employers, and policymakers. Peer counseling, lactation consultation, and formal breastfeeding education during pregnancy appear to increase both initiation and duration of breastfeeding.

Most females are able to produce enough breast milk providing essential nutrients to support infant growth and health. Breastfeeding has many advantages for the infant and the mother (see Box 13.1). Further discussion regarding infant feeding is provided in Chapter 14.

Breast milk provides all the infant needs for about the first 6 months of life to support optimal growth and development, with rare exceptions.[112] Principal reasons given by mothers for stopping breastfeeding is that they perceive the infant is not satisfied by breast milk alone, pain associated with breastfeeding, and returning to onion, garlic, curry, chili peppers, and chocolate, may cause gastrointestinal distress, rash, or irritability in the infant. These foods only need to be omitted if they affect the infant.

Many nonnutritive substances and drugs may be secreted in breast milk. Alcohol may impair milk flow and is transmitted in breast milk in approximately the same proportions as in the mother's blood. Intake should be limited to less than 0.5 g/kg daily.[116] Large amounts of coffee and tea intake may adversely affect the iron content of human milk. Caffeine can be transferred to the infant in breast milk; therefore caffeine intake should be moderate (300 mg).[117]

Because of the risk of medications being passed into breast milk, all drugs, including over-the-counter medications and herbal remedies, should be used cautiously and only if essential. Medications less likely to be secreted into the milk can be prescribed by the health care provider.

MyPlate website (https://www.myplate.gov/life-stages/pregnancy-and-breastfeeding) provides a plethora of health and nutrition information for breastfeeding females. Individualized nutrition guidance is available on the Internet consistent with the *Dietary Guidelines* to assist breastfeeding mothers. Nutrition information is provided for exclusively breastfeeding and partially breastfeeding mothers. Tips are available for eating a balanced diet, healthy weight maintenance or weight loss, physical activity, and the use of dietary supplements.

Dietary assessment of usual food intake by an RDN is suggested, followed by nutrition counseling regarding foods rich in nutrients deficient in the diet. Continued use of the prenatal vitamin or a multivitamin supplement is recommended to ensure an adequate supply of folate if the female may become pregnant again.

🦷 DENTAL CONSIDERATIONS

Assessments
- *Physical:* Socioeconomic status, types of drugs, over-the-counter medications, supplements, and herbals used.
- *Dietary:* Adequacy of calories, nutrients, and fluid intake; alcohol and caffeine intake.

Interventions
- For a postpartum patient, encourage gradual return to prepregnancy weight (maximum weight loss of 4 lb/month for lactating females) through a balanced diet and moderate exercise.
- Encourage lactating females to obtain their nutrients from a well-balanced diet.
- Stress the importance of choosing a nutrient-dense diet utilizing fruits and vegetables, enriched and whole-grain breads and cereals, calcium-rich dairy products, and protein-rich and carbohydrate-rich foods to provide required nutrients.
- Encourage the intake of at least 10 to 12 cups of fluid, preferably water, each day.
- Discuss increasing the intake of nutrient-dense foods to achieve a calorie intake of at least 1800 cal daily.
- Discourage the use of strict weight loss diets and appetite suppressants.
- Emphasize the importance of reduced-fat milk, cheese, or other calcium-rich dairy products.
- Encourage the intake of vitamin D–fortified foods, such as fortified milk or cereal, for females with limited exposure to ultraviolet light.
- To support females during lactation, use the Internet to access *MyPlate* website (https://www.myplate.gov/life-stages/pregnancy-and-breastfeeding) to provide nutrition education.
- For vegans who are breastfeeding, stress the importance of a balanced diet with appropriate supplements, especially vitamin B_{12}, in sufficient quantities. Offer a referral to an RDN.

🌐 NUTRITIONAL DIRECTIONS

- Breastfeeding helps with weight loss.
- Limit the intake of coffee (regular and decaffeinated), other caffeine-containing beverages, and medications. Choose fluids such as juice, milk, and water.
- *MyPlatePlan* (https://www.myplate.gov/myplate-plan) can be an effective tool for improving dietary intake and promoting weight loss during lactation.

Oral Contraceptive Agents

Many nutrients (especially folate, vitamins B_6 [pyridoxine], B_{12} [cobalamin], C, and E, zinc, magnesium, and selenium) are affected by oral contraceptive agents (OCAs),[118] but vitamin deficiencies have been identified with marginal diets only. Low-estrogen preparations currently in the market do not adversely affect the female's vitamin levels as much as earlier preparations. Lower levels of water-soluble vitamins are a result of decreased intestinal absorption and increased metabolism. Low body reserves of B_6 may put females at risk for vitamin B_6 inadequacy during pregnancy upon cessation of OCAs.[119]

Increased amounts of pyridoxine may be indicated because estrogen increases the production of tryptophan which uses pyridoxine in its metabolism. Supplements are appropriate if a deficiency is diagnosed by laboratory evaluation; increasing intake of vitamin B_6-rich foods is appropriate to avoid side effects of excessive amounts. Depression and impaired glucose tolerance attributed to OCAs may be alleviated with pyridoxine supplementation. Since nutrient intake of many females taking OCAs may not be adequate, or they may have an unhealthy lifestyle or poor nutrient absorption, to reduce the side effects of OCAs and prevent vitamin and mineral deficiencies, a multivitamin-mineral supplement may be advisable.[118,120] Progestins can cause weight gain related to increased appetite and altered carbohydrate metabolism. Estrogens may lead to an increase in subcutaneous fat and fluid retention.[121,122]

Use of OCAs is associated with the increased risk of cardiovascular disease (CVD) related to changes in serum lipids.[123] Progestin may cause the elevation of low-density lipoprotein, total cholesterol, and triglyceride levels (discussed in Chapter 6). The net effect on serum lipids depends on the amount and ratio of progestin and estrogens.[124]

Menopause

During different stages of life, hormonal changes have many repercussions on general health. Female hormonal changes may be related to increased incidence of osteoporosis, which may be accompanied by some oral conditions, CVD, and certain cancers that occur later in life.

Genetics, general health, and the age of menarche influence when perimenopause and menopause actually begin (usually in the late 40s). For several years before menopause, a range of symptoms may be experienced, including changes in menstruation, fatigue, night sweats, hot flashes, insomnia, loss of bone density, and mood swings. This cluster of symptoms is called **perimenopause**. **Menopause** (decreased production of estrogen and progesterone by the ovaries, resulting in termination of menses) occurs between the ages of 35 and 58 years. Estrogen production

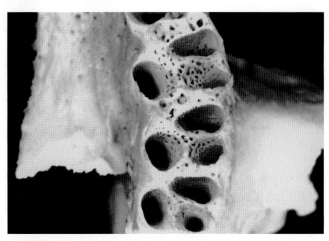

• **Fig. 13.4** Alveoli of the molar area. Note the thinness of the buccal plates over the first molar roots compared with those of the second and third maxillary molars. The third molar alveoli are rarely separated as distinctly as in this specimen. (From Nelson SJ. *Wheeler's Dental Anatomy, Physiology, and Occlusion*.10th ed. St. Louis, MO: Elsevier Saunders; 2015.)

decreases. Loss of beneficial effects of estrogen can cause health and nutrition issues.

Lower estrogen levels affect the natural process of bone turnover, resulting in a decrease of bone mass. Estrogen receptors on the bone-resorbing osteoclasts increase activity in response to the estrogen level, whereas estrogen receptors on the bone-forming osteoblasts decrease their activity.[125] Bone resorption exceeds bone formation, with significant trabecular and cortical bone loss. Rate of bone loss is rapid in early menopause, then slows and gradually decreases for 8 to 10 years after menstruation ceases.[126] This bone loss may result in osteopenia or osteoporosis (discussed in *Health Application 9* in Chapter 9). The alveolar bone provides a potential labile source of calcium; changes in the alveolar process may signify potential diagnosis of osteoporosis (Fig. 13.4).[127] A referral to the health care provider should be offered.

Reduced salivary gland secretion is a possible cause for increased dental caries and may lead to increased prevalence of oral dysesthesia (impairment of the sense of touch) and taste alterations. Senile atrophic gingivitis (abnormally pale gingival tissues) may develop concurrently. Menopausal gingivostomatitis (dry and shiny gingivae and edematous mucosa) results in easily bleeding gingiva that may be abnormally pale to quite erythematous. Postmenopausal females with osteoporosis exhibit an exaggerated response to dental plaque biofilm, including increased bleeding on probing, loss of dentoalveolar bone height, and decreased bone-mineral density of the alveolar crestal and subcrestal bone.[128] Uncontrolled osteoporosis may lead to edentulism; markedly resorbed residual alveolar ridges may be unsuitable for conventional dentures (see Fig. 13.4).

Declines in estrogen and progesterone production are accompanied by unfavorable changes in body composition (increased abdominal fat and decreased lean tissue). Weight gain is a major health concern of postmenopausal females. Weight loss becomes more difficult because body metabolism is lower and physical activity may be reduced.[129] Weight loss during this stage of life often requires greater focus on dietary monitoring, home-prepared meals, and increasing physical activity. Weight loss has been associated with bone-mineral density loss and increased fracture risk that may not recover with weight regain.[130–132] Following intentional weight loss, weight gain frequently follows; even

partial weight regain is associated with increased cardiometabolic risk.[133] Despite the possible need to lose weight, maintaining lean muscle mass is more important to prevent age-related functional and mental declines. Higher levels of protein consumption (up to 2.02 g/kg body weight) along with physical activity are positively associated with maintaining lean muscle mass.[134]

Medically, symptoms of perimenopause and menopause may be treated with hormone replacement therapy (HRT), which consists of low levels of estrogen and progesterone. This treatment is controversial, but when HRT treatment is initiated at the onset of menopause, increased osteoblastic activity may reduce the risk of osteoporosis and promote oral health by inhibiting gingival inflammation, periodontitis, and the consequent loss of teeth.[128] If symptoms significantly affect quality of life, decisions regarding HRT should involve the female's genetic and medical history.[135] Plant-based foods, such as legumes and soybeans, provide phytoestrogens and soluble fiber that may potentially reduce menopausal symptoms (i.e., hot flashes and night sweats) and may regulate blood cholesterol levels.[136,137] Foods containing phytoestrogens include soy products or isoflavone extracts. Herbal supplements that have been effective in the treatment of acute menopausal symptoms include Ginkgo biloba, black cohosh, and flaxseed, but further studies are needed to support their efficacy.[138] Studies acknowledge that soy isoflavone supplements containing a sufficient amount of genistein, derived by extraction or chemical synthesis, alleviate hot flashes and are safe. Approximately 50 to 120 mg/day may be necessary, but further studies are needed to confirm dose, isoflavone form, and treatment duration.[139,140]

Nutritional approaches to reducing menopausal symptoms continue to focus on the quality of dietary choices and healthy weight maintenance. Adequate amounts of calcium, selenium, magnesium, beta-carotene, vitamins D and K, and magnesium are important for protecting bone health.[141] Intake of adequate amounts of fruits, vegetables, and grains, following the *Dietary Guidelines*, are effective in possibly reducing the risk of cancer and CVD. Although a reduction in total energy consumption is necessary to prevent weight gain, adequate protein intake is important—at least three servings of iron-rich foods daily. Physical exercise, including aerobic activity and resistance and weight-bearing exercise, is beneficial for bone and cardiovascular health and weight control.[142,143]

DENTAL CONSIDERATIONS

Assessments

- *Physical:* Age, medical history (including drugs taken), dental history, oral examination, physical activity, oral radiographic findings.
- *Dietary:* Health and nutritional knowledge and skills, adequacy of calcium and vitamin D intake from food and supplements, caffeine intake.

Interventions

- Maintain meticulous daily oral self-care to reduce the risk for periodontal disease resulting from an exaggerated response to plaque biofilm.
- For xerostomia, provide information on preventive strategies, such as home and therapeutic fluoride applications; use of xylitol gum or mints; and minimizing choices of cariogenic snacks and beverages to reduce caries risk (see Chapter 20).
- Patients not prescribed HRT or other medications to deter progressive bone loss may exhibit increased alveolar bone loss; their periodontal condition should be carefully monitored at regular intervals with the use of oral radiographs.

NUTRITIONAL DIRECTIONS

- Encourage a minimum of three servings of low-fat dairy products or foods fortified with calcium and vitamin D to maintain bone mass. Consumption of greater than 90 mg/day of isoflavones in soy products may be effective in increasing bone mass of menopausal females.
- Calcium and vitamin D supplementation beyond the UL is not advisable unless recommended by a health care provider.
- Encourage good sources of lean protein and regular exercise to maintain muscle mass.

- Choose whole grains, vegetables, fruit, low-fat dairy products, and lean meat or soy substitutes to minimize the risk of CVD and to maximize bone health.
- If xerostomia is present, recommend avoidance of alcohol and alcohol-containing products to minimize burning and discomfort in the oral tissues.
- Provide nutritional advice about noncariogenic snack choices.

HEALTH APPLICATION 13

Fetal Alcohol Spectrum Disorder

The Centers for Disease Control and Prevention, American College of Obstetricians and Gynecologists, American Academy of Pediatrics, and March of Dimes, all recommend total abstinence from alcohol intake during pregnancy. There is no safe trimester during pregnancy for alcohol intake. Consumption of alcohol during pregnancy is the leading cause of preventable birth defects and intellectual and neurodevelopmental disabilities.[41,42]

Fetal alcohol syndrome (FAS) is a cluster of birth defects resulting from prenatal alcohol exposure. An infant with FAS exhibits full effects of the alcohol (Box 13.2), characterized by a pattern of minor facial anomalies, prenatal and postnatal growth retardation, and functional or structural central nervous system abnormalities. Fetal alcohol spectrum disorder (FASD) is a combination of irreversible birth defects and behavioral challenges in infants and children whose mothers consumed alcohol during pregnancy. Approximately 2% to 5% of school-age children show signs of prenatal alcohol exposure.[144–146] Worldwide, about 119,000 infants are born each year with fetal alcohol syndrome; approximately 15 per 10,000 people have fetal alcohol syndrome.[147,148] Small amounts of alcohol consumption may be associated with adverse effects, such as spontaneous abortion, growth retardation, cleft palate, or some of the neurologic and behavioral effects of FASD without physical abnormalities. Prenatal alcohol exposure can cause damage to the brain, resulting in significant problems with regulating behavior and optimal thinking and learning. This condition, called fetal alcohol effects, is difficult to diagnose.

A group of experts on FASDs proposed clinical guidelines for diagnosing FASD in 2016.[144] These new guidelines clarify and expand previous guidelines to help clinicians distinguish among the four distinct subtypes of FASD (see Box 13.3), to evaluate facial and physical deformities characteristic of FASD and information about cognitive and/or behavioral impairments seen in different FASD subtypes.

The first trimester, especially the first month, is the most vulnerable time for the fetus because the female may not even be aware of the pregnancy. A recent study reported that 1 in 5 (19.6%) reporting current alcohol use and 1 in 10 (10.5%) reporting binge drinking during the first trimester of pregnancy.[149] The FAS child has specific physiologic deformities (Fig. 13.5), but how alcohol affects the fetus is not fully understood. Accumulation of toxic levels of alcohol may interfere with cell formation. Several nutrients—especially folic acid, magnesium, and zinc—may be involved. The mental and physical abnormalities cannot be reversed.[150]

Even with adequate nutrition, normal development of fetal organs is jeopardized. Other habits that usually accompany alcohol consumption (e.g., smoking, excessive amounts of coffee the "morning after," poor eating habits with little attention to needed nutrients, and perhaps the use of tranquilizers) may also adversely affect the unborn child. Ethanol is a source of energy; chronic alcoholics may have a relatively low intake of protein, essential fats, vitamins, and minerals. Alcohol may impair placental transport of amino acids, calcium, and some vitamins.[84]

Because the brain has a special affinity for alcohol, it is one of the first organs affected. Intellectual impairment is frequently reported in children with FAS. Even at birth, the circumference of the head is small (microcephaly), indicating abnormal brain capacity (i.e., weight of 140 g in an infant with FAS compared with a normal brain weighing 400 g).[151] Fewer brain cells exist, with damaged cells preventing normal functioning; fewer neurons result in disorganized thought. The cognitive ability of the brain is permanently disturbed.[152] The average IQ is 68; maladaptive behaviors are common. Additionally, as a result of fewer total body cells, abnormal weight gain affects normal cell development and growth.[153,154]

Because of global adverse effects of alcohol intake, health care providers should advise pregnant females and females who might become pregnant to abstain from alcohol. Nutritional information and other efforts to improve food intake, such as referral to a social worker for food or monetary resources, are warranted. A multivitamin may need to be recommended for heavy substance abusers who have difficulty changing their habits to improve nutrient intake.

BOX 13.2   Signs of Fetal Alcohol Syndrome

Fetal alcohol syndrome is a cluster or pattern of related problems, not just a single birth defect. The severity of symptoms varies, but the symptoms are irreversible. Signs of fetal alcohol syndrome may include the following:
- Small head circumference and brain size (microcephaly)
- Distinctive facial features: small eyelid openings; eyes close together; a sunken nasal bridge; a short, upturned, undefined nose; an exceptionally thin upper lip; and a smooth skin surface between the nose and upper lip
- Oral cavity: small teeth with faulty enamel, prominent ridges in palate, cleft lip or palate, and small jaws; may have sleep and sucking problems as an infant
- Ears poorly formed and incorrectly positioned; hearing problems

- Heart defects
- Deformities of joints, limbs, and fingers; poor coordination
- Weak skeletal muscles (hypotonia) and poor coordination
- Low birth weight
- Slow physical growth before and after birth
- Vision difficulties, including nearsightedness (myopia)
- Intellectual disabilities and delayed development
- Abnormal behavior such as poor reasoning and judgment, short attention span, hyperactivity, poor impulse control, extreme nervousness and anxiety, and social interaction problems

Adapted from National Center on Birth Defects and Developmental Disabilities, Centers for Disease Control and Prevention. *Fetal Alcohol Spectrum Disorders (FASDs)*. https://www.cdc.gov/ncbddd/fasd/facts.html.

• BOX 13.3   Common Subtypes of Fetal Alcohol Syndrome

- Fetal alcohol syndrome (FAS)—most profoundly affected
- Partial fetal alcohol syndrome—displays some but not all physical/neurodevelopmental characteristics of FAS
- Alcohol-related neurodevelopmental disorder—demonstrates cognitive or behavior impairment with characteristic physical features
- Alcohol-related birth defects—physical malformations linked to maternal drinking with no other symptoms.
- Neurobehavioral Disorder Associated with Prenatal Alcohol Exposure—demonstrates neurodevelopmental, neurobehavioral, or mental health effects of prenatal alcohol exposure with or without cardinal facial dysmorphia and/or significant growth problems.

Adapted from American Academy of Pediatrics. Common Fetal Alcohol Spectrum Disorder Definitions. https://www.aap.org/en/patient-care/fetal-alcohol-spectrum-disorders/common-definitions; National Center on Birth Defects and Developmental Disabilities, Centers for Disease Control and Prevention. *Fetal Alcohol Spectrum Disorders (FASDs)*. https://www.cdc.gov/ncbddd/fasd/facts.html.

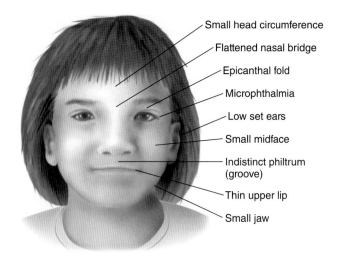

• **Fig. 13.5** Fetal alcohol syndrome. (From Moore M. *Pocket Guide to Nutritional Assessment and Care*. 6th ed. Mosby; 2009.)

◆ CASE APPLICATION FOR THE DENTAL HYGIENIST

Your regular patient, Betty, a 16-year-old, confides to you on her 6-month recare appointment that she is 3 months' pregnant. Even though she and her parents have decided to keep the infant, she has not seen a health care provider yet. Betty indicates that her mother lost a tooth with each child; thus she expects the same thing will happen to her.

Nutritional Assessment

- Knowledge about nutrition during pregnancy
- Special dietary restrictions; food fad practices; ethnic, cultural, or religious customs
- Adequacy of diet, especially calories, protein, calcium, vitamin D, iron, and folate
- Medications (including vitamin supplements), drug, and tobacco use
- Support of parents, living arrangements, and social support
- Psychological status and feelings about the reality of becoming a mother at such a young age

Nutritional Diagnosis

Altered nutrition: less than body requirements related to the lack of nutritional information and weight concerns.

Nutritional Goals

The patient will consume a nutrient-dense diet (based on *MyPlate* website for pregnant and breastfeeding females, https://www.myplate.gov/life-stages/pregnancy-and-breastfeeding) with additional calories during the second and third trimesters, and will verbalize ways to increase protein, iron, calcium, and folate intake.

Nutritional Implementation

Intervention: Encourage Betty to visit a health care provider as soon as possible.

Rationale: Fetal outcome is affected by nutrient intake during pregnancy; birth defects are likely to occur if dietary habits are poor, or if drug use occurs early in the pregnancy. Inadequate prenatal care leads to poor outcomes for the mother and fetus.

Intervention: Clarify nutritional misconceptions by providing written material and discussing the principal nutrients that need to be increased. Provide the name of an RDN with whom she can discuss these concerns.

Rationale: Nutritional requirements are quite high to meet the growth needs of the adolescent and fetus because Betty is still growing and storing nutrients in her own body.

Intervention: Teach Betty about the importance of consuming enough calcium and vitamin D during the pregnancy.

Rationale: Calcium and vitamin D are important in the formation of skeletal tissue and teeth.

Intervention: Discuss fermentable carbohydrates, and determine how frequently Betty consumes them.

Rationale: Fermentable carbohydrates, especially soft foods, stick to teeth, enhance plaque formation, and increase severity of periodontal issues. Parental food selections reflect foods that a child is exposed to and accepts.

Intervention: Talk to Betty about gingivitis during pregnancy, why it occurs, and risks associated with it.

Rationale: Hormonal changes during pregnancy lead to an increased risk of oral problems affecting pregnancy outcome.

Intervention: Discuss increased nutrients requirement during pregnancy. Provide snack ideas (cheese, nuts, yogurt, milkshakes, popcorn, raw vegetables, and fruits) that contain these nutrients.

Rationale: Most teenagers have an inadequate intake of calcium, iron, and vitamins A and D. Adequate intake of calories, protein, calcium, iron, B vitamins, and zinc is essential for a healthy infant and to protect maternal stores.

Intervention: Explain the effects of her nutritional status on the oral development of her infant.

Rationale: Nutrition can determine whether teeth achieve their optimum genetic potential.

Intervention: Explain why she should limit the intake of coffee, tea, and especially carbonated beverages containing caffeine. Explain why she should abstain from alcohol use.

Rationale: Large amounts of caffeine could be responsible for the malformations and increased susceptibility to decay of the primary first molars. Alcohol consumption may cause fetal alcohol spectrum disorder (FASD).

Evaluation

Betty should improve eating habits to consume at least the number of food groups recommended in *MyPlate* website for pregnant and breastfeeding females. Other behaviors, such as decreasing sugar intake, consuming milk and dairy products (for calcium and vitamin D intake), and consuming raw fruits and green leafy vegetables (for folate intake), will increase intake of nutrients needed during pregnancy. Betty has been taking appropriate action toward oral hygiene self-care to prevent or minimize periodontal problems.

◆ Student Readiness

1. Plan food intake for 1 day with two snacks for a pregnant patient who has four new carious lesions. What reasons would you give her for restricting sugar intake?
2. Explain what pica is, and the type of individuals who may be practicing this behavior.
3. Why is it undesirable to lose weight during pregnancy?
4. List five effects on oral development of the fetus when maternal nutrient intake is inadequate.
5. Why is oral health care especially important during pregnancy?
6. Which nutrients may be needed if dietary assessment indicates deficient intake that cannot be corrected by changing eating habits?
7. List advantages of breastfeeding, especially on oral-motor development.

◆ CASE STUDY

A 32-year-old mother of two children (3 years and 6 months old) who is breastfeeding complains of bleeding and sore gums and tongue. She has not visited her health care provider since the birth of her younger child because of financial limitations and lack of time. She has returned to her job as a clerk at a local department store. When questioned about her diet, she reports drinking a cup of coffee on her way to work with 2 teaspoons of added sugar; she usually takes a peanut butter and jelly sandwich and soft drink for lunch; and during the evening, she grabs something fast and easy to eat such as hot dogs, canned soup, crackers, cookies, chips, or soft drinks. She complains of being tired and irritable, and feels this is because of the stress imposed on her by the two children and her work.

1. List probable causes of the mother's symptoms.
2. Discuss how nutrition needs change during pregnancy and lactation.
3. Determine other foods that should be readily available for her, such as cottage cheese, yogurt, nuts, fresh fruit, and raw vegetables.
4. Discuss possible nutrition-related causes of the "bleeding and sore gums and tongue."

References

1. Centers for Disease Control and Prevention. *Preterm Birth.* https://www.cdc.gov/reproductivehealth/maternalinfanthealth/pretermbirth.htm.
2. National Research Council. *Maternal Nutrition and the Course of Pregnancy. Report of the Committee on Maternal Nutrition.* Food and Nutrition Board. National Academy of Sciences; 1970.
3. Board on Children, Youth and Families, Food and Nutrition Board. *Influence of Pregnancy Weight on Maternal and Child Health: Workshop Report.* National Academies Press; 2007.
4. Centers for Disease Control and Prevention. *Preconception Health and Health Care Is Important for All.* https://www.cdc.gov/preconception/overview.html.
5. Stang J, Huffman LG. Position of the Academy of Nutrition and Dietetics: obesity, reproduction, and pregnancy outcomes. *J Acad Nutr Diet.* 2016;116(4):677–691.
6. Hoek A, Wang Z, van Oers AM, Groen H, Cantineau AEP. Effects of preconception weight loss after lifestyle intervention on fertility outcomes and pregnancy complications. *Fertil Steril.* 2022;118(3):456–462.
7. United Nations Population Fund. *State of the World Population. Seeing the Unseen. The Case for Action in the Neglected Crisis of Unintended Pregnancy.* 2022. https://www.unfpa.org/sites/default/files/pub-pdf/EN_SWP22%20report_0.pdf.
8. Paknahad Z, Fallah A, Moravejolahkami AR. Maternal dietary patterns and their association with pregnancy outcomes. *Clin Nutr Res.* 2019;8(1):64–73.
9. American College of Obstetricians and Gynecologists; Society for Maternal-Fetal Medicine Obstetric care consensus no. 8: interpregnancy care. *Obstet Gynecol.* 2019;133(1):e51–e72.
10. Moreno-Fernandez J, Ochoa JJ, Lopez-Frias M, Diaz-Castro J. Impact of early nutrition, physical activity and sleep on the fetal programming of disease in the pregnancy: a narrative review. *Nutrients.* 2020;12(12):3900.
11. Fawcett EJ, Fawcett JM, Mazmanian D. A *meta*-analysis of the worldwide prevalence of pica during pregnancy and the postpartum period. *Int J Gynaecol Obstet.* 2016;133(3):277–283.
12. Miao D, Young SL, Golden CD. A *meta*-analysis of pica and micronutrient status. *Am J Hum Biol.* 2015;27(1):84–93. https://doi.org/10.1002/ajhb.22598.
13. Burke M. *Pica.* Medscape. https://emedicine.medscape.com/article/914765-overview?form=fpf.
14. Office of Disease Prevention and Health Promotion. Increase the proportion of pregnant women who receive early and adequate prenatal care-MICH-08. In: *Healthy People* 2030. United States Department of Health and Human Services. https://health.gov/healthypeople/objectives-and-data/browse-objectives/pregnancy-and-childbirth/increase-proportion-pregnant-women-who-receive-early-and-adequate-prenatal-care-mich-08.
15. Kaya AE, Doğan O, Başbuğ A, et al. An evaluation of the association of reproductive history and multiple births during adolescence with postmenopausal osteoporosis. *Geburtshilfe Frauenheilkd.* 2019;79(3):300–307.
16. Farpour-Lambert NJ, Ells LJ, Martinez de Tejada B, Scott C. Obesity and weight gain in pregnancy and postpartum: an evidence review of lifestyle interventions to inform maternal and child health policies. *Front Endocrinol.* 2018;9:546.
17. Driscoll AK, Gregory ECW. Increases in prepregnancy obesity: United States, 2016–2019. NCHS. *Data Brief.* 2020;392:1–8.
18. Institute of Medicine (IOM) and National Research Council (NRC). *Weight Gain During Pregnancy: Reexamining the Guidelines.* National Academies Press; 2009.
19. Siega-Riz AM, Bodnar LM, Stotland NE, Stang J. *The current understanding of gestational weight gain among women with obesity and the need for future research. NAM Perspectives. Discussion Paper.* National Academy of Medicine; 2019.
20. Sun Y, Shen Z, Zhan Y, et al. Effects of pre-pregnancy body mass index and gestational weight gain on maternal and infant complications. *BMC Pregnancy Childbirth.* 2020;20(1):390.
21. Haugen M, Brantsaeter AL, Winkvist A, et al. Associations of prepregnancy body mass index and gestational weight gain with pregnancy outcome and postpartum weight retention: a prospective observational cohort study. *BMC Pregnancy Childbirth.* 2014;14:201.
22. Division of Reproductive Health, National Center for Chronic Disease Prevention and Health Promotion. *Weight Gain During Pregnancy.* https://www.cdc.gov/reproductivehealth/maternalinfanthealth/pregnancy-weight-gain.htm.
23. American Public Health Association. *Improving Access to Dental Care for Pregnant Women Through Education, Integration of Health Services, Insurance Coverage, An Appropriate Dental Workforce, and Research. Policy No. 20202.* 2020. https://www.apha.org/policies-and-advocacy/public-health-policy-statements/policy-database/2021/01/12/improving-access-to-dental-care-for-pregnant-women.
24. Lee H, Tranby E, Shi L. Dental visits during pregnancy: pregnancy risk assessment monitoring system analysis 2012–2015. *JDR Clin Trans Res.* 2022;7(4):379–388.
25. Rocha JS, Arima L, Chibinski AC, et al. Barriers and facilitators to dental care during pregnancy: a systematic review and *meta*-synthesis of qualitative studies. *Cad Saude Public.* 2018;34(8):e00130817.
26. Anunciação BH, Azevedo MJ, Pereira ML. Knowledge, attitudes, and practices of prenatal care practitioners regarding oral

health in pregnancy—a systematic review. *Int J Gynaecol Obstet.* 2023;162(2):449–461.

27. Geisinger ML, Geurs NC, Bain JL, et al. Oral health education and therapy reduces gingivitis during pregnancy. *J Clin Periodontol.* 2014;41(2):141–148.

28. Bobetsis YA, Graziani F, Gürsoy M, Madianos PN. Periodontal disease and adverse pregnancy outcomes. *Periodontol 2000.* 2020;83(1):154–174.

29. Nannan M, Xiaoping L, Ying J. Periodontal disease in pregnancy and adverse pregnancy outcomes: Progress in related mechanisms and management strategies. *Front Med.* 2022;9:963956.

30. Iheozor-Ejiofor Z, Middleton P, Esposito M, Glenny AM. Treating periodontal disease for preventing adverse birth outcomes in pregnant women. *Cochrane Database Syst Rev.* 2017;6(6): CD005297.

31. Bi WG, Emami E, Luo ZC, Santamaria C, Wei SQ. Effect of periodontal treatment in pregnancy on perinatal outcomes: a systematic review and *meta*-analysis. *J Matern Fetal Neonatal Med.* 2021;34(19):3259–3268.

32. Uppal A, Uppal S, Pinto A, et al. The effectiveness of periodontal disease treatment during pregnancy in reducing the risk of experiencing preterm birth and low birth weight: a *meta*-analysis. *J Am Dent Assoc.* 2010;141(12):1423–1434.

33. Le QA, Eslick GD, Coulton KM, et al. Differential Impact of periodontal treatment strategies during pregnancy on perinatal outcomes: a systematic review and *meta*-analysis. *J Evid Based Dent Pract.* 2022;22(1):101666.

34. Ortiz AC, Fideles SOM, Pomini KT, Buchaim RL. Updates in association of gastroesophageal reflux disease and dental erosion: systematic review. *Expert Rev Gastroenterol Hepatol.* 2021;15(9): 1037–1046.

35. Chandel S, Khan MA, Singh N, Agrawal A, Khare V. The effect of sodium bicarbonate oral rinse on salivary pH and oral microflora: a prospective cohort study. *Natl J Maxillofac Surg.* 2017;8(2):106–109.

36. Rhee J, Kim R, Kim Y, et al. Maternal caffeine consumption during pregnancy and risk of low birth weight: a dose–response *meta*-analysis of observational studies. *PLoS ONE.* 2015;10(7):30132334.

37. Soltani S, Salari-Moghaddam A, Saneei P, et al. Maternal caffeine consumption during pregnancy and risk of low birth weight: a dose-response *meta*-analysis of cohort studies. *Crit Rev Food Sci Nutr.* 2023;63(2):224–233.

38. March of Dimes. *Caffeine in Pregnancy.* https://www.marchofdimes. org/find-support/topics/pregnancy/caffeine-pregnancy.

39. Román-Gálvez MR, Martín-Peláez S, Hernández-Martínez L, et al. Caffeine intake throughout pregnancy, and factors associated with non-compliance with recommendations: a cohort study. *Nutrients.* 2022;14(24):5384.

40. James JE. Maternal caffeine consumption and pregnancy outcomes: a narrative review with implications for advice to mothers and mothers-to-be. *BMJ Evid Based Med.* 2021;26(3):114–115.

41. Bandoli G, Hayes S, Delker E. Low to moderate prenatal alcohol exposure and neurodevelopmental outcomes: a narrative review and methodological considerations. *Alcohol Res.* 2023;43(1):01.

42. Williams JF, Smith VC, Committee on Substance Abuse Fetal alcohol spectrum disorders. *Pediatrics.* 2015;136(5):e1395–e1406.

43. Palatnik A, Moosreiner A, Olivier-Van Stichelen S. Consumption of non-nutritive sweeteners during pregnancy. *Am J Obstet Gynecol.* 2020;223(2):211–218.

44. American Pregnancy Association. *Artificial Sweeteners and Pregnancy.* https://americanpregnancy.org/healthy-pregnancy/is-it-safe/ artificial-sweeteners-and-pregnancy/.

45. Halasa BC, Sylvetsky AC, Conway EM, et al. Non-nutritive sweeteners in human amniotic fluid and cord blood: evidence of transplacental fetal exposure. *Am J Perinatol.* 2023;40(12):1286–1291.

46. United States Food and Drug Administration. *People at Risk of Foodborne Illness.* https://www.fda.gov/food/consumers/people-risk-foodborne-illness.

47. Segado-Arenas A, Atienza-Cuevas L, Broullón-Molanes JR, Rodríguez-González M, Lubián-López SP. Late stillbirth due to listeriosis. *Autops Case Rep.* 2018;8(4):e2018051.

48. United States Food and Drug Administration (FDA). *Listeria From Food Safety for Moms to Be.* https://www.fda.gov/food/ health-educators/listeria-food-safety-moms-be.

49. Centers for Disease Control. *Parasites-Toxoplasmosis.* https://www. cdc.gov/parasites/toxoplasmosis/index.html.

50. Centers for Disease Control and Prevention. *Toxoplasmosis: Pregnancy FAQs.* https://www.cdc.gov/parasites/toxoplasmosis/gen_ info/pregnant.html.

51. Dack K, Fell M, Taylor CM, Havdahl A, Lewis SJ. Prenatal mercury exposure and neurodevelopment up to the age of 5 Years: a systematic review. *Int J Environ Res Public Health.* 2022;19(4):1976.

52. Patel NB, Xu Y, McCandless LC, et al. Very low-level prenatal mercury exposure and behaviors in children: the HOME Study. *Environ Health.* 2019;18(1):4.

53. United States Food and Drug Administration (FDA). *Fish: What Pregnant Women and Parents Should Know.* Draft updated advice by FDA and EPA. http://www.fda.gov/Food/ FoodborneIllnessContaminants/Metals/ucm393070.htm.

54. Mayo Clinic. *Pregnancy and Fish: What's Safe to Eat?* https:// www.mayoclinic.org/healthy-lifestyle/pregnancy-week-by-week/ in-depth/pregnancy-and-fish/art-20044185.

55. Centers for Disease Control and Prevention. *Childhood Lead Poisoning: Pregnant Women.* https://www.cdc.gov/nceh/lead/prevention/pregnant.htm

56. Rísová V. The pathway of lead through the mother's body to the child. *Interdiscip Toxicol.* 2019;12(1):1–6.

57. Centers for Disease Control and Prevention. *Childhood Lead Poisoning Prevention: Health Effects of Lead Exposure.* https://www. cdc.gov/nceh/lead/prevention/health-effects.htm.

58. Khan MI, Ahmed N, Neela PK, Unnisa N. The human genetics of dental anomalies. *Glob Med Genet.* 2022;9(2):76–81.

59. Beckett DM, Broadbent JM, Loch C, et al. Dental consequences of vitamin D deficiency during pregnancy and early infancy-an observational study. *Int J Environ Res Public Health.* 2022;19(4):1932.

60. Kawakubo-Yasukochi T, Hayashi Y, Hirata M. Effects of maternal nutrition on oral health in offspring. *Curr Oral Health Rep.* 2023;10:69–74.

61. Tapalaga G, Bumbu BA, Reddy SR, et al. The impact of prenatal vitamin D on enamel defects and tooth erosion: a systematic review. *Nutrients.* 2023;15(18):3863. https://doi.org/10.3390/ nu15183863.

62. Takahashi R, Ota E, Hoshi K, et al. Fluoride supplementation (with tablets, drops, lozenges or chewing gum) in pregnant women for preventing dental caries in the primary teeth of their children. *Cochrane Database Syst Rev.* 2017;10(10):CD011850.

63. Sebastiani G, Herranz Barbero A, Borrás-Novell C, et al. The effects of vegetarian and vegan diet during pregnancy on the health of mothers and offspring. *Nutrients.* 2019;11(3):557.

64. De-Regil LM, Harding KB, Roche ML. Preconceptional nutrition interventions for adolescent girls and adult women: global guidelines and gaps in evidence and policy with emphasis on micronutrients. *J Nutr.* 2016;146(7):1461S–1470S.

65. Morrison JL, Regnault TR. Nutrition in pregnancy: optimising maternal diet and fetal adaptations to altered nutrient supply. *Nutrients.* 2016;8(6):342.

66. Jebeile H, Mijatovic J, Louie JC, et al. A systematic review and metaanalysis of energy intake and weight gain in pregnancy. *Am J Obstet Gynecol.* 2016;214(4):465–483.

67. Goławski K, Giermaziak W, Ciebiera M, Wojtyła C. Excessive gestational weight gain and pregnancy outcomes. *J Clin Med.* 2023;12(9):3211.

68. Marshall NE, Abrams B, Barbour LA, et al. The importance of nutrition in pregnancy and lactation: lifelong consequences. *Am J Obstet Gynecol.* 2022;226(5):607–632.

69. Donovan S, Dewey K, Novotny R, et al. *Dietary Patterns During Pregnancy and Gestational Weight Gain: A Systematic Review*. United States Department of Agriculture, Food and Nutrition Service, Center for Nutrition Policy and Promotion, Nutrition Evidence Systematic Review; 2020.

70. Nevins JEH, Donovan SM, Snetselaar L, et al. Omega-3 fatty acid dietary supplements consumed during pregnancy and lactation and child neurodevelopment: a systematic review. *J Nutr*. 2021;151(11):3483–3494.

71. Middleton P, Gomersall JC, Gould JF, et al. Omega-3 fatty acid addition during pregnancy. *Cochrane Database Syst Rev*. 2018;11(11):CD003402.

72. Dietary Guidelines Advisory Committee. *Scientific Report of the 2020 Dietary Guidelines Advisory Committee: Advisory Report to the Secretary of Agriculture and the Secretary of Health and Human Services*. United States Department of Agriculture, Agricultural Research Service; 2020.

73. Murphy MM, Higgins KA, Bi X, Barraj LM. Adequacy and Sources of Protein Intake among Pregnant Women in the United States, NHANES 2003–2012. *Nutrients*. 2021;13(3):795. https://doi.org/10.3390/nu13030795.

74. Kovacs CS. Maternal mineral and bone metabolism during pregnancy, lactation, and post-weaning recovery. *Physiol Rev*. 2016;96(2):449–547.

75. Wagner CL, Taylor SN, Dawodu A, Johnson DD, Hollis BW. Vitamin D and its role during pregnancy in attaining optimal health of mother and fetus. *Nutrients*. 2012;4(3):208–230.

76. American College of Obstetrics and Gynecology (ACOG) Committee on Obstetric Practice. Opinion no. 495: vitamin D: Screening and supplementation during pregnancy. *Obstet Gynecol*. 2011;118(1):197–198. Reaffirmed 2021. https://www.acog.org/clinical/clinical-guidance/committee-opinion/articles/2011/07/vitamin-d-screening-and-supplementation-during-pregnancy.

77. Zhang H, Wang S, Tuo L, et al. Relationship between maternal vitamin D levels and adverse outcomes. *Nutrients*. 2022;14(20):4230.

78. Amegah AK, Klevor MK, Wagner CL. Maternal vitamin D insufficiency and risk of adverse pregnancy and birth outcomes: a systematic review and *meta*-analysis of longitudinal studies. *PLoS One*. 2017;12(3):e0173605.

79. Hollis BW, Johnson D, Hulsey TC, Ebeling M, Wagner CL. Vitamin D supplementation during pregnancy: double-blind, randomized clinical trial of safety and effectiveness. *J Bone Miner Res*. 2011;26(10):2341–2357.

80. United States Preventive Services Task Force (USPSTF) Recommendation Statement. Folic acid supplementation for the prevention of neural tube defects. *JAMA*. 2017;317(2):183–189.

81. Crider KS, Qi YP, Devine O, Tinker SC, Berry RJ. Modeling the impact of folic acid fortification and supplementation on red blood cell folate concentrations and predicted neural tube defect risk in the United States: have we reached optimal prevention? *Am J Clin Nutr*. 2018;107(6):1027–1034.

82. United States Food and Drug Administration New Release. *FDA Approves Folic Acid Fortification of Corn Masa Flour*. 2016. http://www.fda.gov/NewsEvents/Newsroom/PressAnnouncements/ucm496104.htm.

83. March of Dimes. *Folic Acid*. https://www.marchofdimes.org/find-support/topics/pregnancy/folic-acid.

84. Institute of Medicine (US) Committee on Nutritional Status During Pregnancy and Lactation. In: 14, Iron nutrition during pregnancy. *Nutrition During Pregnancy: Part I Weight Gain: Part II Nutrient Supplements*. National Academies Press (United States); 1990.

85. Means RT. Iron deficiency and iron deficiency anemia: implications and impact in pregnancy, fetal development, and early childhood parameters. *Nutrients*. 2020;12(2):447.

86. Brannon PM, Taylor CL. Iron supplementation during pregnancy and infancy: uncertainties and implications for research and policy. *Nutrients*. 2017;9(12):1327.

87. Trumbo P, Yates AA, Schlicker S, Poos M. Dietary reference intakes: vitamin A, vitamin K, arsenic, boron, chromium, copper, iodine, iron, manganese, molybdenum, nickel, silicon, vanadium, and zinc. *J Am Diet Assoc*. 2001;101(3):294–301.

88. German KR, Juul SE. Iron and neurodevelopment in preterm infants: a narrative review. *Nutrients*. 2021;13(11):3737.

89. Peña-Rosas JP, De-Regil LM, Dowswell T, Viteri FE. Intermittent oral iron supplementation during pregnancy. *Cochrane Database Syst Rev*. 2012;7(7):CD009997. https://doi.org/10.1002/14651858. CD009997. Update in: *Cochrane Database Syst Rev*. 2015;(10): CD009997.

90. Guideline. *Iron Supplementation in Postpartum Women*. World Health Organization; 2016.

91. Wu L, Sun R, Liu Y, et al. High hemoglobin level is a risk factor for maternal and fetal outcomes of pregnancy in Chinese women: a retrospective cohort study. *BMC Pregnancy Childbirth*. 2022;22(1):290.

92. Panth P, Guerin G, DiMarco NM. A review of iodine status of women of reproductive age in the USA. *Biol Trace Elem Res*. 2019;188(1):208–220.

93. Pearce EN, Lazarus JH, Moreno-Reyes R, Zimmermann MB. Consequences of iodine deficiency and excess in pregnant women: an overview of current knowns and unknowns. *Am J Clin Nutr*. 2016;104(Suppl 3):918S–923S.

94. Biban BG, Lichiardopol C. Iodine deficiency, still a global problem? *Curr Health Sci J*. 2017;43(2):103–111.

95. De Leo S, Pearce EN, Braverman LE. Iodine supplementation in women during preconception, pregnancy, and lactation: current clinical practice by United States Obstetricians and Midwives. *Thyroid*. 2017;27(3):434–439.

96. Council on Environmental Health, et al. Rogan WJ, Paulson JA, et al. Iodine deficiency, pollutant chemicals, and the thyroid: new information on an old problem. *Pediatrics*. 2014;133(6): 1163–1166.

97. Filipowicz D, Szczepanek-Parulska E, Mikulska-Sauermann AA, et al. Iodine deficiency and real-life supplementation ineffectiveness in Polish pregnant women and its impact on thyroid metabolism. *Front Endocrinol (Lausanne)*. 2023;14:1068418.

98. Hardley MT, Chon AH, Mestman J. Iodine-induced fetal hypothyroidism: diagnosis and treatment with intra-amniotic levothyroxine. *Horm Res Paediatr*. 2018;90(6):419–423.

99. Ip P, Ho FKW, Rao N, et al. Impact of nutritional supplements on cognitive development of children in developing countries: a *meta*-analysis. *Sci Rep*. 2017;7(1):10611.

100. Office of Disease Prevention and Health Promotion. Reduce iron deficiency in females aged 12 to 49 years, NWS-17. In: *Healthy People 2030*. United States Department of Health and Human Services. https://health.gov/healthypeople/objectives-and-data/browse-objectives/women.

101. Centers for Disease Control and Prevention. *Reproductive Health: Unintended Pregnancy*. https://www.cdc.gov/reproductivehealth/contraception/unintendedpregnancy/index.htm.

102. Rothman KJ, Moore LL, Singer MR, Nguyen US, Mannino S, Milunsky A. Teratogenicity of high vitamin A intake. *N Engl J Med*. 1995;333(21):1369–1373.

103. National Institutes of Health Office of Dietary Supplements. *Zinc Fact Sheet for Health Professionals*. https://ods.od.nih.gov/factsheets/Zinc-HealthProfessional/.

104. Buhling KJ, Scheuer M, Laakmann E. Recommendation and intake of dietary supplements periconceptional and during pregnancy: results of a nationwide survey of gynaecologists. *Arch Gynecol Obstet*. 2023

105. Kominiarek MA, Rajan P. Nutrition recommendations in pregnancy and lactation. *Med Clin North Am*. 2016;100(6):1199–1215.

106. Centers for Disease Control and Prevention (CDC). *Breastfeeding Report Card in the United States*, 2022. https://www.cdc.gov/breastfeeding/data/reportcard.htm.

107. Office of Disease Prevention and Health Promotion. Increase the proportion of infants who are breastfed exclusively through age 6 months-MICH-15. In: *Healthy People 2030.* United States Department of Health and Human Services. https://health.gov/healthypeople/objectives-and-data/browse-objectives/infants/increase-proportion-infants-who-are-breastfed-exclusively-through-age-6-months-mich-15.

108. Office of Disease Prevention and Health Promotion. Increase the proportion of infants who are breastfed at 1 year-MICH-16. In: *Healthy People 2030.* United States Department of Health and Human Services. https://health.gov/healthypeople/objectives-and-data/browse-objectives/infants/increase-proportion-infants-who-are-breastfed-1-year-mich-16.

109. Li R, Perrine CG, Anstey EH, et al. Breastfeeding trends by race/ethnicity among United States children born from 2009 to 2015. *JAMA Pediatr.* 2019;173(12):e193319.

110. World Health Organization. *Nutrition and Food Safety.* https://www.who.int/teams/nutrition-and-food-safety/food-and-nutrition-actions-in-health-systems/ten-steps-to-successful-breastfeeding.

111. United States Preventive Services Task Force, et al. Bibbins-Domingo K, Grossman DC, et al. Primary care interventions to support breastfeeding: United States Preventive Services Task Force Recommendation Statement. *JAMA.* 2016;316(16):1688–1693.

112. Infant and Young Child Feeding. *Model Chapter for Textbooks for Medical Students and Allied Health Professionals.* World Health Organization; 2009.

113. Peres KG, Nascimento GG, Peres MA, et al. Impact of prolonged breastfeeding on dental caries: a population-based birth cohort study. *Pediatrics.* 2017;140(1):e20162943.

114. Centers for Disease Control and Prevention. *Breastfeeding: Vitamin D.* https://www.cdc.gov/breastfeeding/breastfeeding-special-circumstances/diet-and-micronutrients/vitamin-d.html.

115. Domenici R, Vierucci F. Exclusive breastfeeding and vitamin D supplementation: a positive synergistic effect on prevention of childhood infections? *Int J Environ Res Public Health.* 2022;19(5):2973.

116. Samuel TM, Zhou Q, Giuffrida F, et al. Nutritional and non-nutritional composition of human milk is modulated by maternal, infant, and methodological factors. *Front Nutr.* 2020;7:576133.

117. Centers for Disease Control. *Breastfeeding.* https://www.cdc.gov/breastfeeding/breastfeeding-special-circumstances/diet-and-micronutrients/maternal-diet.html.

118. Palmery M, Saraceno A, Vaiarelli A, et al. Oral contraceptives and changes in nutritional requirements. *Eur Rev Med Pharmacol Sci.* 2013;17(13):1804–1813.

119. Wilson SM, Bivins BN, Russell KA, et al. Oral contraceptive use: impact on folate, vitamin B_6, and vitamin B_{12} status. *Nutr Rev.* 2011;69(10):572–583.

120. Mohammad-Alizadeh-Charandabi S, Mirghafourvand M, Froghy L, et al. The effect of multivitamin supplement on continuation rate and side effects of combined oral contraceptives: a randomised controlled trial. *Eur J Contracept Reprod Health Care.* 2015;20(5):361–371.

121. Lopez LM, Ramesh S, Chen M, et al. Progestin-only contraceptives: effects on weight. *Cochrane Database Syst Rev.* 2016;2016(8):CD008815.

122. Kuryłowicz A. Estrogens in adipose tissue physiology and obesity-related dysfunction. *Biomedicines.* 2023;11(3):690.

123. Fabunmi OA, Dludla PV, Nkambule BB. Investigating cardiovascular risk in premenopausal women on oral contraceptives: systematic review with *meta*-analysis. *Front Cardiovasc Med.* 2023;10:1127104.

124. Knopp RH, Walden CE, Wahl PW, Hoover JJ. Effects of oral contraceptives on lipoprotein triglyceride and cholesterol: relationships to estrogen and progestin potency. *Am J Obstet Gynecol.* 1982;142(6 Pt 2):725–731.

125. Mills EG, Yang L, Nielsen MF, et al. The relationship between bone and reproductive hormones beyond estrogens and androgens. *Endocr Rev.* 2021;42(6):691–719.

126. Clarke BL, Khosla S. Female reproductive system and bone. *Arch Biochem Biophys.* 2010;503(1):118–128.

127. Jonasson G, Rythén M. Alveolar bone loss in osteoporosis: a loaded and cellular affair? *Clin Cosmet Investig Dent.* 2016;8:95–103.

128. Jayusman PA, Nasruddin NS, Baharin B, et al. Overview on postmenopausal osteoporosis and periodontitis: the therapeutic potential of phytoestrogens against alveolar bone loss. *Front Pharmacol.* 2023;14:1120457.

129. Greendale GA, Sternfeld B, Huang M, et al. Changes in body composition and weight during the menopause transition. *JCI Insight.* 2019;4(5):e124865.

130. Compston JE, Wyman A, FitzGerald G, et al. Increase in fracture risk following unintentional weight loss in postmenopausal women: the global longitudinal study of osteoporosis in women. *J Bone Miner Res.* 2016;31(7):1466–1472.

131. Von Thun NL, Sukumar D, Heymsfield SB, et al. Does bone loss begin after weight loss ends? Results 2 years after weight loss or regain in postmenopausal women. *Menopause.* 2014;21(5):501–508.

132. Jiang BC, Villareal DT. Weight loss-induced reduction of bone mineral density in older adults with obesity. *J Nutr Gerontol Geriatr.* 2019;38(1):100–114.

133. Beavers DP, Beavers KM, Lyles MF, et al. Cardiometabolic risk after weight loss and subsequent weight regain in overweight and obese postmenopausal women. *J Gerontol A Biol Sci Med Sci.* 2013;68(6):691–698.

134. Martinez JA, Wertheim BC, Thomson CA, et al. Physical activity modifies the association between dietary protein and lean mass of postmenopausal women. *J Acad Nutr Diet.* 2017;117(2):192–203.

135. Palacios S, Stevenson JC, Schaudig K, Lukasiewicz M, Graziottin A. Hormone therapy for first-line management of menopausal symptoms: practical recommendations. *Womens Health (Lond).* 2019;15:1745506519864009.

136. Barnard ND, Kahleova H, Holtz DN, et al. A dietary intervention for vasomotor symptoms of menopause: a randomized, controlled trial. *Menopause.* 2023;30(1):80–87.

137. Trautwein EA, McKay S. The role of specific components of a plant-based diet in management of dyslipidemia and the impact on cardiovascular risk. *Nutrients.* 2020;12(9):2671.

138. Kargozar R, Azizi H, Salari R. A review of effective herbal medicines in controlling menopausal symptoms. *Electron Physician.* 2017;9(11):5826–5833.

139. Thomas AJ, Ismail R, Taylor-Swanson L, et al. Effects of isoflavones and amino acid therapies for hot flashes and co-occurring symptoms during the menopausal transition and early postmenopause: a systematic review. *Maturitas.* 2014;78(4):263–276.

140. Perna S, Peroni G, Miccono A, et al. Multidimensional effects of soy isoflavone by food or supplements in menopause women: a systematic review and bibliometric analysis. *Nat Prod Commun.* 2016;11(11):1733–1740.

141. Silva TR, Oppermann K, Reis FM, Spritzer PM. Nutrition in menopausal women: a narrative review. *Nutrients.* 2021;13(7):2149.

142. Tong X, Chen X, Zhang S, et al. The effect of exercise on the prevention of osteoporosis and bone angiogenesis. *Biomed Res Int.* 2019;2019:8171897.

143. Wu NN, Tian H, Chen P, et al. Physical exercise and selective autophagy: benefit and risk on cardiovascular health. *Cells.* 2019;8(11):1436.

144. Hoyme HE, Kalberg WO, Elliott AJ, et al. Updated clinical guidelines for diagnosing fetal alcohol spectrum disorders. *Pediatrics.* 2016;138(2):pii:e20154256.

145. Lange S, Probst C, Gmel G, et al. Global prevalence of fetal alcohol spectrum disorder among children and youth: a systematic review and *meta*-analysis. *JAMA Pediatr.* 2017;171(10):948–956.

146. Wozniak JR, Riley EP, Charness ME. Clinical presentation, diagnosis, and management of fetal alcohol spectrum disorder. *Lancet Neurol.* 2019;18(8):760–770.

147. Popova S, Lange S, Probst C, et al. Estimation of national, regional, and global prevalence of alcohol use during pregnancy and fetal alcohol syndrome: a systematic review and *meta*-analysis. *Lancet Glob Health*. 2017;5(3):e290–e299.

148. Hur YM, Choi J, Park S, Oh SS, Kim YJ. Prenatal maternal alcohol exposure: diagnosis and prevention of fetal alcohol syndrome. *Obstet Gynecol Sci*. 2022;65(5):385–394.

149. England LJ, Bennett C, Denny CH, et al. Alcohol use and co-use of other substances among pregnant females aged 12–44 years—United States, 2015–2018. *MMWR Morb Mortal Wkly Rep*. 2020;69(31): 1009–1014.

150. Barve S, Chen SY, Kirpich I, Watson WH, Mcclain C. Development, prevention, and treatment of alcohol-induced organ injury: the role of nutrition. *Alcohol Res*. 2017;38(2):289–302.

151. Treit S, Zhou D, Chudley AE, et al. Relationships between head circumference, brain volume and cognition in children with prenatal alcohol exposure. *PLoS One*. 2016;11(2):e0150370.

152. Granato A, Dering B. Alcohol and the developing brain: why neurons die and how survivors change. *Int J Mol Sci*. 2018;19(10): 2992.

153. Almeida L, Andreu-Fernández V, Navarro-Tapia E, et al. Murine models for the study of fetal alcohol spectrum disorders: an overview. *Front Pediatr*. 2020;8:359.

154. Streissguth AP, Aase JM, Clarren SK, Randels SP, LaDue RA, Smith DF. Fetal alcohol syndrome in adolescents and adults. *JAMA*. 1991;265(15):1961–1967.

▶ Evolve Resources

Please visit http://evolve.elsevier.com/Mallonee/nutritional for additional practice and study support tools.

14

Nutritional Requirements During Growth and Development and Eating Habits Affecting Oral Health

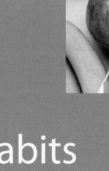

STUDENT LEARNING OUTCOMES

On completion of this chapter, the student will be able to achieve the following learning outcomes:

1. The following are related to the growth and development of infants:
   - Discuss the growth and nutritional requirements of infants.
   - Describe how breast milk and infant formula affect the oral health of infants.
   - Outline the timetable for introducing complementary foods and list reasons for their introduction.
   - Discuss ways to handle typical feeding problems that occur in infants.
   - Discuss oral health concerns and physiologic changes that alter the nutritional status of infants.
2. Discuss dietary recommendations for children older than 2 years of age as described in the *2020-2025 Dietary Guidelines*, *Healthy People 2030*, and *MyPlate* websites.

3. With regard to growth and development of toddlers and preschool children:
   - Discuss the growth and nutritional requirements of toddlers and preschool children.
   - Describe feeding patterns of toddlers and preschool children. Discuss how their feeding patterns relate to their oral health.
4. Describe the nutrition and oral health implications of children with special needs. Discuss the food habits associated with dental care in school-aged children.
5. Discuss the growth and nutrient requirements of adolescents, as well as factors that may affect food choices.
6. Identify effective approaches to nutritional counseling of the adolescent patient.

KEY TERMS

Bruxism	Food jags	Retrognathic
Cleft lip	Hydrolyzed protein	Sealants
Cleft palate	Innate	Suckling
Complementary feeding period	Nonnutritive sucking	
Early childhood caries (ECC)	Overjet	

🔹 TEST YOUR NQ

1. **T/F** Commercial infant formulas have nutrient content for their requirements.
2. **T/F** Fluoride should be provided to all infants from birth if the water supply is not fluoridated.
3. **T/F** Solid foods should be introduced to infants at 6 weeks of age.
4. **T/F** Peanuts and peanut butter should not be given to infants before age 2 to avoid peanut allergy.
5. **T/F** More nutrients are required during adolescence than during any other stage of life.
6. **T/F** Toddlers may refuse to eat anything except one food for several days.
7. **T/F** Breastfed infants do not need any supplements during the first 4 months.
8. **T/F** Bottle-fed infants are less likely to develop malocclusion.
9. **T/F** Children outgrow their need for milk.
10. **T/F** To reduce the risk of plaque biofilm, toddlers and children should not be given snacks.

Proper nutrition during the first 1000 days is a critical period, having a profound impact on an infant's ability to grow, learn, and thrive. The first 1000 days includes nutrition of the mother during pregnancy until the infant reaches age 2 years. During this period, optimal nutrition builds the foundation for brain structure and capacity, lifelong health, and well-being. Achievement of goals established in *Healthy People 2030* will benefit the health of infants and children in the United States, affecting their long-term health status and lifespans.

Infants

An infant's health status, beginning at conception and affecting lifelong well-being, depends on feeding and nurturing the newborn by the mother or caretaker. Infancy is a time of rapid transition from being solely breastfed to introduction of a varied diet consisting of selections from all the food groups daily. The infant is normally able to thrive on human milk or commercially available infant formula, but many physiologic systems are immature at birth. Because of limited stomach capacity, frequent feedings are needed.

Pregnant patients expect the dental hygienist to provide information concerning infant-feeding methods affecting the oral cavity. Practitioners should be prepared to address these issues, basing their advice on scientific evidence. Feeding patterns present during the child's first 2 years create an environment for optimal development of genetically determined factors contributing to oral and general health.[1]

Growth

In infants, toddlers, and children growth is an indicator of nutritional status and health.[2] Nutrition needs change as the child grows. Dental hygienists working with new parents, infants, and children should be familiar with normal growth and developmental patterns associated with adequate nutritional intake.

A healthy breastfed infant is considered the norm for growth patterns in the first year of life.[3,4] Formula-fed infants gain weight more rapidly putting them more at risk of obesity in childhood.[5] The birth weight of an infant doubles in the first 6 months and usually triples by 1 year of age. Length or height increases 50% by 1 year of age. Growth charts developed by the World Health Organization are used for infants and children until age 2 and then Centers for Disease Control and Prevention (CDC) growth charts are used for those age 2 and older (https://www.cdc.gov/growthcharts/who_charts.htm#The%20WHO%20Growth%20Charts).

Nutritional Requirements

Adequate nutrition is more important during infancy and childhood than during any other stage of the life cycle. As might be expected from the rapid growth rate, energy requirements are much higher per pound or kilogram of weight than for an adult: 95 to 83 cal/kg per day between 3 and 12 months of age (energy needs per kg decrease from birth to 12 months) versus 29 to 37 cal/kg per day for adults. Infants have a higher resting metabolic rate and intestinal absorption is relatively inefficient.

Adequate Intake (AI) for protein is 1.52 g/kg daily from birth to 6 months of age, and the Recommended Dietary Allowance (RDA) for older infants is 1 to 1.2 g/kg; this translates to about 8 to 13 g/day (Table 14.1).[6] Recommended protein intakes are based on mean protein intake of breastfed infants. At birth, renal functions are immature; total protein should not exceed 20% of the calories. Breast milk and infant formula provide approximately 50% of calories from fat to meet the high-energy needs.[7]

| TABLE 14.1 | Dietary Reference Intakes (DRI) for Infants Compared With Nutrient Content of Human Breast Milk, Cow's Milk, and Artificial Breast Milk |

Nutrient	DIETARY REFERENCE INTAKE[a] 0–6 Months Old	7–12 Months Old	Human Breast Milk (Per Liter)	Cow's (Whole) Milk[b] (Per Liter)	Average Infant Formula (Per Liter)[b]
Calorie	95 cal/kg (3 months)*[c] 85 cal/kg (6 months)*[c]	83 cal/kg[c]	700 cal	610 cal	660 cal
Protein	9.1 g/day*	13.5 g/day	10 g	33 g	14 g
Fat	31 g/day*	30 g/day*	44 g	32 g	35 g
Cholesterol	ND	ND	140 mg	120 mg	0 mg
Calcium	200 mg/day*	260 mg/day*	320 mg	1230 mg	500 mg
Phosphorus	100 mg/day*	275 mg/day*	140 mg	1010 mg	280 mg
Iron	0.27 mg/day*	**11 mg/day**	0.3 mg	0 mg	12 mg
Sodium	120 mg/day*	370 mg/day*	170 mg	380 mg	180 mg
Potassium	400 mg/day*	700 mg/day*	510 mg	1500 mg	710 mg

Note: Recommended dietary allowances are presented in **bold type** and adequate intakes are followed by an asterisk (*).
[a]Data from National Research Council: *The Guide to Nutrient Requirements.* National Academies Press; 2006; National Research Council. *Dietary Reference Intakes For Calcium and Vitamin D.* National Academies Press; 2011.
[b]Data from U.S. Department of Agriculture (USDA), Agricultural Research Service. *What's in the Foods You Eat Search Tool.* 2019–2020. https://www.ars.usda.gov/northeast-area/beltsville-md-bhnrc/beltsville-human-nutrition-research-center/food-surveys-research-group/docs/whats-in-the-foods-you-eat-search-tool/.
[c]Total energy expenditure.
N/A, Not applicable; *ND,* not determined.

Breast Milk

Human milk, nature's superfood for infants, is the optimal source of appropriate amounts of nutrients to help infants reach their maximum potential (Fig. 14.1). Human milk is very complex, and its exact chemical makeup is unknown. It contains growth factors, hormones, bioactive components, enzymes, bacteria (human breast milk microbiome), and antibodies.[7] The microbiome in breast milk promotes healthy gut colonization of the gastrointestinal tract to aid nutrient absorption and help protect infants from infections and illness.[7] This is especially advantageous because the infant's immune system is not fully developed. Exclusive breastfeeding for at least 6 months is strongly recommended globally to improve cognitive development, decrease risk of obesity,[8] and reduce the incidence of gastrointestinal and respiratory infections, ear infections, and eczema. Long-term benefits of breastfeeding include reduced incidence of chronic health conditions such as hypertension, diabetes, and heart disease.[8] Human breast milk composition varies according to maternal diet, health, and needs of the infant, for example, prematurity.[7]

Breast milk is normally thin, with a slightly bluish color. Breast milk contains substantial amounts of long-chain fatty acids (arachidonic acid [ARA] and docosahexaenoic acid [DHA]), which are important for brain and retinal tissue development.[7] Lipase enzyme inherent in breast milk improves fat digestion. The low mineral and relatively low protein content of human milk is ideal for the infant's immature kidneys. Inherent compounds in human milk promote efficient iron utilization. Iron content of breast milk is low, but the bioavailability is 20% to 50% versus infant formula that is 4% to 7% so supplementation is generally not necessary during the first 4 to 6 months for breastfed infants.

Breast milk is highly recommended for infants at risk for developing food allergies. Breastfeeding for at least 4 months may potentially prevent allergies (especially asthma and eczema), but its role in preventing allergies is controversial.[9,10]

Breast milk provides approximately 0.01 mg/day of fluoride, regardless of drinking water and maternal plasma levels. Despite the low fluoride levels, infants who are breastfed up to 12 months are not at risk of dental caries.[11] As shown in Table 14.2, the American Dental Association and American Academy of Pediatric Dentistry (AAPD) recommend delaying fluoride supplements for all infants until 6 months of age.[12]

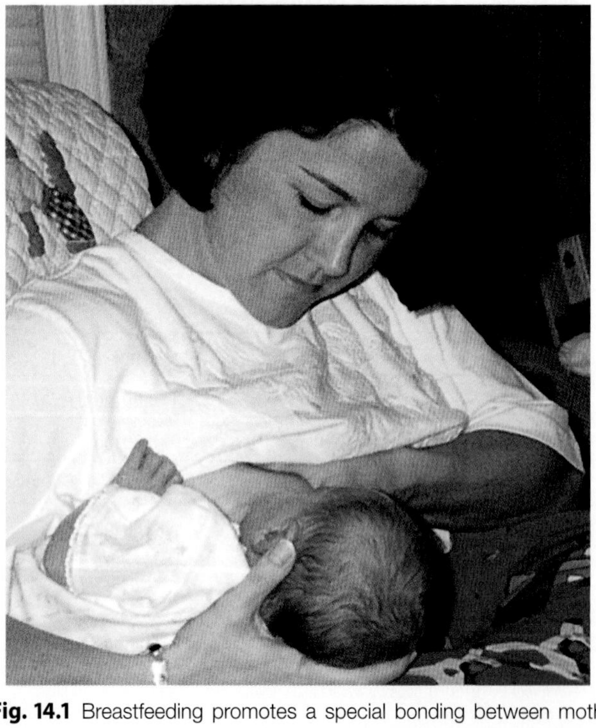

Infant Formula

Although nutrients differ slightly for various brands, all commercial formulas comply with standards set by the Infant Formula Act established in 1980 (see Table 14.1). The US Food and Drug Administration requires that these products meet strict standards. Artificial infant milk formulas duplicate breast milk as closely as technology allows, but the exact composition of breast milk cannot be reproduced, and infant formula cannot match the benefits of breast milk. Infant formulas are continually being modified to ensure that the growth and development of formula-fed infants matches with that of breastfed infants. Adequate nutrients (except for fluoride) are provided in 150 to 180 mL/kg per day in a commercial formula with iron or an appropriate caloric concentration (about 20 cal/oz) until the infant is 4 to 6 months old. Infants given artificial infant milk tend to weigh more than breastfed infants, a negative factor that may put them at greater risk for obesity as adults. However, more research is needed to confirm this association. Breastfed infants develop better control of their milk intake than bottle-fed infants.

Numerous commercial formulas are available to meet different needs and conditions. A health care provider should be consulted regarding any perceived intolerance to artificial breast milk. Almost all formulas are available in different forms; the choice of powdered, concentrated, or ready-to-use is determined by the

• **Fig. 14.1** Breastfeeding promotes a special bonding between mother and infant. (From Lowdermilk DL, Perry SE. Maternity Nursing. 8th ed. Mosby Elsevier; 2011.)

TABLE 14.2 **Fluoride Supplementation**[a]

Age	FLUORIDE ION LEVEL IN DRINKING WATER (PPM)[a]		
	<0.3	0.3–0.6	>0.6
Birth–6 months	None	None	None
6 months–3 years	0.25 mg/day[b]	None	None
3–6 years	0.50 mg/day	0.25 mg/day	None
6–16 years	1.0 mg/day	0.50 mg/day	None

Fluoride Supplement Dosage Schedule—2010.
Approved by the American Dental Association Council on Scientific Affairs.
[a]1.0 ppm = 1 mg/L.
[b]2.2 mg sodium fluoride contains 1 mg fluoride ion.
American Dental Association. Oral Health Topics: Fluoride Supplements. Facts about Fluoride. http://www.ada.org/en/member-center/oral-health-topics/fluoride-supplements#dosage; and American Academy of Pediatric Dentistry (AAPD). Clinical Practice Guidelines Reference Manual. http://www.aapd.org/media/ Policies_Guidelines/G_FluorideTherapy.pdf. From Rozier RG, Adair S, Graham F, et al. Evidencebased clinical recommendations on the prescription of dietary fluoride supplements for caries prevention: a report of the American Dental Association Council on Scientific Affairs. *J Am Dent Assoc.* 2010;141(12):1480–1489.

parent's preference and lifestyle. Some of the types of formulas available include (1) standard cow's milk with and without iron, (2) soy based, (3) hypoallergenic (hydrolyzed protein [protein broken down into amino acids]), (4) reduced lactose or lactose free, (5) elemental formulas, and (6) specialized formulas for special metabolic problems. Other ingredients added to formulas based on new information available include DHA and ARA (natural ingredients of breast milk), added rice (for acid reflux), prebiotics and probiotics, antioxidants, and organic ingredients. When determining which formula to use, parents should discuss any problems or concerns with their health care provider. Formula manufacturers promote products that have no proven benefit; increased regulation of marketing claims by manufacturers is needed to protect consumers and ensure that they make wise decisions.[7]

Fluorosis has been associated with fluoride intake during enamel development; the severity is dependent on dose, duration, and timing of intake. Because of reported cases of fluorosis, no fluoride is added to artificial infant milk, but a small amount is inherently present as a result of some of the ingredients and processing. After 6 months of age, all infants need fluoride supplementation if local drinking water or bottled water contains less than 0.3 parts per million (ppm) of fluoride. Infants receiving breast milk or formula do not need additional water. Most bottled water does not contain fluoride. If bottled water is used for formula dilution, water specially marketed for babies (sometimes called "nursery water") contains appropriate amounts of fluoride. If local water contains too much fluoride, water that contains no or minimal amounts of fluoride—purified, demineralized, deionized, distilled, or reverse osmosis filtered water—are readily available in local stores.

Commercial infant formula is more appropriate for infants than cow or goat milk. Malnutrition has been reported in infants fed home-recipe formulas. This may be related to variations in nutrient composition or unsanitary handling practices that may result in frequent infections or gastrointestinal disorders. In other countries, infants become malnourished and die when food manufacturers fail to include required nutrients or prevent contaminants, or when water mixed with the formula is dirty or contaminated.

Infant formulas should be discontinued by 12 to 14 months of age, and vitamin D–fortified whole milk should be provided until age 2. Low-fat milk is not recommended for children before the age of 2 years. Special toddler formulas are nutritionally safe and do not need refrigeration, but they are unnecessary.

Feeding Practices

Feeding in the first weeks may be every 1 to 3 hours and as the infant stomach grows and they can consume larger amounts at each feeding, they will be able to go longer in between feedings.[13] This feeding pattern gradually evolves, eventually allowing the infant and caregivers to sleep through the night. An infant should never be left alone with a bottle propped during feeding. Propping the bottle leads to overfeeding increasing risk for overweight and obesity.[14] In addition, bottle propping results in pooling of formula in the mouth when the child goes to sleep increasing risk for ear infections and dental caries once the teeth have erupted.[14] In addition, propping the bottle reduces physical contact between the mother and the infant that helps to strengthen bonding.

Oral and Neuromuscular Development

Sucking is more difficult from the breast than from a bottle. Breastfeeding requires the infant to coordinate movement of the lips, tongue, and mandible to extract milk, a process called suckling. Breastfeeding encourages the orofacial development. Infants who are breastfed for at least 6 months are less likely to develop malocclusion—overjet (horizontal projection of upper teeth beyond the lower teeth), crowding (absence of lower arch developmental space), open bite, and posterior crossbite.[15-17] The same effect on decreased risk for the development of malocclusion was found in children breastfed beyond 6 months.[18]

Nonnutritive sucking (sucking on thumb, fingers, or a pacifier), which begins in utero, is normal, giving the child a sense of calm and comfort. It is also important in the development of self-regulation and ability to control emotions. Exclusive breastfeeding appears to diminish the risk of acquiring nonnutritive sucking habits.[19] Nonnutritive sucking is more prevalent in infants who were breastfed less than 6 months versus those exclusively breastfed longer than 6 months.[19] Use of a pacifier is not recommended in infants who are breastfed as it may result in poor breastfeeding outcomes.[20]

Children who engage in nonnutritive sucking daily for more than a year have a higher risk of dental-maxillary anomalies such as anterior open-bite, narrow maxilla with upper protrusion, crossbite; and Class II malocclusion with a possible retrognathic mandible.[21] Prolonged habits altering the orofacial development may lead to orthodontic problems persisting into the permanent dentition.

Introduction of Foods

Good nutrition is essential for the rapid growth and development that occurs during an infant's first year. The complementary feeding period, also called the sensitive period or critical window, occurs around 6 months of age when neither breast milk nor formula adequately meets all the nutrient requirements to promote growth and development.[22] Introduction of complementary foods begins the infant's development of healthy eating and dietary habits.

Introduction of complementary foods is not recommended until 6 months of age but is also dependent on the developmental stage of the infant.[22-24] Developmental readiness for complementary foods includes neuromuscular and gastrointestinal maturation along with the ability to sit without support.[23] Food intake is incredibly complex and impacted by physiological, psychological, and environmental factors. Consuming food (biting, chewing, and swallowing) involves simultaneous coordination of multiple systems. The infant needs to be able to move pureed foods to the back of the mouth for swallowing.[23] If semisolid foods are offered prior to this time, the tongue may force the food out as a reflex action (also called an extrusion reflex).[22]

Development of fine, gross, and oral-motor skills to consume foods correlates with the requirement for additional calories and nutrients. If foods are not added by 6 months of age, undernutrition may result in growth below normal growth curves.[22] Eight teeth normally erupt between 6 and 12 months of age allowing a broader range of nutrient-dense foods and textures to be introduced.

The goal for introducing complementary foods is to promote a pattern of food consumption that matches the child's energy and nutrient needs for ideal growth and development but does not increase risk for becoming overweight. Table 14.3 lists recommendations from Health Canada for feeding infants from birth to 24 months, indicating timing of introduction of supplements

TABLE 14.3   **Key Recommendations of the Joint Statement by Health Canada, Canadian Paediatrics Society, Dietitians of Canada, and Breastfeeding Committee for Canada on Feeding of Infants From Birth to 24 Months**

Birth to 6 Months

1	Exclusive breastfeeding for the first 6 months is considered the standard for infants.
2	Supplemental vitamin D for breastfed infants.
3	Monitor infant growth to assess health and nutrition.
4	Commercial infant formula is the alternative when not breastfeeding. Need careful preparation and storage of the formula to reduce the risks of bacteria-related illness.
5	Feeding changes are unnecessary for most common health conditions in infancy (e.g., colic, constipation, reflux, acute gastroenteritis/diarrhea).
6	The first complementary foods should be iron-rich (e.g., iron-fortified cereal, meat, or meat alternatives).

6–24 Months

1	Breastfeeding is encouraged for up to age 2 years or beyond.
2	It is recommended that infants and young children being breastfed be given a daily vitamin D supplement.
3	Introduction to complementary foods begins at 6 months when signs of physiologic and developmental readiness are observed.
4	First complementary foods should be iron-rich, i.e., meat, meat alternatives, and iron-fortified cereal. Avoid introducing cow's milk until 9 to 12 months of age.
5	Offer a variety of nutritious foods from the family meals, providing a range of textures with a gradual progression.
6	Unless there is a family history of food allergy, common allergenic foods can be introduced at 6 months (consult health care provider).
7	Responsive feeding to promote the development of healthy eating skills. Offer finger foods to promote self-feeding. Encourage use of a cup for fluids.
8	Infant food should be prepared, served, and stored safely.
9	After age 1 year, offer a regular schedule of meals and snacks consistent with Canada's Food Guide.

Adapted from Infant Feeding Joint Working Group. *Nutrition for Healthy Term Infants: Recommendations From Birth to Six Months. A Joint Statement of Health Canada, Canadian Paediatric Society, Dietitians of Canada, and Breastfeeding Committee for Canada.* Updated March 29, 2023. https://www.canada.ca/en/health-canada/services/canada-food-guide/resources/infant-feeding/nutrition-healthy-term-infants-recommendations-birth-six-months.html#a4; Infant Feeding Joint Working Group. *Nutrition for Healthy Term Infants: Recommendations from Six to 24 Months. A Joint Statement of Health Canada, Canadian Paediatric Society, Dietitians of Canada, and Breastfeeding Committee for Canada.* Updated January 19, 2015. https://www.canada.ca/en/health-canada/services/canada-food-guide/resources/infant-feeding/nutrition-healthy-term-infants-recommendations-birth-six-months/6-24-months.html.

and types of appropriate complementary foods. The recommendations from Health Canada mirror recommendations by the World Health Organization and organizations in the United States.[13,22,24,25]

While breastfeeding is encouraged for up to 2 years of age, it is important that complementary foods meet the vitamin, mineral, and nutrient needs of the infant/toddler during the critical developmental stages in the first years of life. A variety of nutrient-dense foods particularly those with iron and zinc should be initiated beginning at 6 months.[24] Table 14.4 indicates the role in growth and development for required nutrients, consequences of deficiency, critical time periods needed, and dietary sources. The consistency of foods offered should progress from pureed to mashed to chopped soft foods to finger foods as the child is developmentally able to safely eat the foods. Developing autonomy in feeding is an important skill that is a part of complementary feeding.[23] Initially the caregiver will provide mashed and pureed foods with a spoon (never in a bottle) and this will progress to the infant developing the psychomotor skills to pick up small foods and feed themselves followed by development of the ability to use a utensil for self-feeding. By age 2 years, the child should have transitioned to eating table foods with the family.[26]

Social and Food Environment

Eating is a social and cultural event in addition to consuming nutrients needed for growth and development. The caregivers (and family) need to be present and engaged with the child during meals by talking to them, making eye contact, and modeling eating behaviors.[22,23,26] It is important to be responsive to the cues from the child in regard to hunger and satiety as the child develops the ability to self-regulate the amount of food consumed.[25,27] Providing a variety of textures, tastes, and different food combinations with minimal distractions during meals is essential.[23–25] Avoid forcing or pressuring an infant or toddler to eat certain foods.[26] It may take 8 to 10 exposures to a food before an infant accepts it.[24] Mismatches or an inability of the caregiver to be responsive to the child's satiety cues can lead to overweight and/or obesity.[27]

Sequence of Introducing Complementary Foods

There is not a particular order in which foods must be introduced, but sources of iron and zinc should be some of the first foods to supplement nutrients not present in significant amounts in breast milk.[24,26] These first foods may include iron-zinc fortified baby cereals mixed with breast milk or infant formula; pureed protein; or dairy foods such as yogurt or cheese.[26] While a variety of foods should be introduced, it is best to start with one food at a time and

TABLE 14.4   The ABCs of Nutrition–Key Nutrients in the First 1000 Days

Role in the Body	Consequences of Deficiency	Vital Time Periods During the First 1000 Days	Dietary Sources[a]

Vitamin A

Critical for vision, supports cell growth and differentiation, plays a key role in the normal formation and maintenance of the heart, lungs, kidneys and other organs, immune function

Damage to the eyes, poor growth, loss of appetite, susceptibility to infections. Vitamin A deficiency is rare in the United States

Pregnancy, infancy, early childhood

Egg yolks, liver, yellow and dark-green leafy vegetables and fruits such as spinach, kale, broccoli, sweet potatoes, pumpkin

Vitamin B6

Essential for normal brain development and function, development of neurotransmitters, chemicals that carry signals from one nerve cell to another, helps the body make the hormones serotonin and norepinephrine which influence mood, and melatonin which regulates the body clock

Muscle weakness, irritability, depression, difficulty concentrating

Pregnancy, infancy, early childhood

Meat, liver, fish, chicken, potatoes and other starchy vegetables, bananas

Vitamin B12

Essential for cell health; aids in the production of DNA, the genetic material in all cells; together with folic acid, helps make red blood cells and helps iron work better in the body

Increased risk of birth defects such as neural tube defects, may contribute to preterm delivery, increased risk of poor cognitive function, failure to thrive

Pregnancy, infancy, early childhood

Meat, fish, poultry, eggs, milk and cheese

Calcium

Bone growth and health, tooth development and function, blood clotting, maintenance of healthy nerves and muscles

Greater risk of rickets, a disease characterized by swollen joints and poor growth, increased risk of bone fractures, increased vulnerability to the adverse effects of lead

Pregnancy, infancy, early childhood

Milk, cheese, yogurt and other dairy products, salmon, calcium-fortified foods

Choline

A critical component of the cell membrane, choline is necessary for the normal function of all cells, critical during pregnancy for the development of the brain, where it can impact neural tube closure and lifelong memory and learning functions

Reduced blood vessel growth in baby's brain in utero, increased risk for brain and spinal-cord defects, nerve and muscle problems, may make folate deficiency more likely

Pregnancy, infancy

Meat, seafood, liver, egg yolks, broccoli and brussels sprouts, breast milk also has high concentrations of choline

Continued

TABLE 14.4   The ABCs of Nutrition–Key Nutrients in the First 1000 Days—Cont'd

Role in the Body	Consequences of Deficiency	Vital Time Periods During the First 1000 Days	Dietary Sources[a]

Vitamin C

Essential to forming collagen, a protein that gives structure to bones, muscle and other connective tissue; plays an important role in immune function and body's ability to resist infections; enhances the absorption of iron

Can lead to scurvy, a serious disease which in infants can cause poor bone growth, bleeding, and anemia, bleeding gums

Pregnancy, infancy, early childhood

Citrus fruits, tomatoes, red and green peppers, broccoli, potatoes

Vitamin D

Critical to bone growth and health, key to a healthy immune system and immune response, promotes calcium absorption

Bones can become thin, brittle or misshapen; causes rickets in children, a disease characterized by swollen joints and poor growth

Pregnancy, infancy, early childhood

Vitamin D is produced by the skin when exposed to sunlight. Food sources of vitamin D include: fortified milk, fish, liver, egg yolks. Breast milk typically contains little vitamin D, and it is recommended that either breastfeeding mothers or breastfeeding infants take a vitamin D supplement

Folate

Essential for the proper development of a baby's brain and spinal cord; required for cell division, growth, and the development of healthy blood cells

Greater risk of neural tube defect—a birth defect in which spinal cord does not close properly, leading to learning disability, paralysis, and babies being born with little to no brain

Before pregnancy, pregnancy

Green leafy vegetables such as spinach and broccoli, beans, certain fruits such as bananas and melons, beef liver, fortified breads and cereals. In 1998 the US FDA began requiring manufacturers to add folic acid to breads, cereals, flours, cornmeals, pastas, rice, and other grain products

Iron

Critical for the proper brain development and function in young children, delivers oxygen to tissues, contributes to regulation of immune function and metabolism

Extreme fatigue and depression, impaired cognitive development, reduced resistance to infection

Pregnancy, infancy, early childhood

Eggs and meat, dark leafy vegetables such as spinach, legumes (e.g., beans, lentils), whole grains, fortified breads and cereals. Full-term, healthy babies typically receive enough iron from their mothers in the third trimester of pregnancy to last for the first 4 months of life. Exclusively breastfed babies may need to receive an iron supplement starting at 4 months.

Vitamin K

Plays a key role in helping the blood clot, preventing excessive bleeding

Increases the risk of uncontrolled bleeding, vitamin K deficiency bleeding can potentially result in gross motor skill deficits; long-term neurologic, cognitive, or developmental problems; organ failure or death

Newborn, early infancy

Because all babies are born vitamin K-deficient, a single injection of vitamin K administered at birth is standard practice in the United States

TABLE 14.4 The ABCs of Nutrition–Key Nutrients in the First 1000 Days—Cont'd

⊏ Role in the Body	⚠ Consequences of Deficiency	🕐 Vital Time Periods During the First 1000 Days	✗ Dietary Sources[a]

LC-PUFAs

⊏ These fats, particularly DHA, play a major role in brain development and health. DHA is a major component of retinal and brain tissues, necessary for the formation of healthy cell membranes and support growth and immunity

⚠ Poor weight gain, lowered immunity, poor attention span, hyperactivity, or irritability, problems learning

🕐 Pregnancy, infancy

✗ Fresh fish and fish oils are ideal sources of LC-PUFAs. Cold water/oily fish such as salmon, mackerel, herring, tuna, sardines, and anchovies are high in LC-PUFAs; as well as some seeds and nuts such as flax seeds and walnuts. Breast milk contains small but significant amounts of LC-PUFAs that are necessary for optimal development of the brain, the retina, and other infant tissues

Protein

⊏ Essential component of all cells in the body, muscle tissue, organs, and neurotransmitters in the brain, critical for proper brain development, regulates metabolism

⚠ Fatigue, increased infections, muscle weakness, failure to thrive

🕐 Pregnancy, infancy, early childhood

✗ Eggs, meat, poultry, fish, legumes (e.g., dry beans, peas, nuts), milk and dairy products

Zinc

⊏ Essential for cell growth and metabolism, supports healthy growth and brain function, immune system, and bone growth

⚠ Decreased fetal movement and heart rate variability during pregnancy, possible increased risk of preterm birth, increased risk of infection, poor growth in children

🕐 Pregnancy, infancy, early childhood

✗ Red meat, poultry, whole grains, milk and dairy products, oysters

[a]In general, healthy, full-term breastfed infants receive an adequate amount of all of these nutrients with the possible exceptions of vitamin D and iron.
DHA, Docosahexaenoic acid; *FDA,* Food and Drug Administration; *LC-PUFAs,* long-chain polyunsaturated fatty acids.
Courtesy 1,000 days, 1020 19th Street NW, Suite 250, Washington, DC 20036. From *The First 1,000 Days: Nourishing America's Future.* 2016. www.thousanddays.org/resource/nourishing-americas-future.

wait to try a new food for 3 to 5 days to observe for any allergic reaction. Emerging evidence suggests that introducing vegetables exclusively for the first two weeks of the complementary feeding period results in the child being more likely to consume or willing to try vegetables.[28] Vegetables prepared in a variety of ways should be introduced early to improve acceptance.[26] An infant's grimace when offered a new food is not a sign of dislike. The infant may be reacting to the texture, temperature of the food, or a new taste and it is not unusual to need to expose them to a new food many times before they accept it. Preference for sweet, salty, and unami flavors is an **innate** (inborn) preference over bitter or sour flavors.[26] However with repeated exposure infants and toddlers can learn to like vegetables and other foods. Fruits (not including fruit juice) without added sugar should be a part of the foods introduced, but it should follow the introduction of other nutrient-dense foods.

The *Dietary Guidelines for Americans 2020–2025* provides Dietary Patterns for toddlers aged 12 through 23 months as well as older children.[24]

Commercial infant food may be used, but foods from the family menu can be pureed or finely chopped. Using foods that the family is eating allows the child to experience the common foods the family eats and is less expensive. Avoid highly processed snack foods marketed for infants and toddlers as they offer few nutrients.

Food Allergy

Foods most commonly causing allergies are cow's milk (including ice cream), eggs, peanuts, tree nuts (e.g., walnuts, almonds, cashews, pistachios, pecans), wheat, soy, fish, and shellfish.[26] Introduction of allergenic foods should be initiated at home rather than at a restaurant or daycare center. Evidence shows that exposure to allergenic foods in the first year reduces the risk of developing allergies to those foods.[26] For instance, exposure to peanuts by 11 months of age resulted in an 81% lower rate of peanut allergy at 60 months of age.[26] International consensus guidelines support the benefits of early peanut introduction to reduce the risk of allergy.[29]

Foods to Limit

Fruit juice should not be introduced before 12 months of age; limited to 4 oz/day in toddlers 1 through 3 years of age; and 4 to 6 oz/day for children 4 to 6 years of age.[26,30] The American Academy of Pediatrics' (AAP) rationale for this recommendation was that juice (1) could interfere with infant's consuming the amount of milk or formula needed; (2) lacks the fiber of whole fruit; (3) is easily overconsumed, possibly contributing to weight concerns; and (4) can increase the risk of dental caries. When fruit juice is provided for children age 1 and older, it should be offered in a cup with a meal to limit caries risk. Too much fruit juice—including apple, pear, and prune—can cause diarrhea and decrease intake of other foods containing essential nutrients for infants and toddlers.

Avoid added sugars as foods or beverages for infants and toddlers.[24,26] Nutrient-dense foods are essential to meet the infant and toddler needs for growth. Early introduction to sweets can also strengthen the lifelong preference for these foods.[24,26] Sugar-sweetened beverages like soda have no place in the infant/toddler diet which may otherwise place them at risk for being overweight or obese along with dental caries.[31,32]

Limit foods high in sodium including processed meats, some commercial toddler foods, and salty snacks.[24,26] Choose food with very limited or no added salt.

Honey should not be given to infants under 12 months of age due to the risk of botulism.[24,26] Unpasteurized foods should also be avoided due to the potential for bacterial contamination.

Supplements

The American Academy of Pediatrics (AAP) and Health Canada recommend that exclusively breastfed infants and partially breastfed infants consuming less than 1000 mL of formula each day receive 400 IU (10 µg) vitamin D supplementation beginning during the first 2 months to prevent rickets and continuing until infants are weaned on consuming 1000 mL/day or more of vitamin D–fortified formula or whole milk.[33,34] Artificial formulas marketed in the United States provide 400 IU or more of vitamin D per 1000 mL. Vitamin D supplements marketed for infants supply 400 IU/day. Despite recommendations, only 40% of American infants meet the guidelines for vitamin D.[35]

Healthy, full-term infants have adequate iron stores at birth for the first 6 months, however, iron-rich complementary foods are recommended beginning at 6 months.[24,26,33] Supplementation prior to 6 months of age should be determined in consultation with the pediatric provider.[24] Iron supplementation (usually ferrous sulfate or ferric ammonium citrate) is ordinarily given as liquid drops.

Fluoride supplementation is recommended for infants older than 6 months and children to increase the strength and acid resistance of developing tooth enamel.[12] Before fluoride supplementation is prescribed, however, the AAPD recommends a caries risk assessment along with an evaluation of dietary sources of fluoride (e.g., fluoridated water).[36] Vitamin supplements containing fluoride may be prescribed by a health care provider or dentist (see Table 14.2).

🦷 DENTAL CONSIDERATIONS

Assessment

- *Physical:* Infant's developmental stage, neuromuscular development, age, lip biting, thumb sucking, tongue thrusting, pacifier use.
- *Dietary:* Parent's knowledge and practices for breastfeeding, bottle feeding, feeding of solid foods, oral care for the infant, source of iron, fluoride intake (drinking water from home, daycare, and school; beverages such as soda, juice, and infant formula; prepared foods, and toothpaste), and use of other supplements.

Interventions

- Avoid recommending sugar-free foods, especially those containing sorbitol, which may cause diarrhea in infants and children.
- Inform parents that supplements containing fluoride should not be consumed with milk; fluoride binds with calcium, decreasing absorption of fluoride.
- Exposure to too much fluoride in the early stages of enamel maturation may alter the structure and cause fluorosis.[37]
- Nonfluoridated or minimally fluoridated water is recommended for reconstituting powdered formulas to reduce risk of fluorosis.[38]

🦷 NUTRITIONAL DIRECTIONS

- Follow the pediatric care provider, *Dietary Guidelines* or CDC guidelines for the preparation of infant formula and storage of infant formula or expressed breast milk.[24,39]
- The rate of growth is faster during infancy than at any other stage of life. Fats, a concentrated source of energy, are needed to support growth (40%–50% of the total calories is recommended).[6] Reduced-fat milk is inappropriate for children younger than 2 years.
- Infant formula beyond 12 months of age is not recommended.[24] Prolonged bottle feeding is associated with overweight,[40] obesity,[41] lower intake of meat, meat alternatives, and fruit,[42] iron deficiency anemia,[43] and early childhood caries.[44]
- Cholesterol intake is important during early developmental stages of infancy.
- Store all vitamin-mineral supplements in a place that is protected from children; many children die each year from accidental iron overdose.[45,46]
- Children younger than 2 years should not consume foods or beverages with added sugars.[24,26]
- Honey is inappropriate for children younger than 1 year of age because of the risk of botulism.[24,26,47]
- Toddlers learn about food by touching and playing with it. Encourage this by offering finger foods when the child can sit alone and pick up items.
- During the first year, habits and preferences are beginning to form. Fostering healthy eating early will promote healthful lifelong eating patterns.[24,26]
- After solid foods are introduced, the goal is to gradually include a variety of foods from all food groups on a daily basis. Offer a variety of vegetables early to increase acceptance.

Oral Health Concerns in Early Childhood

Tooth formation begins before birth and is not completed until about 12 years of age; the structure of the tooth is affected by nutrient intake during this time. A clear relationship has been shown between nutritional deficiency during tooth development and tooth size, tooth formation, time of tooth eruption, and susceptibility to caries.[48] Calcium and vitamin D must be present for proper calcification of dentin and normal enamel. Vitamin D is crucial to tooth development; later deficiency may promote tooth decay.[49]

Dental caries are largely preventable, but they remain the number one chronic disease of children and adolescents. Globally the prevalence of early childhood caries is 48% and ranges from a high of 82% in Oceania to 30% in Africa.[50] In US children aged 2 to 5 years, 23% had dental caries in their primary teeth in 2011–16; 10% of children in this age group had untreated dental caries. Untreated dental caries was 15.1% of Hispanic and 14.8% of African American children had untreated dental caries; 17.2% of 2 to 5 year olds in households below 100% of poverty level had untreated dental caries. The strongest risk factors for early childhood caries include lower parental education, untreated caries, exposure to smoking prenatally or secondhand, high levels of *Streptococcus mutans*, poor oral hygiene, visible plaque biofilm, and frequent consumption of sugar-sweetened foods and beverages.[51,52]

Infant Oral Care

Dental problems can begin early. Children who have caries as infants or toddlers have a much greater probability of subsequent caries in permanent teeth.[53]

Good dental care starts in infancy, before the first tooth emerges. Decay and early loss can damage permanent teeth before they erupt. The infant's gingiva should be cleaned daily with gauze, with a soft infant toothbrush and water, or with an infant tooth cleaner to remove plaque biofilm.

When teeth begin erupting, parents should continue brushing the teeth with a soft infant toothbrush using no more than a smear or rice-size amount of fluoride toothpaste twice daily for children under 3 years. The AAPD recommends a visit to the dentist following eruption of the first tooth, typically around 6 months of age, but no later than age 1 year.[36] The earlier the dental visit, the better the chances of preventing dental problems. When the child is able to expectorate (usually around 3 years old), a pea-sized amount of fluoride toothpaste can be used. Because the child does not have the dexterity to brush the teeth thoroughly, the parent should continue brushing the child's teeth as long as needed.

After the first baby teeth begin to erupt, at-will nighttime feedings should be avoided. Infants and toddlers should not be given a bottle or sippy cup of milk or juice in bed. If the infant is given a bottle in bed, it should contain only water. Children should be offered a cup beginning at age 6 months and gradually weaned from the bottle or breast by 12 to 18 months of age.[54] Prolonged bottle feeding may result in dental caries, poor nutritional intake, and risk for overweight and obesity.[54]

Between meals, the sippy cup should contain only water. Sugar-sweetened beverages and fruit juice should not be given to children younger than 12 months of age[24,30] and in very limited amounts thereafter as it increases the risk of early childhood caries and overweight/obesity.

Early Childhood Caries

Early childhood caries (ECC) is the presence of one or more decayed, missing (resulting from caries), or filled tooth surfaces in any primary tooth in a child younger than 6 years old.[55,56] ECC affects more than 600 million children globally.[56] ECC, the term currently used, replaces the terms *nursing bottle caries* and *baby bottle tooth decay* and is characterized by early rampant decay associated with a number of risk factors including inappropriate feeding practices (Fig. 14.2). Any sign of smooth surface caries in children younger than age 3 years is indicative of S-ECC

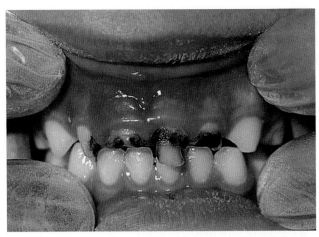

• **Fig. 14.2** Early childhood caries. (From Swartz MH. *Textbook of Physical Diagnosis, History, and Examination*. 7th ed. Saunders Elsevier; 2014.)

(severe early childhood caries), which is a serious public health problem, especially prevalent in lower socioeconomic groups.[55] ECC may compromise food intake and lead to failure to thrive; pain and infection may lead to emergency room visits and need for treatment under general anesthesia; impact ability to learn and contribute to missed school days; and a lower oral health related quality of life.[55] Because ECC is preventable, health care professionals need to provide anticipatory guidance with regular preventive visits beginning at 6 months of age to prevent the disease.

Contributing Factors

Diet is one of the primary etiologic factor in the caries process. However, only advising parents to "avoid sugar or sweets" has limitations in preventing caries because the dietary factors involved in the caries process are more complex than simply avoiding added sugars. The primary contributing factor to ECC are acid producing bacteria including *S. mutans* and Lactobacillus.[55] However research on the microbiome of children with ECC is ongoing so other bacteria may be identified as efforts are made to develop saliva testing to identify children at risk.[55,57] Colonization of *S. mutans* occurs only after the infant's teeth erupt. Infection with the pathogen *S. mutans* is transmitted through vertical transmission from the caregiver to the infant[58] and through horizontal transmission from siblings and playmates.[59] Kissing and sharing utensils or other objects contaminated with saliva are contributing factors. However, whether ECC develops depends on many factors including frequent or prolonged exposure to a fermentable carbohydrate such as infant formula, breast milk, and juice (Box 14.1).[58] Acid produced by bacteria leads to demineralization of enamel. Allowing an infant to go to bed at night or at naptime with a bottle, on-demand breastfeeding, and adding sweet beverages to bottles or sippy cups are risk factors for ECC.[52] Breast milk and infant formula are equally cariogenic.

As the child sleeps, cleansing action of saliva is diminished because of reduced salivary flow. The ultimate effect is poor clearance of the cariogenic liquid pooled in the mouth. Also, the natural or artificial nipple rests on the palate during sucking, allowing the liquid to pool around the maxillary incisors. The position of the tongue covers and protects the mandibular incisors. Because the disease state follows the eruption pattern, maxillary incisors are affected, followed by first molars and then canines.

• BOX 14.1 **Sources of Fermentable Carbohydrates for Infants**

Liquids
- Cow's milk, plain and flavored
- Breast milk
- Formula
- Fruit juices and drinks
- Syrup added to water
- Any sugar-sweetened beverages

Other Sources
- Some infant foods
- Flavored yogurt
- Liquid medication
- Use of sweets to comfort or reward infant or relieve constipation, such as a pacifier dipped in honey or corn syrup
- Infant cereals, teething biscuits, crackers, puffs
- Dry cereals
- Arrowroot biscuits and other cookies
- Fruits

Nutritional Advice

Parents must understand their role in preventing childhood dental disease. Begin anticipatory guidance as soon as the dental team is apprised of the pregnancy. During the initial visit with the child no later than 12 months of age, the goal is to establish a dental home to set the stage for early prevention of oral disease. The early visits are an opportunity to educate parents and provide developmentally appropriate anticipatory guidance that includes controlling oral bacteria and appropriate feeding practices.[36]

🔹 DENTAL CONSIDERATIONS

Assessment
- *Physical:* Cursory oral examination to detect decalcification or carious lesions in teeth; frequency of daily biofilm removal; destructive habits such as lip biting, thumb sucking, tongue thrusting, or pacifier use.
- *Dietary:* Parental knowledge of ECC and what causes it; parental preferences for sweets; sharing of utensils contaminated with saliva; use of bottle propping, especially at night, or continuous use of a sippy cup throughout the day; dipping the bottle nipple or pacifier in honey or molasses; continued use of the bottle after age 1 year; and appropriate fluoride consumption.

Interventions
- Recommend routine dental visits and provide guidance to parents on feeding practices and nutritional needs.
- Teach parents to clean the infant's gingiva after feeding with a clean cloth. A soft infant toothbrush and water can be used when the infant has several teeth.
- If the water supply is optimally fluoridated, encourage using a smear or rice-sized amount of toothpaste until the child learns to expectorate.
- Discuss possible future problems of rampant decay in an infant (discomfort, dental anxiety/fear, infection, cost, tongue-thrust habit).
- Educate expectant parents and parents of infants about techniques for preventing ECC, that is, avoid bottle propping; not using the bottle or sippy cup as a pacifier at bedtime or throughout the day; and not putting sugar-sweetened beverages or fruit juice in the bottle. Use other methods instead of a bottle at bedtime to calm the child, such as rubbing the child's back, rocking in a chair, singing to the child, or providing a favorite stuffed toy.

- Parents should be advised to avoid saliva-sharing practices, such as sharing a spoon when tasting food, to prevent transmission of caries-causing bacteria (*S. mutans*) to the infant.
- Educate parents about risk factors and prevention of ECC (1) to identify early white spot lesions in a young child, (2) encourage parents to have treatment for any active caries, and (3) avoidance of sweets to comfort or reward the infant.
- Explain the importance of primary teeth (appearance, speech, ability to eat). Patients may be under the false impression that because primary teeth fall out, they serve no purpose.
- Discuss the role of carbohydrates (including those present in fruit juice and milk) in the decay process.

🔹 NUTRITIONAL DIRECTIONS

- Do not let the infant suck the bottle unattended.
- Avoid putting fruit juice or other carbohydrate-containing beverages in a bottle. Offer juice in a cup.
- If a fluoride supplement is recommended, tablets should be thoroughly chewed and swished between the teeth before swallowing. The child should not eat or drink for 30 minutes after taking the supplement and should avoid milk products for 1 hour because calcium may interfere with bioavailability of fluoride.
- Limit the child's access to a bottle or sippy cup containing milk, juice, or any sugar-sweetened beverage.
- Home filtration systems may remove fluoride; thus filtered and treated water should be tested to measure fluoride content. Most state health departments assess the fluoride content of water for a minimal fee.
- During the first year, foods that require chewing should be added based on the number of erupted teeth.
- Wean infants from the bottle soon after the first birthday.

Cleft Palate and Cleft Lip

One of the most common birth defects in the United States is **cleft lip** or **cleft palate**, or cleft lip/palate, a malformation in which parts of the upper lip or palate fail to grow together. National data for the prevalence of cleft lip or palate is incomprehensive as data is only available from 11 states. Based on this limited data, approximately 1 of 2800 live births is born with cleft lip with or without cleft palate.[60] Scientists believe numerous factors, including drugs, heredity, and folic acid deficiency, may cause this malformation.

When feeding the infant with a cleft palate, with or without a cleft lip, the main priority is to ensure adequate nutrition. Because of the opening between the roof of the mouth and the floor of the nasal cavity, negative pressure needed for sucking cannot be created (see Figs. 14.3 and 14.4A). However, breastfeeding sometimes can be successful; the infant adapts by squeezing or chewing the nipple. Breastfeeding may promote better growth than spoon-feeding following surgery for cleft palate.[61]

The infant is held in a semi-upright position to prevent formula from entering the nose. Squeezable bottles appear easier to use than rigid feeding bottles.[61,62] Other feeding difficulties include nasal regurgitation, excessive air intake, and frequent burping. As soon as possible, spoon-feeding is introduced. In severe cases, a prosthesis is made when the child is older (see Fig. 14.4B). Length of time needed for feedings to provide adequate nutrients can be exhaustive for both mother and infant. Special feeding devices available are recommended when lengthy feedings are necessary (Box 14.2).

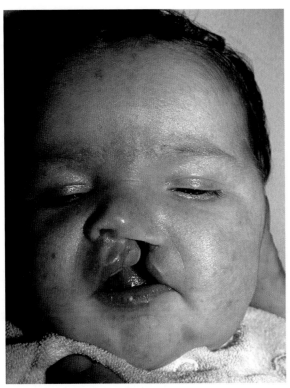

• **Fig. 14.3** Cleft lip/palate. (From Kaban L, Troulis M. *Pediatric Oral and Maxillofacial Surgery*. Saunders Elsevier; 2004.)

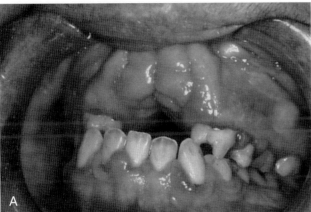

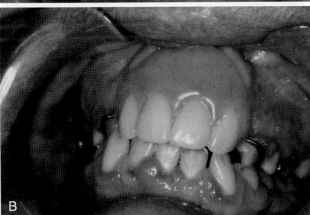

• **Fig. 14.4** (A) Cleft palate. (B) Cleft palate with removable prosthesis. (Courtesy Kathleen B. Muzzin, Texas A&M University School of Dentistry, Dallas, TX.)

• **BOX 14.2** | **Suggestions for Feeding an Infant With Cleft Palate**

- Breastfeeding can be difficult for the infant with cleft palate so the mother should keep the infant in a more upright position at a 45-degree angle to prevent choking. Alternative feeding positions may be necessary such as a modified football method.
- If it is not possible for the infant to breastfeed, breast milk can be expressed and delivered through bottle.
- Nipples for bottle feeding should be soft plastic so little pressure is needed to express milk. A crosscut "X" in the nipple can help with expressing milk more easily.
- Feed every few hours with feeding sessions lasting no more than 30 min
- Burp frequently to aid in releasing excessive air intake.
- Prior to repair of a cleft palate, the infant will need to transition from bottle feeding to spoon-feeding to prevent injury to the site of the surgical repair.

Typically, cereals are the first food introduced and then new nutrient-dense foods can be introduced as recommended for any infant. However, citrus and other acidic foods may be irritating to the tissue around the cleft or to a healing repair.

- Caregivers will need support from an interprofessional team to help manage feeding challenges successfully.

Mink van der Molen AB, van Breugel JMM, Janssen NG, et al. Clinical practice guidelines on the treatment of patients with cleft lip, alveolus, and palate: an executive summary. *J Clin Med*. 2021;10(21):4813. doi:10.3390/jcm10214813. From Kumar Jindal M, Khan SY. How to feed cleft patient? *Int J Clin Pediatr Dent*. 2013;6(2):100–103. doi:10.5005/jp-journals-10005-1198.

Babies born with cleft lip, with or without cleft palate, have no greater risk for health problems and death than infants born with no disability, but they have increased rates of dental abnormalities, including supernumerary, missing, or malformed teeth.[63]

⬡ DENTAL CONSIDERATIONS

Assessment
- *Physical:* Cleft palate/lip, aspiration.
- *Dietary:* Feeding technique and past experiences in feeding infants.

Interventions
- Explain that the principal problem is a lack of normal suction and, by modifying feeding techniques, the infant can obtain adequate nutrients.
- Feed the infant slowly at a 60- to 80-degree angle to provide nutrients while minimizing risks.

⬡ NUTRITIONAL DIRECTIONS

- Introduce spoon-feeding as soon as possible.
- Oral skills develop after surgery to correct the problem.
- Acidic and spicy foods may irritate delicate tissue in the cleft area.
- Young children with cleft palate are at increased risk for choking on foods that may slip into the trachea.
- Because of increased incidence of enamel hypoplasia[64] meticulous oral hygiene practices and limited cariogenic food or liquids is recommended to reduce risk for carious lesions at these sites.
- Refer parents to local support groups and to the American Cleft Palate Association for literature and support.

Children Older Than 2 Years of Age: *Dietary Guidelines 2020–2025* and *Healthy People 2030*

Healthy eating and physical activity patterns optimize normal growth and development, promote cognitive development, and reduce risk for future health problems. Consuming appropriate amounts of nutrients can be best achieved by considering the child's whole diet pattern, using principally nutrient-dense food from each of the main food groups. The Healthy U.S.-Style Dietary Pattern is recommended for choosing foods for meals[24]: (1) select a mix of foods from the five food groups—vegetables, fruits, grains, dairy, and quality protein sources, including lean meats, fish, nuts, seeds, and eggs; (2) offer a variety of food experiences; (3) avoid highly processed foods; (4) avoid high sodium foods and added sugars; and (5) offer appropriate portions.

The general consensus is that most children's diets "need improvement" or are "poor" and are below the recommendations indicated in the Dietary Reference Intakes (DRIs Table 14.5).

TABLE 14.5   Daily Nutritional Goals for Vitamins and Minerals Based on Dietary Reference Intakes for Age-Sex Groups

	Source of Goal	Female 4–8	Male 4–8	Female 9–13	Male 9–13	Female 14–18	Male 14–18
Calorie level(s) assessed		1200	1400–1600	1600	1800	1800	2200, 2800, 3200
Minerals							
Calcium (mg)	RDA	1000	1000	1300	1300	1300	1300
Iron (mg)	RDA	10	10	8	8	15	11
Magnesium (mg)	RDA	130	130	240	240	360	410
Phosphorus (mg)	RDA	500	500	1200	1250	1250	1250
Potassium (mg)	AI[a]	3800	3800	4500	4500	4700	4700
Sodium (mg)	UL	1900	1900	2200	2200	2300	2300
Zinc (mg)	RDA	5	5	8	8	9	11
Copper (mcg)	RDA	440	440	700	700	890	890
Manganese (mg)	AI[a]	1.5	1.5	1.6	1.9	1.6	2.2
Selenium (mcg)	RDA	30	30	40	40	55	55
Vitamins							
Vitamin A (mg) RAE	RDA	400	400	600	600	700	900
Vitamin E (mg) AT	RDA	7	7	11	11	15	15
Vitamin D, IU	RDA	600	600	600	600	600	600
Vitamin C (mg)	RDA	25	25	45	45	65	75
Thiamin (mg)	RDA	0.6	0.6	0.9	0.9	1.0	1.2
Riboflavin (mg)	RDA	0.6	0.6	0.9	0.9	1.0	1.3
Niacin (mg)	RDA	8	8	12	12	14	16
Vitamin B_6 (mg)	RDA	0.6	0.6	1.0	1.0	1.2	1.3
Vitamin B_{12} (mcg)	RDA	1.2	1.2	1.8	1.8	12.4	2.4
Choline (mg)	AI[a]	250	250	375	375	400	550
Vitamin K (mcg)	AI[a]	55	55	60	60	75	75
Folate (mcg DFE)	RDA	200	200	300	300	400	400

[a]*AI*, Adequate intake; *AT*, α-tocopherol; *DFE*, dietary folate equivalents; *RAE*, retinol activity equivalents; *RDA*, recommended dietary allowance; *UL*, tolerable upper intake level.
From Institute of Medicine. *Dietary Reference Intakes: The Essential Guide to Nutrient Requirements.* National Academies Press; 2006; Institute of Medicine. *Dietary Reference Intakes for Calcium and Vitamin D.* National Academies Press; 2010. U.S. Department of Health and Human Services and U.S. Department of Agriculture. *2020-2025 Dietary Guidelines for Americans.* 9th ed. https://www.dietaryguidelines.gov/.

For children aged 2 to 17 years, the Healthy Eating Index–2010 scores ranged from 44.6% to 49.6% out of an ideal score of 100% in 2015 to 2016.[65,66] The Healthy Eating Index measures the quality of diets based on the *Dietary Guidelines*. Dairy and protein food groups scored highest (approximately 85%). The estimated number of children 2 to 5 years of age with poor diet quality was 39.8% and this increased with age to 66.6% in those aged 12 to 19 years.[65] Despite these findings, there were modest improvements in intake of the food groups.[65] Intake of vegetables (especially dark greens and beans), replacing refined grains with whole grains, and substituting seafood for some meat and poultry along with reducing foods with high sodium are still necessary. Prevalent and persistent childhood nutritional concerns include energy balance, excessive intakes of saturated fats, added sugar, and sodium.

Children 3 to 5 years of age generally meet physical activity guidelines. Physical activity decreases for most children after age 7 years, partially due to more nonacademic screen time and increases the risk of being overweight or obese.[67–69] Underconsumed nutrients of public health concern include calcium, potassium, magnesium, dietary fiber, and vitamin D (nutrients contributed from dairy foods, vegetables, fruits, seafood, and whole grains).[41] Intake of many of these nutrients decreases with age; intake of teenagers, especially girls, is notably lower than intake of younger children. Also of concern are excessive amounts of several nutrients; sodium, total and saturated fat, added sugars, and total caloric intake are significantly above amounts recommended in the *Dietary Guidelines* and the Acceptable Macronutrient Distribution (AMDR) (Box 14.3). The rationale behind the AAP recommendations to limit fruit juice consumption to 8 oz/day for children 7 to 18 years of age is to encourage whole fruit consumption for the benefit of fiber intake and because of the longer time to consume the same amount of calories as opposed to juice consumption.[30]

Healthy People 2030 objectives directly linked to weight and food and nutrition consumption for children age 2 years through adolescence are shown in Table 14.6. Some 2030 objectives are new so only baseline data is available. Existing objectives either worsened or had little or no detectable changes with the exception of success in reducing sodium intake and increasing vitamin D intake.[70] The key message of *Dietary Guidelines* (variety, moderation, and balance in food choices) applies to childhood nutrition. The rationale for providing dietary recommendations and guidelines for children older than 2 years are to (1) provide adequate calories and nutrients to support growth and development and ensure genetic potential, and (2) reduce risk of diet-related chronic diseases later in life. Children's diets containing adequate energy and 25% to 35% of total energy from fat have positive effects on health later in life.

Due to the increasing prevalence of childhood obesity, children and adolescents are experiencing co-morbidities formerly seen primarily in adults such as Type 2 diabetes, hypertension, and high cholesterol.[71] While the US Preventive Health Services Task Force does not recommend screening of all children and adolescents, it does support targeted screening of children and adolescents with a family history of hypercholesterolemia (high cholesterol) or premature CVD.[72,73] Another measure of health

---

• BOX 14.3 Acceptable Macronutrient Distribution Ranges (AMDRs) for Children and Adolescents

AMDRs as a percentage of energy intake for carbohydrates, fat, and protein are as follows:

- Carbohydrates—45%–65% of total calories for ages 2–18 years
- Fat—30%–40% of calories for ages 1–3 years, and 25%–35% of calories for ages 4–18 years
- Protein—5%–20% for ages 1–3 years, and 10%–30% for ages 4–18 years

  Added sugars should not exceed 10% of total calories (to ensure sufficient intake of essential micronutrients).

  Consumption of saturated fat should be less than 10% of calories per day beginning at age 2 years.

  Nutritional goals for total fiber are as follows:

- Children ages 1–3 years: 14 g/day (M/F)
- Children ages 4–8 years: 17 g/day (F)/20 g/day (M)
- Children ages 9–13 years: 22 g/day (F)/25 g/day (M)
- Adolescents ages 14–18 years: 25 g/day (F)/31 g/day (M)

Data adapted from U.S. Department of Agriculture, U.S. Department of Health and Human Services. *Dietary Guidelines for Americans.* 9th ed. 2020. dietaryguidelines.gov

---

TABLE 14.6 *Healthy People 2030* Objectives for Children Over Age 2 Years

Objective	Progress (☺ ☹)
Reduce the proportion of children and adolescents with obesity.	☹
Eliminate very low food security in children	☹
Increase contribution of intake from	
• fruits	☺
• total vegetables	☺
• dark-green vegetables, red and orange vegetables, beans and peas	☹
• whole grains	☺
• increase vitamin D consumption	☺
Increase calcium intake.	☹
Reduce consumption of calories from	
• saturated fat	☹
• added sugars	☹
Increase intake of potassium	☹
Reduce consumption of sodium	☺

From Office of Disease Prevention and Health Promotion. *Healthy People 2030.* U.S. Department of Health and Human Services. https://health.gov/healthypeople/objectives-and-data.

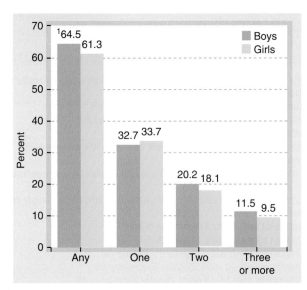

• **Fig. 14.5** Percentage of youth aged 2–19 years who consumed sugar-sweetened beverages on a given day, by number of beverages and sex: United States, 2011–14. [1]Significantly different from girls, $P < .05$.

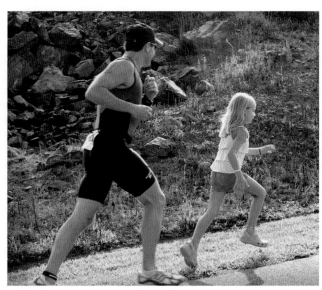

• **Fig. 14.6** Parents should encourage individual physical activities and model these behaviors. (Courtesy Sara Birkemeier, Raleigh, NC.)

is CVH (cardiovascular health) scores which range from 0 to 100 and those with higher scores are at greater risk for poor cardiovascular health. In children 2 to 19 years of age the CVH based on diet, physical activity and body mass index was 65.5 suggesting cardiovascular health was not optimal.[74] Avoiding obesity by balancing energy intake, making healthy choices following the healthy dietary patterns in the *Dietary Guidelines*, and regular physical activity in childhood is central to a lifetime of cardiovascular health.

The *Dietary Guidelines* recommend less than 10% of total energy intake from added sugars, which would mean between 120 and 200 cal or 30 to 40 g of sugar daily. Consumption beyond these levels puts the child/adolescent at risk of exceeding energy needs leading to obesity and/or replacing healthy options putting them at risk for inadequate nutrient intake and dental caries. As shown in Fig. 14.5, almost two-thirds of US youth consumed at least one sugar-sweetened beverage on a given day and including children aged 1 to 5 years, 57% consumed a sugar-sweetened beverage at least once in the preceding week.[75,76]

While the visual image of the five food groups for *MyPlate* website appears the same for all ages, the portion size differs for adults, adolescents, and children. The MyPlate.gov website provides many resources to help provide parents, caregivers, and teens information about appropriate portion sizes based on age, sex, height, weight, and physical activity. The *Dietary Guidelines* also provide guidance on healthy eating patterns to maintain a healthy weight and reduce risk of chronic disease.

About 18% of energy comes from junk food for children aged 2 to 19 years.[65] One in five calories consumed by children is from junk food.[65] Junk foods that children consume come primarily from grocery stores (73%) with about 8% from restaurants.[65] To address healthy eating, the National Restaurant Association created the Kids LiveWell Program to help parents make healthier choices from kids' menu items.[77]

Physical activity is important for bone mineralization, growth, and cardiovascular health. Parents should encourage individual physical activities and model them for the children (Fig. 14.6). Children should be given the opportunity to participate in a variety of activities, from walking to jumping rope to competitive sports. Activity is important in helping manage weight and reduce the risk for CVD, diabetes, and high blood pressure.

The Physical Activity Guidelines for Americans advocates preschool children to have at least 3 hours of physical activity throughout the day.[78] The recommendation is for 1 hour or more of physical activity daily for children 6 to 17 years old. The 60 or more minutes of physical activity daily for older children should include each of the following at least 3 days a week: (1) either moderate- or vigorous-intensity aerobic activity, (2) muscle-strengthening activity, and (3) bone-strengthening activities.[78]

By ensuring that at least half of the grain servings are whole grains, as recommended in the *Dietary Guidelines*, fiber and other nutrient guidelines can be met. Current intakes of whole grains and vegetables are below recommendations in all age groups.[24] The *Dietary Guidelines* and *MyPlate* website promote increasing fruit and vegetable consumption to five or more servings daily. To increase fiber intake, fresh fruits are recommended over fruit juice.

Because of the high calcium requirement to increase bone mineral density in children, milk and dairy products are essential components. Calcium and vitamin D levels were established to achieve optimal bone mineral health to decrease the risk of osteoporosis later in life. Average dairy intake is below recommended levels in children aged 2 years and over, and continues to worsen in teenagers.[24] Dairy and fortified alternatives should be encouraged because they contain nutrients needed for overall health and accrual of adequate bone mass.[24]

Utilizing the ChooseMyPlate Website

The *MyPlate* website (http://www.ChooseMyPlate.gov) provides guidance for healthy food choices and an active, healthy lifestyle for all life stages. The website has resources for parents, children, and teens providing information to help make healthy eating choices. As discussed in Chapter 1, and depicted in Fig. 1.4, the plate divides foods into five major food groups: grains, vegetables, fruits, dairy, and proteins. As children grow, needs may differ from those in the *MyPlate* website guide. A doctor, nurse, or RDN should be consulted about a child's nutritional needs and how to best meet them if problems such as lethargy, undernutrition, excess weight gain, or symptoms of any chronic disease, are observed.

ChooseMyPlate.gov website (https://www.myplate.gov/life-stages) provides guidelines, tips, and resources for preschoolers, kids, and teens to help improve health and well-being. This website provides information about appropriate foods and portion sizes and suggestions for meal patterns or snacks. Additionally, age-appropriate activities for preschoolers and school-age children include cooking skills, games, activity sheets, videos, and songs. Getting children involved in food preparation and cooking early increases their kitchen responsibilities.

These activities help children and teens become more aware of the connection between their food choices and feeling healthy and their ability to participate in physical activities, thus providing a fun way to learn about nutritional needs. The website can also be helpful for teachers to plan activities and classroom materials. It also offers cell phone apps including *Shop Simple with MyPlate* and *Start Simple with MyPlate*.[79]

Toddler and Preschool Children

Growth

After the child reaches 1 year of age, the growth spurt slows. A toddler gains approximately 4 to 6 lb until the age of 2 years, and height doubles by age 4 years. In a normally growing child, height increases parallel to the weight. Children grow approximately 2 to 3 inches a year and gain around 5 lb a year. One-half of adult height is achieved by 2½ to 3 years of age.

Nutrient Requirements

The caloric requirement for infants/toddlers from 12 months to 2 years of age is 700 to 1000 calories/day to support growth and development.[24] It is essential that foods consumed by young children are nutrient dense because they are unable to eat large quantities. The Dietary Guidelines provide food patterns for this age group to help caregivers plan healthy diets for them.[24] Added sugars are to be avoided, yet estimates are that the added sugar accounts for 104 calories/day in infants/toddlers 12 months to 2 years of age.[24] This might not sound like much for an adult, but for a toddler with a calorie budget of 700 to 1000 calories, it is significant. Even snacks need to be carefully planned to choose nutrient-dense options. Healthy snacks can contribute vital nutrients, but snacks are frequently energy-dense foods and beverages with added sugars, saturated fat, and sodium.[24]

Energy intake of preschool children has trended higher since 1989 to 1991, especially in families of Hispanic origin, with low income and low educational levels.[80] Higher energy intake has resulted in overweight being pandemic even in young children (see *Health Application 14*), and eating patterns established at this age may impact lifelong health. By striving toward healthy eating and physically active habits, children may achieve healthful weights, possibly preventing lifetime risks of chronic health problems.

During the past 30 years, the nutritional status of children in the United States has improved, with few nutrient deficiencies observed. The estimated number of children 2 to 5 years of age with poor diet quality was 39.8%.[65] Poor diet quality and nutritional status of children (as measured by growth rate and biochemical indices) are more prevalent in lower socioeconomic groups with food insecurity.[66]

Anemia remains a public health concern among young (less than 2 years old) low-income children. Among children aged 1 to 2 years, 13.5% were iron deficient and 2.7% had iron deficiency anemia.[81] The incidence of anemia usually declines with age and is observed more often in households that are food insecure.[82] Iron-rich foods, such as meat, and fresh fruits and vegetables containing vitamin C to enhance iron absorption, are expensive compared with calorically dense foods such as chips or candy. Milk is a poor source of iron and large amounts of milk impair iron absorption. While iron is important for brain development, the evidence about the effect on cognitive and psychomotor abilities needs more research.[83]

As mentioned earlier, research studies note that ensuring vitamin D sufficiency throughout childhood and during the time of maximal bone mineral accrual seems particularly warranted. The prevalence of vitamin D insufficiency (<75 nmol/L or <30 ng/mL) in the United States was 47% to 56% in infants and 16% in children.[84] Depending on vitamin D intake and amount of sun exposure, a supplement may be needed.

Food-Related Behaviors

Lifelong habits and food attitudes are formed during preschool years that, to some extent, affect health throughout life.[23,24] A variety of foods should be available that provide the needed nutrients. Basic understanding of the nutrient content of foods, the role of foods in health, and food-related behaviors for these age groups is important for parents and caregivers to promote food habits conducive to adequate nutrient intake. Healthful eating produces benefits in cognitive and physical performance, fitness, psychological well-being, and energy level.

Parental attitudes and food preferences, eating habits, and food choices are influential factors in the child's food preferences.[85] Choosing a variety of healthy food is more effective than telling a child what to eat. Foods disliked by one or both parents may not be served often or at all; children tend to enjoy foods preferred by their parents. Providing fruits for snacks and serving vegetables at mealtime may affect a young child's eating patterns for life.

When planning menus, parents must consider the child's food preferences, but parents must maintain control over the options. Without appropriate guidance, young children do not independently make healthy food choices; the parents' role is to offer nutritious foods and role model eating the foods. Children can choose how much or even whether they will eat the food provided. Parenting style impacts feeding practices and ultimately the risk for obesity. Authoritarian parenting styles and responsive feeding are associated with maintaining a healthy weight.[86] Feeding problems can result when either the parent or the child crosses this line of responsibility (i.e., the parent bribes or forces the child to eat, or the child is allowed to tell the parent what to prepare). Family mealtime is essential for children's nutrition, health, and overall well-being. Family meals have benefits in regard to diet quality.[87]

Toddlers (1 to 3 Years Old)

Food preferences are formed in these early years so it is critical to introduce a variety of flavors and textures.[26] During the second year of life, toddlers develop fine motor skills while learning to feed themselves, but skills and capabilities do not occur at exactly the same time for every child. Although this is a messy learning process, this transitional period stabilizes by age 2 years. Finger feeding may be preferred to spoon-feeding; some finger foods should be provided at every meal. A toddler can manipulate a cup by about 12 months of age.[13] Rotary chewing skills develop in the second year. Until then, finely chopped meats are accepted more readily minimizing the risk of choking.

Caregivers are responsible for familiarizing the toddler with new foods; deciding on the types of foods offered; frequency of foods offered; amount of food; responding to the child's cues for hunger and satiety (responsive feeding); serving as role models for eating; and managing the eating environment (e.g., family meals, limit distractions).[26] Eating on a regular schedule each day is desirable and helps control appetite.[26] Regular meals also help to avoid fatigue, which can lead to an overly emotional situation that interferes with appetite. Tired children eat poorly. If the child has been very active, a short rest period before the meal improves intake.

Three meals and 2 to 3 snacks a day are recommended. Small amounts of food should be offered for each.[13] Serving sizes should be based on appetite, but initially about 1 tbsp of food can be offered for each year of age. The amount of liquids consumed can result in a poor appetite for foods, or more food is consumed in addition to the calories provided in liquid form.

Food jags (may eat only one or just a few foods for several days) in toddlers and children are common and may be a way to assert independence. Parents should continue to offer a variety of healthy foods and let the child decide what and how much to eat.[26] Do not pressure the child to eat or show signs of frustration which may prolong or even lead to more problematic picky eating behaviors.[26]

Appetites can be erratic and unpredictable which is normal and may relate to the current growth rate of the child.[13,26] When well-balanced meals are provided, caloric intake at any given meal varies greatly, but compensation at subsequent meals is normal.[26] If sufficient amounts are not eaten at the meal, parents should be sure the child is not drinking too many liquids before meals and provide nutrient-dense snacks. Snacks can contribute significantly to adequate nutrient intake (Box 14.4).

Until age 4 years, children are more at risk for choking on food because they are learning to chew and the primary dentition has not fully erupted. Foods most likely to cause choking include: (1) small nuts and seeds, such as peanuts; (2) round, firm, smooth foods such as grapes, hard candy, hot dogs, and round candies; (3) dry or hard foods, such as raw carrots, cookies, pieces of pretzels, potato chips, and popcorn; and (4) sticky or tough foods such as chewing gum, raisins, chewy fruit snacks, tough meat, and caramel candy.[26,88] To prevent choking, closely supervise children at all times while eating and do not allow walking, playing, talking, laughing, crying, or lying down while they are eating.

Safe levels of caffeine intake for children are unknown. Estimates are that the average intake of caffeine in 2- to 8-year-old children is approximately 15 to 30 mg/day and comes primarily from soda.[89,90] However, there are concerns of access to energy drinks and possible overdose so caffeine should be minimized and ideally avoided.

• BOX 14.4   Healthy Snack Choices

- Cut-up fresh vegetables with low-fat dip or salad dressing
- Air-popped popcorn with a sprinkle of parmesan cheese
- Fresh fruit[a]
- Frozen fruit (grapes, bananas)[a]
- Nuts
- Low-fat cheese (sticks, strings, cubes, or slices)
- Low-fat cottage cheese or yogurt
- Peanut butter on apple slices[a] or celery sticks
- Pretzels[a]
- Baked chips[a]
- Hard-boiled eggs
- Animal crackers[a]
- Graham crackers[a]
- Sliced turkey or chicken
- Dry, low-sugar cereal[a]
- Rice cakes[a]
- Low-fat pudding[a]
- Sugar-free gelatin with fruit
- Mini bagels[a]
- Pickles
- Frozen juice bars[a]

[a]Cariogenic potential. Encourage tooth-brushing after snacks.

Preschool Children (4–6 Years Old)

Preschoolers are relatively independent at the table and can feed themselves. More frequent family meals have shown positive associations with children developing positive health behaviors and eating a better quality diet.[91] Parents should be aware of the developmental stage of their child and focus on positive non-mealtime activities. Conversation and role modeling can reinforce appropriate eating behavior and promote intake of a variety of foods.

To encourage children to try new foods, let them choose new foods at the grocery store. Engage children in growing vegetables and helping to prepare them in the kitchen. Encourage children to help with preparation for meals like washing vegetables, helping to measure ingredients or setting the table. Offer children the option to choose and pair foods they like with new foods. Remember that new foods may need to be offered more than a dozen times before they are accepted. Even after they have accepted a food, preschool children may not eat it every time it is served. The USDA MyPlate for Life Stages (https://www.myplate.gov/life-stages) has many resources for parents and caregivers.

Because preschool children still enjoy eating with their fingers, cutting fruits and vegetables into small pieces increases their acceptance. Cutting foods into fun shapes can make them more appealing, for instance, use a cookie cutter to cut their peanut butter sandwich into a shape they love like a unicorn. Preschoolers generally prefer their foods separate; casseroles and stews may not be well-accepted. Nutrient-dense snacks may supplement meals to meet daily nutrient intake (see Box 14.5). The body uses food more effectively and energy levels are more consistent when children "refuel" every 2 to 4 hours. The number of snacks varies, depending on the family schedule, and the child's activity and hunger levels.

● DENTAL CONSIDERATIONS

Assessment

- *Physical:* Socioeconomic level, child's age, and child's developmental level.
- *Dietary:* Eating environment, frequency of meals and snacks, quantity of foods consumed, adequacy of intake, parental beliefs and food preferences.

Interventions

- Encourage eating meals at regular times and family meals. Serve food shortly after being seated to avoid restless behavior.
- Evaluate and assess children's diets at regular intervals.
- Growth charts are available on the *MyPlate* website for children that can be used by parents to ensure appropriate growth rates.
- Stress the importance of providing adequate amounts of protein; vitamins A, C, and D; calcium; phosphorus; and fluoride during formation and calcification of teeth.
- If sufficient amounts are not eaten, provide nutrient-dense snacks, as shown in Box 14.4.
- Consider parents' attitudes, cultures, beliefs, fears, and educational levels when developing and providing oral health education.
- Help parents clarify any misconceptions about providing healthy food options to their child.
- Recommendations for fluoride usage should be determined by need, based on caries risk assessment.
- Encourage the use of fluoridated toothpastes for children older than 2 to 3 years.
- Encourage parents to assume responsibility for the child's oral health care and model good oral health behaviors.
- Refer low-income patients to government or local social programs (e.g., Women, Infants, and Children [WIC] program, Supplemental Nutrition Assistance Program [SNAP]) for which they may be eligible.

- Minimize the use of processed foods that contain added sugars, sodium, and fat.
- Water is the ideal beverage between meals; omitting sugar-sweetened beverages (sodas and fruit juice) helps prevent risk of excess weight gain by limiting extra calories and dental caries by lowering the frequency of tooth exposure to sugar.
- Offer children whole fruits rather than fruit juices or fruit drinks and limit fruit juice to 6 oz/day.
- By offering a wide variety of foods to toddlers who are healthy and growing appropriately, parents need not be overly concerned about risk of nutrient deficiency.
- Teach the child to use an age-appropriate rice-size smear or pea-size amount of toothpaste to limit the amount accidentally swallowed.
- Ensure that the child receives a dental examination every 6 to 12 months; topical fluoride may be applied if the water supply is not fluoridated. The dental team determines an appropriate fluoride regimen for each child.
- The goal for parents/caregivers is to prevent caries by minimizing intake of cariogenic foods and manage plaque biofilm formation.

● NUTRITIONAL DIRECTIONS

- Small amounts of new foods should be served with foods the child likes and recognizes. It may take offering a new food many times before it is accepted. The child should be encouraged to help with selecting food at the grocery store, growing it in the garden, and preparing meals which may increase acceptance of the new food.
- Risk of heart disease begins in childhood; a reduction of dietary fats (especially saturated) after the second birthday is recommended to reduce the risk of CVD. However, restriction of fat intake could compromise a child's growth and development.
- Until age 6 years, a good rule of thumb for a serving size is one-half an adult portion. Food, especially sweet foods, should not be used as a bribe or reward.
- Teach children to recognize their hunger and satiety cues rather than expecting them to clean their plate. Children who are told to "clean your plate" may be at increased risk of obesity.[92]
- Diet and lifestyle choices during early childhood affect lifelong eating patterns and impact later disease risk.
- Successful childhood feeding may be best accomplished by providing a variety of healthful foods and allowing children to eat without coercion.
- Provide nutrient-dense healthy snacks, but prevent the child from grazing throughout the day to ensure a good appetite at meal time.
- Encourage dairy products for children to support bone health and reduce the risk for prepubertal fractures.
- Family meals are encouraged to develop healthy food behaviors and good diet quality.
- Provide a wide variety of vegetables and fruits daily, especially dark-green, leafy, and deep yellow vegetables and colorful fruits.

● BOX 14.5 Help Children Maintain a Healthy Body Weight

- Develop and model healthy eating patterns with a focus on nutrient-rich choices.
- Encourage adequate sleep.
- Start the day in a positive way with breakfast. Breakfast helps spread the calories throughout the day and helps avoid mid-morning unhealthy snacks.
- Set guidelines for the amount of time that children spend watching television, playing video games, or playing on electronic devices.
- Set goals for physical activity; plan family activities involving physical activity. Instead of watching TV, go hiking or biking, wash the car, or walk around a mall. Offer choices and let children decide.
- Eat meals together as a family and eat at the table, not in front of a television. Eat slowly and enjoy the food. Eating at home with family often translates into a healthier diet.
- Avoid using food as a reward or punishment. Spend some quality time together; take a walk or go on a long bike ride.
- Focus on positive goals. Allow children to determine goals they want to achieve, such as being able to swim five laps in a specified time.
- Do not be too restrictive; focus on moderation. Children should not be placed on restrictive diets unless ordered by a pediatrician (for medical reasons). Encourage kid-sized portions. Sweets and fast foods should be curtailed, but they can be used sparingly.
- Children need food for growth, development, and energy, but if they are forced to clean their plates, they are doing their bodies a disservice.
- Make eating a family activity. Involve children in meal planning, grocery shopping, and meal preparation. This helps them learn about healthy eating and gives them a role in decision making.
- Keep healthy snacks on hand. Good options include fresh, frozen, or canned fruits and vegetables; low-fat cheese, yogurt, or frozen fruit juice bars.
- Monitor what children drink. High-energy drinks provide a lot of sugar with little health benefit.
- Stock the refrigerator and pantry with nutrient-dense healthy foods; do not purchase foods they should not eat.
- Make small changes as a family. Menu changes should be implemented for all family members. Begin parking the car a little farther away or eating fast food less often.
- Focus on small, gradual changes in eating and activity patterns. This helps form habits that can last a lifetime.
- Get active. Plan activities involving the whole family, such as skating, hiking, or biking. Make an after-dinner walk a regular part of the family's evening.

Attention-Deficit/Hyperactivity Disorder

Attention-deficit/hyperactivity disorder (ADHD) is the most common neurobehavioral disorder of childhood and for about half of children this persists into adulthood.[93,94] ADHD also co-occurs with developmental disorders such as autism.[94] Hyperactivity is characterized by chronic age-inappropriate behaviors, including inattention, impulsiveness, hyperactivity, restlessness, and problems in social interaction and academic performance. Research continues into the etiology of ADHD, but usually both genetic factors and environmental factors (e.g., heavy metals, prenatal exposure to maternal smoking, childhood exposure to secondhand smoke) are involved.[95] Nutritional factors include low maternal vitamin D levels, lower blood levels of omega-3 fatty acids, and a very small increase in ADHD with exposure to artificial food dyes.[95] A common misconception is that sugar causes hyperactivity, or ADHD, in children, but evidence fails to support this belief.[96]

Evidence suggests a healthy diet pattern like those recommended by the Dietary Guidelines for Americans are protective against ADHD.[97] Limiting processed foods will also aid reduce intake of artificial dyes. A diet rich in omega-3 fatty acids would also be prudent.

Children With Special Needs

Developmental conditions, such as intellectual disabilities, cerebral palsy, Down syndrome, and autism spectrum disorder may have significant implications for oral health. Issues affecting oral health can include chewing, swallowing, drooling, gastroesophageal reflux, behavioral problems, and difficulty performing oral self-care.[98]

Children with cerebral palsy and Down syndrome may practice bruxism. Bruxism is involuntary grinding or clenching of teeth, which results in abnormal wear patterns on teeth and joint or neuromuscular problems. Malocclusion, dental malformation (e.g., enamel defects), and delayed tooth eruption may also occur.[98] Children with cerebral palsy, Down syndrome, and intellectual disabilities are likely to have abnormal sensory input and muscle tone. Difficulties with sucking, swallowing, spoon-feeding skills, chewing, and independent feeding are common. Oral habits such as tongue thrust, mouth breathing, and food pouching associated with many of these conditions may result in delayed oral clearance of food increasing caries risk.[98] Dental problems may become exaggerated in the child as a result of difficulty in maintaining good oral hygiene, the child's unique dietary habits and patterns, and the effect of prescribed medications. Such problems include oral infections, dental caries, and periodontal disease.

Treatment by an interprofessional team of health care providers, including a dental hygienist, is individualized depending on the child's potential capabilities and skills. Nutritional intervention for feeding-skill difficulties involves assistance from a registered dietitian nutritionist (RDN) and occupational therapist in planning a diet easiest for the child to eat and meets nutritional needs.

⬧ DENTAL CONSIDERATIONS

Assessment
- *Physical:* Condition of the oral cavity, presence of dental caries, plaque biofilm, abnormal oral-motor habits, such as tongue thrust, bruxism, oral-motor development, medications.
- *Dietary:* Intake of fermentable carbohydrates, frequency of snacking, calcium and vitamin D intake, sources of fluoride, pica (consumption of non-food items such as paper, dirt, and cigarette butts).

Interventions
- Prior to the first visit, talk or meet virtually through telehealth with the parent/caregiver to gather medical/dental history and identify what has worked and what has not worked to make the dental visit a positive experience for the child.
- Behaviors that are rewarded will increase in frequency. Provide reinforcement throughout the dental procedure by verbally praising desirable behavior and tangible rewards (stickers, baseball cards). Provide appropriate recommendations or referrals.
- These children are less likely to maintain good oral hygiene; schedule more frequent recare appointments.

⬧ NUTRITIONAL DIRECTIONS

- Provide nutritious snacks, such as cheese cubes, string cheese, or raw vegetables. Fibrous foods promote salivary flow, increasing the buffering capacity of saliva. However, if the child has chewing or swallowing difficulties, the snack choices may need to be adjusted.
- Vitamin D–fortified milk and cheeses not only provide nutrients needed for healthy teeth but also are cariostatic.
- Provide an opportunity to brush the teeth after eating; if brushing is not possible, rinse with water.
- Inappropriate dietary habits and unhealthy food preferences developed during childhood have lifelong implications.
- Limit sticky carbohydrate foods—such as candies, cookies, crackers, pastries, potato chips, and raisins—between meals. Frequently choosing these at snack time may contribute to dental caries risk.

School-Age Children (7–12 Years Old)

The middle childhood years continue to be an important period for the formation of eating habits. New activities and friends begin to influence choices and broaden the child's horizon. Students who consume an adequate amount of fruit, vegetables, milk, protein, fiber, and other components of a healthy diet are more likely to perform better in school and maintain good nutrition practices that affect lifelong health. The child exposed to different foods and food patterns usually enjoys more foods. New ideas experienced with friends and at school may affect food choices at home.

The healthy eating index scores decline from 61 in toddlers and young children to 52 in 9 to 13 year olds.[24] This age group exceeds recommended limits for added sugars, saturated fat, and sodium.[24] Average vegetable, fruit, dairy, and whole grain intake are below recommendations while refined grains are above recommendations for daily food group intakes.[24] Protein intake tends to be close to or slightly below the recommendations.

Family meals can be an opportunity to offer healthy choices. Nutrients available from family dinner meals are significantly associated with the child's overall dietary intake.[87,91] Encourage children to help make grocery lists, choose meals for the family menu, and assist with the preparation and cooking of meals. Stocking the kitchen with healthy snacks may encourage healthy eating.

School breakfast and lunches can improve dietary quality when the child is away from home.[99] During the COVID-19 pandemic, universal school meals were made available showing improvements in food security and academic performance.[100] Some states such as California, Colorado, Maine, Minnesota, New Mexico, and Vermont have passed legislation for universal school meals and other states may follow.

Minimize availability of foods with added sugars, refined grains, high sodium, or saturated fat. Children may still access these foods from peers, vending machines, and school bake sales, but modeling healthy habits at home can help children build lifelong habits. Ultimately children need to be educated to make healthy choices, the *MyPlate* website (https://www.myplate.gov/life-stages/kids) has games/apps and activities to engage children.

Dental Caries in School-Age Children

According to the CDC, trends in the prevalence of untreated tooth caries in the permanent teeth of children have improved, but 13.2% of children between 5 and 19 years still have untreated caries.[101] The odds of untreated dental caries were greater based on family income, access to care, and race/ethnicity.[102] Untreated dental disease can lead to pain, infection, school absences, and poor academic performance.[103] In addition, children could experience feelings of embarrassment, withdrawal, and anxiety.

This age range generally marks exfoliation of all or most of the primary teeth and the eruption of most permanent teeth. Systemic fluoride is effective before eruption and during the mineralization phase of erupting teeth. When 1 ppm of fluoride in drinking water is present during tooth formation, the caries rate is reduced 26% in permanent teeth.[104] To provide maximum protection, systemic fluoride is recommended through age 16 years for children in nonfluoridated or inadequately fluoridated areas. Application of topical fluoride (professionally and self-applied) becomes as effective as systemic fluoride for school-age children. Topical administration of fluoride (dentifrices, rinses, gels, fluoride supplements, varnishes, and fluoridated water) can help in the reduction of tooth decay.[105] For early carious lesions, silver diamine is also effective in arresting caries.[105]

Application of sealants (a clear or shaded plastic material applied to occlusal surfaces of permanent teeth) acts as a barrier protecting caries-prone areas of teeth from plaque biofilm and acid.[105] However, even oral self-care, fluoride toothpaste, and sealants cannot completely prevent caries due to other risk factors.

Another factor in caries formation is food selection and patterns of consumption (e.g., frequency). Cariogenicity of food is influenced by the presence of fermentable carbohydrates, physical properties, and frequency of consumption (see Chapter 18). While evidence is conflicting in regard to xylitol preventing caries, the use of sugar-free chewing gum containing xylitol has been shown to reduce levels of harmful *S. mutans* bacteria in plaque biofilm which may aid in reducing caries risk.[106–108]

● DENTAL CONSIDERATIONS

Assessment
- *Physical:* Schoolwork or emotional difficulties, activity level, sports interests.
- *Dietary:* Nutrient and fluid intake, appetite, food preferences and eating patterns, child's and parent's beliefs about nutrition.

Interventions
- Evaluate sources of fluoride to ensure optimal intake to protect erupting and newly erupted teeth while minimizing excessive intake and risk for fluorosis.
- Use a motivational interviewing approach for children and parents to encourage behavior change in regard to oral hygiene habits for caries prevention.
- Antimicrobial agents, such as chlorhexidine, can be used to control existing plaque biofilm and formation of new plaque biofilm by controlling bacteria and limiting acid production.
- Ask low-income parents/caregivers about access to food, as food insecurity is a concern for many families. In addition, explore whether the child is participating in government child nutrition programs (e.g., National School Lunch, School Breakfast, Summer Food Service, and Special Milk).

● NUTRITIONAL DIRECTIONS

- Cutting foods into shapes (smiley faces, stars, or animals) often creates interest in the food or snack. Engaging children in helping by using cookie cutters can make it more fun for kids.
- Children involved in meal preparation are more likely to eat the food they prepare, and to be aware of what is in the food.
- Have nutritious foods available for snacks (see Box 14.4).
- Encourage healthy choices for meals and snacks. Refer to the MyPlate website for many resources.
- Encourage appropriate oral hygiene techniques.

Adolescents

Growth and Nutrient Requirements

Major biological, social, psychological, and cognitive changes occur during adolescence. Because of these changes and rapid growth rates, American teenagers are considered to be at nutritional risk due to Healthy Eating Index of 51 (on a scale of 100), consuming inadequate amounts of vegetables, fruits, dairy, and whole grains along with the excess saturated fat, sodium, and added sugars places them at risk for developing chronic diseases (e.g., diabetes, obesity, and cardiovascular disease).[24] Declining fitness levels are another contributing factor for chronic diseases. The guidelines for the youth are 60 minutes of physical activity per day, yet among high school students, only 29% met this guideline.[78]

The gap between the *Dietary Guidelines* and intake of adolescents places them at risk of nutrient inadequacies at a time of rapid growth and development.[24] Growth of long bones, secondary sexual maturation, and fat and muscle deposition create increased nutrient requirements.

Although the Dietary Reference Intakes (DRIs) provide nutrient recommendations based on chronological age, nutrient needs closely parallel physical development. Adolescent girls need to increase their energy intake sooner and decrease it more quickly than boys because of earlier onset of puberty and lower total body weight after entering adulthood. Adolescent boys have greater nutritional needs than adolescent girls because of growth rates and body composition changes (see Table 14.5). An active 18-year-old boy requires approximately 3200 cal compared with about 2400 cal for an 18-year-old girl.[24] However, teens need to be careful of amounts and frequency of eating when their rapid growth rate levels off and/or with changes in activity level.

In 14 to 18 year olds, on average, males meet the recommendations for total protein intake, but females fall below the *Dietary Guidelines*.[24] The protein intake may also fall below recommended amounts due to fad diets for weight loss, increased needs due to chronic illness, or restrictive diets (e.g., vegan/strict vegetarian). If total calorie intake is inadequate for growth, dietary protein may be used to meet energy needs and would not be available for needed growth and repair. In addition, low protein intake may impact bone development and bone mass.[109]

The need for calcium, vitamin D, and iron is of particular importance throughout childhood. Adolescents are particularly vulnerable to inadequate calcium and vitamin D intake at a time when teens are building bone mass. Peak bone mass on average is reached at 18.8 years in females and 20.5 years in males with peak mineral content reached much earlier at 14.8 years in females and 16.5 years in males.[110] Inadequate intake can affect fracture risk in adolescence as well as development of osteoporosis later in life. Health care providers should educate teenagers about the importance of bone health, achieving maximum bone density, and maintaining strong bones. Daily calcium intake of 1300 mg/day and vitamin D intake of 600 IU (15 µg)/day in addition to adequate protein and exercise during adolescence promotes building of bone mineral density. However, average calcium intake is below recommendations in males with an average of 1105 and 822 mg/day in females 12 to 19 years of age.[111] Vitamin D intake is also well below recommendations at 5.2 µg/day in males and 3.5 µg/day in females.[111] The American Academy of Pediatrics discourages recommendation of supplements in adolescents and advises health care providers to encourage food sources of nutrients to support bone and overall health.[112] The MyPlate website (https://www.myplate.gov/life-stages/teens) has many resources for teens to support them in making healthy choices.

Increased iron is required because of the expansion of blood volume, and increase in red blood cell mass and muscle mass. The average iron intake for males 12 to 19 years of age is 15.8 mg/day and for females, it is 12.2 mg/day. While males exceed the RDA of 11 mg/day, females are below the RDA of 15 mg/day. The higher RDA for girls is to replace iron losses associated with menstruation which puts them at higher risk for iron deficiency. Low iron levels may have critical effects on neurodevelopment in adolescence which may have implications for cognition and learning.[113] Risk for inadequate iron levels include disordered eating, vegan and other restrictive eating patterns, and participation in sports with high training loads (e.g., endurance and resistance training).[114–116] Identifying teens at risk for iron deficiency anemia is essential and dietary changes to include foods rich in iron along with iron supplementation may be indicated to decrease the prevalence of anemia in this age group.[117]

Factors Influencing Eating Habits

Eating is an important part of socialization and exerting one's independence. Food choices are influenced by complex external factors, such as family, peers, mass media, social media, economic and sociocultural factors, and internal factors, such as physiologic needs, body image, self-concept, food preferences, and personal values and beliefs about health and nutrition.[118,119] Probably the strongest influential factor among teenagers is peer pressure including through social media.[118]

Increasing numbers of adolescents are overweight or obese (21.2% or 1 in 5) (see *Health Application 14*).[120] Adolescents are often obsessed with their body image and a desire to change their body shape.[118] Girls are more likely to be dissatisfied and try to lose weight with fad diets and other unsafe weight-loss methods while boys may think they are too thin and want to "bulk up."[118] Restrictive eating is not recommended for adolescents because of the rapid physical and mental development they are undergoing along with the risk for developing disordered eating behaviors that persist into adulthood.[118] Social media increasingly fuels disordered eating promoted by adolescent and celebrity influencers.[119] A discussion of problems associated with eating disorders is presented in Chapter 17. Boys may misuse anabolic steroids both to lose weight and to increase muscle mass which put them at danger of adverse health effects during a time when their body and brain are developing.[121] Lifestyle modifications including diet and exercise following the *Dietary Guidelines* are the initial focus of weight management. The dental hygienist can support the adolescent in making healthy choices.

In order to meet the *Dietary Guidelines* for a healthy eating pattern, nutrient-dense food choices need to be 85% of total calories.[24] The percentage of energy from junk food consumption in children is high accounting for 1 in 5 calories.[122] In particular, adolescents consume more than twice the added sugars consumed by younger children.[123] In 2015 to 2018 children 12 to 19 years old consumed nearly 39% of total calories/day from added sugars.[123] The leading source was sweetened beverages accounting for nearly 51% of added sugars.[123] Potential health problems that may occur as a result of high intake of sugar-sweetened beverages (SSBs) include, but are not limited to overweight, obesity, cardiovascular risk, and dental caries.[31,124,125] The American Academy of Pediatrics continues to advocate for public policies to reduce marketing and access in schools to sugar-sweetened beverages.[126]

In adolescents, commonly consumed SSBs are sports and energy drinks with large amounts of sugar, caffeine, and other stimulant substances.[127,128] While sports drinks in moderation may be appropriate for some athletes for hydration and electrolyte replacement, stimulant-containing energy drinks have no place in the diets of children under age 12 years.[127] Children and adolescents may experience adverse effects from consuming energy drinks which may include dehydration, cardiovascular effects (i.e. irregular heartbeat), anxiety, and insomnia.[129,130]

High-intensity sweetened (nonnutritive, diet or low-calorie) beverages have gained popularity among children and adolescents. Approximately 25% of children report consuming nonnutritive sweeteners at least once daily.[131] While nonnutritive sweeteners may reduce caries risk, they may still result in tooth enamel erosion.[132]

Adolescents have more access to food outside the home with junk food readily available from fast food outlets, vending machines, grocery stores, convenience stores, and restaurants.[122] These foods tend to be of lower diet quality because of increased amounts of saturated fat, added sugar, and sodium. A recent study showed the HEI (Healthy Index Score) for food consumed from restaurants was slightly worse in 2017–18 versus 2003–04.[65] In adolescents, 97% exceed the guidelines for average sodium intake, saturated fat (82%–84%), and added sugars (77%–80%) so these are the areas where the dental hygienist can focus on recommending changes. Fast foods can be consumed in moderation as a part of an overall healthy eating pattern. Looking for healthy options at restaurants can help minimize excess calories, sodium, saturated fat, and added sugars.

Despite the availability of school breakfasts, skipping breakfast tends to increase with age. Skipping breakfast has been associated with a lower diet quality and risk for being overweight or obese.[133] In addition, breakfast may improve school performance on cognitive tasks.[134]

Nutritional Advice

Adolescence is a time for becoming more independent and making decisions which includes making food choices. The MyPlate.gov website provides information targeted at this population in the life stages section which provides resources to encourage teens to take charge of their health. Many factors may impact their food choices such as availability (including food security), personal preferences, cost, peer pressure, marketing/advertising, sports, etc. By presenting nutrition and health information in terms relevant to adolescent lifestyles and personal interests, dental professionals can help teenagers understand how current eating and exercise habits affect their current and future health. Refer to Chapter 21 for guidance about ways to approach nutrition education.

DENTAL CONSIDERATIONS

Assessment

- *Physical:* Activity level, growth spurt, use of illicit drugs, use of tobacco products, body image, self-efficacy, influence of peer pressure, stress level.
- *Dietary:* Adequacy of nutrient intake based on *MyPlate* website; amount and frequency of sodas and energy drinks; use of fast foods, convenience foods, or vending machine foods; food preferences and personal values and beliefs about health and nutrition; dietary and nutritional supplements; breakfast; and alcohol intake.

Interventions

- Encourage use of calcium and vitamin D–rich foods.

- Praise good eating patterns; collaboratively work with adolescents to modify food choices and suggest substitutions.
- Determine the frequency, quantity, and form of cariogenic foods.
- Encourage a smoking cessation program for adolescents who smoke or vape (see Chapter 19, *Health Application 19*).
- Provide knowledge to teens regarding risks of using smokeless tobacco and other tobacco products.
- Encourage parents to promote healthy dietary behavior and provide healthy choices that can contribute to oral health and appropriate weight gain.

NUTRITIONAL DIRECTIONS

- Teenagers should be knowledgeable of long-term risks and benefits of good nutrition, but the best approach is to focus on short-term benefits of eating well.
- Restriction of calorie intake during rapid growth periods compromises lean body mass accumulation despite a seemingly adequate protein intake.
- Intense physical activity can cause increased urinary loss of calcium and red blood cell destruction. Referral to an RDN may be needed to ensure adequate nutritional intake.
- Snacking can have a positive influence on overall nutritional and health status of the teenager. Kitchens should be stocked with nutritious snack foods (see Box 14.4) to encourage good eating habits.
- Water and low-fat or fat-free milk are the most healthful beverages; moderate use of 100% fruit juice has health benefits as well.

- Routine ingestion of sports drinks, energy drinks, and soda with added sugars can lead to dental caries.
- Use of dietary supplements by most adolescents is not needed.
- An inadequate intake of calcium and vitamin D during childhood or adolescence results in not achieving the genetically predetermined peak height and bone mass.
- Children and adolescents who skip breakfast, miss the opportunity to consume a nutrient-rich meal; unhealthful dietary behaviors may have an adverse effect on body weight.
- An adolescent with light skin needs to spend about 5 to 10 minutes in the sun with only a part of the body exposed (arms or legs) two or three times a week to produce enough vitamin D; a person of color needs to spend 15 to 30 minutes. Additionally, calcium intake should be adequate (3 cups of milk or equivalent milk products).

HEALTH APPLICATION 14

Childhood and Adolescent Obesity

Childhood obesity is the greatest challenge to child health in the 21st century, and children born since 1980 may be the first generation worldwide to have shorter life expectancy than their parents as a direct consequence of the obesity epidemic.[135,136] Childhood obesity, similar to adult obesity, is a complex disease caused by an imbalance between calorie intake and output. About one in five children is obese (19.7%).[137] Prevalence of obesity in Hispanic and non–Hispanic Black children is about one in four (26.2 and 24.8% respectively).[137]

The Centers for Disease Control and Prevention recommends that World Health Organization growth standards be used to monitor growth for infants and children from birth to age 2 years. BMI charts are appropriate for boys and girls older than 2 years of age. Because children grow in spurts and frequently grow in height for a while, followed by an increase in muscle mass and adiposity before growing taller again, the BMI is a screening tool used to detect potential weight problems. While BMI has limitations, the American Academy of Pediatrics recommends it for screening of children who are overweight or obese.[138] Overweight has been defined as a BMI that is greater than or equal to the 85th but less than or equal to the 95th percentiles for age and sex. Obesity is greater than or equal to the 95th percentile and extremely obese is a BMI of greater than or equal to 120%. Children with a high BMI do not necessarily manifest clinical complications or health risks related to increased body fat. A high BMI is a cue that more in-depth assessment of the child is needed to assess health status.

The complex factors related to obesity include genetic predisposition, environmental (e.g., easy access to junk food, food insecurity, advertising of unhealthy foods), behavioral (e.g., screen time, sedentary behavior, sleep), and metabolic factors (e.g., hormone signaling of hunger and satiety).[136] Obesity is considered a chronic disease and not merely a result of lack of willpower.

Obesity in children can potentially cause significant physiologic and psychosocial complications leading to negative health consequences.

Health problems associated with childhood obesity include diabetes; high cholesterol and hypertension, which are risk factors for CVD; sleep apnea (interrupted breathing while sleeping); and liver disease.[138] In addition, research demonstrates that childhood overweight and obesity adversely affect adult morbidity and mortality.[135] Oral health implications for childhood obesity include an increased risk for dental caries and tooth erosion.[139–141] Higher levels of plaque biofilm and gingivitis are also associated with obesity in children and adolescents.[142,143]

The US Preventive Services Task Force (USPSTF) regards the prevalence and problems of obesity in childhood as being serious, and recommend all health care providers screen children over 6 years old and adolescents, and refer them to comprehensive, intensive behavioral interventions to promote improvements in weight status.[144] Given dental providers are not experts in the complex area of obesity, our role is to support a healthy dietary pattern consistent with the *Dietary Guidelines* and refer the patient to a health care provider for further guidance.

Obesity is an important issue for all health care professionals to discuss with their patients. Obesity is a systemic problem, not isolated from oral health. The topic is a difficult subject to discuss even in a clinical setting, however, having the discussion has been shown to result in the effective treatment.[145] A focus on a nonstigmatizing approach is the best with first asking permission to discuss BMI or weight, use of person-first language, and more neutral terminology like unhealthy weight or gaining excess weight.[138] Words like obese, overweight, and chubby may be perceived as negative or offensive. Despite all efforts, this discussion may still result in strong emotions such as anger. While the health care provider should validate how the parent or patient is feeling, the focus should be on the child's general and oral health. Treatment of obesity for any child or adolescent requires the expertise of many health care disciplines.

Continued

◆ HEALTH APPLICATION 14—CONT'D

Childhood and Adolescent Obesity

Perhaps more devastating to an overweight child are adverse childhood experiences such as weight stigma, weight bias, and weight-related bullying.[136] Overweight children often experience decreased social involvement, poor body image, low self-esteem, depression, and impaired school performance.[136] All these things may lead to increased risk for eating disorders and unhealthy approaches to weight loss.[136] Children and adolescents want to fit in with peers and having a different appearance can lead to the negative psychosocial consequences previously discussed.

Although the cause of the childhood obesity epidemic is multifaceted, factors driving this phenomenon include rapid changes in modern food selections and activity levels of children superimposed onto genetic and metabolic predispositions for weight gain. The problems of American children eating too many high-calorie fast foods and snacks along with being inactive are well recognized as contributing factors. The problem will not be resolved by any single action; rather, concerted action is needed across many disciplines, sectors, and settings, such as childcare facilities, communities, health care professionals, and schools.

Primary prevention of overweight and obesity in children and adolescents should be the first goal. Components of prevention are for parents/caregivers to model health eating patterns; be physically active as a family; establish consistent sleep routines; and replace screen time with family time (Box 14.5).[146]

For obese children and adolescents, the American Academy of Pediatrics guidelines and USPSTF recommend intensive behavior and lifestyle intervention.[138] In young children, the focus is parents and caregivers with attention to the child's development abilities. In adolescents, the focus is on autonomy, preferences, and self-image.[138] Research shows the greatest factor for success is "dose" or contact hours for the intervention.[138] Motivational interviewing is used as a part of the interventions. In severe obesity (BMI≥35 kg/m^2) bariatric surgery for weight loss is safe and effective, and results in improvement or remission of chronic conditions such as diabetes.[138] Ultimately self-management is critical to the success of maintenance of weight loss. Barriers to treatment can be policies impacting payment for services for the intervention and long-term coordinated care by the medical team.[138]

While oral health care professionals are well-positioned to support patients in making healthy choices and screening for overweight and obesity, research suggests barriers include lack of time, limited knowledge, and fear of offending the patient.[147] Despite these concerns, the role of dental providers is to support the parents and patient in making lifestyle modifications to prevent and manage chronic diseases including obesity. This includes nutrition counseling for healthy dietary patterns particularly in regard to reduction of added sugars along with encouraging being physically active.

◆ CASE APPLICATION FOR THE DENTAL HYGIENIST

A mother brings her 3-year-old son in because of the need for a routine oral examination required by the Head Start program he is attending. She knows that he has some white spots on his front teeth, but he will not allow her to brush his teeth and she does not routinely check to see if he has brushed his teeth. He is still using a sippy cup but gave up the bottle at age 18 months.

Nutritional Assessment
- Willingness to seek nutritional information
- Desire for increased knowledge about healthy dietary patterns
- Knowledge of community resources
- Cultural or religious influences
- Knowledge regarding the *Dietary Guidelines* and *MyPlate* website

Nutritional Diagnosis
Health-seeking behaviors related to lack of knowledge concerning optimal nutrition practices in relation to dental health.

Nutritional Goals
The parent verbalizes correct information concerning the importance of oral hygiene and foods and beverages affecting the oral cavity; is aware of snacks that do not promote dental caries; is able to read food labels; and can name the food groups in *MyPlate* website, the number of servings needed for the child, and portion sizes from each group.

Nutritional Implementation
Intervention: Ask the parent to write down everything the child ate yesterday from the time he got up in the morning until the office visit.
Rationale: This will help tailor the information provided to the needs of the patient. You especially need to know the child's access to the sippy cup during the day, what beverage is in the cup, and whether he goes to bed with it.
Intervention: (1) Encourage intake of a variety of foods, using the *MyPlate* website. Review the number of servings needed and what consists of a serving size. (2) Recommend substituting fresh fruit for juices and limiting fruit juice to 4 to 6 oz daily. (3) Instruct her to avoid products that contain fermentable carbohydrates, such as cookies, crackers, or cereal, between meals.
Rationale: It is the total dietary pattern along with the variety that promotes optimal nutrition. Providing the minimal number of servings prevents nutritional deficiencies in healthy individuals. Certain foods, although they may be wholesome and nutritious, may not be advisable for oral health.

Intervention: (1) Explain how to read labels for carbohydrate content. The name of most sugars ends in "-ose." (2) Emphasize moderation of sugar intake. (3) Explain that "diet" and "sugar free" do not mean that the product is low in calories or low in cariogenic potential. (4) Explain the relationship between carbohydrate and the caries process; emphasize the importance of proper oral hygiene after its use.
Rationale: Refined sugar contains calories and no other nutrients but is acceptable when used in items that contain appreciable amounts of other nutrients (e.g., a pudding would provide more nutrients than a gelatin dessert or carbonated beverage).
Intervention: Consider having the mother bring a food the children often eats and (1) Review the label with the mother to help her understand how to use it, (2) determine a serving size, and (3) explain the types of carbohydrates.
Rationale: Knowledge increases compliance and allows the mom to make informed choices regarding food selections.
Intervention: Discuss the importance of three regular mealtimes and two to three healthy snacks and avoidance of grazing.
Rationale: Adequate nutrients are important for growth and health of the child; only nutrient-dense snacks should be offered to a 3-year-old to obtain adequate nutrients. Assist the child in tooth brushing after meals and snacks.
Intervention: Ask the mother how she feels about being able to implement the changes. If she feels overwhelmed, ask her to choose one change to implement until the next visit.
Rationale: This will give you the opportunity to empathize with her about the difficulties of changing food habits and perhaps make further suggestions for implementing changes.
Intervention: Refer the patient to governmental programs for which she may be eligible—WIC, food stamps, or expanded nutrition programs.
Rationale: These agencies may help in providing healthful foods and provide practical guidelines through newsletters, workshops, and written materials to improve health.

Evaluation
To determine effectiveness of care, have the parent read labels; have the parent state the number of servings and portion sizes needed for her son. Additionally, the parent should be able to plan a menu using foods recommended and to state how to obtain or use community information and support. The parent should be able to indicate how changes in food choices will not only improve overall health but also maintain health of the oral cavity and ensure optimal growth of her son with minimal or no problems in the oral cavity.

◆ Student Readiness

1. Plan meals for 1 day for a family with a 2-year-old toddler, a 10-year-old boy, and a 15-year-old girl.
2. Discuss feeding an infant from birth to 12 months.
3. What is considered normal weight for a newborn?
4. Create an outline for discussing ECC with an expectant parent.
5. A mother wants to know why snacks are needed and which ones to give her preschooler to lessen the risk of developing dental caries. What would you tell her? Provide a list of specific suggestions and food choices for the mother.
6. A mother states that because her child is hyperactive, she is going to eliminate all sugar. What is a good response to this statement?
7. List barriers for not being able to decrease the use of fast food restaurants. List healthier choices available at favorite fast food restaurants.

◆ CASE STUDY

Mrs. C. is at her 6-month recall visit and talks about her 6-month-old daughter, Jennifer. Jennifer weighed 7 lb at birth and now weighs 15 lb. She was bottle fed from birth. At 3 months, Mrs. C. introduced cereals, but Jennifer has resisted all attempts to increase her solid food intake. She is allowed to go to sleep with a bottle propped in her crib at the daycare center.

1. What additional assessment data do you need?
2. Is Jennifer's weight gain within the expected range?
3. How much should she gain in the next 6 months?
4. What potential oral health issue may result from the current feeding practice?
5. The dental hygienist encourages Jennifer's mother to discontinue the habit of putting her in bed with a bottle and to request that the daycare center does the same. Why?
6. The health care provider recommends solid foods be introduced gradually to Jennifer. What foods should be introduced first?
7. When will Jennifer be old enough for finger foods?
8. Why should honey be withheld until 1 year of age?
9. Why would the dental hygienist want to assess Mrs. C's dietary intake?

◆ CASE STUDY

R.J. is a 16-year-old boy who has complained to you about pain from dental caries. He is active in athletics in school and has a part-time job. He is 6 feet, 4 inches tall and weighs 190 lb. You determine from his dietary history that his appetite is very good, and his nutrient intake is adequate except for vegetables. Snacking, principally soft drinks, candy, and cookies, constitutes almost 50% of his total caloric intake.

1. How would you advise R.J.? What motivational factors would you consider for him?
2. What are some dental nutritional diagnoses and goals, and interventions for R.J.?
3. What further data are needed for a complete assessment?
4. When having R.J. choose better snack options, what are some that you would recommend?
5. How do you think R.J. will feel about your suggestions?

◆ CASE STUDY

Norma returns for a 6-month recall visit. Since her last checkup, this 17-year-old girl has developed 12 new dental caries in the mandibular anterior teeth. Norma's parents are in their 50 s. Her father has lost numerous teeth as a result of periodontal disease, and her mother is completely edentulous. Norma has no medical problems other than rhinitis (inflammation of the nasal mucous membranes secondary to allergies), which causes her to breathe through her mouth much of the time. The oral examination showed normal color and tone of the oral mucosa, tongue, and gingiva. She reports eating a varied, well-balanced diet, except for fruit and vegetable intake. Because of the dryness in her mouth, she relies heavily on cough drops and chewing gum.

1. What is a possible cause of these new dental caries?
2. What suggestions would you give her to relieve mouth dryness?
3. Based on her dietary habits, what nutrient(s) may be inadequate?

References

1. Taveras EM, Perkins ME, Boudreau AA, et al. Twelve-month outcomes of the first 1000 days program on infant weight status. *Pediatrics*. 2021;148(2):e2020046706.
2. World Health Organization. *Malnutrition in Children*. https://www.who.int/data/nutrition/nlis/info/malnutrition-in-children
3. World Health Organization. *WHO Child Growth Charts*. 2010. https://www.cdc.gov/growthcharts/who_charts.htm
4. Centers for Disease Control and Prevention, National Center for Health Statistics. *CDC Growth Charts*. 2022. https://www.cdc.gov/growthcharts/cdc_charts.htm
5. Centers for Disease Control and Prevention, Division of Nutrition, Physical Activity, and Obesity. *Infant Growth Patterns*. 2022. https://www.cdc.gov/nccdphp/dnpao/growthcharts/who/using/growth_patterns.htm
6. National Academy of Medicine. *Dietary Reference Intakes for Energy, Carbohydrate, Fiber, Fat, Fatty Acids, Cholesterol, Protein, and Amino Acids*. National Academies Press; 2005.
7. Kim SY, Yi DY. Components of human breast milk: from macronutrient to microbiome and microRNA. *Clin Exp Pediatr*. 2020;63(8):301–309.
8. Binns C, Lee M, Low WY. The long-term public health benefits of breastfeeding. *Asia Pac J Public Health*. 2016;28(1):7–14.
9. Lodge CJ, Tan DJ, Lau MXZ, et al. Breastfeeding and asthma and allergies: a systematic review and *meta*-analysis. *Acta Paediatr*. 2015;104(467):38–53.
10. Miliku K, Azad MB. Breastfeeding and the developmental origins of asthma: current evidence, possible mechanisms, and future research priorities. *Nutrients*. 2018;10(8):995.
11. Tham R, Bowatte G, Dharmage SC, et al. Breastfeeding and the risk of dental caries: a systematic review and *meta*-analysis. *Acta Paediatr*. 2015;104(467):62–84.
12. Rozier RG, Adair S, Graham F, et al. Evidence-based clinical recommendations on the prescription of dietary fluoride supplements for caries prevention: a report of the American Dental Association Council on Scientific Affairs. *J Am Dent Assoc*. 2010;141(12):1480.
13. Centers for Disease Control and Prevention. *Infant and Toddler Nutrition*. Centers for Disease Control and Prevention; 2022. https://www.cdc.gov/nutrition/infantandtoddlernutrition/index.html
14. Cheng H, Chen R, Milosevic M, Rossiter C, Arora A, Denney-Wilson E. Interventions targeting bottle and formula feeding in the prevention and treatment of early childhood caries, overweight and obesity: an integrative review. *Int J Environ Res Public Health*. 2021;18(23):12304.
15. Doğramacı EJ, Rossi-Fedele G, Dreyer CW. Malocclusions in young children: does breast-feeding really reduce the risk? A systematic review and *meta*-analysis. *J Am Dent Assoc*. 2017;148(8):566–574.e6.

16. Thomaz EBAF, Alves CMC, Gomes E, Silva LF, et al. Breastfeeding versus bottle feeding on malocclusion in children: a *meta*-analysis study. *J Hum Lact*. 2018;34(4):768–788.

17. Abate A, Cavagnetto D, Fama A, Maspero C, Farronato G. Relationship between breastfeeding and malocclusion: a systematic review of the literature. *Nutrients*. 2020;12(12):3688. https://doi.org/10.3390/nu12123688.

18. Sum FHKMH, Zhang L, Ling HTB, et al. Association of breastfeeding and three-dimensional dental arch relationships in primary dentition. *BMC Oral Health*. 2015;15:30.

19. Lopes TSP, Moura L, de FA, de D, Lima MCMP. Breastfeeding and sucking habits in children enrolled in a mother-child health program. *BMC Res Notes*. 2014;7:362.

20. Buccini GDS, Pérez-Escamilla R, Paulino LM, Araújo CL, Venancio SI. Pacifier use and interruption of exclusive breastfeeding: systematic review and *meta*-analysis. *Matern Child Nutr*. 2017;13(3):e12384.

21. Ling HTB, Sum FHKMH, Zhang L, et al. The association between nutritive, non-nutritive sucking habits and primary dental occlusion. *BMC Oral Health*. 2018;18(1):145.

22. World Health Organization. Complementary feeding. In: *Infant and Young Child Feeding: Model Chapter for Textbooks for Medical Students and Allied Health Professionals*. World Health Organization; 2009. https://www.ncbi.nlm.nih.gov/books/NBK148957/.

23. Lutter CK, Grummer-Strawn L, Rogers L. Complementary feeding of infants and young children 6 to 23 months of age. *Nutr Rev*. 2021;79(8):825–846.

24. U.S. Department of Agriculture, U.S. Department of Health and Human Services. *Dietary Guidelines for Americans*. 9th ed. 2020. dietaryguidelines.gov

25. Robert Wood Johnson Foundation. Healthy Eating Research: Tips for Families. https://healthyeatingresearch.org/tips-for-families/

26. Perez-Escamilla R, Segura-Perez S, Lott M. *Feeding Guidelines for Infants and Young Toddlers: A Responsive Parenting Approach*. Healthy Eating Research; 2017. https://healthyeatingresearch.org/wp-content/uploads/2017/02/her_feeding_guidelines_report_021416-1.pdf

27. Bergamini M, Simeone G, Verga MC, et al. Complementary feeding caregivers' practices and growth, risk of overweight/obesity, and other non-communicable diseases: a systematic review and *meta*-analysis. *Nutrients*. 2022;14(13):2646.

28. Bell LK, Gardner C, Tian EJ, et al. Supporting strategies for enhancing vegetable liking in the early years of life: an umbrella review of systematic reviews. *Am J Clin Nutr*. 2021;113(5):1282–1300.

29. Fleischer DM, Sicherer S, Greenhawt M, et al. Consensus communication on early peanut introduction and prevention of peanut allergy in high-risk infants. *Pediatr Dermatol*. 2016;33(1):103–106.

30. Heyman MB, Abrams SA, Section on Gastroenterology, Hepatology, and Nutrition, et al. Fruit juice in infants, children, and adolescents: current recommendations. *Pediatrics*. 2017;139(6):e20170967.

31. Abbasalizad Farhangi M, Mohammadi Tofigh A, Jahangiri L, Nikniaz Z, Nikniaz L. Sugar-sweetened beverages intake and the risk of obesity in children: an updated systematic review and dose-response *meta*-analysis. *Pediatr Obes*. 2022;17(8):e12914.

32. Bernabé E, Ballantyne H, Longbottom C, Pitts NB. Early introduction of sugar-sweetened beverages and caries trajectories from age 12 to 48 months. *J Dent Res*. 2020;99(8):898–906.

33. Infant Feeding Joint Working Group. *Nutrition for Healthy Term Infants: Recommendations From Birth to Six Months. A Joint Statement of Health Canada, Canadian Paediatric Society, Dietitians of Canada, and Breastfeeding Committee for Canada*. 2012. https://www.canada.ca/en/health-canada/services/canada-food-guide/resources/infant-feeding/nutrition-healthy-term-infants-recommendations-birth-six-months.html

34. Wagner CL, Greer FR, American Academy of Pediatrics Section on Breastfeeding, American Academy of Pediatrics Committee on Nutrition Prevention of rickets and vitamin D deficiency in infants, children, and adolescents. *Pediatrics*. 2008;122(5):1142–1152.

35. Simon AE, Ahrens KA. Adherence to vitamin D intake guidelines in the United States. *Pediatrics*. 2020;145(6):e20193574.

36. American Academy of Pediatric Dentistry. *Periodicity of Examination, Preventive Dental Services, Anticipatory Guidance/Counseling, and Oral Treatment for Infants, Children, and Adolescents*. AAPD; 2022:253–265. https://www.aapd.org/research/oral-health-policies--recommendations/periodicity-of-examination-preventive-dental-services-anticipatory-guidance-counseling-and-oral-treatment-for-infants-children-and-adolescents/.

37. Den Besten PK. Mechanism and timing of fluoride effects on developing enamel. *J Public Health Dent*. 1999;59(4):247–251.

38. Centers for Disease Control and Prevention, Division of Oral Health. Infant formula. In: *FAQs | Community Water Fluoridation*. Division of Oral Health, CDC; 2018. https://www.cdc.gov/fluoridation/faqs/infant-formula.html

39. Centers for Disease Control and Prevention. *Infant Formula Preparation and Storage*. 2022. https://www.cdc.gov/nutrition/downloads/prepare-store-powered-infant-formula-508.pdf

40. Bonuck K, Kahn R, Schechter C. Is late bottle-weaning associated with overweight in young children? Analysis of NHANES III data. *Clin Pediatr (Phila)*. 2004;43(6):535–540.

41. Gooze RA, Anderson SE, Whitaker RC. Prolonged bottle use and obesity at 5.5 years of age in US children. *J Pediatr*. 2011;159(3):431–436.

42. Yeung S, Chan R, Li L, Leung S, Woo J. Bottle milk feeding and its association with food group consumption, growth and socio-demographic characteristics in Chinese young children. *Matern Child Nutr*. 2017;13(3):e12341.

43. Bonuck KA, Kahn R. Prolonged bottle use and its association with iron deficiency anemia and overweight: a preliminary study. *Clin Pediatr (Phila)*. 2002;41(8):603–607.

44. Peres KG, Nascimento GG, Peres MA, et al. Impact of prolonged breastfeeding on dental caries: a population-based birth cohort study. *Pediatrics*. 2017;140(1):e20162943.

45. Bateman DN, Eagling V, Sandilands EA, et al. Iron overdose epidemiology, clinical features and iron concentration-effect relationships: the UK experience 2008-2017. *Clin Toxicol (Phila)*. 2018;56(11):1098–1106.

46. Yuen HW, Becker W. *Iron toxicity*. StatPearls. StatPearls Publishing; 2023. http://www.ncbi.nlm.nih.gov/books/NBK459224/.

47. Infant Feeding Joint Working Group. *Nutrition for Healthy Term Infants: Recommendations from Six to 24 Months. A Joint Statement of Health Canada, Canadian Paediatric Society, Dietitians of Canada, and Breastfeeding Committee for Canada*. 2014. https://www.canada.ca/en/health-canada/services/canada-food-guide/resources/infant-feeding/nutrition-healthy-term-infants-recommendations-birth-six-months/6-24-months.html

48. Psoter WJ, Reid BC, Katz RV. Malnutrition and dental caries: a review of the literature. *Caries Res*. 2005;39(6):441–447.

49. Rigo L, Bidinotto AB, Hugo FN, Neves M, Hilgert JB. Untreated caries and serum vitamin D levels in children and youth of the United States: NHANES 2013-2014. *Braz Dent J*. 2023;34(1):99–106.

50. Uribe SE, Innes N, Maldupa I. The global prevalence of early childhood caries: a systematic review with *meta*-analysis using the WHO diagnostic criteria. *International Journal of Paediatric Dentistry*. 2021;31(6):817–830.

51. Kirthiga M, Murugan M, Saikia A, Kirubakaran R. Risk factors for early childhood caries: a systematic review and *meta*-analysis of case control and cohort studies. *Pediatr Dent*. 2019;41(2):95–112.

52. Lam PPY, Chua H, Ekambaram M, Lo ECM, Yiu CKY. Risk predictors of early childhood caries increment-a systematic review and *meta*-analysis. *J Evid Based Dent Pract*. 2022;22(3):101732.

53. Kazeminia M, Abdi A, Shohaimi S, et al. Dental caries in primary and permanent teeth in children's worldwide, 1995 to 2019: a systematic review and *meta*-analysis. *Head Face Med*. 2020;16:22.

54. American Academy of Pediatrics. *From Bottle to Cup: Helping Your Child Make a Healthy Transition*. HealthyChildren.org; 2023. https://www.healthychildren.org/English/ages-stages/baby/feeding-nutrition/Pages/Discontinuing-the-Bottle.aspx

55. American Academy of Pediatric Dentistry. *Policy on Early Childhood Caries (ECC): Consequences and Preventive Strategies*. AAPD; 2022:90–93.

56. Pitts N, Baez R, Diaz-Guallory C, et al. Early childhood caries: IAPD Bangkok Declaration. *Int J Paediatr Dent*. 2019;29(3):384–386.

57. Dashper SG, Mitchell HL, Lê Cao KA, et al. Temporal development of the oral microbiome and prediction of early childhood caries. *Sci Rep*. 2019;9:19732.

58. da Silva Bastos V, de A, Freitas-Fernandes LB, Fidalgo TK, da S, et al. Mother-to-child transmission of Streptococcus mutans: a systematic review and *meta*-analysis. *J Dent*. 2015;43(2):181–191.

59. Manchanda S, Sardana D, Liu P, Lee GHM, Lo ECM, Yiu CKY. Horizontal transmission of Streptococcus mutans in children and its association with dental caries: a systematic review and *meta*-analysis. *Pediatr Dent*. 2021;43(1):1E–12E.

60. Centers for Disease Control and Prevention. *Facts About Cleft Lip and Cleft Palate*. Centers for Disease Control and Prevention; 2022. https://www.cdc.gov/ncbddd/birthdefects/cleftlip.html

61. Bessell A, Hooper L, Shaw WC, Reilly S, Reid J, Glenny AM. Feeding interventions for growth and development in infants with cleft lip, cleft palate or cleft lip and palate. *Cochrane Database Syst Rev*. 2011;2011(2):CD003315.

62. Kumar Jindal M, Khan SY. How to feed cleft patient? *Int J Clin Pediatr Dent*. 2013;6(2):100–103.

63. Berg E, Haaland ØA, Feragen KB, et al. Health status among adults born with an oral cleft in Norway. *JAMA Pediatr*. 2016;170(11):1063–1070.

64. Lavôr JR, Lacerda RHW, Modesto A, Vieira AR. Maxillary incisor enamel defects in individuals born with cleft lip/palate. *PLoS One*. 2020;15(12):e0244506.

65. Liu J, Rehm CD, Onopa J, Mozaffarian D. Trends in diet quality among youth in the United States, 1999-2016. *JAMA*. 2020;323(12):1161–1174.

66. Jun S, Cowan AE, Dodd KW, et al. Association of food insecurity with dietary intakes and nutritional biomarkers among US children, National Health and Nutrition Examination Survey (NHANES) 2011-2016. *Am J Clin Nutr*. 2021;114(3):1059–1069.

67. Bourke M, Haddara A, Loh A, Carson V, Breau B, Tucker P. Adherence to the World Health Organization's physical activity recommendation in preschool-aged children: a systematic review and *meta*-analysis of accelerometer studies. *Int J Behav Nutr Phys Act*. 2023;20(1):52.

68. Cooper AR, Goodman A, Page AS, et al. Objectively measured physical activity and sedentary time in youth: the International Children's Accelerometry Database (ICAD). *Int J Behav Nutr Phys Act*. 2015;12:113.

69. van Ekris E, Wijndaele K, Altenburg TM, et al. Tracking of total sedentary time and sedentary patterns in youth: a pooled analysis using the International Children's Accelerometry Database (ICAD). *Int J Behav Nutr Phys Act*. 2020;17:65.

70. USDHHS, Office of Disease Prevention and Health Promotion. *Healthy People 2030*. https://health.gov/healthypeople

71. Di Bonito P, Pacifico L, Licenziati MR, et al. Elevated blood pressure, cardiometabolic risk and target organ damage in youth with overweight and obesity. *Nutr Metab Cardiovasc Dis*. 2020;30(10):1840–1847.

72. Guirguis-Blake JM, Evans CV, Coppola EL, Redmond N, Perdue LA. Screening for lipid disorders in children and adolescents: updated evidence report and systematic review for the US Preventive Services Task Force. *JAMA*. 2023;330(3):261.

73. US Preventive Services Task Force, et al.Barry MJ, Nicholson WK, et al. Screening for lipid disorders in children and adolescents: US Preventive Services Task Force recommendation statement. *JAMA*. 2023;330(3):253.

74. Lloyd-Jones DM, Ning H, Labarthe D, et al. Status of cardiovascular health in US adults and children using the American Heart Association's New "Life's Essential 8" Metrics: prevalence estimates from the National Health and Nutrition Examination Survey (NHANES), 2013 through 2018. *Circulation*. 2022;146(11):822–835.

75. Rosinger A, Park S. Sugar-sweetened beverage consumption among U.S. youth, 2011–2014. *NCHS Data Brief*. 2017;271:1–8.

76. Hamner HC. Fruit, vegetable, and sugar-sweetened beverage intake among young children, by state—United States 2021. *MMWR Morb Mortal Wkly Rep*. 2023;72(7):165–170.

77. National Restaurant Association. *Updates to Kids Livewell: White Paper on Updated Nutrition Criteria 2021*. 2021. https://restaurant.org/getmedia/8bbc70ec-aa58-411d-8f57-d0bf794917cd/kids-livewell-whitepaper.pdf

78. U.S. Department of Health and Human Services. *Physical Activity Guidelines for Americans Midcourse Report: Strategies to Increase Physical Activity in Youth*. USDHHS; 2012:48. https://health.gov/our-work/nutrition-physical-activity/physical-activity-guidelines/previous-guidelines/2008-physical-activity-guidelines.

79. USDA MyPlate. *Preschoolers*. https://www.myplate.gov/life-stages/preschoolers

80. Slining MM, Mathias KC, Popkin BM. Trends in food and beverage sources among US children and adolescents: 1989-2010. *J Acad Nutr Diet*. 2013;113(12):1683–1694.

81. Gupta PM, Perrine CG, Mei Z, Scanlon KS. Iron, anemia, and iron deficiency anemia among young children in the United States. *Nutrients*. 2016;8(6):330.

82. Office of Dietary Supplements. *Iron: Fact Sheet for Health Professionals*. https://ods.od.nih.gov/factsheets/Iron-HealthProfessional/

83. McCann S, Perapoch Amadó M, Moore SE. The role of iron in brain development: a systematic review. *Nutrients*. 2020;12(7):2001.

84. Palacios C, Gonzalez L. Is vitamin D deficiency a major global public health problem? *J Steroid Biochem Mol Biol*. 2014;144PA:138–145.

85. Costa A, Oliveira A. Parental feeding practices and children's eating behaviours: an overview of their complex relationship. *Healthcare*. 2023;11(3):400.

86. Shloim N, Edelson LR, Martin N, Hetherington MM. Parenting styles, feeding styles, feeding practices, and weight status in 4-12 year-old children: a systematic review of the literature. *Front Psychol*. 2015;6:1849.

87. Glanz K, Metcalfe JJ, Folta SC, Brown A, Fiese B. Diet and health benefits associated with in-home eating and sharing meals at home: a systematic review. *Int J Environ Res Public Health*. 2021;18(4):1577.

88. Centers for Disease Control and Prevention. *Choking Hazards*. Centers for Disease Control and Prevention; 2022. https://www.cdc.gov/nutrition/infantandtoddlernutrition/foods-and-drinks/choking-hazards.html

89. Branum AM, Rossen LM, Schoendorf KC. Trends in caffeine intake among US children and adolescents. *Pediatrics*. 2014;133(3):386–393.

90. Drewnowski A, Rehm CD. Sources of caffeine in diets of US children and adults: trends by beverage type and purchase location. *Nutrients*. 2016;8(3):154.

91. Robson SM, McCullough MB, Rex S, Munafò MR, Taylor G. Family meal frequency, diet, and family functioning: a systematic review with *meta*-analyses. *J Nutr Educ Behav*. 2020;52(5):553–564.

92. Pietrobelli A, Agosti M, MeNu Group. Nutrition in the first 1000 days: ten practices to minimize obesity emerging from published science. *Int J Environ Res Public Health*. 2017;14(12):1491.

93. Song P, Zha M, Yang Q, Zhang Y, Li X, Rudan I. The prevalence of adult attention-deficit hyperactivity disorder: a global systematic review and *meta*-analysis. *J Glob Health*. 2021;11:04009.

94. Rajaprakash M, Leppert ML. Attention-deficit/hyperactivity disorder. *Pediatr Rev*. 2022;43(3):135–147.

95. Faraone SV, Banaschewski T, Coghill D, et al. The World Federation of ADHD International Consensus Statement: 208 evidence-based conclusions about the disorder. *Neurosci Biobehav Rev*. 2021;128:789–818.

96. Farsad-Naeimi A, Asjodi F, Omidian M, et al. Sugar consumption, sugar sweetened beverages and attention deficit hyperactivity

disorder: a systematic review and *meta*-analysis. *Complement Ther Med.* 2020;53:102512.

97. Del-Ponte B, Quinte GC, Cruz S, Grellert M, Santos IS. Dietary patterns and attention deficit/hyperactivity disorder (ADHD): a systematic review and *meta*-analysis. *Journal of Affective Disorders.* 2019;252:160–173.

98. National Institute of Dental and Craniofacial Research. *Developmental Disabilities & Oral Health.* 2020. https://www.nidcr.nih.gov/health-info/developmental-disabilities

99. Mansfield JL, Savaiano DA. Effect of school wellness policies and the Healthy, Hunger-Free Kids Act on food-consumption behaviors of students, 2006-2016: a systematic review. *Nutr Rev.* 2017;75(7):533–552.

100. Cohen JFW, Hecht AA, McLoughlin GM, Turner L, Schwartz MB. Universal school meals and associations with student participation, attendance, academic performance, diet quality, food security, and body mass index: a systematic review. *Nutrients.* 2021;13(3):911.

101. Centers for Disease Control and Prevention. *FastStats: Oral and Dental Health.* 2023. https://www.cdc.gov/nchs/fastats/dental.htm

102. Gupta N, Vujicic M, Yarbrough C, Harrison B. Disparities in untreated caries among children and adults in the U.S., 2011–2014. *BMC Oral Health.* 2018;18(1):30.

103. Ruff RR, Senthi S, Susser SR, Tsutsui A. Oral health, academic performance, and school absenteeism in children and adolescents: a systematic review and *meta*-analysis. *J Am Dent Assoc.* 2019;150(2):111–121.e4.

104. Iheozor-Ejiofor Z, Worthington HV, Walsh T, et al. Water fluoridation for the prevention of dental caries. *Cochrane Database Syst Rev.* 2015(6).

105. Cabalén MB, Molina GF, Bono A, Burrow MF. Nonrestorative caries treatment: a systematic review update. *Int Dent J.* 2022;72(6):746–764.

106. Janakiram C, Deepan Kumar CV, Joseph J. Xylitol in preventing dental caries: a systematic review and *meta*-analyses. *J Nat Sci Biol Med.* 2017;8(1):16–21.

107. Nasseripour M, Newton JT, Warburton F, et al. A systematic review and meta-analysis of the role of sugar-free chewing gum on Streptococcus mutans. *BMC Oral Health.* 2021;21(1):217.

108. Riley P, Moore D, Ahmed F, Sharif MO, Worthington HV. Xylitol-containing products for preventing dental caries in children and adults. *Cochrane Database Syst Rev.* 2015;2015(3):CD010743.

109. Chevalley T, Rizzoli R. Acquisition of peak bone mass. *Best Pract Res Clin Endocrinol Metab.* 2022;36(2):101616.

110. Baxter-Jones AD, Faulkner RA, Forwood MR, Mirwald RL, Bailey DA. Bone mineral accrual from 8 to 30 years of age: an estimation of peak bone mass. *J Bone Miner Res.* 2011;26(8):1729–1739.

111. Agricultural Research Service, USDA. *What We Eat in America, NHANES 2017-2020.* Food Surveys Research Group; 2022. https://www.ars.usda.gov/ARSUserFiles/80400530/pdf/1720/Table_1_NIN_GEN_1720.pdf

112. Golden NH, Abrams SA, Committee on Nutrition, et al. ικbone health in children and adolescents. *Pediatrics.* 2014;134(4):e1229–e1243.

113. Larsen B, Baller EB, Boucher AA, et al. Development of iron status measures during youth: associations with sex, neighborhood socioeconomic status, cognitive performance, and brain structure. *Am J Clin Nutr.* 2023;118(1):121–131.

114. Damian MT, Vulturar R, Login CC, Damian L, Chis A, Bojan A. Anemia in sports: a narrative review. *Life.* 2021;11(9):987.

115. Rudloff S, Bührer C, Jochum F, et al. Vegetarian diets in childhood and adolescence. *Mol Cell Pediatr.* 2019;6:4.

116. Pettersson C, Svedlund A, Wallengren O, Swolin-Eide D, Paulson Karlsson G, Ellegård L. Dietary intake and nutritional status in adolescents and young adults with anorexia nervosa: a 3-year follow-up study. *Clin Nutr.* 2021;40(10):5391–5398.

117. da Silva Lopes K, Yamaji N, Rahman MO, et al. Nutrition-specific interventions for preventing and controlling anaemia throughout the life cycle: an overview of systematic reviews. *Cochrane Database Syst Rev.* 2021;9(9):CD013092.

118. Daly AN, O'Sullivan EJ, Kearney JM. Considerations for health and food choice in adolescents. *Proc Nutr Soc.* 2022;81(1):75–86.

119. Kucharczuk AJ, Oliver TL, Dowdell EB. Social media's influence on adolescents' food choices: a mixed studies systematic literature review. *Appetite.* 2022;168:105765.

120. National Institute of Diabetes and Digestive and Kidney Diseases. *Overweight & Obesity Statistics.* National Institute of Diabetes and Digestive and Kidney Diseases; 2021. https://www.niddk.nih.gov/health-information/health-statistics/overweight-obesity

121. Jampel JD, Murray SB, Griffiths S, Blashill AJ. Self-perceived weight and anabolic steroid misuse among US adolescent boys. *J Adolesc Health.* 2016;58(4):397–402.

122. Liu J, Lee Y, Micha R, Li Y, Mozaffarian D. Trends in junk food consumption among US children and adults, 2001-2018. *Am J Clin Nutr.* 2021;114(3):1039–1048.

123. Park S, Zhao L, Lee SH, et al. Children and adolescents in the United States with usual high added sugars intake: characteristics, eating occasions, and top sources, 2015–2018. *Nutrients.* 2023;15(2):274.

124. Pitchika V, Standl M, Harris C, et al. Association of sugar-sweetened drinks with caries in 10- and 15-year-olds. *BMC Oral Health.* 2020;20(1):81.

125. Vos MB, Kaar JL, Welsh JA, et al. Added sugars and cardiovascular disease risk in children: a scientific statement from the American Heart Association. *Circulation.* 2017;135(19):e1017–e1034.

126. Muth ND, Dietz WH, Magge SN, et al. Public policies to reduce sugary drink consumption in children and adolescents. *Pediatrics.* 2019;143(4):e20190282.

127. Jagim AR, Harty PS, Tinsley GM, et al. International society of sports nutrition position stand: energy drinks and energy shots. *J Int Soc Sports Nutr.* 2023;20(1):2171314.

128. Hardy LL, Bell J, Bauman A, Mihrshahi S. Association between adolescents' consumption of total and different types of sugar-sweetened beverages with oral health impacts and weight status. *Australian and New Zealand Journal of Public Health.* 2018;42(1):22–26.

129. Moussa M, Hansz K, Rasmussen M, et al. Cardiovascular effects of energy drinks in the pediatric population. *Pediatr Emerg Care.* 2021;37(11):578–582.

130. Centers for Disease Control and Prevention. *Energy Drinks.* 2022. https://www.cdc.gov/healthyschools/nutrition/energy.htm

131. Sylvetsky AC, Jin Y, Clark EJ, Welsh JA, Rother KI, Talegawkar SA. Consumption of low-calorie sweeteners among children and adults in the United States. *J Acad Nutr Diet.* 2017;117(3):441–448.e2.

132. Samman M, Kaye E, Cabral H, Scott T, Sohn W. Dental erosion: effect of diet drink consumption on permanent dentition. *JDR Clin Trans Res.* 2022;7(4):425–434.

133. Ricotti R, Caputo M, Monzani A, et al. Breakfast skipping, weight, cardiometabolic risk, and nutrition quality in children and adolescents: a systematic review of randomized controlled and intervention longitudinal trials. *Nutrients.* 2021;13(10):3331.

134. Peña-Jorquera H, Campos-Núñez V, Sadarangani KP, Ferrari G, Jorquera-Aguilera C, Cristi-Montero C. Breakfast: a crucial meal for adolescents' cognitive performance according to their nutritional status. The Cogni-Action Project. *Nutrients.* 2021;13(4):1320.

135. Lindberg L, Danielsson P, Persson M, Marcus C, Hagman E. Association of childhood obesity with risk of early all-cause and cause-specific mortality: a Swedish prospective cohort study. *PLoS Med.* 2020;17(3):e1003078.

136. Haqq AM, Kebbe M, Tan Q, Manco M, Salas XR. Complexity and stigma of pediatric obesity. *Child Obes.* 2021;17(4):229–240.

137. Bryan S, Afful J, Carroll M, et al. *NHSR 158. National Health and Nutrition Examination Survey 2017–March 2020 Pre-Pandemic Data Files.* National Center for Health Statistics (U.S.); 2021:21.

138. Hampl SE, Hassink SG, Skinner AC, et al. Clinical practice guideline for the evaluation and treatment of children and adolescents with obesity. *Pediatrics*. 2023;151(2):e2022060640.

139. Manohar N, Hayen A, Fahey P, Arora A. Obesity and dental caries in early childhood: a systematic review and *meta*-analyses. *Obes Rev*. 2020;21(3):e12960.

140. Piovesan ÉTde A, Leal SC, Bernabé E. The relationship between obesity and childhood dental caries in the United States. *Int J Environ Res Public Health*. 2022;19(23):16160.

141. Mohamed RN, Basha S, Al-Thomali Y, AlZahrani FS, Ashour AA, Almutair NE. Dental erosion prevalence and its association with obesity among children with and without special healthcare needs. *Oral Health Prev Dent*. 2021;19(1):579–586.

142. Schmidt J, Vogel M, Poulain T, et al. Association of oral health conditions in adolescents with social factors and obesity. *Int J Environ Res Public Health*. 2022;19(5):2905.

143. Marro F, De Smedt S, Rajasekharan S, Martens L, Bottenberg P, Jacquet W. Associations between obesity, dental caries, erosive tooth wear and periodontal disease in adolescents: a case-control study. *Eur Arch Paediatr Dent*. 2021;22(1):99–108.

144. US Preventive Services Task Force, et al.Grossman DC, Bibbins-Domingo K, et al. Screening for obesity in children and Adolescents: US Preventive Services Task Force Recommendation Statement. *JAMA*. 2017;317(23):2417–2426.

145. McPherson AC, Hamilton J, Kingsnorth S, et al. Communicating with children and families about obesity and weight-related topics: a scoping review of best practices. *Obes Rev*. 2017;18(2):164–182.

146. Centers for Disease Control and Prevention. *Prevent Childhood Obesity*. Centers for Disease Control and Prevention; 2023. https://www.cdc.gov/nccdphp/dnpao/features/childhood-obesity/index.html

147. Greenberg BL, Glick M, Tavares M. Addressing obesity in the dental setting: What can be learned from oral health care professionals' efforts to screen for medical conditions. *J Public Health Dent*. 2017;77(Suppl 1):S67–S78.

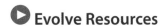 **Evolve Resources**

Please visit http://evolve.elsevier.com/Mallonee/nutritional for additional practice and study support tools.

15

Nutritional Requirements for Older Adults and Eating Habits Affecting Oral Health

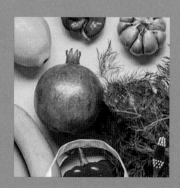

STUDENT LEARNING OBJECTIVES

On completion of this chapter, the student will be able to achieve the following learning outcomes:

1. Identify oral nutritional problems typically observed in older adults.
2. Predict physiologic changes that may alter an older individual's nutritional status.
3. Name socioeconomic and psychological factors influencing food intake of older patients.
4. Explain why nutrient requirements of older patients differ from younger patients.
5. Describe typical eating patterns of older adults, relate *Dietary Guidelines* and *MyPlate* to the diet of an older adult, and suggest implementation of dietary changes to provide optimum nutrient intake for older patients.

KEY TERMS

Age-related macular degeneration
Alternative medicine
Atrophic gastritis
Botanical
Complementary medicine
Denture stomatitis
Dysphagia

Genomics
Herb
Homeopathy
Homeostatic mechanisms
Hypogeusia
Incontinence
Naturopathy

Nocturia
Polypharmacy
Quality of life
Sarcopenia
Spices

◆ TEST YOUR NQ

1. **T/F** Normal physiologic changes occurring in older adults do not affect nutritional requirements.
2. **T/F** Nutritional requirements for a 50-year-old patient are different from those for an 81-year-old patient.
3. **T/F** Food selection is highly correlated with dentition.
4. **T/F** Edentulous patients should puree their food.
5. **T/F** Dehydration is seldom observed in older adults.
6. **T/F** Older adults need more vitamins D and B_{12} than individuals younger than 51 years of age.
7. **T/F** Healthy older females require increased amounts of iron.
8. **T/F** Energy requirements decrease with age.
9. **T/F** Self-medication with vitamins is a healthy practice for older adults.
10. **T/F** Exercise is of no benefit to older adults.

Major shifts in the age of the US population are affecting health care needs. Compared with the year 2000, when more than 35 million people were aged 65 years and older (13% of the population), this group is expected to increase to approximately 74 million by 2030 (21% of the population). The 85-years-and-older group is the fastest growing segment of the older population (Fig. 15.1) This group which increased to 2% of the population in 2020 is projected to increase to 5% by 2060.[1] US life expectancy may rise to over 80 by 2030.

Genetics accounts for about 20% to 30% of an individual's lifespan, with the rest attributed to diet and lifestyle choices. Individual healthy lifestyle choices (never smoking, moderate alcohol consumption, physical activity, and regularly choosing a healthy diet) are moderately associated with successful aging; their combined impact is substantial. Improved medical care from infancy has improved Americans' lifespan, but it is important to

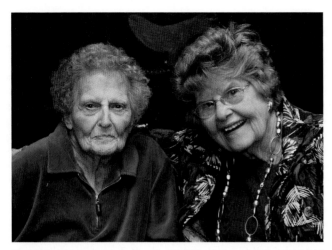

• **Fig. 15.1** Relatives celebrating their 100th (*left*) and 90th (*right*) birthdays. Life expectancy is higher for baby boomers than for the current older population. (Courtsey D2 Studios, http://www.d2studios.net.)

increase the quality of the older years by adopting healthy lifestyles and consistently choosing nutrient-dense foods.

Quality of life is defined by the World Health Organization as individuals' perception of their position in life in the context of the culture and value systems in which they live and in relation to their goals, expectations, standards, and concerns.[2] Oral health impacts systemic health. Therefore, oral care is an important consideration in maintaining quality of life. Whereas people were once disabled by conditions such as poor vision and cardiovascular disease (CVD), which are now more treatable, currently degenerative conditions, such as Alzheimer disease and dementia, are plaguing older individuals. By age 85 years, 50% of older adults will have dementia, which may impact function and nutritional status.[3]

The *Dietary Guidelines* recognize that the health and nutritional status of people older than 50 years needs special consideration; changes in food habits are needed to adjust to physical and metabolic changes that occur with aging. It is never too late to make lifestyle changes to improve one's health, longevity, and quality of life.

General Health Status

The most common nutritional disorder in older individuals is obesity. The prevalence of obesity is about 42% for adults aged 60 and older.[4] More males than females are overweight, but more females than males are obese. Obesity is more common among African Americans and slightly higher among Hispanic Americans than among non-Hispanic Whites.[5]

Obesity causes serious medical complications, impairing quality of life by exacerbating the age-related decline in physical function and cognitive disability. Approximately 95% of older Americans have at least one noncommunicable chronic disease, and 80% have been diagnosed with two or more chronic conditions.[6] Obesity contributes to some chronic conditions commonly seen in older adults, including CVD, diabetes, lung disease, arthritis, and Alzheimer's disease. Most of these conditions increase the risk of poor nutritional status. Routine nutritional care for older adults can help prevent or manage chronic diseases.

Malnutrition is another nutrition-related problem diagnosed in older adults admitted to hospitals and long-term care facilities,

and in those with serious medical problems. Malnutrition is associated with impaired immune response, impaired muscle and respiratory function, delayed wound healing, overall increased complications, longer rehabilitation, longer hospitalizations, and increased mortality. Factors considered to be contributing causes of older individuals being at risk of malnutrition include less education and lower income; being housebound or unable to purchase food; multiple medications; physical disabilities, depression, and other mental challenges; recent drastic lifestyle changes, such as death of spouse; and lacking regularly cooked meals. Identifying individuals at nutritional risk is critical to cost-effectiveness for the health care system and to assist older patients in maintaining their independence and personal well-being. Food choices are also related to oral problems; thus a dental assessment should include questions regarding food intake and oral problems affecting intake.

Dietary restrictions associated with management of chronic diseases, such as diabetes, renal disease, or CVD, can be confusing, especially if more than one condition exists. Improper food selection or fear of choosing unhealthy foods may be a factor for inadequate nutrition. The result of certain treatments can affect eating by creating loss of appetite, nausea and vomiting, diarrhea or constipation, xerostomia, or changes in the taste of food, for example, chemotherapy.

Prescription use, polypharmacy (use of at least five or more prescriptions), and supplement use, are prevalent. Approximately 36% of older adults take five or more prescriptions; 88% take at least one prescription medication; almost 64% are taking dietary supplements.[7] Some of these drugs depress appetite, interfere with nutrient absorption, and affect cognitive abilities. Classes of medications that place older adults at risk include (1) diuretics, (2) opioid painkillers, (3) tranquilizers, (4) antidepressants, (5) statins, (6) oral hypoglycemics, and (7) antacids and anticholinergics. Although drug-nutrient interactions can compromise anyone's nutritional status, these problems are amplified in older adults. Physiologic and pathophysiologic changes, such as decreased hepatic and renal clearance, result in greater variability and less predictability of a drug's effects.

Physiologic Factors Influencing Nutritional Needs and Status

Aging significantly impacts body composition. Many organ functions decline with age. These physiologic changes can substantially influence nutritional requirements of older adults by affecting absorption, transportation, metabolism, and excretion of nutrients. With aging, the body is less able to correct nutrient imbalances, such as increasing absorption when intake is decreased. Physiologic balance may be upset by disease; physical and mental challenges; and environmental, economic, and social disabilities. However, chronological age and functional capacity do not always correlate. Older individuals differ from one another in physiologic and health status more than any other age group, meaning that chronologic status is not useful in predicting physiologic abilities and health status.

Impairment of visual, auditory, and olfactory sensory organs is common. Poor vision makes food preparation difficult, even hazardous in some cases, and may be responsible for senior citizens not identifying contaminated foods, a potential cause of foodborne illness. Poor hearing increases isolation and decreases socialization.

Oral Cavity

Oral health problems (e.g., chewing, swallowing, compromised dentition) are indicators of nutritional risk and may be primary contributors to malnutrition. Persistent oral health problems are associated with impaired intake of certain foods and nutrients. A progressive decline in gustatory and olfactory sensitivity affects food choices and quantity because "nothing tastes good." Olfactory and taste receptors are affected by impaired chewing and swallowing.

Some conditions and certain medications also lead to deterioration of taste sensitivity. Hypogeusia (loss of taste) may be associated with certain disorders rather than being a normal component of the aging process. Older adults may confuse taste sensations, describing sour foods as metallic and salty foods as tasteless. Many people gradually begin to lose their sense of smell around age 60 years, a condition called anosmia. This is considered as normal as we get older.[8] As a consequence of anosmia and hypogeusia, foods may be overly seasoned with salt or sugar. Losses in salt or sugar perception make it difficult to comply with low-sodium or diabetes guidelines. Other seasonings and spices can help replace the taste of salt or sugar.

Xerostomia, a common complaint among older adults, compromises oral processing of foods. Most individuals requiring polypharmacy report problems with xerostomia. A lack of saliva affects both the oral preparatory and oral phases of swallowing, thus leading to impaired bolus formation and oropharyngeal bolus transport. Xerostomia increases the risk for oral disease because antimicrobial components and minerals in saliva help rebuild tooth enamel after acid-producing, decay-causing bacterial attacks. Crunchy foods stimulate saliva flow, but foods such as raw vegetables and crispy fruits are less likely to be consumed. Hard candy or gum may be used to stimulate saliva flow and relieve the dryness. However, frequent exposure to fermentable carbohydrate promotes root caries and reduces intake of nutrient-dense foods (see Chapter 20 for further discussion of xerostomia).

Recession of gingival tissues exposes root surfaces of teeth to the oral environment; this process increases with aging. The lack of a protective enamel layer on the root, surface roughness of roots, and demineralization related to a lower pH, make the area highly susceptible to dental caries. The prevalence of root caries, further discussed in Chapter 20, is much higher in older adults than in younger individuals. Data from 2015–16 shows that 29.1%, of adults age 75 years and older had root caries.[9]

Both osteoporosis and periodontitis are the diseases characterized by bone resorption. Periodontitis involves inflammatory bone loss in alveolar cortical bone supporting the teeth. A negative calcium balance results in calcium loss from the maxilla and mandible, which are primarily trabecular bone. Age-related bone loss affecting alveolar bone results in tooth loss and edentulism. Low bone-mineral density and osteoporosis/osteopenia are both risk factors for tooth loss, especially prevalent in postmenopausal females.[10] More than half of individuals older than 65 years have periodontitis.[11] Periodontal disease increases the likelihood of weight loss in older adults; the more extensive and severe the disease, the greater the weight loss.[12] This condition is partially responsible for the loss of teeth; control of periodontal disease can significantly reduce tooth loss.

The prevalence of edentulism is nearly twice as high among people aged 85 years and over (31%) as in people aged 65 to 74 years (15%).[1] Edentulism is not inevitable with advancing age; however, its prevalence among adults older than age 50 has decreased significantly. Hispanic Americans and African Americans have the highest rates of edentulism, possibly due to lack of receiving annual oral health services. More seniors with lower incomes are edentulous than those in higher income brackets.[1]

The quality of chewing, or chewing ability, is affected by the number of teeth in functional occlusion. Tooth loss adversely affects chewing ability, causing difficulties in forming a bolus. A larger bolus size interferes with optimal swallowing, leading to additional swallowing abnormalities in the oral preparatory stage.[13,14] Patients with periodontal conditions, edentulous areas, and/or patients who wear dentures tend to alter food choices to reduce chewing or because of fear of choking. Tooth loss may be an early indicator of accelerated aging.[15] Weight changes can be a reason for an ill-fitting dental appliance. Normally, alveolar bone is maintained in response to occlusal forces associated with chewing. If severe mandibular resorption occurs, it is very difficult to construct a well-fitting dental prosthesis. Treatment with mandibular implant-supported dentures has a significant positive effect on both bite force and masticatory performance.[16]

Tooth loss, edentulous status, and conventional dentures reflect differences in healthy behaviors, attitudes toward oral health, and dental care. Nutrient intakes of patients with compromised dentition can fall below minimum requirements, increasing risk of malnutrition in older adults.[17,18] Even the loss of a few teeth can affect nutrient quality of the diet; individuals have difficulty managing high-fiber fruits and vegetables, especially raw apples and carrots, tossed salads, and dietary fiber.[17]

Compromised dental status also negatively affects animal protein intake. Nutrient intake decreases as the total number of teeth decreases, which may result in an inadequate amount of total protein, magnesium, zinc, vitamins B_1, B_6, and C, niacin, folate, pantothenic acid, and beta-carotene.[17]

Denture stomatitis may affect between 20% and 80% of partial and complete denture wearers.[19] Dental stomatitis is traumatization and chronic inflammation of mucus membranes supporting a removable denture. While many risk factors contribute to the etiology of denture stomatitis, *Candida albicans* is indicated as a prime culprit. Any condition that allows proliferation of candida and possibly affects immune function of the host may result in irritation of the mucus membranes. A high sugar intake increases the risk of denture stomatitis as the sugar stimulates growth of *Candida*. This may be as significant as poor denture hygiene in the development of denture stomatitis. Other nutritional factors frequently implicated as increasing risk include dietary deficiencies (iron, folate, vitamin B_{12}) and xerostomia.[20]

Gastrointestinal Tract

Changes in esophageal motility and deterioration of nerve function may cause dysphagia (difficulty with swallowing). This frequently observed disorder increases risk of aspiration pneumonia and morbidity; individuals with swallowing problems eat slowly and may be unable to consume adequate amounts.

Atrophic gastritis, a chronic stomach inflammation with atrophy of the mucous membrane and glands and diminished hydrochloric acid production, is frequently observed in older patients. Diminished hydrochloric acid secretion may affect calcium, iron, and vitamin B_{12} absorption. Additionally, lack of acid permits overgrowth of bacteria that may compromise vitamin B_{12} availability.

Constipation may be a consequence of altered gastrointestinal motility, loss of bowel muscle tone, medications, inadequate food and fluid intake, low-fiber diet, and inactivity. Additional causes include chronic laxative use and some medications, especially analgesics, antihypertensives, and narcotics. Problems with constipation may be averted by increasing fiber-containing foods, fluid intake, and activity level.

Hydration Status

Decreased thirst sensations are associated with aging; dehydration occurs more frequently in older adults. Fluid intake may not increase automatically to offset increased water losses from the compromised kidney. As a result of poor fluid intake, susceptibility to caries is increased.

Homeostatic mechanisms indicate the body's ability to correct imbalances, such as decreased nutrient intake accompanied by an increase in nutrient absorption or efficiency of use. Certain chronic illnesses (heart and kidney disease) lead to impairment of various homeostatic mechanisms controlling water balance. Fever, which can lead to mild dehydration in healthy individuals, may result in severe dehydration in older adults. Other seemingly mild stresses, such as the presence of infection or diarrhea or use of diuretics, can upset the normal homeostasis of an older individual.

Water is the single most important substance consumed. Regardless of the setting in which older adults are living, at home or in long-term care, dehydration or inadequate fluid intake is a common disorder.[21,22] Dehydration is one of the primary causes of confusion in older patients and can occur because of the kidney's inability to concentrate urine, changes in thirst sensation, changes in functional status, side effects of medications, and lack of mobility.[21] Dehydration can lead to loose-fitting dentures. The condition frequently results in hospitalization as a result of fecal impaction, cognitive impairment, and overall functional decline.[23]

Musculoskeletal System

Two nutrition-related conditions encountered by older persons involving the musculoskeletal system are osteoporosis and sarcopenia; thus maintaining bone health and muscle mass are primary concerns. As discussed in Chapter 9, *Health Application 9*, osteoporosis or shortening and outward bowing of the spine may develop. Trabecular bone loss may be associated with physical inactivity, unavailability of calcium (inadequate dietary intake, imbalance in calcium-to-phosphorus ratio, and decreased calcium absorption), changes in hormones affecting calcium metabolism, lack of vitamin D, or altered vitamin D metabolism associated with impaired renal function. Bone loss increases susceptibility to fractures, which can result in disability.[24,25]

Sarcopenia is the loss of skeletal muscle mass (unintentional), strength (loss of muscle), and physical performance related to aging. The older person may become weak and frail, creating functional problems that further contribute to sarcopenia. If enough muscle is lost, it can be debilitating. This complex multifaceted process is also observed in persons who have been physically inactive throughout their lives. Individuals with dependent ambulatory status experience a higher prevalence of sarcopenia compared with ambulatory patients.[26] Functional decline inevitably leads to frailty, reduced mobility, falls, fractures, and mortality. Hospital stays are longer and functional recovery is often incomplete even after rehabilitation.[27] Impaired dentition is significantly associated with sarcopenia.[28,29]

Sarcopenia can even occur in an obese person (body mass index [BMI] $> 27\,kg/m^2$; called sarcopenic obesity). These individuals are at a heightened disadvantage with the loss of muscle strength needing to support increased body weight[30] The prevalence of sarcopenic obesity differs substantially among studies because of the lack of a standard definition.

Inactivity is responsible for loss of muscle strength and balance. Physical activity can help ameliorate some chronic health problems, yet only 15% of people ages 65 to 74 years and 5% of those 85 years old and over meet the physical guidelines.[31] An active lifestyle also helps improve physiologic well-being, and relieves symptoms of depression and anxiety. Box 15.1 lists some benefits of physical activity. Many older adults can be motivated to make changes to prevent or delay a decline in health and an increase in disability if information is presented with an understandable rationale.

The *Physical Activity Guidelines for Americans* (see Chapter 1) addressing older adults may help to deter sarcopenia.[32] Older adults unable to do 150 minutes of moderate-intensity aerobic activity a week because of chronic conditions should be as physically active as their abilities and conditions allow. Older

---

• **BOX 15.1** **Health Benefits of Physical Activity**

Strong Evidence
- Lower risk of early death
- Lower risk of cardiovascular disease
- Lower risk of stroke
- Lower risk of adverse blood lipid profile
- Lower risk of type 2 diabetes
- Lower risk of metabolic syndrome
- Lower risk of colon cancer
- Lower risk of breast cancer
- Prevention of weight gain
- Weight loss, particularly when combined with reduced calorie intake
- Improved cardiorespiratory and muscular fitness
- Prevention of falls
- Reduced depression
- Better cognitive function (for older adults)

Moderate to Strong Evidence
- Better functional health (for older adults)
- Reduced abdominal obesity

Moderate Evidence
- Lower risk of hip fracture
- Lower risk of lung cancer
- Lower risk of endometrial cancer
- Weight maintenance after weight loss
- Increased bone density
- Improved sleep quality

Note: The Advisory Committee rated the evidence of health benefits of physical activity as strong, moderate, or weak. To do so, the Committee considered the type, number, and quality of studies available, as well as consistency of findings across studies that addressed each outcome. The Committee also considered evidence for causality and *dose-response* in assigning the strength-of-evidence rating.

From United States Department of Health and Human Services. *Physical Activity Guidelines for Americans*. 2nd ed. United States Department of Health and Human Services; 2018. https://health.gov/sites/default/files/2019-09/Physical_Activity_Guidelines_2nd_edition.pdf.

adults with chronic conditions should understand whether and how their conditions affect their ability to safely participate in regular physical activities. Exercises that maintain or improve balance are recommended. Walking and other moderate exercise are linked to lower stroke and heart attack risk even for people in their 70s.[33] Physical activity (walking, swimming, or dancing) may improve quality of life for older adults by maintaining their independence longer, improving longevity, and increasing brain function and boosting memory.[34,35] The more physical activity older adults do, the greater the health benefit.[36] Optimizing physical activity should be encouraged for all adults—not just when symptoms of physical or cognitive decline appear.

With aging, intra-abdominal fat increases more than subcutaneous or total body fat, and peripheral muscle declines more than central muscle mass.[37] As musculature shrinks, fat tissue accumulates. When older people reduce their food intake without exercising, they lose more lean muscle mass and less fat compared to those who exercise while dieting.[38]

Even with no increase in weight, fat stores replace lean muscle mass as we age. Low protein intake contributes to muscle loss and a negative nitrogen balance that evokes muscle breakdown. Maintaining muscle is essential to reduce the risk of falling.[39]

Diminished sense of taste and smell, rapid satiety, poor oral health, decreased metabolism, gastrointestinal changes, and dementia—all increasingly common with aging—result in decreasing food intake and increased adiposity (caused by fatigue and lack of activity). This can create a vicious cycle that leads to more gain in fat and more muscle loss, eventually resulting in functional consequences (e.g., disability), reduced quality of life, and early death.

Although many consider sarcopenia to be inevitable with aging, it can vary based on risk factors that may increase incidence. High-protein foods stimulate muscle protein synthesis, even in older adults. Protein use may be impaired, but this can be overcome by consuming high-quality protein at each meal. Resistance exercise combined with adequate consumption of protein stimulates maximum anabolic response and may help older individuals yield a greater muscle protein synthesis response. A diet that consists of high-quality protein foods with adequate amounts of fruits and vegetables has been shown to reduce risk of sarcopenia.[40–42] Protein supplementation has not consistently shown benefits on muscle mass and function. Maintaining appropriate blood levels of vitamin D may also aid in retaining muscle strength and physical performance.[43,44] Muscle mass can be preserved by increasing physical activity. Less lean body mass results in a decreased basal metabolic rate (Fig. 15.2). As we age, the basal metabolic rate declines and the body burns fewer calories than during earlier years; thus less food is needed to prevent weight gain. Less intake of vital proteins inhibits healing after a physiologic injury or insult and contributes to the declining function of many organ systems.[45]

Socioeconomic and Psychological Factors

Many changes occur affecting food intake of older adults (Fig. 15.3). Most retired people live on fixed incomes significantly lower than when they were employed. In 2020, approximately 7.1% (5.5 million) adults age 60 and over were faced

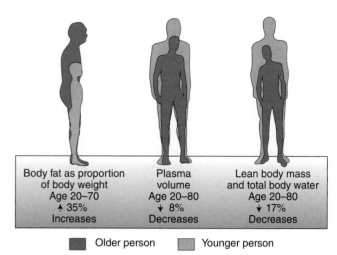

• **Fig. 15.2** Changes in the body with aging. Younger person, age 20 years. Older person, age 80 years. (Redrawn from Vestal RE. Drugs and the Elderly, NIH Publication No. 79–1449. United States Department of Health, Education, and Welfare, 1979.)

with the threat of food insecurity; with the greatest impact among Black and Hispanic seniors. From 2020 to 2021, the fraction of older adults experiencing the threat of food insecurity increased by 35% and 90% for those with very low food security [46] Inflation, failing health, and medical bills (especially cost of medications) can have a devastating effect on fixed incomes. The food budget frequently is affected and is a risk factor for inadequate nutrition. Fresh fruit and vegetable choices may be curtailed because of their high cost and limited shelf life. Title III Nutrition Programs for the Elderly (congregate dining and Meals-on-Wheels) are available to improve nutritional and health status of older patients and possibly prevent or postpone more expensive services of long-term care institutions. Nutritious meals are furnished at a minimal charge to older adults or free for those who qualify. These programs have been proven to improve dietary intakes of recipients whose diets were previously below the Recommended Dietary Allowance (RDA).[47]

An inability to drive or lack of access to transportation affects use of health services and availability of food. Approximately 27% of noninstitutionalized individuals older than age 65 years live alone; this percentage increases with age. More females than males live alone; among females 75 years and older, this proportion increases to 43%.[48] Individuals who live with another person and are socially active tend to consume a larger variety of foods. An inactive person who lives alone may lack motivation to prepare well-balanced meals, especially if the appetite is poor.

Apathy and depression can predispose older individuals to decreased appetite and interest in food. Depression is difficult to distinguish from symptoms related to stresses of later life, such as illness and changes in lifestyle. Some older individuals may consider depression as a natural, inevitable component of aging and may not seek treatment. Deterioration in oral health and oral health–related problems increase the risk of depressive symptoms among older adults, signifying the importance of maintaining good oral health as a determinant of subjective quality of life.[49]

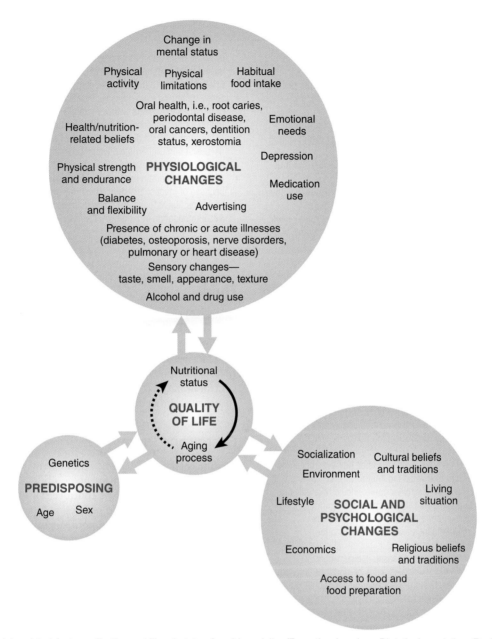

• **Fig. 15.3** Multiple interrelated factors affecting nutritional status for older adults. (From the American Dietetic Association. Position of the American Dietetic Association: Nutrition, aging, and the continuum of care. *J Am Diet Assoc.* 2000;100(5):580–594.)

DENTAL CONSIDERATIONS

Assessment
- *Physical:* Blood pressure; diagnosis of chronic disease, dentures, swallowing process, xerostomia, condition of oral cavity and gingiva; educational level; financial, socioeconomic, mental, and psychological status; types of medications taken, including over-the-counter drugs, herbal supplements, and aspirin use.
- *Dietary:* Screen for nutritional health; motivation to eat and drink; beliefs and attitudes toward foods or products to delay the aging process.

Interventions
- Osteoporosis and periodontal disease both require interdisciplinary approaches for their prevention and management.
- Encourage new denture wearers to swallow liquids with the dentures first, then to chew soft foods, and, last to bite and masticate regular foods. It is

easier to master complex masticatory movements in this order, and the mouth is protected from becoming sore. New denture wearers need to eat slowly, chew food longer, and cut raw fibrous foods such as apples and carrots into bite-size pieces.
- For edentulous patients, inquire about the preferred texture of food. Do not assume that edentulous patients require pureed foods; because of lack of visual appeal and flavor, appetite may be affected if only pureed foods are offered.
- Sweet sensitivity declines with age, leading to a compensatory increase in desire to choose foods containing sugar and possibly other carbohydrate foods.
- Normal swallowing is closely associated with chewing ability and ample saliva secretion.
- Adequate oral care, provision of dentures, prevention of tooth loss, and working with a speech pathologist on swallowing exercises may have positive effects on general health in elderly adults.

Continued

DENTAL CONSIDERATIONS   CONT'D

- Without adequate oral care, general health including swallowing, will steadily worsen.
- Improvement for problems associated with swallowing disorders related to xerostomia can be managed with oral moisturizers, lubricants, and careful use of fluids during mealtime.
- Tooth brushing may increase salivary flow for those with medication-induced dry mouth; mechanical stimulation of the salivary glands during tooth brushing may promote salivary flow.[50]
- Well-fitted dentures are effective in increasing chewing ability and thus improve food intake and oral health–related quality of life.
- Teach older patients about appropriate oral hygiene techniques to minimize gingival recession, followed by a fluoride regimen.
- Assess the fit of a denture or any prosthesis. The dental team may need to make recommendations for adjusting the prosthesis for a better fit or

refer the older patient to a physician or registered dietitian nutritionist for assessment and management of unintentional weight changes.
- Encourage older patients to eat slowly and chew their food well.
- Often, health care providers recommend lemon glycerin swabs to moisten oral tissues in patients with xerostomia. This may be detrimental to the mouth for two reasons: (1) lemon is an acid and may cause decalcification of the teeth, and (2) glycerin is a form of alcohol that can further dry oral tissues. A better alternative would be to moisten a swab with water and apply it to the dry mucosa.
- Avoidance of certain food groups (fresh fruits and vegetables, and meats) because of masticatory difficulties may aggravate other nutrition-related problems; these foods are major sources of vitamins and minerals. Recommendation of a daily multivitamin should be considered.

NUTRITIONAL DIRECTIONS

- Factors that slow the aging process include regular physical activity, abstinence from smoking, and getting adequate sleep. Physical activity enhances muscle strength and preserves muscle mass.
- Preventing and controlling oral disease to achieve good oral health is essential to healthy aging.
- Less muscle tissue and a lower activity level result in a reduced calorie requirement.
- If xerostomia is present, use artificial saliva products (oral moisturizers), sugar-free gum or hard candies (preferably containing xylitol); practice frequent oral hygiene care; and drink adequate noncariogenic fluids.
- For compromised natural dentition or xerostomia, include fluids, sauces, or gravies with each meal to make chewing easier. However, beverage consumption should not interfere with food intake.
- Because of decreased stomach acid, older adults should take calcium citrate with vitamin D supplements between meals for optimal absorption or use calcium carbonate supplements with meals.
- Low calcium intake is related to increased risk of tooth loss.
- Moderate physical activity, such as walking, is beneficial in preventing or slowing the progression of chronic diseases in older adults.[31]
- Adults aged 65 and older, need 30 minutes a day of moderate-intensity activity such as brisk walking. Exercise may also improve balance and coordination to reduce the likelihood of falling. Physical activity should include moderate-intensity aerobic activity, muscle-strengthening activity, flexibility, and balance.[32,51]

Nutrient Requirements

Dietary Reference Intakes

In 1997, the Dietary Reference Intakes (DRIs) added recommendations for individuals 51 to 70 years old and individuals older than 70 years. Metabolism to maintain body functions requires all the same nutrients, but the requirements for most micronutrients are increased because of the effects of aging on absorption, use, and excretion. With few exceptions, the recommended nutrient amounts for both groups are the same. Energy needs are lower for older individuals because of declining basal metabolism and activity level. Recommendations for several nutrients differ from those for adults 31 to 50 years old, including fiber, calcium, chromium, iron (for females), and vitamins D and B$_6$ (Table 15.1).

Fluids

In normal situations, at least eight glasses of fluids per day is recommended. Fluid intake is of particular concern because of susceptibility to fluid imbalances secondary to physiologic changes. An older patient may intentionally restrict fluids because of nocturia (excessive urination at night), incontinence (inability to control urinary excretion), pain associated with movement related to arthritis, or having to request assistance to go to the toilet.

Energy and Protein

Despite the fact that calorie requirements are less, energy balance is usually recommended for older adults. Clinical recommendation of weight loss remains controversial because of the potential for loss of lean muscle and physical function. If intentional calorie deficit to lose weight (and consequently fatty tissue) is accompanied by routine exercise to maintain physical fitness, mobility and walking speed can improve. While overweight and obesity are associated with a higher risk of CVD and weight loss is normally recommended, physical activity may be more beneficial for cardiovascular health than losing weight.[52] Weight loss, even with intentional calorie restriction and improved health indices, will not necessarily increase the lifespan in humans.

Calorie needs decrease with age, but protein needs do not. Older adults tend to consume less protein than younger adults, primarily due to reduced energy needs. Protein intake may be compromised because of illness, debilitating injuries, depressed appetite, or difficulty eating. Approximately one-third of adults over age 50 fail to meet the RDA for protein; close to 10% of older females fail to meet even the Estimated Average Requirements (EAR) for protein (0.66 g protein/kg/day).[53–55] Despite what is indicated in the RDAs, protein needs are proportional to body weight, not energy intake. Essential amino acid requirement is increased for older adults to produce a positive response in muscle protein synthesis and metabolism and stimulate bone protein metabolism. Protein also plays a pivotal role in maintenance of bone health by increasing calcium absorption and muscle strength and mass, thereby benefiting the skeleton.

The percentage of protein from animal sources providing all the essential amino acids predicts the probability of meeting the RDA. Older persons who consume higher percentages of protein can lose weight with less age-related reduction in lean tissue mass.[53] Regular moderate physical activity at any age increases

TABLE 15.1   Dietary Reference Intakes for Selected Nutrients for Older Adults

Nutrients	AGE 51–70 YEARS		AGE OLDER THAN 70 YEARS	
	Males	Females	Males	Females
Protein (g)	56	46	56	46
Carbohydrate (g)	130	130	130	130
Fiber (g)	30*	21*	30*	21*
Fat-Soluble Vitamins				
Vitamin A (µg)	900	700	900	700
Vitamin E (mg)	15	15	15	15
Vitamin D (µg/IU)[a]	15/600	15/600	20/800	20/800
Vitamin K (µg)	120*	120*	90*	90*
Water-Soluble Vitamins				
Ascorbic acid (mg)	90	75	90	75
Folate (µg)	400	400	400	400
Niacin (mg)	16	14	16	14
Riboflavin (mg)	1.3	1.1	1.3	1.1
Thiamin (mg)	1.2	1.1	1.2	1.1
Vitamin B_6 (mg)	1.7	1.5	1.7	1.5
Vitamin B_{12} (µg)[a]	2.4	2.4	2.4	2.4
Biotin (mg)	30*	30*	30*	30*
Choline (mg)	550*	550*	550*	550*
Minerals				
Calcium (mg)	1000	1200	1200	1200
Phosphorus (mg)	700	700	700	700
Iodine (µg)	150	150	150	150
Iron (mg)	8	8	8	8
Magnesium (mg)	420	320	420	320
Zinc (mg)	11	8	11	8
Selenium (µg)	55	55	55	55

[a]1 µg cholecalciferol = 40 IU vitamin D.

Note: Recommended Dietary Allowances (RDAs) are presented in bold type and Adequate Intakes (AIs) are followed by an asterisk (*).

Data from Institute of Medicine, Food and Nutrition Board. *Dietary Reference Intakes for Calcium and Vitamin D.* National Academies Press; 2011; Institute of Medicine, Food and Nutrition Board. *Dietary Reference Intakes for Vitamin C, Vitamin E, Selenium, and Carotenoids.* National Academies Press; 2000; Institute of Medicine, Food and Nutrition Board. *Dietary Reference Intakes for Calcium, Phosphorus, Magnesium, Vitamin D, and Fluoride.* National Academies Press; 1997; Institute of Medicine, Food and Nutrition Board. *Dietary Reference Intakes for Vitamin A, Vitamin K, Arsenic, Boron, Chromium, Copper, Iodine, Iron, Manganese, Molybdenum, Nickel, Silicon, Vanadium, and Zinc.* National Academies Press; 2001. Institute of Medicine. *Dietary Reference Intakes for Energy, Carbohydrate, Fiber, Fat, Fatty Acids, Cholesterol, Protein, and Amino Acids.* The National Academies Press; 2005; National Academies of Sciences, Engineering, and Medicine. *2023 Dietary Reference Intakes for Energy.* The National Academies Press; 2023.

the body's need for protein; thus protein intake slightly above the RDA (1.0 g/day) may be needed for increasing bone-mineral density and muscle mass. Protein intakes above the RDAs have been supported by several expert groups (Box 15.2). Approximately 25 to 30 g (or slightly more than 3 oz of meat) of high-quality protein will maximize muscle protein synthesis, but this amount of protein is needed three times a day rather than consuming most of the protein at one meal.[56–58]

Vitamins and Minerals

Older patients (especially females) more commonly have a negative calcium balance and lost bone mass, leading to osteoporosis and spontaneous fractures. Inadequate calcium intake is one possible reason for this, but genetic, hormonal, and environmental factors are also important.[59] Decreased physical activity contributes to calcium loss over the years. The RDA of 1200 mg of calcium

• BOX 15.2   Recommended Protein Intakes

Routinely active adults: 1.2–2.0 g/kg[a]
Healthy older adults: 1.0–1.2 g/kg[bc]
Older adults with acute or chronic disease: 1.2–1.5 g/kg[b]
Older adults with severe illness/marked malnutrition: up to 2 g/kg[b]

[a]From Thomas DT, Erdman KA, Burke LM. Position of the Academy of Nutrition and Dietetics, Dietitians of Canada, and the American College of Sports Medicine. Nutrition and athletic performance. *J Acad Nutr Diet.* 2016;116(3):501–528

[b]From Bauer JM, Diekmann R. Protein and older persons. *Clin Geriatr Med.* 2015;31(3):327–338; Deutz NE, Bauer JM, Barazzoni R, et al. Protein intake and exercise for optimal muscle function with aging: recommendations from the ESPEN Expert Group. *Clin Nutr.* 2014;33(6):929–936.

[c]From English KL, Paddon-Jones D. Protecting muscle mass and function in older adults during bed rest. *Curr Opin Clin Nutr Metab Care.* 2010;13(1):34–39.

for everyone older than age 70 years is higher than for younger adults so as to maintain bone mass and reduce risk of osteoporosis. Calcium supplements may not be as effective for remodeling bone matrix unless adequate protein (at least 1.0 g/kg) is available. [60,61] Calcium absorption, healthy bone density, and physical function, all require adequate vitamin D levels.

To prevent problems with bone mineralization, the recommendation for vitamin D intake is higher for individuals over 70 years—20 µg/day (800 IU). It is important to ensure that patients receive adequate calcium in addition to vitamin D. Low vitamin D levels are linked to muscle weakness, loss of bone strength, and falls and fractures. Prevalence of vitamin D deficiency in Americans is a public health concern because of its effects on quality of life. Vitamin D insufficiency may occur in older adults because aging skin cannot synthesize vitamin D as efficiently, homebound or institutionalized individuals are less likely to spend much time outdoors, and vitamin D intakes may be inadequate. A deficiency may also be the result of reduced production of vitamin D_3 by the skin as a result of covering the skin and using sunscreen. Other causes of vitamin D deficiency include dietary insufficiency, malabsorption, kidney disease, and use of glucocorticoids.

As many as half of older adults in the United States could be vitamin D deficient as evidenced by the numbers of hip fractures. The RDAs may be adequate for most of older individuals, but these amounts may not be adequate for high-risk seniors—those who are obese, have osteoporosis, have limited sun exposure, or experience malabsorption. For these individuals, the International Osteoporosis Foundation recommends checking status by measuring serum 25-OHD (1,25-dihydroxyvitamin D3) level. Measurement of serum 25-OHD should not be routine but is indicated for those individuals with notable risk factors [62] In vitamin D insufficiency in older individuals, supplementation reduces bone loss. Supplementation with vitamin D may reduce risk of falls only in older people whose serum vitamin D levels are low; higher levels of vitamin D seem to promote falls.[63] Muscle performance also is improved, which reduces the risk of falling and fracture risk. Current evidence by the US Preventive Services Task Force is inconclusive about the overall benefit of vitamin D, calcium or combined supplementation in the prevention of fractures.[64]

Physiologic requirements for vitamins B_6 and B_{12} are increased to prevent a decline in cognitive function and physical mobility associated with aging; B_6 has also been shown to reduce risk of CVD.[65,66] Economic factors and chewing problems may negatively affect meat consumption, thus negatively affecting vitamins B_6 and B_{12} intake. Neurologic symptoms similar to dementia may

result from deficiencies of vitamins B_6 and B_{12} when intake is reported to be marginal.[65]

Cobalamin (vitamin B_{12}) may be less available in older adults because of atrophic gastritis, **hypochlorhydria**, and bacterial overgrowth. Decreased absorption of vitamin B_{12} due to reduced hydrochloric acid production, or adverse effects of medications such as metformin, proton-pump inhibitors, and histamine H2 blockers, is common among older adults. Choosing foods fortified with vitamin B_{12} or taking a vitamin B_{12}–containing supplement is recommended to meet the RDAs. Symptoms such as cognitive decline, confusion, disorientation, and neurologic problems may improve in individuals treated with vitamin B_{12}.[67] Literature suggests that high doses of oral vitamin B_{12} may be as effective as intramuscular injections in treating symptoms of deficiency and neurological symptoms in some older adults.[67] Megaloblastic anemia occurs only in severely vitamin B_{12}–depleted individuals.

Folate is a nutrient that may be lacking in the older adult diet due to underconsumption of fruits and vegetables. Optimal folate levels have been shown to help prevent damage to blood vessels and reduce risk of atherosclerosis.[68] Supplements may result in elevated folate concentrations. High intake of folate can mask a deficiency of vitamin B12. High serum levels of folate can contribute to cognitive decline and impaired function.[69,70]

Dietary mineral intake, especially sodium, may need to be adjusted based on the patient's physiologic status. Excess or even normal dietary levels can have deleterious consequences in certain diseases, particularly hypertension or congestive heart failure. Rigid and severe restrictions may seriously affect food acceptance. Individualization is crucial; changes in intake should be under the guidance of a primary care provider or registered dietitian nutritionist.

Aging may negatively affect absorption of magnesium from foods, and the kidneys may increase excretion. Some older adults need medications that interact with magnesium (especially diuretics and long-term prescriptions for proton-pump inhibitor drugs). Higher magnesium intake to offset aging physiologic changes is associated with better physical performance. This is observed more readily in older females.[71] Dark green leafy vegetables and whole grains are good dietary sources.

Older adults generally have a weakened immune system, making them more susceptible to infection. Adequate amounts of zinc may play an important role in improving their immune system, susceptibility to infections, and decrease the severity of illnesses.[72]

Eating Patterns

Deficiencies

Compared with younger age groups, the diets of Americans 65–74 years rate better on average with regard to higher consumption of vegetables and lower sodium (Fig. 15.4). As with most Americans, the prevalence of low-energy-dense diets are more likely to provide inadequate amounts of nutrients. Most adults age 65 and older consume more calories from refined grains, added sugars, and saturated fats, and fail to meet the RDA for many nutrients. The choice of soft foods can result in a decrease in protein and more simple carbohydrate intake. Inadequate monetary resources to purchase meat products may result in less protein consumption.

Dairy products, fruits, and vegetables are frequently lacking, especially for individuals living alone. Eating more fruits and vegetables can help ward off frailty. In a study of participants with ages ranging from 69 to 82 years, those who consumed three

Average diet quality scores[a] using the Healthy Eating Index-2015 for the population age 65 and over, by age group, 2015–2016

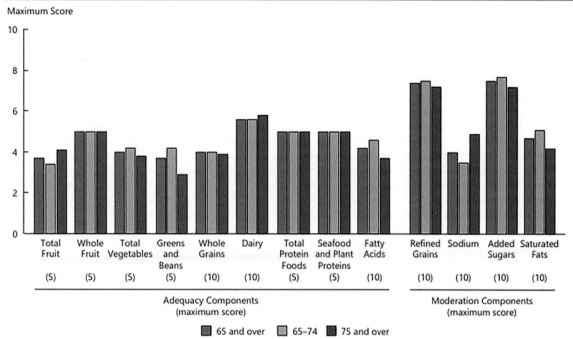

[a]Calculated using the population ratio method.

NOTE: The Healthy Eating Index-2015 (HEI-2015) is a measure of diet quality with 13 components used to assess how well a set of foods aligns with the key recommendations of the 2015–2020 Dietary Guidelines for Americans.[27] Intakes equal to or better than the standards set for each component are assigned a maximum score. Maximum HEI-2015 component scores range from 5 to 10 points. Scores for intakes between the minimum and maximum standards are scored proportionately. Scores for each component are summed to create a total maximum HEI-2015 score of 100 points. Nine of the 13 components assess adequacy components. The remaining four components assess dietary components that should be consumed in moderation. For the adequacy components, higher scores reflect higher intakes. For the moderation components, higher scores reflect lower intakes because lower intakes are more desirable. A higher total score indicates a diet that aligns better with the Dietary Guidelines. HEI-2015 total and component scores reflect usual dietary intakes among older adults in the United States. This tool was developed by the U.S. Department of Agriculture, Center for Nutrition Policy and Promotion and the U.S. Department of Health and Human Services, National Cancer Institute. The bars represent the actual scores obtained for each component. The maximum scores possible for each component are included in parentheses under each category. Total HEI scores are available in Table 24.

Reference population: These data refer to the resident noninstitutionalized population.

SOURCE: From National Center for Health Statistics, What We Eat in America, National Health and Nutrition Examination Survey (2015–2016).

• **Fig. 15.4** Healthy Eating Index–2015 average diet quality scores for population 65 and over, by age group, 2015–16.

servings of fruit and two servings of vegetables daily were at 69% lower risk of developing frailty.[73] Older individuals at highest risk of consuming minimal amounts of fruits and vegetables are those who are socially isolated, have missing pairs of posterior teeth, have poor self-reported health, and are obese.[74] Additionally, lactose intolerance may contribute to inadequate dairy intake (see Chapter 4, *Health Application 4*).

Snacks and Nutritional Supplements

Older adults have lower energy needs but increased nutrient needs in comparison to young adults. Nutrient-dense snacks may ensure consumption of adequate amounts of calories and protein for those experiencing weight loss. Underweight is a recognized risk factor for disease and disability. Between-meal snacks can be used to offset some nutrient deficits.

Milk-based food supplements, such as an instant breakfast mix, are economical and can help prevent nutrient deficiencies. Liquid supplements can augment overall nutrient intake to maintain nutritional status. Commercial liquid nutrition supplements, such as

Ensure (Abbott Nutrition), Boost (Nestle) and powder supplement Sustacal (Nestlè Health Science), that can be added to liquids, are more convenient and may be preferred. These supplements, when used routinely, may produce a small but consistent weight gain, but there is no evidence that liquid supplements affect important clinical outcomes, such as quality of life, mood, functional status, or survival. These beverages are primarily "liquid candy" nutrition shakes, resembling a multivitamin in a bottle.[75] Oral nutritional supplements can be recommended for acutely ill patients who are malnourished. Referral to the health care provider or registered dietitian nutritionist (RDN) is appropriate for these patients.

Food Safety

Foodborne illness can be very serious for older patients. Many older adults are more susceptible to foodborne illness because of a compromised immune system (placing them at risk for infections), decreased secretion of gastric hydrochloric acid, and reduced smell and taste. Food poisoning is caused by food contaminated with pathogenic bacteria, toxins, viruses, or parasites.

Dietary Guidelines and MyPlate Website for Older Adults

During 2015 to 2016, Americans aged 75 years and over met the *Dietary Guidelines* for whole fruits; Americans between the age of 65 and 75 years met the recommendations for total protein foods (see Fig. 15.4). Older Americans need to better align with the *Dietary Guidelines* by increasing dietary intakes of whole grains, vegetables and legumes, fat-free or low-fat milk products, and foods and beverages lower in sodium and that have fewer calories from solid fats and added sugars. Fruits and vegetables are also smart choices for maintaining a healthy weight because they are nutrient-dense, containing fiber, vitamins, minerals and phytonutrients.[76] Incorporating colorful fruits and vegetables such as berries, peaches, and peppers into a diet can help combat gradual weight gain.

Dietary patterns, as exemplified on the *MyPlate* website and the Mediterranean diet, higher in nutrient-rich, plant-based foods such as leafy green vegetables, berries and fruits, whole grains, nuts, olive oil, legumes and seafood while limiting red and/or processed meats, sugar-sweetened foods and drinks, refined grains, and added salt are generally associated with lower risk of age-related cognitive decline and dementia, muscle and physical deterioration and may improve quality of life and increase the lifespan.[77–82] Whereas only five servings of fruits and vegetables are recommended in the *Dietary Guidelines*, doubling that amount, or 10 servings of produce daily, may help increase the lifespan by preventing CVD, cancer, and premature mortality.[83]

The updated version of *MyPlate for Older Adults*, based on the *Dietary Guidelines* and *MyPlate* website, focuses on the unique needs associated with the aging process (see Fig. 15.5). *MyPlate for Older Adults* emphasizes nutrient-dense food choices and the importance of fruits and vegetables, healthy oils, and herbs and spices to reduce the need for salt. Further guidelines for implementation and understanding are given in Box 15.3. The groupings on this plate are slightly different than the USDA version: (1) icons of many bright-colored fruits and vegetables (fresh, frozen, dried, canned) occupy half of the plate; (2) whole, enriched, and fortified grains cover one-fourth of the plate; (3) protein sources, including nuts, beans, fish, lean meat, poultry cover one-fourth of the plate; and (4) fat-free and low-fat dairy products such as milk, cheese, and yogurts are on the top right side of the plate along with other beverages (e.g., water, coffee, tea, soup). In the center of the plate are icons depicting heart-healthy fats, for example, liquid vegetable oils and soft spreads. Figures below the plate are a reminder of the importance of staying active. The accompanying website spotlights herbs and spices as a replacement for salt to lower sodium intake.

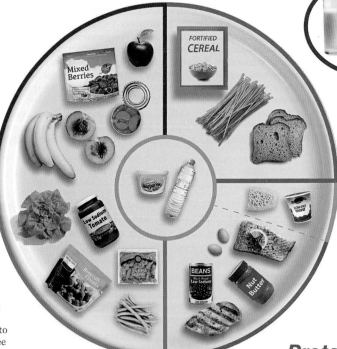

MyPlate for Older Adults

Fruits & Vegetables

Whole fruits and vegetables are rich in important nutrients and fiber. Choose fruits and vegetables with deeply colored flesh. Choose canned varieties that are packed in their own juices or low-sodium.

Healthy Oils

Liquid vegetable oils and soft margarines provide important fatty acids and some fat-soluble vitamins.

Herbs & Spices

Use a variety of herbs and spices to enhance flavor of foods and reduce the need to add salt.

Fluids

Drink plenty of fluids. Fluids can come from water, tea, coffee, soups, and fruits and vegetables.

Grains

Whole grain and fortified foods are good sources of fiber and B vitamins.

Dairy

Fat-free and low-fat milk, cheeses and yogurts provide protein, calcium and other important nutrients.

Protein

Protein rich foods provide many important nutrients. Choose a variety including nuts, beans, fish, lean meat and poultry.

Remember to Stay Active!

• **Fig. 15.5** *MyPlate for Older Adults*. (From Tufts University. 2022. https://hnrca.tufts.edu/myplate/about/download-myplate.)

• BOX 15.3   Strategies to Shift

Older adults can begin by making small shifts in food and beverage choices to improve their overall eating pattern, and then continue to build on them. Making small changes and sticking with them is the best approach to long-term improvements in eating habits. Before making major dietary changes, talk with a primary health care provider.

When selecting foods:

- Buy a variety of fresh, frozen, or no-salt-added canned vegetables and fruit packed in its own juices so that they are readily available for eating as is or adding to sauces, soups, and salads.
- Choose reduced-sodium varieties of beans, salad dressings, and baked products, as available.
- If only varieties packed in sugary syrup or salty fluids are available, rinse them before serving.
- Dried fruit and unsalted nuts make good portable snacks.
- When food is not prepared at home, try to identify, in advance, nearby restaurants and other food outlets that offer options consistent with healthy dietary patterns. When in doubt, ask the restaurant for information. Chain restaurants may post nutrition information on their website and sometimes have it available in the restaurant, and many restaurants allow some customization of entrées to better fit into a healthy dietary pattern.

Adapted from Updated nutrition for older adults. *Tufts Health Nutr Lett.* 2016;34(3):4–5.

Eating should be an enjoyable routine and, whenever possible, mealtimes should involve social interaction. Shifting toward healthier food choices can decrease risk for developing chronic diseases such as diabetes, hypertension and heart disease, neurodegenerative diseases, obesity, and early death.[84]

Vitamin-Mineral Supplements

Frequently food choices of older adults are not as well balanced as they should be or sometimes less food is consumed. Natural foods are the best source of vitamins and minerals; thus if additional food is needed for adequacy, nutrient-dense snacks should be encouraged. Because of impaired absorption of nutrients and reduced food intake, daily multivitamin-mineral supplementation at 100% of the RDA levels may be helpful in protecting against a decline in immune response and preventing anemia. Because of increased need for calcium, vitamins D and B_{12} in the older adult accompanied by poor dietary intake and decreased calorie requirements, a vitamin and/or mineral supplement may prevent deterioration of cognition and nutritional status.

A discussion with a health care provider such as medical doctor or registered dietitian nutritionist, about the need for nutritional supplements may be in order. The following recommendations about dietary supplements should be considered in combination with the individual's regular food intake with a goal of ensuring nutrients in the amounts listed in Table 15.1.

- Calcium: The recommended upper limit for calcium intake for those aged 51 years and older is 2000 mg/day. Females over age 50 years need 1200 mg (milligrams) each day. Males need 1000 mg between age 51 and 70 years and 1200 mg after 70 years. For better absorption, supplements should be taken in two 600-mg doses. Calcium not only keeps bones healthy, but also helps muscles function properly and normalizes blood pressure.
- Vitamin D: 600 IU (International Units) for people age 51 to 70 years and 800 IU for those over 70 years, but no more than 4000 IU each day. This should be taken with calcium to increase calcium absorption. This amount should not be increased without a recommendation from the health care provider.
- Vitamin B_{12}: Because of reduced absorption of vitamin B_{12} as we age, it is recommended to consume 2.4 µg daily, which may help improve cognitive function and symptoms of depression and prevent pernicious anemia.
- Omega-3 fatty acids: People who do not eat fish at least weekly may benefit from a fish oil supplement (300 mg of omega-3 fatty acid).

Over 70% of adults aged 60 years and over 25% of adults aged 60 years and over report regular use of dietary (vitamin-mineral) supplements with 25% of them reporting they are taking four or more supplements daily. Many use supplements to maintain a healthy life or prevent a disease/medical problem because they know their eating patterns are not ideal or because a health care professional recommended them.[85] Although it is common to take dietary supplements, doing so in combination with already consuming a nutrient-dense diet can result in exceeding the upper limit for one or more nutrients.

Age-related macular degeneration is a deterioration in the central area of the retina (back of the eye) in which lesions lead to loss of central vision. Evidence suggests that a diet rich in lutein and zeaxanthin (carotenoid vitamins, related to beta-carotene and vitamin A) and diets rich in fatty fish, such as salmon may reduce the risk and progression of age-related macular degeneration.[86] Evidence suggests that taking vitamin E, beta-carotene, or antioxidant supplements may prevent age-related macular degeneration. Findings showed that zinc and carotenoid supplements improved visual acuity. Beta-carotene demonstrated the ability to prevent progression of age-related macular degeneration.[87] These vitamin supplements are generally recognized as safe but can have harmful effects; clear evidence of benefit is needed before recommending them. Referral to the health care provider or an RDN is necessary to assess the need for supplements.

DENTAL CONSIDERATIONS

Assessment

- *Physical:* Visual appraisal of weight status; dry mucous membranes.
- *Dietary:* Adequacy of nutrients and fluid intake based on the *MyPlate for Older Adults*; multivitamin/mineral/herbal use.

Interventions

- To prevent dehydration, encourage older patients to use caffeine in moderation and to take medications with 8 oz of fluid. Encourage nutrient-dense foods, especially for older patients whose calorie expenditure is low.
- Discuss economical fruit, vegetable, and meat selections (see Chapter 16).
- Older patients who have had an unintentional weight change of 10% (loss or gain) in 6 months should be referred to a health care provider.

- Although absorption of vitamin B_{12} from vitamin supplements or fortified foods is not affected by atrophic gastritis, it is recommended that adults over 51 years meet the RDA for B_{12} to ensure optimum intake. Suggest enriched or fortified cereals to increase intake of iron and vitamin B_{12}.
- Encourage consumption of a vitamin C–rich food daily.
- Review economical sources of folate and cooking practices to retain folate.
- Vitamin supplements providing more than 100% of the RDA should be taken only in cases of specific need or if recommended by a health care provider.
- Encourage wise selections of convenience foods. Explain how to read food labels to make selections appropriate for restricted diets or to provide a well-balanced, nutrient-dense diet.

NUTRITIONAL DIRECTIONS

- Keep healthy snacks on hand, such as cheese, hard-boiled eggs, low-fat milk products, natural peanut butter, and fresh fruit or canned fruit with no added sugar.
- A well-balanced, nutrient-dense diet following the *MyPlate for Older Adults* or the Mediterranean style diet may delay symptoms of aging.
- Consume 2 to 4 oz of lean meat or other protein source at each meal.
- Adequate vitamin D levels are important; consult your health care provider before self-medicating with vitamin D.
- Lack of vitamin B_{12} can cause a decline in cognition and impaired balance.
- Nutrition counseling by an RDN can provide information on consuming adequate amounts of high-quality protein on a limited budget and offer alternatives to eating problems.
- Nonfat or low-fat milk is the best source of calcium and vitamin D.
- Dietary intake should strive to optimize immune function and reduce risk of disease.
- Calcium supplements should also contain vitamin D to enhance calcium absorption.

- Adequate fluid intake is beneficial for preventing and treating constipation. Soups, juices, milk products, decaffeinated soft drinks, and decaffeinated tea and coffee can enhance fluid intake.
- The vitamin B_{12} fortified in breakfast cereals or supplements is better absorbed than the form present in animal foods.
- Consult your health care provider or RDN to find out whether supplements are needed.
- Contact your health care provider or an RDN when food choices are limited over a period of time because of illness, chewing problems, lack of appetite, or inability to shop for or prepare food.
- Use of vitamin-mineral supplements does not eliminate the need to consume a nutritionally balanced diet, and supplements do not protect against development of chronic diseases associated with inappropriate food intake.
- Excess supplementation of vitamins and minerals may cause more problems with hypervitaminosis and detrimental effects on other nutrients. Zinc supplements can result in copper imbalance and reduce high-density lipoprotein cholesterol levels. Consult your health care provider or RDN.
- Heed food safety guidelines to ensure that foods do not cause illness.

 HEALTH APPLICATION 15

Complementary and Alternative Medicine and Botanical Supplements

Complementary and alternative medicine (CAM) is using diverse medical and health care systems and products, generally not considered part of conventional medicine. Complementary medicine utilizes CAM medicine together with conventional medicine, such as using acupuncture to alleviate pain. Alternative medicine pertains to use of CAM in place of conventional medicine. CAM practices often utilize herbal medicines and other "natural products." Many are available over the counter as dietary supplements. Interest in and use of CAM products have grown considerably in the past few decades. People have many reasons for turning to alternative medicine including dissatisfaction with mainstream medicine.

Medical systems that have evolved from different cultures apart from conventional or Western medicine include homeopathy (treatment of diseases with minute doses of drugs that cause symptoms of a disease in healthy people to cure similar symptoms in sick people) and naturopathy (support of the body's inherent ability to maintain and restore health, using noninvasive treatments with minimal use of surgery and drugs). Theoretically, if a certain substance causes a symptom in a healthy person, a very small amount of the same substance may cure the symptoms. The National Center for Complementary and Alternative Medicine (NCCAM), part of the National Institutes of Health (NIH), notes that most rigorous clinical trials and systematic analyses of research on homeopathy have concluded that "there is little evidence to support homeopathy as an effective treatment for any specific condition."[88] In general, homeopathic medicines are benign because, being so dilute they are unlikely to cause harm if used properly.

As with any medical treatment, risks are associated with CAM therapies. Several general-principle precautions to help minimize risks are: (1) "natural" does not always mean "safe"; (2) herbal supplements may contain dozens of compounds and some active ingredients may not be known; (3) ingredients indicated on the label and actual ingredients in the product may be different; (4) some active ingredients may be lower or higher than indicated on the label; (5) the product may be contaminated with other herbs, pesticides, or metals; (6) some dietary supplements may interact with medications or nutrients, and may have their own side effects; and (7) inform all health care providers about use of any complementary and alternative practices. Most important, homeopathy should not be used as a replacement for proven conventional care or to postpone seeing a health care provider about a medical problem.

A botanical is a plant or plant part valued for its medicinal or therapeutic properties, flavor, and/or scent. Herbs are leafy green parts of a plant, whereas spices are from any other part of the plant that can be used for seasoning—seeds, fruits, flowers, bark, or roots. Herbs are a subset of botanicals. Botanical dietary supplements, also called herbal medicines or herbal supplements have been used for centuries in attempts to maintain or improve health.

Many medications, prescription and over the counter, are actually based on naturally occurring active ingredients in plants. Until sometime in the 1970s, most medications were derived from herbs. These medications using natural substances have been thoroughly researched to verify benefits and adverse outcomes with standard quantities of active ingredients. Many natural plant materials are too toxic for human consumption.

In the 1990s the German Commission E, generally acknowledged as Europe's leading regulatory authority for evaluating therapeutic activities of herbs and the equivalent of the US Food and Drug Administration in the United States, published *The Complete German Commission E Monographs— Therapeutic Guide to Herbal Medicines*. In 1998 the National Center for Complementary and Alternative Medicine (NCCAM), already stated earlier in Health Application, was established to provide scientifically based information about CAM and herbs. About the same time, more publications focusing primarily on herbs popular in the United States were written to help health care professionals and consumers make informed decisions about herbal use and their interactions with medications.

Research-based information about specific CAM treatments and herbs is available on the NCCAM website: https://nccam.nih.gov/. NCCAM's Herbs at a Glance, a link on the same website, provides updated reliable information about more than 50 botanicals—research, potential side effects and cautions, and resources for more information. Box 15.4 shows the type of information found on the website for Ginkgo, a product that is used by many older adults. This herb is promoted to improve numerous conditions, but scientific evidence for efficacy for many of these uses is inconclusive.

Because herbs are not actual nutrients, when used for health benefits, they are considered CAMs or dietary supplements. The Dietary Supplement Health and Education Act (1994) discussed in *Health Application 11, Vitamin and Mineral Supplements* applies to herbal supplements. Herbs are not innocuous; most Americans are unaware of the potential toxicity of herbs. Consumers can purchase as much as they want of any of these products. Many people believe that "natural" products are safe and harmless.

HEALTH APPLICATION 15

Complementary and Alternative Medicine and Botanical Supplements—cont'd

Many botanicals provide a large array of phytochemicals, antioxidants, and biologically active compounds. Herbal supplements do not have to be tested for safety and effectiveness before they are marketed. Some botanicals have been evaluated in scientific studies, but the amount of scientific evidence supporting various botanical ingredients varies widely. In the amounts currently used, no negative side effects are expected. Some of the biologically active compounds have been identified and characterized, and many have unknown actions.

Herbal supplements are available in many forms—as fresh or dried products, liquid or solid extracts, tablets, capsules, powders, and teas. The form of the herb determines its potency. For instance, ginkgo seed and ginkgo leaves have different safety and clinical application profiles. Consumption of the seeds is associated with seizures and can be fatal; the active ingredients in *Ginkgo biloba* leaves (flavonoids) reduce clotting time and may be effective in improving cognitive disorders. The active compound is extracted from the plant by using a solvent such as water, fat, oil, or alcohol.

In the United States, dietary supplements are not required to be standardized. Standardization is a process manufacturers use to ensure that all batches are consistent with regard to specific chemicals. Standardization is a measure of quality control that is dependent on the manufacturer, supplier, and others in the production process. Herbs are living organisms comprised of thousands of ingredients, and the proportions may differ dramatically between two plants. Due to different growing conditions—such as the weather, amount of sun, level of soil acidity, and rainfall—known compounds present in herbs can vary significantly. The degree of accuracy between label statements and actual content is unreliable. Some products have been found to contain toxic substances.

Popular herbs do not contain any known, single active ingredients. Therefore determining the effectiveness of a given herbal batch is almost impossible. Even names of botanicals can be confusing because of different names for the same herb—ginkgo (*G. biloba*) has a pharmacopeial name of ginkgo folium; other names include duck foot tree, maidenhair tree, and silver apricot.

Emerging evidence indicates that commonly used botanicals (herbs and spices) may help protect against certain chronic conditions, such as cancer, diabetes, and heart disease. Of particular concern is the fact that one-third of older adults use CAM, and approximately 36% failed to discuss this practice with their primary care physicians.[89,90] The greatest health risk in the use of CAM and botanical medicines is the potential of the product interacting with prescribed medications. It is very important for the health care provider to be aware of any use of CAM and/or botanical medicines.

• BOX 15.4 Ginkgo

This fact sheet provides basic information about ginkgo—common names, usefulness and safety, and resources for more information.
Common Names: ginkgo, *Ginkgo biloba*, fossil tree, maidenhair tree, Japanese silver apricot, baiguo, yinhsing
Latin Name: *Ginkgo biloba*

Background

- Ginkgo, one of the oldest living tree species in the world, has a long history in traditional Chinese medicine. Members of the royal court were given ginkgo nuts for senility. Other historical uses for gingko were for asthma, bronchitis, and kidney and bladder disorders.
- Today, the extract from gingko leaves is used as a dietary supplement for many conditions, including dementia, eye problems, intermittent claudication (leg pain caused by narrowing arteries), tinnitus, and other health problems.
- Ginkgo is made into tablets, capsules, extracts, tea, and cosmetics.

How Much Do We Know?

- There have been a lot of studies on the possible health effects and risks of people using ginkgo.

What Have We Learned?

- There is no conclusive evidence that ginkgo is helpful for any health condition.
- Ginkgo does not help prevent or slow dementia or cognitive decline according to studies, including the long-term Ginkgo Evaluation Memory Study, for which more than 3000 older adults enrolled, and was funded in part by the National Center for Complementary and Integrative Health (NCCIH).
- There is no strong evidence that ginkgo helps with memory enhancement in healthy people, blood pressure, intermittent claudication, tinnitus, age-related macular degeneration, the risk of having a heart attack or stroke, or with other conditions.
- Ongoing NCCIH-funded research is looking at whether a compound in ginkgo may help with diabetes.

What Do We Know About Safety?

- For many healthy adults, ginkgo appears to be safe when taken by mouth in moderate amounts.
- Side effects of ginkgo may include headache, stomach upset, and allergic skin reactions. If you are older, have a known bleeding risk, or are pregnant, you should be cautious about ginkgo possibly increasing your risk of bleeding.
- In a 2013 research study, rodents given ginkgo had an increased risk of developing liver and thyroid cancer at the end of the 2-year tests.
- Ginkgo may interact with some conventional medications, including anticoagulants (blood thinners), research reviews show.
- Eating fresh (raw) or roasted ginkgo seeds can be poisonous and have serious side effects.

Keep in Mind

- Tell all your health care providers about any complementary or integrative health approaches you use. Give them a full picture of what you do to manage your health. This will help ensure coordinated and safe care.

For More Information

- Using Dietary Supplements Wisely (https://nccih.nih.gov/health/supplements/wiseuse.htm)
- *Ginkgo* (https://www.niehs.nih.gov/health/materials/botanical_dietary_supplements_program_ntp_508.pdf)
- Know the Science: How Medications and Supplements Can Interact (https://nccih.nih.gov/health/know-science/how-medications-supplements-interact)
- Know the Science: 9 Questions To Help You Make Sense of Health Research (https://nccih.nih.gov/health/know-science/make-sense-health-research)

From National Center for Complementary and Integrative Health, National Institutes of Health. *Ginkgo*. https://www.nccih.nih.gov/health/ginkgo.

◆ CASE APPLICATION FOR THE DENTAL HYGIENIST

A 75-year-old edentulous patient is not eating because he states that he has difficulty chewing and food does not taste good. He reports that he dislikes a lot of red meat and milk. He has lost 14 lb since his last recare appointment (usual weight 170 lb).

Nutritional Assessment

- Height; weight; appropriateness of BMI; significant weight changes, especially loss
- Nutrient and fluid intake in relation to DRIs
- Medications
- Alterations in taste, smell, or vision
- Support group, significant others, living arrangements, social support
- Psychological status

Nutritional Diagnosis

Altered nutrition: less than body requirements related to taste changes and chewing difficulty.

Nutritional Goals

The patient will consume a well-balanced diet (based on the *MyPlate for Older Adults*) and verbalize ways to increase protein and calcium intake and exercise.

Nutritional Implementation

Intervention: Encourage small, frequent meals.
Rationale: This helps the older patient consume adequate amounts of nutrients by decreasing fatigue and feelings of fullness that may occur with larger meals.
Intervention: Suggest use of spices such as pepper, thyme, and basil.
Rationale: These spices may improve the taste of foods because the older patient's ability to detect tastes is altered.
Intervention: Encourage fluids with meals.
Rationale: Drinking fluids with meals makes chewing and swallowing easier.
Intervention: Examine and question about the fit of the prosthesis. Clinically, conduct an intraoral and extraoral examination, especially noting any deviations from normal of the underlying tissue.
Rationale: The weight change may have created a loose-fitting denture and ultimately difficulty in chewing. An ill-fitting denture may also result in weight loss.

Intervention: Teach the patient to perform an oral self-examination.
Rationale: The patient also can identify oral problems earlier for more effective treatment.
Intervention: Emphasize use of eggs, turkey, chicken, fish, tenderized meat in marinades (e.g., wine or vinegar), and soy products, such as tofu.
Rationale: Because he does not like red meats, the patient may obtain needed protein in a more acceptable manner with these options.
Intervention: Emphasize the use of low-fat or nonfat dairy products, such as yogurt, cream cheese, cheese, or frozen yogurt.
Rationale: His dislike of milk lessens the likelihood of his choosing milk; these foods are alternatives to supply the needed calcium.
Intervention: Encourage adding powdered milk to soups, sauces, cereals, and casseroles.
Rationale: These are methods to increase protein and calcium consumption.
Intervention: Encourage the patient to walk outdoors for 10 to 20 minutes daily and eat foods that require more chewing, such as lettuce salads, raw carrots, cabbage, and apples.
Rationale: Physical activity is important to maintain bone density in the mandible and throughout the body. Available dietary calcium is better absorbed because it is dependent on vitamin D, which can be obtained through sunshine.
Intervention: Suggest mixing meat with vegetables.
Rationale: Because he enjoys vegetables, this form may be more palatable for him and would enhance protein intake.
Intervention: Refer the patient to Meals-on-Wheels or another federally funded program (e.g., food stamps), community meals centers, or church-sponsored centers.
Rationale: Anorexia may be a result of a lack of socialization during mealtimes.

Evaluation

The patient should be eating adequate amounts of fruits, vegetables, grains, and protein servings using *MyPlate for Older Adults* as a guide and steadily gaining weight until desired body weight is achieved. Other behaviors, such as consuming yogurt, eggs, fish, and dry milk in foods, will increase calcium and protein intake. Referral to an RDN is indicated to assist the patient in getting back to a healthy weight.

◆ Student Readiness

1. Plan a day's menus for an older edentulous patient.
2. What are some vitamin and mineral deficiencies that might influence cognitive status of older patients?
3. Discuss reasons older patients might not eat adequately.
4. Schedule a visit with a senior group meal program such as a Congregate meal program. Review the menu with an RDN and discuss beneficial effects of the program's various activities.
5. List nutritional interventions to help a healthy older patient with full dentures to eat a well-balanced diet.
6. Why are older individuals prone to dehydration? How can dehydration affect oral status?
7. Describe procedures for encouraging adequate food intake for new denture wearers.
8. What are some suggestions you could make for a patient experiencing xerostomia?
9. Name three differences in *MyPlate* and *MyPlate for Older Adults*.

◆ CASE STUDY

A 75-year-old male widowed for 2 years is seen in the health care clinic for decreased intake and a weight loss of 6 lb in the past year. He states that nothing tastes good. He is on a fixed income from Social Security. His current weight is 130 lb, and his height is 5 feet, 7 inches. He is edentulous and refuses to get dentures because he feels he is "too old."

He fixes a bologna sandwich occasionally, but mostly eats frozen food dinners. He thinks meats and fruits are too expensive to buy and states, "They spoil before I can eat them." He eats overcooked vegetables in the summer because a neighbor shares fresh produce from his garden. He does not want to use any community resources because he objects to "a handout."

1. How would you explain why "food does not taste good"?
2. What psychological and social factors may influence his dietary patterns?
3. What are some practical ways to increase protein and calcium in his diet?
4. How could you address his attitude of not wanting to accept "a handout"?
5. What medical and dental information should you assess on this male to determine nutritional status?
6. What are the strengths and weaknesses of his diet?

References

1. Federal Interagency Forum on Aging-Related Statistics. *Older Americans 2020: Key Indicators of Well-Being. Federal Interagency Forum on Aging-Related Statistics.* United States Government Printing Office; 2020. https://agingstats.gov/docs/LatestReport/OA20_508_10142020.pdf. Accessed September 17, 2023.

2. World Health Organization Quality of Life Group (WHOQOL). *WHOQOL Measuring Quality of Life.* World Health Organization; 2012. https://www.who.int/tools/whoqol.

3. Cleveland Clinic. *Dementia.* https://my.clevelandclinic.org/health/diseases/9170-dementia.

4. Centers for Disease Control. *Adult Obesity Facts.* https://www.cdc.gov/obesity/data/adult.html#:~:text=The%20obesity%20prevalence%20w%2039.8,adults%20aged%2060%20and%20older.

5. National Institute of Health. National Institute of Diabetes and Digestive and Kidney Diseases. *Overweight and Obesity Statistics.* https://www.niddk.nih.gov/health-information/health-statistics/overweight-obesity.

6. National Council on Aging. *Get the Facts on Chronic Disease Self-Management.* https://www.ncoa.org/article/get-the-facts-on-chronic-disease-self-management.

7. Qato DM, Wilder J, Schumm LP, et al. Changes in prescription and over-the-counter medication and dietary supplement use among older adults in the United States, 2005 vs. 2011. *JAMA Intern Med.* 2016;176(4):473–482.

8. Kondo K, Kikuta S, Ueha R, Suzukawa K, Yamasoba T. Age-related olfactory dysfunction: epidemiology, pathophysiology, and clinical management. *Front Aging Neurosci.* 2020;12:208. https://doi.org/10.3389/fnagi.2020.00208.

9. U.S. Department of Health and Human Services. *Healthy People 2030. Oral Conditions.* https://health.gov/healthypeople/objectives-and-data/browse-objectives/oral-conditions.

10. Goyal L, Goyal T, Gupta ND. Osteoporosis and periodontitis in postmenopausal women: a systematic review. *J Midlife Health.* 2017;8(4):151–158.

11. Eke PI, Thornton-Evans GO, Wei L, Borgnakke WS, Dye BA, Genco RJ. Periodontitis in United States adults: National Health and Nutrition Examination Survey 2009–2014. *J Am Dent Assoc.* 2018;149(7):576–588.e6.

12. Velázquez-Olmedo LB, Borges-Yáñez SA, Andrade Palos P, García-Peña C, Gutiérrez-Robledo LM, Sánchez-García S. Oral health condition and development of frailty over a 12-month period in community-dwelling older adults. *BMC Oral Health.* 2021;21(1):355. https://doi.org/10.1186/s12903-021-01718-6.

13. Okamoto N, Morikawa M, Yanagi M, et al. Association of tooth loss with development of swallowing problems in community-dwelling independent elderly population: the Fujiwara-kyo Study. *J Gerontol A Biol Sci Med Sci.* 2015;70(12):1548–1554.

14. Furuta M, Takeuchi K, Adachi M, et al. Tooth loss, swallowing dysfunction and mortality in Japanese older adults receiving home care services. *Geriatr Gerontol Int.* 2018;18(6):873–880.

15. Xu KH, Li L, Jia SL, et al. Association of tooth loss and diet quality with acceleration of aging: evidence from NHANES. *Am J Med.* 2023;136(8):773–779.e4.

16. Kumar A, Karthik KVGC, Sunkala L, et al. Evaluation of the mean bite force and masticatory performance of maxillary and mandibular complete dentures vs mandibular implant-supported over denture. *J Contemp Dent Pract.* 2022;23(5):513–519.

17. Shen J, Qian S, Huang L, et al. Association of the number of natural teeth with dietary diversity and nutritional status in older adults: a cross-sectional study in China. *J Clin Periodontol.* 2023;50(2):242–251.

18. Moynihan P, Varghese R. Impact of wearing dentures on dietary intake, nutritional status, and eating: a systematic review. *JDR Clin Trans Res.* 2022;7(4):334–351.

19. McReynolds DE, Moorthy A, Moneley JO, Jabra-Rizk MA, Sultan AS. Denture stomatitis--An interdisciplinary clinical review. *J Prosthodont.* 2023;32(7):560–570.

20. Puryer J. Denture stomatitis—a clinical update. *Dent Update.* 2016;43(6):529–535.

21. Katz B, Airaghi K, Davy B. Does hydration status influence executive function? A systematic review. *J Acad Nutr Diet.* 2021;121(7):1284–1305.e1.

22. Marra MV, Simmons SF, Shotwell MS, et al. Elevated serum osmolality and total water deficit indicate impaired hydration status in residents of long-term care facilities regardless of low or high body mass index. *J Acad Nutr Diet.* 2016;116(5):828–836.

23. Li S, Xiao X, Zhang X. Hydration status in older adults: current knowledge and future challenges. *Nutrients.* 2023;15(11):2609.

24. Sözen T, Özışık L, Başaran NÇ. An overview and management of osteoporosis. *Eur J Rheumatol.* 2017;4(1):46–56. https://doi.org/10.5152/eurjrheum.2016.048.

25. NIH Consensus Development Panel on Osteoporosis Prevention. Diagnosis, and Therapy. Osteoporosis prevention, diagnosis, and therapy. *JAMA.* 2001;285:785–795.

26. Maeda K, Shamoto H, Wakabayashi H, et al. Sarcopenia is highly prevalent in older medical patients with mobility limitation. *Nutr Clin Pract.* 2017;32(1):110–115.

27. Landi F, Calvani R, Ortolani E, et al. The association between sarcopenia and functional outcomes among older patients with hip fracture undergoing in-hospital rehabilitation. *Osteoporos Int.* 2017;28(5):1569–1576.

28. Han CH, Chung JH. Association between sarcopenia and tooth loss. *Ann Geriatr Med Res.* 2018;22(3):145–150.

29. Iwasaki M, Kimura Y, Ogawa H, et al. The association between dentition status and sarcopenia in Japanese adults aged ≥75 years. *J Oral Rehabil.* 2017;44(1):51–58.

30. Batsis JA, Villareal DT. Sarcopenic obesity in older adults: aetiology, epidemiology and treatment strategies. *Nat Rev Endocrinol.* 2018;14(9):513–537.

31. United States Department of Health and Human Services. *Physical Activity Guidelines for Americans Midcourse Report: Implementation Strategies for Older Adults.* United States Department of Health and Human Services; 2023 https://health.gov/sites/default/files/2023–06/PAG_MidcourseReport_508c_final.pdf.

32. United States Department of Health and Human Services. *Physical Activity Guidelines for Americans.* 2nd ed. United States Department of Health and Human Services; 2018. https://health.gov/sites/default/files/2019–09/Physical_Activity_Guidelines_2nd_edition.pdf.

33. Ciumărnean L, Milaciu MV, Negrean V, et al. Cardiovascular risk factors and physical activity for the prevention of cardiovascular diseases in the elderly. *Int J Environ Res Public Health.* 2021;19(1):207.

34. Hayes SM, Hayes JP, Williams VJ, et al. FMRI activity during associative encoding is correlated with cardiorespiratory fitness and source memory performance in older adults. *Cortex.* 2017; pii: S0010–9452(17)30005–9.

35. Wong MYC, Ou KL, Chung PK, Chui KYK, Zhang CQ. The relationship between physical activity, physical health, and mental health among older Chinese adults: a scoping review. *Front Public Health.* 2023;10:914548.

36. Langhammer B, Bergland A, Rydwik E. The importance of physical activity exercise among older people. *Biomed Res Int.* 2018;2018:7856823.

37. Ponti F, Santoro A, Mercatelli D, et al. Aging and imaging assessment of body composition: from fat to facts. *Front Endocrinol (Lausanne).* 2020;10:861.

38. American Physiological Society. Older people who diet without exercising lose valuable muscle mass. *ScienceDaily.* 2008. http://www.sciencedaily.com/releases/2008/09/080917095349.htm.

39. Coelho-Junior HJ, Marzetti E, Picca A, Cesari M, Uchida MC, Calvani R. Protein Intake and Frailty: A Matter of Quantity, Quality, and Timing. *Nutrients.* 2020;12(10):2915.

40. Liao CD, Tsauo JY, Wu YT, et al. Effects of protein supplementation combined with resistance exercise on body composition and physical function in older adults: a systematic review and *meta*-analysis. *Am J Clin Nutr.* 2017;106(4):1078–1091.

41. Nazri NSM, Vanoh D, Soo KL. Natural food for sarcopenia: a narrative review. *Malays J Med Sci.* 2022;29(4):28–42. https://doi.org/10.21315/mjms2022.29.4.4. Epub 2022 Aug 29.

42. Ganapathy A, Nieves JW. Nutrition and sarcopenia—what do we know? *Nutrients.* 2020;12(6):1755. https://doi.org/10.3390/nu12061755.

43. Verlaan S, Maier AB, Bauer JM, et al. Sufficient levels of 25-hydroxyvitamin D and protein intake required to increase muscle mass in sarcopenic older adults—the PROVIDE study. *Clin Nutr.* 2017 pii: S0261–5614(17)30010–9. [Epub ahead of print].

44. Uchitomi R, Oyabu M, Kamei Y. Vitamin D and sarcopenia: potential of vitamin D supplementation in sarcopenia prevention and treatment. *Nutrients.* 2020;12(10):3189.

45. Wang X, Yu Z, Zhou S, Shen S, Chen W. The effect of a compound protein on wound healing and nutritional status. *Evid Based Complement Altern Med.* 2022;2022:4231516.

46. Ziliak J.P., Gundersen C. *The State of Senior Hunger in American in 2021: An Annual Report.* 2023. https://www.feedingamerica.org/sites/default/files/2023–04/State%20of%20Senior%20Hunger%20in%202021.pdf.

47. Gearan E, Niland K. Mathmatica Research. Older American Act Title III-D Nutrition Services Program: key food sources of sodium, saturated fat, empty calories and refined grains in the diets of program participants. Administration for Community Living. *Adm Aging Issue Brief.* 2019. https://acl.gov/sites/default/files/programs/2019-01/AoA_Issue_Brief_Food_Sources.pdf.

48. Department of Health and Human Services. *Administration for Community Living, Administration on Aging. 2021 Profile of Older Americans.* 2022. https://acl.gov/sites/default/files/Profile%20of%20OA/2021%20Profile%20of%20OA/2021ProfileOlderAmericans_508.pdf.

49. Park KE, Lee H, Kwon YD, Kim S. Association between changes in oral health-related quality of life and depressive symptoms in the Korean elderly population. *Int J Public Health.* 2023;68:1605403.

50. Affoo RH, Trottier K, Garrick R, et al. The effects of tooth brushing on whole salivary flow rate in older adults. *Biomed Res Int.* 2018;2018:3904139.

51. Centers for Disease Control. *How Much Physical Activity Do Older Adults Need?* https://www.cdc.gov/physicalactivity/basics/older_adults/index.htm#:~:text=Adults%20aged%2065%20and%20older,hiking%2C%20jogging%2C%20or%20running.

52. Koolhaas CM, Dhana K, Schoufour JD, et al. Impact of physical activity on the association of overweight and obesity with cardiovascular disease: the Rotterdam Study. *Eur J Prev Cardiol.* 2017;24(9):934–941.

53. Krok-Schoen JL, Archdeacon Price A, Luo M, Kelly OJ, Taylor CA. Low dietary protein intakes and associated dietary patterns and functional limitations in an aging population: a NHANES analysis. *J Nutr Health Aging.* 2019;23(4):338–347.

54. Wolfe RR, Miller SL. The recommended dietary allowance of protein: a misunderstood concept. *JAMA.* 2008;299:2891–2893.

55. Houston D.K., Nicklas B.J., Ding J., et al. Dietary protein intake is associated with lean mass change in older, community-dwelling adults: the Health, Aging, and Body Composition (Health ABC) study. *Am J Clin Nutr.* 2008; 87:150–155.

56. Porter Starr KN, Pieper CF, Orenduff MC, et al. Improved function with enhanced protein intake per meal: a pilot study of weight reduction in frail, obese older adults. *J Gerontol A Biol Sci Med Sci.* 2016;71(10):1369–1375.

57. Gaytán-González A, Ocampo-Alfaro MJ, Torres-Naranjo F, et al. The consumption of two or three meals per day with adequate protein content is associated with lower risk of physical disability in Mexican adults aged 60 years and older. *Geriatrics (Basel).* 2020;5(1):1.

58. Bauer J, Biolo G, Cederholm T, et al. Evidence-based recommendations for optimal dietary protein intake in older people: a position paper from the PROT-AGE Study Group. *J Am Med Dir Assoc.* 2013;14(8):542–559.

59. Management of osteoporosis in postmenopausal women. the 2021 position statement of The North American Menopause Society. *Menopause.* 2021;28(9):973–997.

60. Kerstetter J, O'Brien K, Insogna K. Dietary protein affects intestinal calcium absorption. *Am J Clin Nutr.* 1998;68:859–865.

61. Zittermann A, Schmidt A, Haardt J, et al. Protein intake and bone health: an umbrella review of systematic reviews for the evidence-based guideline of the German Nutrition Society. *Osteoporos Int.* 2023;34:1335–1353.

62. International Osteoporosis Foundation. *Vitamin D.* https://www.osteoporosis.foundation/health-professionals/prevention/nutrition/vitamin-d.

63. Thanapluetiwong S, Chewcharat A, Takkavatakarn K, Praditpornsilpa K, Eiam-Ong S, Susantitaphong P. Vitamin D supplement on prevention of fall and fracture: a *meta*-analysis of randomized controlled trials. *Med (Baltim).* 2020;99(34):e21506.

64. United States Preventive Services Task Force. Vitamin D, calcium, or combined supplementation for the primary prevention of fractures in community-dwelling older adults: recommendation statement. *Am J Phys.* 2018;98(4). https://www.aafp.org/pubs/afp/issues/2018/0815/od2.pdf.

65. Wang Z, Zhu W, Xing Y, Jia J, Tang Y. B vitamins and prevention of cognitive decline and incident dementia: a systematic review and *meta*-analysis. *Nutr Rev.* 2022;80(4):931–949. https://doi.org/10.1093/nutrit/nuab057.

66. Yang D, Liu Y, Wang Y, Ma Y, Bai J, Yu C. Association of serum vitamin B6 with all-cause and cause-specific mortality in a prospective study. *Nutrients.* 2021;13(9):2977.

67. Wang H, Li L, Qin LL, et al. Oral vitamin B_{12} versus intramuscular vitamin B_{12} for vitamin B_{12} deficiency. *Cochrane Database Syst Rev.* 2018;3(3):CD004655. https://doi.org/10.1002/14651858.CD004655.pub3.

68. Wei T, Liu J, Zhang D, et al. The relationship between nutrition and atherosclerosis. *Front Bioeng Biotechnol.* 2021;9:635504.

69. Fan Y, Liu W, Chen S, et al. Association between high serum tetrahydrofolate and low cognitive functions in the United States: a cross-sectional study. *J Alzheimers Dis.* 2022;89(1):163–179.

70. Bailey RL, Jun S, Murphy L, et al. High folic acid or folate combined with low vitamin B-12 status: potential but inconsistent association with cognitive function in a nationally representative cross-sectional sample of United States older adults participating in the NHANES. *Am J Clin Nutr.* 2020;112(6):1547–1557. https://doi.org/10.1093/ajcn/nqaa239.

71. Arias-Fernández L, Struijk EA, Caballero FF, et al. Prospective association between dietary magnesium intake and physical performance in older women and men. *Eur J Nutr.* 2022 Aug;61(5):2365–2373.

72. Fantacone ML, Lowry MB, Uesugi SL, et al. The effect of a multivitamin and mineral supplement on immune function in healthy older adults: a double-blind, randomized, controlled trial. *Nutrients.* 2020;12(8):2447.

73. Kojima G, Taniguchi Y, Urano T. Fruit and vegetable consumption and incident frailty in older adults: a systematic review and *meta*-analysis. *J Frailty Aging.* 2022;11(1):45–50.

74. Kossioni AE. The association of poor oral health parameters with malnutrition in older adults: a review considering the potential implications for cognitive impairment. *Nutrients.* 2018;10(11):1709.

75. AGS Choosing Wisely Workgroup. American Geriatrics Society identifies five things that healthcare providers and patients should question. *J Am Geriatr Soc.* 2013;61(4):622–631.

76. Lee SH, Moore LV, Park S, Harris DM, Blanck HM. Adults Meeting Fruit and Vegetable Intake Recommendations—United States, 2019. *MMWR Morb Mortal Wkly Rep.* 2022;71:1–9.

77. Masana MF, Koyanagi A, Haro JM, et al. N-3 fatty acids, Mediterranean diet and cognitive function in normal aging: a systematic review. *Exp Gerontol.* 2017;91:39–50.

78. Yannakoulia M, Ntanasi E, Anastasiou CA, et al. Frailty and nutrition: from epidemiological and clinical evidence to potential mechanisms. *Metabolism.* 2017;68:64–76.

79. Shlisky J, Bloom DE, Beaudreault AR, et al. Nutritional considerations for healthy aging and reduction in age-related chronic disease. *Adv Nutr.* 2017;8(1):17–26.

80. Guasch-Ferré M, Willett WC. The Mediterranean diet and health: a comprehensive overview. *J Intern Med.* 2021;290(3):549–566.

81. Miller MG, Thangthaeng N, Poulose SM, et al. Role of fruits, nuts, and vegetables in maintaining cognitive health. *Exp Gerontol.* 2017;94:24–28.

82. Coelho-Júnior HJ, Trichopoulou A, Panza F. Cross-sectional and longitudinal associations between adherence to Mediterranean diet with physical performance and cognitive function in older adults: a systematic review and *meta*-analysis. *Ageing Res Rev.* 2021;70:101395.

83. Aune D, Giovannucci E, Boffetta P, et al. Fruit and vegetable intake and the risk of cardiovascular disease, total cancer and all-cause mortality—a systematic review and dose–response *meta*-analysis of prospective studies. *Int J Epidemiol.* 2017;46(3):1029–1056.

84. Sotos-Prieto M, Bhupathiraju SN, Mattei J, et al. Association of changes in diet quality with total and cause-specific mortality. *N Engl J Med.* 2017;377:143–153.

85. Mishra S, Gahche JJ, Ogden CL, et al. *Dietary supplement use in the United States: National Health and Nutrition Examination Survey, 2017–March 2020. National Health Statistics Reports; No 183.* National Center for Health Statistics; 2023.

86. Eisenhauer B, Natoli S, Liew G, Flood VM. Lutein and Zeaxanthin-Food Sources, Bioavailability and Dietary Variety in Age-Related Macular Degeneration Protection. *Nutrients.* 2017;9(2):120.

87. Li SS, Wang HH, Zhang D. Efficacy of different nutrients in age-related macular degeneration: A systematic review and network *meta*-analysis. *Semin Ophthalmol.* 2022;37(4):515–523.

88. National Institutes of Health (NIH), National Center for Complementary and Integrative Health (NCCIH). *Homeopathy: What You Need to Know.* https://nccih.nih.gov/health/homeopathy.

89. Johnson PJ, Jou J, Rockwood TH, Upchurch DM. Perceived benefits of using complementary and alternative medicine by race/ethnicity among midlife and older adults in the United States. *J Aging Health.* 2019;31(8):1376–1397.

90. Golden J, Kenyon-Pesce L, Robison J, Grady J, Guerrera MP. Disclosure of complementary and alternative medicine use among older adults: a cross-sectional study. *Gerontol Geriatr Med.* 2023;9 23337214231179839.

▶ Evolve Resources

Please visit http://evolve.elsevier.com/Mallonee/nutritional for additional practice and study support tools.

16

Food Factors Affecting Health

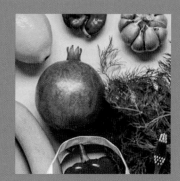

STUDENT LEARNING OBJECTIVES

On completion of this chapter, the student will be able to achieve the following learning objectives:

1. Discuss health care disparities and how they relate to oral health.
2. Regarding (or with regard to) food patterns:
   - Explain how a patient can obtain adequate nutrients from different cultural food patterns.
   - Identify reasons for food patterns.
   - Respect cultural and religious food patterns while providing nutritional recommendations for patients.
3. Pertaining to food budgets:
   - Explain to a patient how to prepare and store food to retain nutrient value.

- Inform patients of ways to make economical food purchases.
- Explain to a patient how food processing, convenience foods, and fast foods affect overall intake.
- Discuss reasons why food additives are used.
4. Describe food fads, and list reasons why health quackery can be dangerous. Also, identify common themes of health fraud or scams and why they are inconsistent with evidence-based research.
5. Provide referrals for nutritional resources, and describe the role of dental hygienists in combating nutrition fads and misinformation.

KEY TERMS

Chelation therapy
Detoxification
Dietary acculturation
Evidence-based
Foodborne illness
Food deserts

Food fad
Food insecurity
Food patterns
Food quackery
Hunger
Irradiated foods

Meta-analysis
Observational studies
Organic
Stable nutrients
Systematic reviews
Very low food security

⬡ TEST YOUR NQ

1. **T/F** Religion can affect food patterns.
2. **T/F** Adults usually avoid the foods they ate during childhood.
3. **T/F** The nutritional content of food is the most important reason for an individual's food choices.
4. **T/F** Most consumers spend about 25% of their income on food.
5. **T/F** Fad diets are usually well-balanced and nutritious.
6. **T/F** Organic foods are more nutritious.
7. **T/F** All food processing is detrimental to the nutritional quality of foods.
8. **T/F** Fast foods are usually a good source of protein.
9. **T/F** Food additives improve the nutritional value of foods.
10. **T/F** Individual food preferences do not ordinarily influence nutritional adequacy of the diet.

Health Care Equity and Disparities

Health care equity is a serious problem in the United States and leads to health disparities for many groups, especially for racial/ethnic minorities and low-income groups. The Centers for Disease Control and Prevention (CDC) reports that quality of health care in the United States varies according to the patient's income, race and ethnicity, resulting in health care disparities.[1] By 2060, 55.7% of the American population may consist of ethnic minorities in contrast to 38.7% in 2016.[2] Many racial and ethnic minorities may come from different cultural backgrounds with a variety of health beliefs and practices. Health literacy is a social determinant of health and includes an understanding of how to access health information and services to make informed decisions.[3] In addition, language may present a barrier to health literacy.

Health professionals need to be able to provide health care to accommodate different cultural beliefs. A diverse health care workforce and cultural competence of health care providers contributes to reducing racial and ethnic disparities in health and health care. Cultural competency requires a dedication of dental professionals to understand and serve others and be responsive to a variety of cultural and health beliefs to improve health outcomes. Additionally, they should be familiar with health problems common among the racial and ethnic groups served most frequently in their community, whether they be Black, Asians, Hispanics/Latinos, Native American/Alaskan Natives, Native Hawaiian/Pacific Islanders, or low socioeconomic groups.

Dietary Patterns

Dietary patterns are generally developed during childhood and reflect the family's lifestyle and its ethnic or cultural traditions and customs, religious, personal preferences, geographic location, budget constraints, and psychological components.[4] All of these influence one's attitudes, feelings, and beliefs about food. However, cultural and economic factors typically have the greatest influence on food choices.

Nutritional value is secondary, especially if a food has established social, religious, or economic status. For example, kale is one of the most nutritious vegetables (based on nutrient density) available in the United States but is a less-popular vegetable. On the other hand, the tomato, the most commonly eaten vegetable, rates comparatively low as a source of vitamins and minerals.

Cultural Traditions and Customs

Because of growing diversity in the United States and other countries, dietary needs unique to cultures have a direct impact on the national health. One of the most interesting and visible ways that cultural identity is expressed is through an individual's food choices.[5,6] In many cultures, food has social and religious or ceremonial roles.[7]

Many cultures have brought a rich heritage of various **food patterns** to the United States, resulting in distinct and discrete patterns of food consumption. Cultural dietary patterns establish the foundation for a child's lifelong eating patterns regarding meal times and frequency of eating, foods acceptable for specific meals, preparation methods, likes and dislikes, foods suitable for specific members of a group or specific time of day, table manners, the social role of foods and eating, and attitudes toward eating and health (Fig. 16.1).

American diets have become more homogeneous because of transportation, advertising, mobility, new methods of production, changes in income distribution, and appreciation of one another's heritage. While food preferences are influenced by diverse cultures, some regional food patterns are still evident—few

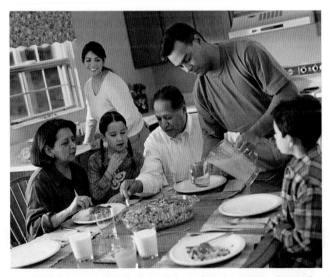

• **Fig. 16.1** An extended family eating a dinner together. (From Food and Nutrition Service, United States Department of Agriculture and Food and Nutrition Information Center, National Agricultural Library. *SNAP-Ed Connections: Photo Gallery*. https://snaped.fns.usda.gov/extended-family-eating-dinner-together.)

people in northern states would routinely choose grits and many Southerners might not choose lentils.

Status and Symbolic Influences

Cultures often regard a food differently. For example, beef is regarded as a high-status food among some people in the United States, but some Hindus from India consider cows sacred and do not eat beef. The choice of different foods is influenced by religious beliefs, preferences, availability, cost, cultural values, and traditions.

Because of the cultural meanings of food, food and eating evoke emotion, feelings of comfort, cultural identity and can be a symbol of acceptance.[6,7] Foods sometimes become symbolic because of religious connotations. Food may also be used as a reward. After a child has fallen, a mother may give the child ice cream or candy to help forget the pain and stop crying. Food may also be withheld for bad behavior.

Working with Patients with Different Food Patterns

Respect for Other Eating Patterns

As a part of gathering medical, dental, and psychosocial history, the dental hygienists must also explore health beliefs and behaviors which include cultural food beliefs. It is essential to put aside our own beliefs, bias, and assumptions.[7] Cultural sensitivity and competence is the ability to discover each patient's cultural and ethnic preferences and effectively adapt interventions.

Even when the patient information is gathered, an analysis of the situation is needed to identify individual habits and preferences. Information should be obtained regarding food habits using open-ended questions rather than leading questions to get an authentic response from the patient. For example, "Tell me everything you had to eat or drink when you got up this morning" might elicit a different response than the leading question, "What did you eat for breakfast this morning?"

Changing Behavior

Knowledge of food preferences and attitudes is important for recognizing and respecting differences that may impact the recommendations provided to the patient. An empathetic, observant dental hygienist understands and is aware of unique characteristics of local cultures and treats each patient with respect while attempting to promote healthy dietary patterns.

Cultural food patterns have contributed to survival of the group in a particular environment. People have a remarkable ability to obtain a nutritious diet out of available foodstuffs. Some eating patterns that seem unusual may actually be beneficial to improve or preserve nutritional value, such as fermenting vegetables for sauerkraut or kimchi.

Food patterns of other countries in some instances are nutritionally superior or at least comparable to "ordinary" American traditions. When people relocate, they retain their traditional food patterns only if their native foods are available in a new location at an affordable price. Finding native foods that were the basis of their family traditional food pattern may be a challenge. This can have a negative impact on new immigrant's cultural identity and well-being, and it is referred to as cultural food insecurity.[6]

Foods from the country of origin, which were cheapest at "home," may be very expensive or possibly unavailable at the new location. Immigrants may find their culturally preferred foods easily in urban areas because many Americans are interested in exotic and ethnic cuisines, increasing availability of ethnic foods in supermarkets and ethnic restaurants. If the location is a rural, less populated area, finding native foods may be more difficult.

Each food, food-related behavior, and tradition can be categorized as beneficial, neutral, or potentially harmful. A food that is beneficial promotes health by contributing necessary nutrients. Neutral foods are not especially beneficial but are not harmful to health. Foods are not usually harmful, but customs affecting nutritional content of the food may be potentially harmful. Efforts should be made to alter only those patterns negatively affecting nutritional value or health. For example, because many water-soluble vitamins are destroyed by heat, the practice of cooking foods (especially vegetables) for long periods is discouraged unless the liquids are consumed.

Food patterns are generally deeply ingrained, contribute to psychological stability, and are hard to change. If dietary changes are indicated for health or dental reasons, suggest minimal alterations in the patient's normal patterns and, if possible, present the information with options consistent with established food habits. Rather than indicating that a patient needs to stop eating a food that is a part of the cultural heritage, talk about portion control of the food. Health care workers who do not address individual patient needs are ineffective, and patients feeling uncomfortable with the information will not use it.

Cultural patterns tend to be used more consistently by older family members. First-generation immigrants are still rooted in their homeland and may prefer traditional foods. Dental professionals should learn about cultural and ethnic foods for immigrants in the area so they can assist in suggesting alternatives or similar types of foods. Gradually, the diet conforms to food resources of the new location, a process called **dietary acculturation**. This is not always a good thing because the diet quality of the US diet is lower than many of the immigrant's native countries.[8] Second-generation Americans are raised without that direct cultural connection, and their parents, often struggling with new foods themselves, may not have the knowledge to educate their children about healthy American dietary patterns.

It is impossible to cover the dietary practices of all cultures and religions in this text. This USDA website: Culture and Food has links to many resources https://www.nutrition.gov/topics/shopping-cooking-and-meal-planning/culture-and-food. Fig. 16.2 is a food guide for Mexico. The Canadian Food Guide was presented in Chapter 1 (see Fig. 1.7). https://www.myplate.gov/website.

Religious Dietary Rules

Religious beliefs affect eating pattern which have symbolic meanings to food and drink. Religions with dietary rules include Judaism, Hinduism, Islam, Catholicism, Seventh Day Adventist, Sikhism, and Orthodox churches. For example, Hindus hold cows as sacred and many avoid eating meat fish, and eggs.[9] While many dietary rules do not result in any nutritional problems and some vegetarian diets may be beneficial, there is some risk of deficiencies in the dietary patterns that are strictly vegan (e.g., vitamin B12 and iron) and for those restricting dairy (e.g., calcium and vitamin D).[9]

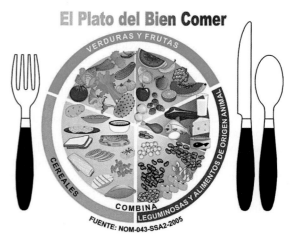

• **Fig. 16.2** Mexican food guide. (From Mahan LK, Escott-Stump S, Raymond JL. *Krause's Food and the Nutrition Care Process*. 13th ed. Saunders; 2012.)

DENTAL CONSIDERATIONS

- Be aware of cultural or religious beliefs to adapt recommendations to fit with the patient's belief system to increase compliance.
- The increasing ethnic and cultural diversity of the United States presents new challenges to health professionals in offering culturally sensitive interventions to improve the health of their patients.
- When working with patients who have strong cultural ties, maintain a sensitive, nonjudgmental, and respectful perspective of their preferences.
- A strong accent or lack of English proficiency is not indicative of educational level or intelligence.
- Patients are more likely to disclose crucial information to an open-minded dental hygienist who avoids cultural biases.
- Allow patients from different cultures the time needed to respond and explore options for using pictures and/or an interpreter to add with communication.
- Patients are more receptive to minor changes in the diet pattern. The key is to make small changes.
- Identify advantages and disadvantages for each cultural food pattern in your area.
- Use an understanding of ethnic food habits to encourage or incorporate beneficial practices into the patient's diet.
- Compliance is improved when a patient has input into changes in food choices, understands why changes are indicated, and feels responsible for following any suggestions.
- Individuals from all cultures have unique tastes and preferences and it is important to understand that this can be connected to their cultural identity. Avoid bias, but open-mindedly.
- In many cases, dietary acculturation to American food practices adopted by immigrants have been deleterious to their health by contributing to the same chronic diseases typical in the United States.

NUTRITIONAL DIRECTIONS

- Dietary patterns and attitudes internalized during childhood promote a sense of stability, comfort, and security for adults.
- An adequate diet can be planned incorporating most cultural and religious beliefs. The *Dietary Guidelines* and *MyPlate* are flexible and created to adapt to various cultural dietary patterns and traditions.

Food Budgets

Foods available in the home are primarily the result of food shopping behaviors and budget. If nutrient-dense healthful foods are not purchased, they cannot be consumed. Likewise, if more energy-dense foods are purchased, they compete with more healthful choices. Many Americans are anxious about food prices increasing by 9.9% in 2022 and predicted to rise by another 5.9% in 2023.[10] Fluctuating prices from year to year reflect supply and demand both within the United States and internationally. Evidence that poor or fair health status and malnutrition increase as income level decreases, is discussed in *Health Application 16*.

The average American family spends approximately 11% of its disposable income on food; families at the poverty level may spend 31%.[11] Based on US Department of Agriculture (USDA) food plans for 2023, the monthly cost of food for a family of four ranges between $822 (low-cost plan) and $1243 (liberal food plan).[12]

In 2021 Americans spent more on food away from home (56%) than for foods purchased for the home.[11] In general, a large proportion of the food dollar is spent on processed foods. A general awareness of food costs can help patients stretch their food dollar to make healthy choices. Box 16.1 provides some basic principles for managing a food budget.

The controversy continues about whether healthy eating is too expensive, particularly for low-income individuals and families.[13-16] The average cost per person of a healthy diet in 2021 was $3.22 per day, and 1.4% or 4 million individuals in the United States were unable to afford a healthy diet.[15] Unfortunately diets with more ultra and highly processed foods are less expensive than those with minimally processed foods so careful planning and use of food dollars is critical to stay within a budget and maximize diet quality (see Box 16.1).[14,16] Vegetables followed by fruit and protein recommendations tend to be the most challenging components of the *Dietary Guidelines* and *MyPlate* to meet, particularly for low-income individuals and families.[17] Minimizing purchasing of food with low nutrient quality like soft drinks and other sugar-sweetened beverages, sweets can help to preserve food dollars for healthy options. Another way to reduce food costs is to prepare meals at home.[18] In one study, the monthly spending for food was reduced by $261 to $330 and improved diet quality.[18] Foods prepared away from home are higher in calories from saturated fat, sodium, and refined grains with large portion sizes.[18,19]

Based on the *Dietary Guidelines*, food choices of low-income households are affected not only by available food dollars, but also personal (education level) and neighborhood factors (e.g., food deserts). **Food deserts** are located in lower-income inner-city and rural areas with few supermarkets; numerous small stores stock limited nutritious food items, particularly fruits and vegetables, at affordable prices. Low-income shoppers spend less on food purchases despite the fact that food prices are higher where they are compelled to shop. Without transportation, low-income consumers are often limited to shopping close to where they live or they must spend money for travel or delivery services. Lack of availability of a variety of produce and poor quality are deterrents to eating healthier for very-low-income consumers. Small, low-income-area grocery stores may inconsistently stock whole grains, low-fat cheeses, lean ground beef, and larger package sizes. In addition, the educational level of consumers impacts food purchases.

Individuals with lower levels of education and living in rural areas or food deserts were more likely to have lower diet quality

---

• BOX 16.1   Basic Principles for Economical Food Purchases

1. Take inventory of the food you have on hand before going to the grocery store.
2. Plan weekly or monthly menus using the *MyPlate* website as a guideline.
3. Plan menus around seasonal foods or weekly specials.
4. Prepare a shopping list based on the menu and stick to it. Be sure to plan for using leftovers to minimize food waste. Be organized and limit the number of trips to the grocery store. Know your food prices and check warehouse stores, co-ops, and other grocery stores with lower priced items. Avoid shopping at convenience stores where selection is limited and prices are high.
5. Never shop when hungry.
6. Shop alone when possible, bringing children and other family members may increase the chances of impulse purchases.
7. Rely on minimal servings of meats. On the average, purchase 1 lb ground beef or turkey for four people. When purchasing steaks, check the weight; most would serve at least two people.
8. Use meat substitutes (e.g., legumes, nuts, peanut butter, and cheese) several times each week.
9. Serve appropriate portion sizes of whole grains, cereals, and pasta products (6–11 servings per day).
10. Prepare most foods from scratch rather than buying preprepared or convenience items, such as frozen pizza.
11. Limit highly processed foods that are expensive or have low nutrient density (e.g., carbonated beverages and chips). Replace these foods with fresh fruits and vegetables.
12. Avoid impulse buying, and be prepared to make substitutions if a similar item is a better buy.
13. Purchase store brands, which are usually less expensive and equal in quality and taste to well-advertised national brands.
14. Read labels to determine nutritive value and compare with similar products.
15. Compare unit prices. If available, the price per unit (e.g., ounce) stated on the shelf below the grocery item facilitates comparing various sizes.
16. Buy larger sizes (which are usually cheaper per serving) if the food will be eaten before it spoils, but purchase individual serving sizes of products such as low-fat yogurt, if portion control is important.
17. Avoid purchasing high-energy snack foods and breakfast cereals with a high sugar content.
18. Do most of your shopping around the perimeter of the store, where seasonal items and basic essentials such as fresh meat, milk, and eggs are located. Highly processed foods line the inner supermarket shelves.
19. Frozen meats, vegetables, and fruits may be cheaper and just as nutritious.
20. Plan to use highly perishable items, such as fresh fish or strawberries, as soon as possible after purchasing.
21. Use dating information on products to select the freshest foods. Do not let food in the pantry or refrigerator go to waste, but do not dispose of items just because they are past their "Best if used by" date without checking to see if the product is good.
22. Pay attention at the checkout counter to be sure that the advertised price or the price indicated on the shelf is what is charged.
23. Visit Nutrition on a Budget https://www.nutrition.gov/topics/food-security-and-access/nutrition-budget for more resources and tips.

---

than those of higher-income households.[20] Low-income negatively impacts all dietary components particularly sugar-sweetened beverages and processed meats.[20] This suggests the complexity of the challenges with access to a healthy diet.

In 2021, the Supplemental Nutrition Assistance Program (SNAP) benefit allotment had a significant update based on a revised Thrifty Food Plan, but effective use of these food dollars requires knowledge, planning, and access so these remain ongoing challenges for low-income families.[21] The Thrifty Food Plan is based on a family of four and provides a guide to the weekly amounts of foods and beverages consistent with a healthy diet.[21] In 2023, the Thrifty Food Plan estimated a monthly cost of $975.80.[22]

On the basis of nutrient density, spinach, liver, turkey, canned tuna, lentils/beans, nonfat and low-fat milk, cottage cheese, tofu, eggs, and fresh carrots are usually the most economical foods. Buying seasonal, homegrown fruits and vegetables is more economical. Generally, more of the food dollar should be spent for fruits, vegetables, whole grain products, low-fat milk, and dry beans; less is needed for meats and high-sugar, high-fat food items (e.g., candy, sugar-sweetened beverages, and chips).

Maintaining Optimal Nutrition During Food Preparation

From the time the produce is harvested, nutrient content begins to degrade. Harvesting, processing, and cooking food means nutrient losses are occurring, but good handling processes, such as chilling or freezing, minimize losses and bacterial growth.

Methods of Preparation

In many instances, cooking enhances palatability, increases digestibility of food, and destroys pathogenic organisms. However, cooking also affects nutritional value of food. Nutrients most likely to be lost during food preparation are the water-soluble vitamins (C, thiamin, riboflavin, niacin, folate, B_6, and B_{12}). Minerals may also be affected but to a lesser degree than vitamins. Interestingly, cooked vegetables retain more vitamin E and beta-carotene than raw vegetables.[23] Following a few guidelines can help preserve nutrients during cooking (Box 16.2) and the *MyPlate* website has tips for healthy food preparation.

Adding large amounts of fats during the cooking process, as in frying, is discouraged. Methods of preparing meats, such as broiling or cooking on a grill, are recommended to lessen natural fat content. Meats cooked to the well-done stage contain less fat. To remove fats during cooking, meats can be boiled; microwaved; or roasted or broiled on a rack. Air frying without added fat is another option for healthier food preparation.[24] Absorption of fat-soluble vitamins requires availability of a small amount of fat; that is, absorption of vitamins A, D, E, and K from a vegetable salad is enhanced with a salad dressing, meat, or some other food containing small amounts of fat.

Cooking increases digestibility of protein in meats. Cooking generally softens cellulose in fresh produce. Total volume and bulk of the food decrease; thus a greater quantity of these low-calorie foods can be eaten. Stir frying is a traditional Asian technique that is a highly recommended method and has the added benefit of being quick. Bite-sized pieces of food are cooked very briefly over high heat with or without a small amount of vegetable oil. Vegetables retain their nutrient value, color, and crispness.

A microwave oven is another timesaver because of shorter cooking times. Research suggests microwaving retains the most vitamin C of any cooking method.[23] Generally there is good retention of vitamins with microwave cooking, especially if a minimal amount of water is added.

• BOX 16.2   Guidelines for Preserving Nutrients During Preparation

1. Prepare fresh produce as near to serving time as possible to prevent deterioration of many nutrients when they are exposed to air. Refrigerate within 2 h of cutting or peeling.
2. Do not soak fruits and vegetables that have been cut to prevent loss of water-soluble vitamins and some minerals (especially potassium) into the water. If cut-up fruits and vegetables are soaked in water, use the water in food preparation.
3. Scrub fruits and vegetables rather than peeling them to increase fiber and nutrient intake. When necessary, peel as thinly as possible to maintain nutrients.
4. Boil nonconsumable peelings and portions of vegetables in water and incorporate in soup stock or gravies. This is a very rich source of potassium and water-soluble vitamins.
5. Leave produce whole or in large pieces so that less surface area is available for oxidation of nutrients.
6. Carotenoids—such as beta-carotene, lycopene, and lutein—are more easily absorbed when vegetables are cooked rather than raw.
7. Store any fruits or vegetables that have been cut or otherwise processed, such as fruit juice, in airtight containers. Container size should be appropriate for the amount to be stored to prevent excessive oxidation from air inside the container.
8. Quick-cooking methods rather than extended cooking times are usually best to retain the B complex and C vitamins. Boiling removes water-soluble vitamins; thus quick steaming or sautéing is recommended to reduce loss into the cooking medium unless the liquid is also consumed (e.g., in soups or incorporated into a gravy).
9. A covered pan minimizes cooking time by increasing the temperature inside.
10. Use the least amount of liquid possible in cooking. Serve vegetables as soon as they are prepared.
11. Do not use baking soda when cooking vegetables.

Food Sanitation and Safety

Food carefully chosen for nutritional value may be adversely affected by handling techniques and preparation for consumption. Foodborne illness affects about one in six Americans, contributing to 3000 deaths every year.[25] Of the 31 pathogens known to cause foodborne illness, six account for most of the illnesses, hospitalizations, and deaths annually—*Campylobacter, Escherichia coli, Listeria monocytogenes, Salmonella, Vibrio,* and *Yersinia*.[25] In recent years, progress has been made in significantly reducing foodborne infections caused by *E. coli, Listeria, Salmonella,* and *Campylobacter*; infections from *Campylobacter* and *Salmonella* caused the most illnesses. The official statistics are probably underestimates, because many foodborne infections are not reported or are not identified.

For most people, the illness resolves on its own, but these illnesses can be fatal for young children, pregnant females, older adults, and those with weakened immune systems.[26] Illness caused by *Listeria* can result in miscarriage, fetal death, or severe illness or death of a newborn (see Chapter 13).

A food safety survey conducted in 2019 indicated most respondents thought that food poisoning was not common from food prepared at home; only 6%–9% thought raw vegetables could have germs present in themselves.[27] Most foodborne illnesses can be prevented by following safe food-handling and preparation recommendations and by avoiding consumption of raw or undercooked foods of animal origin such as eggs, ground beef, and poultry; unpasteurized milk, cheese, and juices; and raw or undercooked oysters.

The *Dietary Guidelines* provide food safety principles and guidance in general terms to reduce the risk of foodborne illness: *Clean* (handwashing, food preparation surfaces, and food), *Separate* (to prevent cross-contamination), *Cook* (to recommended safe temperature), and *Chill* (to maintain foods at a safe temperature). Edibles must be handled with care to prevent contamination with foodborne organisms, and some foods—especially meat, poultry, and eggs—must be cooked to sufficiently high temperatures to kill microorganisms naturally present in them. When foods remain in the "Danger Zone" (between 40°F and 140°F), bacteria can multiply rapidly, causing a single bacterium to multiply to 17 million in 12 hours. Box 16.3 lists some specific guidelines for handling food.

In recent years, nationwide recalls by the Food and Drug Administration (FDA) of food products have included meats, peanut butter, vegetables, salad, snacks, fast foods, and dessert items, causing thousands of illnesses and even a few deaths. In addition to processed foods, fresh meat, eggs, fruits, and vegetables may have harmful microbes leading to foodborne illness.[28] Contrary to popular opinion, pathogens that cause illness are odorless, colorless, and invisible. Therefore smelling, tasting, or looking at food is not a good gauge of whether it may be contaminated. Spoilage bacteria evidenced by slimy films on lunch meat, soggy edges on vegetables, or sticky chicken are not as toxic as pathogens.

Due to concern over the possibility of terrorist acts to contaminate the food supply, the US FDA authorized suspicious food to be detained with the Public Health Security and Bioterrorism Preparedness and Response Act of 2002 (Bioterrorism Act). The FDA Food Safety Modernization Act was signed into law in early 2010 and is slowly being implemented with regulations, processes, and systems developed based on science-based standards. These regulations encompassing growing, harvesting, and packing produce strengthen oversight of imported foods and require food producers to identify possible hazards and take steps to prevent outbreaks of foodborne illness. The Act enables the FDA to better protect public health by focusing on preventing food safety problems rather than reacting to problems after they occur. Imported foods have to comply with the same standards as domestic foods.

The FDA acknowledges that to progress in this battle against foodborne illness, reform of behaviors is needed. The FDA teamed with the Partnership for Food Safety Education to provide consumers and food safety educators with information to implement safe food-handling practices. The website for Fight Bac! (http://www.fightbac.org/) provides free resources regarding food safety basics, food poisoning, and food safety education to help prevent this unnecessary illness.

Most people feel that foods with a "sell by" or "use by" date somehow goes bad after that date. The "sell by" date tells the store how long to display the product for sale and the "use by" is the date recommended to use the product at peak quality.[29] These confusing labels have led to an estimated 30% of the food supply being wasted.[29] Food Safety and Inspection Service has issued new guidance aimed at reducing food waste by encouraging food manufacturers and retailers to use a "Best if used by" date label. This terminology does not indicate a safety date but a guideline for enjoying the best flavor or quality.

Processed Foods

When the word "processed" is used, consumers often make the mistake of assuming that the food is automatically unhealthy and

---

• BOX 16.3 Safe Sanitary Kitchen Guidelines

Shopping
- Wash reusable grocery bags.
- Purchase pasteurized juice and milk to avoid harmful bacteria.

Storage
- Use an appliance thermometer to ensure that the refrigerator temperature is between 40°F and 32°F and freezer is 0°F or below.
- Refrigerate or freeze meat, poultry, eggs, and other perishables as soon as possible.
- Refrigerate perishable goods within 2 hours.
- Cook or freeze fresh meat and poultry within 2 days.
- Wrap meat securely to prevent meat juices from cross-contaminating other food.

Thawing
- Defrost meats in the refrigerator or the microwave.

Preparation
- Wash your hands with soap and water for at least 20 seconds before preparing meals and handling any foods.
- Keep kitchen countertops, refrigerator, cookware, and cutlery clean. Disinfect countertops, sink, and cutting boards with a weak chlorine (1 tsp household bleach in 1 gallon water) solution.
- Avoid cross-contamination by keeping fresh produce away from uncooked meats.
- Never use the same utensils or cutting surfaces for preparing meats and vegetables. Use different cutting boards for fresh produce, dairy products, poultry, fish, and meats. Wash with a weak chlorine solution after using. Marinate meats and poultry in a covered container.
- Wash fruits and vegetables.

Cooking
- Use a food thermometer to ensure that meats are cooked to appropriate temperature—beef, pork, veal, and lamb at 160°F; turkey and chicken at 165°F; ham at 140°F; fish at 145°F; leftovers at 165°F.

Serving
- Hot foods should be held at 140°F or warmer and cold foods should be 40°F or colder.
- Keep foods hot in chafing dishes or slow cookers. Keep cold food cold by placing bowls in ice baths or using smaller serving dishes that are replaced frequently.
- Perishable food should not be left at room temperature for more than 2 hours.

Leftovers
- Discard foods left at room temperature for more than 2 hours.
- Refrigerate leftovers to 40°F or below within 2 hours of serving. Seal leftovers in an airtight, clean container labeled with the expiration date.
- Leftovers should be eaten within 3–4 days.
- Reheat leftovers to 165°F.

Adapted from USDA, Food Safety and Inspection Service. *Keep Food Safe! Food Safety Basics.* 2016. https://www.fsis.usda.gov/food-safety/safe-food-handling-and-preparation/food-safety-basics/steps-keep-food-safe.

should be avoided. Actually, everything that is done to a food after harvesting to prepare for consumption is food processing, whether it occurs at home or by the food manufacturer. Food processing is a method used since ancient times to preserve and improve foods. Processed foods are not always unhealthy and may be beneficial, both nutritionally and for convenience. Active, mobile lifestyles and an increasing number of females working full-time or part-time outside the home have led to a continued increase in availability and consumption of processed foods. Although growing one's own food and making foods from "scratch" can give consumers control over how food is handled and what is added, this is not feasible for most Americans.

Effect of Processing on Nutrients

Many consumers have been misled in assuming that nutrient content of our food supply has deteriorated. Based on studies conducted by the USDA, nutrient changes are mixed—some nutrients have gone down whereas others have improved.

Nutrient content of foods can be affected by the way food is handled—that is, the type of processing to which the food is subjected (e.g., milling, cooking, freezing, canning, dehydration)— and how it is stored. In general, most minerals, carbohydrates, lipids, proteins, and vitamin K and niacin are stable nutrients. Nutrients are considered stable if at least 85% of the original level is retained during processing and storage. B-vitamins and ascorbic acid are most likely to be destroyed or depleted by processing, storage, and method of food preparation.

Manufacturers involved in food processing attempt to maintain optimal qualities of taste, freshness, safety, cost, and value— five traits important in consumer choices. Food processing has both advantages and disadvantages. The milling process removes the bran coat of grains. Removal of the high lipid-containing bran produces a more stable grain, increasing its shelf life. Nutritionally, however, this results in a reduction of fiber and loss of B-vitamins and iron.[30] Enrichment replaces some nutrients (thiamin, riboflavin, niacin, folic acid, and iron) lost in processing, but not all of them (see Chapter 1, Table 1.5). Without the enrichment and fortification processes, many American diets would be deficient in nutrient intake of vitamins A, C, and D; and thiamin, iron, and folate.[31]

Fresh fruits and vegetables have a higher nutritive value and better taste immediately after harvest but rapidly deteriorate if transported through long distances or improperly stored.[32] Frozen foods packed immediately after harvesting are frequently higher in nutritive value than their fresh counterparts available in the supermarket and refrigerated more than 5 days.[32] In the initial processing of canned vegetables, there are losses of water-soluble vitamins, but then the nutrient content remains stable during storage.[32] Depending on storage and cooking of fresh or frozen vegetables, canned foods may have an equal or higher nutritional content and be a good value. In addition, some canned foods, especially tomatoes, tuna, and salmon, are cheaper and as nutritious as their counterpart fresh products.

The most negative effect of food processing has been the addition of ingredients that enhance taste and desirability of the product—sweeteners, salt, and artificial colors and flavors. Because of the way foods are processed quickly and transported rapidly, fresh produce is available year round, harmful microorganisms are reduced, maximum efficiency in production results in reduced costs, and foods are fortified or enriched with nutrients.

Highly (HPFs) and ultra-processed foods (UPFs) are usually less nutritious than the fresh form (i.e., potato chips are less nutritious than a baked potato; a handful of corn chips does not compare to a sweet ear of freshly picked corn). In addition, higher intake of HPFs and UPFs are associated with higher risk for chronic disease (e.g., obesity, diabetes), risk of mortality, and oral disease (e.g., dental caries and periodontal disease).[33–37] Consumers are free to choose foods that are minimally processed and thus healthier, or ready-to-eat foods that may contain less-desirable ingredients (Fig. 16.3). Reading nutrition and ingredient labels is important. Avoid processed foods that reduce a food's nutritional value or add ingredients that should be avoided—added sugar, sodium, or saturated or *trans* fats. Choose whole foods with a minimum amount of processing.

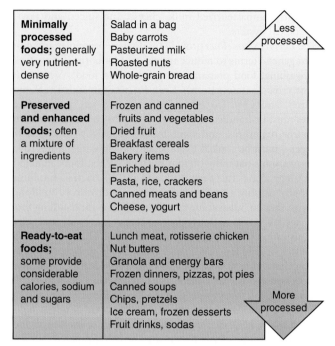

Minimally processed foods; generally very nutrient-dense	Salad in a bag Baby carrots Pasteurized milk Roasted nuts Whole-grain bread	Less processed
Preserved and enhanced foods; often a mixture of ingredients	Frozen and canned fruits and vegetables Dried fruit Breakfast cereals Bakery items Enriched bread Pasta, rice, crackers Canned meats and beans Cheese, yogurt	
Ready-to-eat foods; some provide considerable calories, sodium and sugars	Lunch meat, rotisserie chicken Nut butters Granola and energy bars Frozen dinners, pizzas, pot pies Canned soups Chips, pretzels Ice cream, frozen desserts Fruit drinks, sodas	More processed

• **Fig. 16.3** How do I make sure that I am eating "healthy" processed foods? The chart shows the range of processed foods available. Minimally processed foods are similar to, and sometimes even more nutritious than, the same foods in their unprocessed form. Although the ready-to-eat category contains some foods that are high in calories and nutrient poor, this category also includes convenient, ready-to-eat meals and snacks that provide a significant source of nutrients. (From Dairy Council of California. *Processed Foods: A Range, Not a Dichotomy.* 2012. http://www.healthy-eating.org/Portals/0/Documents/Health%20Wellness/White%20Papers/ProcessedFoods_72dpi.pdf.)

Convenience Foods

Convenience foods are usually popular because they save time in meal preparation, planning, purchasing, and cleanup. The variety of foods available has also expanded. Convenience foods prepared by food manufacturers may cost more because of extra handling and packaging. Convenience foods also contain more preservatives, sodium, and fat than home-cooked products. On the positive side, foods that are convenient can actually increase the likelihood that the consumer will eat a healthier diet.

Irradiated Foods

Foods treated with controlled amounts of ionized radiation for a prescribed period to kill spoilage-causing and disease-causing bacteria, and molds in meats and produce are known as irradiated foods.[38] This process, which breaks down DNA molecules of harmful organisms without significantly increasing the temperature of the food, is often called "cold pasteurization." Irradiation can extend the period of ripeness of fruits and vegetables, prolong the freshness of many foods, and prevent certain foodborne illnesses. Washing fresh fruits and vegetables can reduce risk of food contamination, but irradiation kills bacteria that are beyond the reach of conventional chemical sanitizers, such as inside the leaves of curly spinach and lettuce. At the low doses of radiation allowed, nutrient losses are either not measurable or are insignificant.[15] Foods have been safely irradiated in the United States for more than 30 years, and the World Health Organization endorses the safety of irradiated food.[38] The process is carefully controlled and monitored by numerous government organizations; irradiated foods bear the label shown in Fig. 16.4.

Organic Foods

The sharp rise in consumer demand for organic food outpaces domestic supply. Certified organic sales were an estimated $11.2 billion in 2021.[39] Sales were greatest in California followed by Washington, and Pennsylvania.[39] Crops like fruits and vegetables accounted for 54% of sales while livestock, poultry and related products accounted for 46% of sales.[39] Organic foods received significant price premiums over conventionally grown products. Average organic prices for 17 produces was 20% over conventionally produced products for over two-thirds of the items.[40]

This rapid growth in purchase of certified organics is driven by factors affecting consumer buying behaviors which include being health conscious, knowledge about organic food, availability, subjective norms (perceived social pressure), and price.[41] Consumers indicate other reasons for choosing organic foods because they are more environment friendly, use more humane treatment of animals, and less antibiotic-resistant bacteria.

In 2002, the USDA passed regulations defining organic food and permitting use of a seal (Fig. 16.5) for foods meeting specific standards. Organic certification regulates how these foods are grown, handled, and processed. Foods labeled organic are grown without *synthetic* pesticides, growth hormones, antibiotics, or genetic engineering. Organic farmers are allowed to use pesticides approved by the National Organic Standards Board that are naturally occurring chemicals, principally animal and crop wastes; botanical, biologic, or nonsynthetic pest controls; or specific synthetic materials that quickly degrade when exposed to oxygen and sunlight. Contamination with the dangerous bacterium *E. coli* does not differ between organic and conventional produce.

Animals raised by organic producers cannot be given antibiotics to stimulate growth; thus organic meats, poultry, milk, or eggs do not contain any residue of these drugs.[42] New standards became effective in 2011 requiring that all organic animals have year-round outdoor access, ruminant animals must graze on pasture land during the entire grazing season, and at least 30% of their dry nutrition must be from the pasture while they are grazing.[42] Beef and lamb must come from animals that were not confined during the finishing period (when animals are usually fattened on grain). The USDA states that organic agriculture is meant "to protect natural resources, conserve biodiversity, and use only approved substances," but the "organic" label does not have any bearing on the healthfulness of a product.[43]

Food manufacturers voluntarily provide information to the USDA about substances and practices used in food production, including how nonorganic and organic foods are kept separate. The USDA is responsible for inspecting the agricultural site annually and certifying a producer. Products labeled "Made with Organic Ingredients" must contain at least 70% organic ingredients.[42] A product containing more than 5% of the allowable pesticide tolerance level established by the Environmental Protection Agency (EPA) cannot be labeled organic.

Whether organic foods are more nutritious than conventional foods has been a point of contention for years. While there are numerous studies of individual organic foods, that is, eggs, tomatoes, the current evidence is not adequate to verify health benefits of consuming a diet of organic foods.[44,45] In observational studies, there have been associations between organic foods and reduced incidence of some conditions, but more long-term research is needed high quality study design to verify an effect.

Despite lack of strong evidence of health benefits of organic foods, a persistent belief is that a benefit of organic foods is that they do not contain pesticides. However, organic foods may not be pesticide free.[46] The amount and type of chemical pesticides permitted in agricultural use have been restricted since 1996. Pesticides in the US food supply have decreased significantly with approximately 99% of the products sampled in 2021 showing residues below the EPA tolerances and 24% had no detectable residue.[47] Currently allowed pesticides metabolize quickly and are not stored in the body; a few days after ingesting a pesticide, it is completely absent from the body.

Several measures can be taken to ensure minimal intake of questionable chemicals other than purchasing only organic products, as described in Box 16.4. Blanching, boiling, canning, frying, juicing, peeling, and washing fruits and vegetables reduces pesticide residues. Even after washing fruits and vegetables, some foods still contain higher levels of pesticide residue than others. Annually, the Environmental Working Group analyzes conventionally grown products for pesticide residue (see Box 16.4). Buying locally produced fresh vegetables and fruits in season is helpful because fewer pesticides are used when long storage periods and long-distance shipping are not required.

Another consumer concern relates to the use of antibiotics in animals and residue. Beginning in June 2023, the FDA updated guidelines that described policy direction regarding the judicious use of medically important antibiotics in animals.[48] Nonorganic animals do not contain antibiotic residues because FDA regulations prohibit farmers from giving feed with antibiotics to conventionally raised animals during a "withdrawal time" before slaughter. This length of time is specific to the antibiotic used to ensure that the drug is not present in the animal's system before the meat or milk enters the food supply. Tests rarely detect traces of antibiotics or other drugs in conventionally produced meat, poultry, milk, or eggs.

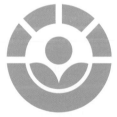

• **Fig. 16.4** Official package label for irradiated foods. (Courtesy United States Food and Drug Administration [FDA]. https://www.fda.gov/Food/ResourcesForYou/Consumers/ucm261680.htm.)

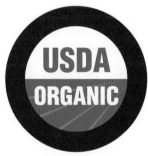

• **Fig. 16.5** Official USDA organic seal. (From United States Department of Agriculture. *Agricultural Marketing Service.* https://www.ams.usda.gov/sites/default/files/media/Organic4colorsealJPG.jpg.)

• BOX 16.4   Facts About Pesticides

1. Both traditional and organic food production may use pesticides.
2. Pesticide residue levels on both traditional and organic produce are well below the maximum amount allowed by the Environmental Protection Agency.
3. Eat a variety of fruits and vegetables to minimize exposure to a single pesticide.
4. Wash fruits and vegetables under running water prior to eating or cutting.
5. Scrub firm fruits and vegetables such as carrots and melons.
6. Discard the outer leaves of leafy vegetables like lettuce.
7. The benefits of consuming fruits and vegetables outweigh any risks from the amount of pesticide from these foods.
8. Evidence does not support health benefits of organic foods over conventionally grown foods.
9. To help avoid any possibility of consuming unhealthy amounts of pesticides, the Environmental Working Group (EWG) analyzes conventionally grown produce annually and has listed the following as the Dirty Dozen for 2023 (indicating that they tested positive for a number of pesticide residues and contained higher concentrations of pesticides than other produce)[2]: Strawberries; spinach; kale, collard and mustard greens; peaches; pears; nectarines; apples; grapes; bell and hot peppers; cherries; blueberries; and green beans.
10. The EWG also lists the following as having the least amount of pesticide residue (relatively few pesticides detected on them, and low total concentrations of pesticide residues): avocadoes, sweet corn, pineapple, onions, papaya, sweet peas (frozen), asparagus, honeydew, melon, kiwi, cabbage, mushrooms, mangoes, sweet potatoes, watermelon, and carrots.[2]

Organic food generally comes at a premium cost for many reasons, including higher production and labor costs, lower yields, and high demand. Organic products cost approximately 158% to 92% more than conventional products. However, this varies depending on the organic product and region of the United States.[49]

The food industry has developed many new organic products that are not healthful choices. For instance, a jelly bean is all sugar and not a healthful food choice, whether it is 100% organic or not. To know whether a product is healthy, read food labels (nutrition and ingredient labels) to determine levels of calories, saturated fat, sugar, and sodium, as well as protein, fiber, and vitamins and minerals. An organic cracker may be made with wheat flour, but if whole grain is not the first ingredient, the cracker is inconsistent with the *Dietary Guidelines*. Organic foods to avoid include sweetened beverages, crackers, candy, energy bars, and chips. These foods are high in calories and are not nutrient dense. When deciding whether the additional cost for organic food is worth it, remember it is premature to say that either organic or conventional foods are superior with respect to safety or health benefit and ultimately make choices consistent with the *Dietary Guidelines* and the *MyPlate* website.

Fast Foods and Other Food Establishments

Fast foods have become an integral part of the American fast-paced lifestyle with 33.6% of every food dollar being spent on eating out.[11] Providing nutrition information at restaurants is one avenue for educating consumers about what they are eating. The Patient Protection and Affordable Care Act (2010) authorized the FDA to establish uniform requirements for chain restaurants with 20 or more locations to post the number of calories in each

---

• BOX 16.5   Options for Healthful Eating Away From Home

Compare the nutrition numbers (calories, fat, and sodium) for your favorite items between fast food chains. Many restaurants have nutrition information for the menu online. Some simple switches that may be more healthful include:

- Instead of a quarter-pound cheeseburger, opt for a regular hamburger without cheese, potentially saving 280 calories, 9 g saturated fat, and 1.5 *trans* fat, and 630 mg sodium.
- Instead of a salad topped with crispy fried chicken, substitute with grilled chicken, potentially saving 160 calories, 2 g saturated fat, and 170 mg sodium.
- Instead of a fried-fish sandwich, order a veggie burger, potentially saving 110 calories, 2 g saturated fat, and 330 mg sodium.
- Instead of a sausage and cheese breakfast muffin, substitute oatmeal with maple and fruit, potentially saving 10 calories, 3.5 g saturated fat, and 590 mg sodium.
- Instead of a caramel mocha coffee drink, order a regular coffee (add nonnutritive sweetener and low-fat creamer if desired), potentially saving up to 320 calories, 7 g saturated fat, and 170 mg sodium.

From Tufts University. Fast Food: Why It Pays to Compare. *Health Nutr Lett.* 2015.

---

standard menu item.[50] Restaurants must also provide nutrition information upon request.[50] Menu labeling will ensure that customers can process the calorie information when they are deciding what to eat at the point of purchase.

Nutritional analyses by fast food chains, full-service, and fast-casual restaurants show that less than 10% of them met the American Heart Association criteria for a "heart-healthy meal."[51] Entrees at full-service restaurants had the highest number of calories, sodium, and saturated fat.[51] Nutrition information for restaurant menus can often be found online and can allow for advance planning to make healthy choices. In addition, the *MyPlate* website provides tips for dining out.

Concerns with frequent consumption of fast food include: (1) The calorie count of a large-sized bundled meal (cheeseburger, french fries, and sugar-sweetened beverage) represents 65% to 80% of a 2000 calories per day meal pattern; (2) sodium content 63% to 91% of the 2300 mg per day recommendation; and (3) more than 100% of the recommendation for added sugar per day. Fast foods are also a source of highly processed and UPFs which have implications for chronic diseases including obesity, diabetes, and cardiovascular disease.[52,53]

The impact of fast foods on nutritional status depends on how frequently they are consumed, composition of each item selected, and other foods eaten during the day. Wise choices are possible when an individual's nutritional needs and nutrient content of menu items are known. New menu items and reduced-portion sizes by several fast food chains simplify decisions to choose healthier foods, but consumers need to comparison shop (Box 16.5).

While some consumers say labeling is helpful, others find it confusing or disregard the information. Numerous reviews have shown that menu labeling in restaurants and fast food establishments has had no significant impact on consumers' food choices in the long term.[54–56]

Food Additives

The use of food additives is regulated by law. During the 1950s, the Delaney Clause (Food Additive Amendment) was added to prohibit use of any food additive that is carcinogenic in humans or animals.[57] Additives deemed to be harmless were labeled "generally recognized as safe" (GRAS). These substances met certain specifications of safety under what might be called a "grandfather clause"—in other words, they are generally recognized by experts as safe, based on their use in foods for years without any known occurrence of health problems.[57]

In 1960 similar regulations were passed for color additives. Colors currently in use were required to undergo further testing to continue being marketed. Since then, approximately 90 of the original 200 color additives have been classified as safe and continue to be added to foods.

In 2016 the FDA issued regulations to strengthen oversight of substances added to human and animal food.[57] Before a newly proposed additive can be marketed, it must undergo strict testing to establish its safety for the intended purpose; safe use of ingredients must be widely recognized by qualified experts. Safety levels of additives established by FDA limit the quantity and use of the additive. Currently, additives are specific, well-known substances meeting specifications for purity, and have been shown to be free from harmful effects in amounts commonly used. All preservatives used in food products must be declared in the ingredient list on the food label. Preservatives cannot be used to conceal damage or inferiority, make the food appear better than it is, or adversely affect nutritive value of the food. "Safe" is defined as "a reasonable certainty" in the minds of competent scientists that the substance is not harmful under intended conditions of use. However, some people experience allergic reactions to food additives, just as allergies to natural foods can occur.

Almost all food additives (99%) are derived from plants, animals, or minerals or are synthetically produced to be identical to the natural chemical substance.[58] In many instances, a compound may have benefits in a food, and so it may be added to other food to achieve a similar effect. For instance, calcium propionate in Swiss cheese was observed to retard mold; therefore it was added to bread to inhibit mold growth.

Despite being GRAS, concerns have emerged about some food additives. For instance, several synthetic food colorings have been associated with adverse effects on behavior in children with and without preexisting behavioral disorders, but more research is needed.[59] Meats processed using sodium nitrite/nitrate have been associated with an increased risk of bladder, thyroid, and stomach cancer with higher intake.[60]

The use of food additives makes many foods more readily available by preventing spoilage and keeping food wholesome and appealing. Complicated chemical names found on labels can be intimidating. Many food manufacturers are abandoning artificial preservatives and chemical additives due to consumer concerns and attitudes. Even names of vitamins on labels (e.g., thiamin mononitrate or cyanocobalamin) can cause apprehension for consumers unfamiliar with the terms. Food additives have the following benefits (Table 16.1):

1. They improve nutritional value. Enrichment and fortification have helped reduce malnutrition in the United States. Nutrients added help ensure adequate intake of vitamins or minerals. All added nutrients must be listed on product labels.
2. They maintain wholesomeness and palatability of foods. Bacterial contamination can cause foodborne illnesses. Preservatives retard spoilage caused by mold, air, bacteria, fungi, or yeast and preserve natural color and flavor. Antioxidants prevent oxidation of fats and oils, fruits, and vegetables.[58]

3. They maintain product consistency. Emulsifiers enable particles to mix and prevent separation. Stabilizers and thickeners contribute to a smooth, uniform texture.
4. They provide leavening or control pH. Leavening agents, such as yeast and baking powder, are used to make foods light in texture and to cause baked goods to rise.
5. They enhance flavor and appearance. These substances are the most widely used and the most controversial additives. Included in this category are coloring agents, natural and synthetic flavors, spices, flavor enhancers, and sweeteners. Sugar, corn syrup, and salt are used in the largest amounts. Without these additives, foods are less appealing, a factor that influences selection and nutrient intake.

DENTAL CONSIDERATIONS

- Emphasize following the recommendations on how to retain nutrients during preparation that are listed in Box 16.2.
- Clarify any misinformation about use of organic foods, but respect patients' beliefs and assist them in obtaining economical products that are acceptable to them.

NUTRITIONAL DIRECTIONS

- Products stored at room temperature should be kept in cool, dry areas in airtight containers.
- Regular ground beef is more economical than ground round, and total fat content can be significantly reduced by using a low-fat cooking method and rinsing crumbled ground beef after cooking.
- Organic foods cost more but are not more nutritious or significantly different in taste. Fresh, locally or home grown produce is ideal.
- Organic produce may not look as attractive and unblemished as traditionally grown produce; organically processed foods have a shorter shelf life than products containing preservatives.
- The terms "natural" and "organic" were used interchangeably in the past to describe food that was minimally processed and free of artificial additives or preservatives; however, consumers should be aware that only products with an organic label have met USDA standards. Legally, use of terms such as "natural" or "all-natural" can mean anything the manufacturer wants them to mean.
- Food additives are tested before they can be used. They are considered safe, but should be consumed in moderation. Cumulative amounts of additives such as added sweeteners or sodium (from many different sources) may be undesirable. Choosing fresh foods is usually ideal; these foods usually have fewer additives.
- Populations consuming large amounts of fruits and vegetables, even with the use of fertilizers and pesticides, have a lower rates of colorectal, breast, and lung cancer.[61]
- Eat a wide variety of fruits and vegetables to limit exposure to any one type of pesticide residue.
- Purchase only fruits and vegetables subject to USDA regulations. Imported produce is not grown under the same regulations as those enforced by the USDA.
- Buying organic foods should be a personal choice, based on availability, price, appearance, and taste, as well as personal values of the consumer. The most important factor is eating a wide variety of fruits and vegetables.

TABLE 16.1   Guide to Food Additives

Type or Function	Commonly Used Additives	Food Usage
Vitamins and minerals improve nutritive value of foods	Vitamin A acetate and palmitate; vitamin D, D$_2$ and D$_3$; potassium iodide (iodine); thiamin mononitrate (vitamin B$_1$), riboflavin (vitamin B$_2$), niacin and niacinamide (vitamin B$_3$), folic acid (folacin); ferrous sulfate and ferrous citrate (iron); ascorbic acid/sodium ascorbate (vitamin C)	Milk, margarine; iodized salt; enriched or fortified breakfast cereals, macaroni, pastas, breads, flour; fruit juices and fruit drinks, cured meats, cereals
Preservatives maintain wholesomeness and palatability of foods	BHA; tocopherols (vitamin E)	Cereals, chewing gum, potato chips, vegetable oils
Antioxidants prevent unsaturated fats and oils, flavorings, and colorings from oxidation, which would result in rancidity, flavor changes, and loss of color	Citric acid, ascorbic acid (vitamin C), propyl gallate, erythorbic acid	Instant potatoes, fruit drinks, sherbet, cured meats, vegetable oils, meat products
Other preservatives control growth of mold, bacteria, and yeast	Sodium benzoate, calcium (or sodium) propionate and potassium sorbate, sulfites, sodium nitrite/nitrate, sorbic acid	Pickles, preserves, fruit juice; breads, rolls, pies, cakes; dried fruit, frozen potatoes, wines; bacon, ham, frankfurters, luncheon meats, smoked fish, cheese
Processing aids product consistency and texture; emulsifiers keep oil and water mixed together with uniform dispersion of tiny particles	Monoglycerides and diglycerides, lecithin, polysorbate 60	Baked goods, margarine, candy, peanut butter; frozen desserts, imitation dairy products
Stabilizers (other processing aids) help maintain smooth texture and uniform color and flavor	Alginate and propylene glycol alginate; carrageenan	Ice cream, cheese, yogurt; jelly, chocolate milk, artificial breast milk
Thickeners (more processing aids) provide desired thickness or gel	Various gums (arabic, guar, xanthan), casein/sodium caseinate, pectin, gelatin, starch/modified starch	Beverages, salad dressing, cottage cheese, frozen pudding; ice cream, sherbet, coffee creamers; jelly; powdered dessert mixes, yogurt, cheese spreads; soup, gravy, baby food
Acids and bases control the pH of many foods and may act as buffers or neutralizing agents or as leavening agents	Citric acid and sodium citrate, fumaric acid, lactic acid, phosphoric acid, sodium bicarbonate	Frozen desserts, fruit drinks, carbonated beverages, candy; pudding, pie fillings, gelatin desserts; olives, cheese, powdered foods and drinks, instant potatoes, cured meats; breads, pastries, baked goods
Colorings, cosmetic additives in natural and synthetic forms, enhance the appearance of foods	Beta-carotene, caramel color, artificial colors, ferrous gluconate	Margarine, shortening, nondairy whiteners; carbonated beverages, candy; baked goods, cherries in fruit cocktail, gelatin desserts; sausage, black olives
Flavoring agents, cosmetic additives available in natural and synthetic forms, enhance flavors	Artificial and natural flavoring, HVP, vanillin (substitute for vanilla), MSG, quinine, salt (sodium chloride)	Carbonated beverages, candy, breakfast cereals, gelatin desserts; instant soups, frankfurters, sauce mixes, beef stew; ice cream, baked goods, chocolate; tonic water, bitter lemon; soup, potato chips, crackers
Sweeteners are cosmetic additives used to increase sweetness	Dextrose (corn syrup, glucose), high-fructose corn syrup, invert sugar, sugar (sucrose), lactose	Candy, toppings, syrups, snack foods, imitation dairy foods; soft drinks, processed sweetened foods; whipped topping mix, breakfast pastry
Alternative sweeteners are cosmetic additives replacing sugar in products to reduce calories or to reduce risk of dental decay	Acesulfame-K, aspartame, mannitol, saccharin, sorbitol, sucralose	Baked goods, chewing gum, gelatin desserts, soft drinks, drink mixes, frozen desserts, chewing gum, low-calorie foods; "diet" products; candy, shredded coconut
Other additives needed for processed foods to be prepared, stored, and shipped include anticaking agents; humectants; curing agents; sequestrants; and firming, bleaching, and maturing agents	Calcium (or sodium) stearyl lactylate, EDTA, glycerin	Bread dough, cake fillings, processed egg whites; salad dressing, margarine, processed fruits and vegetables, canned shellfish; marshmallows, candy, fudge, baked goods

BHA, Butylated hydroxyanisole; *EDTA*, ethylenediamine tetraacetic acid; *HVP*, hydrolyzed vegetable protein; *MSG*, monosodium glutamate.

Food Fads and Misinformation

Nutrition is a very popular subject, but even with all the current knowledge, it is no easier to understand today than it was in 1938:

> More food notions flourish in the United States than in any other civilized country on earth, and most of them are wrong. They thrive in the minds of the same people who talk about their operations; and like all mythology, they are a blend of fear, coincidence, and advertising (p. 144).[62]

As consumers' interest in nutrition increases, misinformation and misconceptions surrounding the subject continue to confuse. Purveyors of nutrition misinformation capitalize on fears and hopes by exaggerating and oversimplifying health virtues or curative properties of foods. Too few consumers understand the effects of various nutrients on the body and how nutrients are used, opening the door to food faddism or nutrition quackery.

Food fad is a generic term describing nutrition misconceptions and trends, characterized by exaggerated beliefs about the value of nutrition for health and disease. A food fad may be based on a fact or fallacy. People often begin a diet or believe claims for specific foods or supplements on the basis of something they read or hear without investigating its validity or effectiveness. Some fad diets are nutritionally inadequate and can lead to serious deficiencies. A fad is sometimes harmful because a specific therapy is substituted for advice of a health care provider and consumers delay medical treatment.

Fad diets are prevalent in the United States as Americans continue to search for a magic formula to lose weight and defy the aging process. According to promoters of weight loss diets, specific foods or food combinations facilitate weight loss, implying that a specific food or combination of foods oxidizes body fat, increases metabolic rate, or inhibits voluntary food intake.[63] Some diets may be deficient in essential nutrients and/or encourage excess intake of nutrients related to chronic disease (e.g., saturated fat).[63] Other benefits, such as rapid weight loss, may not be long-lasting.

Fad diets may promise to melt away fat with an immediate weight loss of several pounds, without exercise or limiting food intake.[63] Diets consistent with the *Dietary Guidelines* and *MyPlate* website along with adequate physical activity are desirable and more effective in the long term.

Food quackery is the promotion of nutrition-related products or services having questionable safety and/or effectiveness for claims made. These claims or promises may be due to ignorance, delusion, misconception, or deliberate deception. The question of why people turn to quackery instead of legitimate health professionals is multifactorial. In part many people do not trust the experts in nutrition and turn to social media and the Internet for information from celebrities and "influencer's" which often provide misinformation and disinformation (false information) that fits with what the individual wants to hear for a "quick fix."[64] Part of the issue is lack of nutrition literacy along with the plethora of individuals who call themselves nutritionists who have no formal training or licensure.[64]

Numerous unproven theories and procedures abound regarding food allergies and intolerances, ranging from fraudulent diagnostic testing to treatment with diets and supplements not shown to be effective in scientific studies. An example of false health claims is for caffeine supplements which include "reduces the perceived effort," "gives energy," and "improve immune function."[65] Caregivers and individuals with autism are bombarded by non–evidence-based treatment from chelation therapy to gluten-free casein-free diets.[66] Be cautious of recommendations for vitamin or mineral doses more than the RDAs or over the tolerable upper intake levels for the nutrient. Only certain conditions require doses beyond the RDAs, and a legitimate medical source should monitor the effects (see Chapter 11, *Health Application 11*). Careful review of best evidence is important to prevent harm from following restrictive diets or taking unproven vitamin or herbal supplements.

Juicing or detoxification diets/treatments or "cleanses" have been popular for weight loss. Because detoxification diets are extremely restrictive, there is a risk of severe energy restriction and inadequate nutritional intake.[67] In addition, supplement or other aids used as part of detoxification treatment may contain illegal, potentially harmful ingredients.[68] Detoxification may include juicing; colon cleansing; laxatives resulting in severe diarrhea; chelation therapy; removal of all amalgam (silver) fillings; supplements; and large amounts of water or herbal tea that results in imbalances in electrolytes.[68] During the detoxification diet/treatment, individuals may experience side effects of fatigue, malaise, aches and pains, emotional duress, headaches, and allergies. There is no evidence for the value of detoxification diets or treatment.[67]

Juicing is often a component of detoxification diets/treatment. The diet typically is 2 to 21 days and juices are used to replace all meals.[69] While juice contains most of the vitamins, minerals, and phytonutrients found in the whole fruit, the fiber in whole fruits and vegetables are lost in juicing. There is no evidence to support health benefits of juicing and there have been reports of kidney stones and renal failure due to oxalate crystals.[69] Oxylates are naturally occurring in many vegetables, but juicing concentrates them beyond normal levels.

The removal of mercury fillings is based on the concept that mercury in amalgam causes numerous health problems; thus fillings are removed to prevent or treat disease. Although it is indisputable that mercury can be toxic, scientific evaluation generally indicates mercury levels in people with fillings is significantly below levels that cause toxic symptoms.

Some detoxification diets include dietary and herbal supplements. The FDA only monitors supplements aftermarket meaning that they mainly respond if a supplement causes harm or makes unfounded health claims. Herbal supplements should be approached with caution. The benefit of herbs, including herbal teas and other plant-based formulations, in most cases have little evidence to support claims. Herbal products may be contaminated or contain alternative plant products not listed on the label. Deaths and severe health problems—including CVD, cirrhosis, and renal failure—have occurred from use of some herbal preparations in the United States.

Identifying Sources of Nutrition Misinformation

With the prolific amount of information disseminated on the news and on social media, it has become increasingly difficult to distinguish valid nutrition information on which to base one's decisions. Even within the medical and nutrition professions, recommendations have occasionally done an about face, causing confusion for consumers. Medical scientists and academics must publish their research to advance our knowledge; medical organizations must release health recommendations to remain relevant.

News organizations feel they must report on new research and recommendations as they are released. The news media often have a poor understanding of research methods and statistics, seldom reporting the extent and limitations of information or important nuances of a research study. In addition, they may report on research findings before the study has completed, peer review with a panel of experts.[70] Frequently, reporters are anxious to publish before the competition and may prematurely report on a study without fully checking out the story. In addition, the news generally reports medical findings as "facts" which results in confusing the consumer.

Some guidelines shared in 1994 remain relevant today and suggest the media keep in mind the way results are reported to help prevent misinterpretation of scientific studies.[71] The guidelines include: (1) an *association* between two events is not the same as a cause and effect; (2) each study's findings should be consider preliminary (or the piece of a puzzle) as further research is needed to add to what is known; (3) results of a study can be by chance or can be true in one population, but not another; and (4) the way that a scientific result is framed can greatly affect its impact.[71]

Sometimes it is hard to separate what is truly a medical certainty from what is merely scientific conjecture. Why so much confusion among scientists and physicians? Recommendations are needed; sometimes a theory works for one group, so it is anticipated that it will work for other groups as well. Sometimes recommendations fail because high-quality research behind them is lacking. Observational trials or epidemiologic studies are not proof that a recommendation works for everyone. Sometimes, there are unintended consequences of recommendations because of many unknowns. For instance, the recommendation to follow a low-fat diet may have resulted in more consumption of refined carbohydrate and UPFs to reduce fat intake.[72]

Very likely, some of the things in this text you have been taught may be contradictory to what you thought or were previously taught. Just remember, nutrition should be based on science, not opinions. Nutrition is a relatively young science (the word *vitamin* was first used in 1911). Nutrition is not a science of breakthroughs; it is evolution, not revolution. Confusion comes from constantly evolving new evidence being added to the existing body of research. However, the medical and nutrition community recommend the same foundational lifestyle changes (physical activity, do not smoke, drink in moderation, and so on) and following healthy dietary patterns consistent with the *Dietary Guidelines*, despite the public looking for a quick fix.

The factors just mentioned cause confusion even within the health care field. Therefore it is easy to understand how unscrupulous health promoters can get away with lies and fake products. If the label on a dietary supplement makes false or misleading claims about treating, preventing, or curing a disease, the FDA can take action.[73] However, dietary supplements can be legally promoted in the media, social media, and on the Internet as long as the message does not suggest the product treats or cures a disease. While the FDA is primarily involved in any harmful effects postmarketing of a supplement, supplement manufacturers who market products interstate must register and list the product with the FDA at least 75 days prior to marketing.[73]

Consumer interest in health and nutrition information is high as consumers are taking more responsibility for their own health care. The American culture is bombarded with nutrition information—television and radio talk shows, podcasts, commercials, infomercials, magazines, newspapers, books, Internet, social media, family and friends, and health care providers. People are frequently influenced by testimonials from celebrities, sports figures, fitness experts, and others without nutrition expertise touting a nutritional product.

The Internet and social media are an unregulated source of nutrition information and disinformation.[64,74] Information may be presented as fact, but the validity or credibility of information on websites and social media, especially those with products

to sell, should be verified before making a purchase. Videos on social media networks such as TikTok, Instagram and YouTube may contain testimonials from people sometimes referred to as "influencers" who are compensated for promoting products.

A popular tactic is to discredit the interpretation of scientific research by the medical community and governmental agencies. Inaccurate information is based on misunderstanding and misrepresentation. Evaluating nutrition information for its legitimacy and validity can be tedious. Health care professionals, regardless of where the nutrition information is presented—on the Internet, on television, on podcasts, in print, or any other media—should evaluate the findings in light of well-established nutrition principles.

The best way to begin a search on the Internet is to go to credible websites of trusted health organizations with names you recognize, universities, and state and national government agencies and offices. The Food and Nutrition Science Alliance is a partnership of several professional nutrition science associations, including the Academy of Nutrition and Dietetics, American College of Nutrition, American Society for Nutrition, and the Institute of Food Technologists who have combined their efforts to help debunk the junk advice. The information provided in Box 16.6 is helpful for evaluating oral or written claims.

Dental professionals and consumers can begin by checking credentials of the person making a questionable claim. Most articles appearing in established medical and scientific journals were submitted to a board of peer scientists for evaluation before publication. If peer reviewers consider conclusions to be well-supported by the research, it is published for others to read. A single study never proves a theory; it may provide definitive findings but provokes more questions needing further studies. A single study usually serves as another piece of the puzzle.

When evaluating individual studies, consideration must be given to the number of participants and length of the study and other pertinent information, as described in Box 16.6. For instance, the Nurses' Health Study that began in 1976 has involved almost 122,000 females aged 30 to 55 years and is still ongoing. This study, funded by the National Institutes of Health to investigate potential long-term consequences of oral contraceptives, has limitations in its credibility because professionally trained health care workers may have different values and practices than a cross-cultural sample of females.

Many types of studies—epidemiologic, case control, placebo controlled, randomized, crossover design, double blind, clinical trials, or interventions—together help provide conclusive information. The gold standard is "**evidence-based**," a term used for medical practices that have been thoroughly evaluated in rigorous well-designed research. Interventions used in randomized, placebo controlled studies are evaluated based on risks and benefits revealed during clinical trials. Experts review data from numerous studies to determine whether treatment can be recognized as safe or effective. The Cochrane Collaboration is dedicated to creating systematic reviews of peer-reviewed studies. The Academy of Nutrition and Dietetics also maintains an evidenced-based library of nutrition-related studies.

Meta-analysis combines all relevant studies from independent sources using a statistical technique, most often used to assess clinical effectiveness of health care interventions. **Systematic reviews** also provide reliable information based on all relevant published and unpublished evidences, selecting studies for inclusion, assessing the quality and bias of each study, then compiling the findings and interpreting them to present a balanced and impartial

• BOX 16.6   Debunk the Junk

The following are 10 red flags to help separate plausible but incorrect nutrition advice from the good stuff.

1. *Recommendations that promise a quick fix.* Ignore any product (sometimes foods, supplements, or pills) that promises fast results. Scientific studies about the effectiveness of the product are usually conducted by the manufacturer; thus the data is biased. Scientific literature does not use terms such as "amazing," "exclusive," "cure," or "long life." Quick-fix product claims are also peppered with medical jargon to further mislead the consumer. Serious medical problems cannot be cured with remedies marketed by mail order, social media, or on the Internet. In short, do not allow these companies to manipulate you.

2. *Warnings of danger from a single nutrient or food pattern.* One particular thing is not responsible for being overweight or unhealthy (fat makes you fat, carbohydrates are toxic, sugar is white death). Typically, it is a combination of factors and/or lack of exercise. Sometimes people adopt an all-or-nothing approach, swinging from paleo to vegan. Too much of any one thing in the diet is unhealthy, but it will not be the sole reason for weight gain.

3. *Claims sound too good to be true.* Scrutinize the science behind the recommendation to determine whether the recommendation is worth following or just wishful thinking. Study the label on the product. (1) The instructions on the label should clarify the product's benefits. (2) Advertisements or promotional material should agree with the product label. Unsubstantiated false claims are usually found in books, television, brochures, infomercials, social media, and promotional materials. Beware of "cures" for serious diseases and products claiming to cure multiple health problems. Symptoms of many illnesses are similar, and a misdiagnosis can be hazardous if the condition is not being treated appropriately. A proper diagnosis requires an assessment, including a physical examination, by a health professional. Delaying treatment may allow progression of the disease beyond help.

4. *Oversimplified conclusions drawn from complicated research.* Many consumers want a study to conclude with black-and-white answers, but most science is very complicated, requiring critical thinking and more investigating to understand it. A study will take into account previous research on the subject. Good scientific studies have limitations that scientists acknowledge, inviting further research to cover these areas.

5. *Recommendations based on a single study.* Be wary of any recommendations from a single study, especially if the conclusion is contrary to everything else that has been published. Be a skeptic; do not ignore studies that go against prevailing wisdom. Compare findings with all the published literature on the subject, not just the most recent.

6. *Statements contradicted by well-respected scientific institutions.* For a nutrition statement that seems too good to be true, too simplistic, or claims to be a quick fix, definitely verify what reputable scientific organizations have to say. If it sounds too good to be true, it probably is. A list of credible government agencies and nutrition organizations are listed along with their websites throughout this text.

7. *Lists of "good" and "bad" foods.* Lists are problematic because foods are not all good or all bad. Balance, variety, and moderation are all necessary. An occasional candy bar can be okay, and not every vegetable consumed has to be chock full of antioxidants and vitamins. The key, though, is moderation, and balance. Indulge on occasion, but ensure that you eat healthful well-balanced meals regularly.

8. *Recommendations made to market a product.* If the health article, YouTube video, or social media post ends with a sales pitch for a supplement or if all the studies referenced at the end are by the author, the quackery alarm should sound. Be cautious and ensure findings are not inconsistent with other research. Investigate information based on testimonials or case histories or promoted by movie stars, sports figures, or any celebrity. This is not scientific evidence. The FDA cannot regulate a testimonial about a product.

9. *Recommendations based on studies that are not peer reviewed.* Research published in a peer-reviewed journal mean that a group of outside reviewers who are experts on the topic have deemed the research well-conducted, the results credible, and the findings significant. Peer review is necessary in science for reliability and accuracy.

10. *Recommendations from studies that ignore differences among individuals or groups.* Nutrition is not a "one size fits all" science. A study making broad generalizations is not reliable. The results of a study on bone health conducted using teen-age athletes would not be applicable to older females experiencing osteoporosis.

Adapted from redOrbit. *Food and Nutrition Science Alliance Gives 10 Bits of Advice on Junk Science.* 2023. http://www.redorbit.com/news/health/1113214063/debunk-the-junk-science-in-nutrition-081714/; Flaherty J. Debunk the Junk. *TuftsNow.* 2014. http://now.tufts.edu/articles/debunk-junk.

---

summary while defining limitations of the evidence. Meta-analysis studies and systematic reviews have been given a lot of prestige because they were considered a concise synopsis of multiple studies with reliable conclusions. However, they are currently being produced in massive amounts as a result of software that streamlines the process and may be biased with vested interests for the entities funding the review. Instead of promoting evidence-based medicine and health care findings, they may be redundant and misleading, with methodological flaws.[75,76]

Observational studies are epidemiologic research studies with no type of intervention or experiment. These may be used to discover possible relationships between lifestyle and diseases. For instance, "people who love ice cream are obese" may survey thousands of participants, but does not clearly determine a cause.

◆ DENTAL CONSIDERATIONS

- Assess patients' use of food fads, economic level, educational level, and the nutrient adequacy of any fad diet undertaken.
- If a patient restricts food choices because of a food fad or belief, ensuring nutrient adequacy is more difficult. A thorough assessment and evaluation by the dental hygienist may indicate risk for a nutritional insufficiency or deficiency. Referral to a registered dietitian nutritionist (RDN) may be needed.
- Encourage patients to choose a variety of foods to ensure a balanced intake and decrease amounts consumed of any particular food to minimize risk of excessive contaminants from any one source. For instance, consumption of fish is encouraged because of beneficial substances to prevent CVD. However, fish, especially large fish such as swordfish, shark, mackerel, tilefish, and tuna, contain methylmercury so that eating too much fish has the potential to cause neurologic problems.
- Provide patients with positive advice based on a broad knowledge base and understanding of nutritional concepts and current research findings.
- Answer any questions about therapies, products, or treatments that a patient may be contemplating or refer the patient to a reliable source.
- Speak out to protect the public from misinformation.
- Do not offer remedies unless they have been shown to be safe and effective in evidence-based sources.
- If a patient is using or contemplating using a food fad or diet you are unfamiliar with, do not hesitate to consult an RDN.

⊙ NUTRITIONAL DIRECTIONS

- Although some fads are physically harmless, they may create an economic hardship for individuals with limited income because the foods or supplements may be expensive.
- Results of fad diets can be devastating and have even led to death.

Referrals for Nutritional Resources

Frequently, patients need special assistance for nutrition due to financial problems. About 10.2% (13.5 million) households experienced food insecurity in 2021 and of these about 56% participated in one of the three largest nutrition assistance programs.[77] A variety of governmental programs available may help with access to food, assist with food budgeting, teach basic nutrition and meal planning, or help clarify nutrition misconceptions. The federal government administers several nutrition programs through the USDA and the US Department of Health and Human Services.

The SNAP (formerly the Food Stamp Program) is the cornerstone for nutrition safety in the United States. This federal assistance program is available to individuals with incomes up to 130% of the federal poverty level. The program, designed to help low-income households purchase nutritious food, is based on family income and household size. Local offices that administer the program are widely distributed throughout the United States. The program was initially designed to boost food consumption and energy intake. Barriers to accessing SNAP benefits may include frustration about the process of applying for and maintaining benefits; feelings of embarrassment and stigma; and cultural beliefs.[78]

The COVID-19 pandemic and economic impact on families led to increases in funding for food and nutrition programs. The number of SNAP participants was 41.2 million in 2022, down slightly from 41.6 million in 2021.[47] SNAP program benefits serve as a safety net and are critically important to help feed families in need. The average benefit per person in 2022 was $230.88/month.[77] Without good money management skills, the monthly food allowance runs out before the end of the month. The program is meant to supplement a household's food budget; it is not intended to be the total food budget. Eating healthy on the SNAP program is challenging but doable—a back-to-basics style of eating. The Thrifty Food Plan as previously mentioned may be a resource for patient. Because most people who qualify for SNAP have less education, however, it is very difficult for them to keep healthful food on the table all month.

Because poor diets exert heavy costs in medical expenditures and lost productivity, measures for promoting healthful food choices could yield considerable benefits. State governments and health advocates recognize that additional modifications are needed to reinforce nutrition education, restrict foods allowed with food stamp benefits, and expand benefits to encourage purchases of more healthful foods, such as fruit and vegetables.

While the program is intended to improve the nutritional and health status of families needing assistance, recipients can use the Electronic Benefit Card to buy any foods sold in participating grocery stores, with the exception of prepared hot foods. However, research suggests SNAP participants have lower diet quality and higher sugar-sweetened beverage intake suggesting the need for more education and support in making healthy choices.[79]

The Special Supplemental Food Program for Women, Infants, and Children (WIC) is designed to prevent nutritional problems in this high-risk, low-income group. The WIC program is available to pregnant and lactating females, infants, and children up to 5 years old who are considered to be at nutritional risk. Some of the criteria for nutritional risk are evidence of iron deficiency, inadequate weight gain during pregnancy, teenage pregnancy, failure to thrive, poor growth patterns, and inadequate dietary patterns. In addition to supplemental foods, nutrition education and referrals are provided to sources for health care. Studies of the WIC program have shown positive effects on lower risk for preterm birth or low birth weight; reduced infant mortality; improved iron status; improved growth and development of infants and children; and increased childhood immunizations.[80]

Thirty-nine percent of all infants in the United States are WIC recipients.[81] WIC food packages were updated in 2022 based on the National Academy of Science, Engineering, and Medicine and the *Dietary Guidelines*.[82] Food packages for mothers and infants include formula (for infants not being breastfed), fruit juice, reduced fat and skim milk, breakfast cereal, cheese, eggs, fruits and vegetables (vouchers), canned fish, legumes or peanut butter.[81] Foods allowed must meet nutritional standards by providing a specific amount of fiber, iron, zinc, vitamin C, or vitamin D.

School breakfast and lunch programs provide nutritious meals for children at school to increase food security and reduce hunger. Some states provide universal free lunch and breakfast and in other states, students have to meet income guidelines for reduced and free meals. Nutritional standards for school lunch require that lunch provide at least one-third, and breakfast at least one-fourth, of the RDAs for children. Children participating in the school lunch program had higher diet quality with higher intake of fruits, vegetables, and milk product than those who did not.[83] Along with this, those who participated in school meal programs met or exceeded requirements for vitamin, A, C, D, E along with calcium, copper, magnesium, phosphorus, and zinc when compared with children who did not participate.[83]

New guidelines for overhauling the school food program were implemented beginning in 2012 with ongoing updates.[84] These requirements are more consistent with the healthy diet pattern recommendations of the *Dietary Guidelines* with a focus on providing fruit, more vegetables variety, whole grains, meat/meat alternatives and milk.[84] Schools are encouraged to make substitutions based on cultural and religious preferences. Milk must be fat free or low fat (1%) (plain or flavored). More whole fruit is required at both meals. Dark-green vegetables, red/orange vegetables, beans/peas (legumes), and starchy vegetables (1/2 cup equivalent) must be offered at least weekly. Fruits and vegetables are not interchangeable. All grains must be whole grain. The food waste has been of concern so *offer versus serve* was implemented beginning in 2015 to allow children to decline food they will not eat.[84] In addition, schools can be innovative to make food more appealing such as offering taste testing before offering new foods, creating marketing, Farm to School activities, and self-serve salad bars.[84]

The Expanded Food and Nutrition Education Program was designed to help lower socioeconomic groups with education to reduce nutrition insecurity. The Expanded Food and Nutrition Education Program (EFNEP) is available through county extension services of land-grant universities and assists with knowledge to make healthier food choices, increases management of food resources (meal planning, budgeting, shopping, and food preparation), food safety, and increases physical activity. Outcomes show improved diets and nutrition practices, ability to better use food dollars, increase in physical activity, and improved ability to manage good safety.[85]

There are a number of nutrition programs for seniors administered by the USDA (e.g., SNAP, Senior Farmer's Market Nutrition

Program, and Commodity Supplemental Good Program) and the Agency on Aging Older Americans Act Nutrition Services (Congregate Nutrition program and Meals on Wheels). The purpose of this program is to improve reduce hunger, food insecurity, and maintain nutrition and health status of older adults.[86] In addition, the goal is to offer participants opportunities to socialize to prevent isolation. The Older Americans Nutrition Services programs provide a range of services (including social services) through approximately 5,000 nutrition service providers and serve more than 2 million older adult participants. The meals are required to be consistent with the *Dietary Guidelines* and provide at least one-third of the DRIs. For congregate meal participants, 70%–80% felt the meals helped them continue to live independently, improved their health, and helped them eat healthier.[86] For those receiving home delivered meals, 75% to 85% reported the meals helped them continue to live independently and eat healthier.[86]

Local health-related organizations furnish free or inexpensive literature, audiovisual material, and health-oriented programs on various topics. Dental hygienists can identify patients or families with nutritional needs, provide appropriate referrals, and help them find resources (Table 16.2).

In addition to federal nutrition assistance programs, state and local health departments usually have various programs to provide nutrition services. Health departments and county hospitals are excellent resources for information about various programs available.

The Area Information Center (2-1-1) maintains comprehensive databases of resources, including federal, state, and local government agencies, and community-based and private nonprofit organizations. "Information and Referral Services" is a national dialing code to link people in need of assistance with appropriate providers of services in their community.

Head Start is a preschool educational program for low-income families. Children are furnished breakfast, lunch, and snacks, and nutrition education is available for parents.

Locally funded food agencies and faith-based organizations increasingly provide direct access to meals and assistance through food banks and food pantries. Food pantries, which usually do not base eligibility for benefits on income status, currently serve millions of Americans. Feeding America (feedingamerica.org) allows searching for local sources of food and groceries and resources to help with applying for SNAP. Feeding America reports that in 2022, 49 million people or one in six Americans received charitable food assistance (e.g., food banks, food panties, meals).[87]

● DENTAL CONSIDERATIONS

- Identify patients needing food assistance and refer them to appropriate sources.
- If calories, sodium, and fat should be restricted, encourage limiting visits to fast food establishments or suggest appropriate fast food selections (e.g., salads or baked chicken).
- Low-income households must allocate a higher proportion of both their income and time to planning, purchasing, and preparing food if they wish to consume nutritious meals.
- When recommending foods to patients, consider the income level. Suggesting steak or lobster as a protein source for low-income patients is inappropriate.

● NUTRITIONAL DIRECTIONS

- Protein sources are generally the most expensive budget items; however, it is unnecessary to buy choice quality grades of meat for good nutrition. ("Select" and "standard" are more economical grades of meat.) Plant-based protein can also be more cost-effective.
- Discuss guidelines for economical food purchases (see Box 16.1) to help low-income patients modify food purchases.
- Health care professionals, including dental hygienists, can encourage communities and food banks to focus on more nutritious food, such as fresh fruits and vegetables.

Role of Dental Hygienists

What role can the dental hygienist play in combating nutrition fads and misinformation? Natalie Van Cleve stated in 1938, when times were different but widespread misinformation on diet was just as prevalent as today[88]:

> It is the duty of all professions active in the field of food and nutrition to cooperate in clarifying any misconceptions of the laity. If the [health care providers] do not know their vitamins, the patients will find a radio announcer who does.

Health care providers, dental hygienists, and even RDNs have sometimes promoted nutrition misinformation by failing to apply their knowledge, misunderstanding, or inaccurately informing how nutrients are used, or marketing products in the office such as supplements without adequate evidence. The dental professional is in a unique position to identify misinformation and disinformation and guide patients to credible sources of information. There are many legitimate resources including governmental and professional organizations. Many legitimate medical journals are also available on the Internet. In addition, the dental professional can make referrals to appropriate resources and agencies. Patients may benefit by ventilating feelings and beliefs about food "handouts."

Dental professionals also need to be aware of cultural health beliefs that may impact nutrition choices and try to make recommendations consistent with the patient's beliefs and national guidelines (*Dietary Guidelines* and *MyPlate website*). Understanding the basics of behavior change and using best practices to deliver patient education is essential.

In regard to access to adequate food, identify those at risk for food insecurity and help patients recognize that having inadequate funds for food is not a sign of failure. Stigma tends to surround asking for help, but 60% of American adults live below the poverty line for at least one year.[89] Adequate food is foundational to staying healthy so an individual is ready for employment when the opportunity comes. If the patient is a parent or caregiver, it is important to stress benefits children would receive (e.g., increased growth, learning, productivity) by participating. Dental professionals can also help by serving at community food resource centers or food donation drives.

TABLE 16.2   **Referral Chart for Community Nutrition Resources**

Population Group	Risk Factor	Referral Source[a]	Contact[b]
Pregnant and lactating females	Low income	Supplemental Nutrition Assistance Program (SNAP)	State food stamp hotline number available at https://www.fns.usda.gov/contact-us 1-800-221-5689
	Anemia, inadequate weight gain, age-related risk factor, inadequate health care, or lack of food and nutrition information	Women, Infants and Children (WIC)	State WIC Program Contacts https://www.fns.usda.gov/wic/program-contacts
		Expanded Food and Nutrition Education Program (EFNEP)	Land-grant universities (may be called Extension Service) https://landgrantimpacts.org/extension-institutions/
Infants	Low birth weight, failure to thrive, or poor growth patterns	Prenatal education	City, county, or state health department Call 1-800-311-BABY (1-800-311-2229) to be connected with local health department For information in Spanish, call 1-800-504-7081
	Inadequate health care	WIC Program	State WIC Program Contacts https://www.fns.usda.gov/wic/program-contacts
Children	Poor growth patterns or overweight, inadequate diet, or anemia	WIC Program (up to 5 years old)	State WIC Program Contacts https://www.fns.usda.gov/wic/program-contacts
	Low income	Children and Youth Project (up to 18 years old)	State Health Department
		Head Start (preschool)	Find Head Start in your area https://eclkc.ohs.acf.hhs.gov/center-locator
		School Lunch	School Lunch Program Contacts https://www.fns.usda.gov/nslp/program-contacts
		School Breakfast	School Breakfast Program Contacts https://www.fns.usda.gov/sbp/program-contacts
Family Based Programs	Overweight and obese children with focus on the family	CDC: Family Health Weight Programs	Resources available at https://www.cdc.gov/obesity/strategies/family-healthy-weight-programs.html
Older adult	Low income	SNAP	SNAP State Directory of Resources available at https://www.fns.usda.gov/snap/state-directory
		Congregate meal sites	State and local agencies on aging
	Homebound	Meals on Wheels	Locations available at https://www.mealsonwheelsamerica.org/find-meals
General adult	Obesity	CDC: Healthy Weight, Nutrition, and Physical Activity	Many resources available at https://www.cdc.gov/healthyweight/index.html
	Cardiovascular disease, hypertension, and hyperlipidemia	American Heart Association	Resources available at https://www.heart.org/en/
	Diabetes	American Diabetes Association	Many resources available at: https://diabetes.org/healthy-living
	Low income	SNAP	SNAP State Directory of Resources available at https://www.fns.usda.gov/snap/state-directory
	Reliable food and nutrition information	EFNEP	Land-grant universities (may be called Extension Service) https://landgrantimpacts.org/extension-institutions/
	General consumer information for all populations	Community nutrition groups and community cooperatives	Local groups
		Academy of Nutrition and Dietetics (AND)	Available at http://www.eatright.org
		Center for Science in the Public Interest	Available at http://www.cspinet.org
		United States Department of Health and Human Services	Available at https://www.hhs.gov
		MyHealthfinder	Available at https://health.gov/myhealthfinder
		MedlinePlus	Hosted by the National Library of Medicine Available at https://medlineplus.gov/

[a]This is only a partial listing. Programs may vary in different parts of the United States.
[b]Call 2-1-1 for free access to health and human services information and referrals in local communities.

◆ HEALTH APPLICATION 16

Food Insecurity in the United States

Food security—that is, access to enough food for an active, healthy life by all family members at all times—is a universal dimension of household and personal well-being and considered a fundamental requirement for a healthy, well-nourished population. However, food insecurity and hunger continue to exist in the United States. Hunger, or an uneasy or painful sensation caused by lack of food, typically precedes food insecurity. Food insecurity refers to the lack of access to enough food to meet basic needs fully at some time during the year because of insufficient funds or resources for food. Food insecurity means having to decide which bills to pay—food, housing, heat, electricity, water, transportation, childcare, or health care. Food insecurity remains a public health concern in the United States, particularly among low-income, urban, ethnically diverse families. Food insecurity is usually recurrent or transient but not chronic, and may involve a low-quality diet that is monotonous and lacking in nutrients. Approximately 10.2% of US households were food insecure sometime during 2021 with 3.8% having very low food security.[90] Prevalence of food insecurity in America increased and remained high between 2007 and 2014 when it finally began to decrease (Fig. 16.6).

In 2015, the typical food secure household spent more on food than the typical food insecure household of the same size and household composition.[91] About 56% of food insecure households participated in one or more of the three largest federal food and nutrition assistance programs during the month prior to the 2021 survey.[91] In 2021, approximately 3.8% of households (7 million) experienced very low food security (at times during the year, food intake of household members was reduced and normal eating patterns were disrupted because of insufficient funds or other resources to obtain food; Fig. 16.7).[91] Hunger rates decrease as income increases, but food insecurity is not exclusive to very-low-income families.

Rates of food insecurity are substantially higher than the national average for households with children headed by a single female (24.3%) or a single male (16.2%).[91] All households with children had higher levels of food insecurity (Fig. 16.8).[91] African American and Hispanic households had rates of food insecurity more than twice those of non-Hispanic White households. Nearly half of American children live in homes that at some point receive governmental nutrition programs.[91]

A work-limiting disability substantially increases the risk of food insecurity for low-income families. In addition to the disabled individual being unable to work and incur burdensome medical costs and other expenses, an adult caretaker may be restricted in work opportunities and hours. Over 6 million people in the United States maintain a home and may even work full-time, but live below the poverty level.[92] (In 2023 the federal poverty guideline was an annual income less than $30,000 for a family of four in the 48 contiguous states.)

Several factors may account for food insecurity—the state of the American economy; unemployment rate; and the changing composition of the US population, particularly households headed by a single female. People who are unemployed for a long period deplete their assets, exhaust unemployment insurance, and turn to SNAP for help. Households attempt to avoid food insecurity by using various food-based and household coping strategies, such as eating less preferred foods, limiting portion sizes, skipping meals, borrowing money to buy food, maternal buffering (a mother limits her eating so that children have enough food), delaying or making partial payments for bills.[93]

Food bank use has increased and tends to be used more by those who have severe food insecurity.[94] Diet quality can be inconsistent and does not meet the Dietary Guidelines due to limited variety of food options.[94] Individuals who use food banks tend to have intake of energy, fruits and vegetables, dairy, meat, and micronutrients (e.g., calcium and iron).[94] These facilities would like to improve the quality of foods that they provide but are dependent on donations of food or money. Emergency food providers serve a diverse population with different reasons for needing assistance. These providers are especially helpful for people during a short-term setback, such as an unexpected emergency medical bill; others need emergency kitchens to receive a hot meal or supplement food stamps.

Food insecurity may cause a variety of negative health outcomes for everyone affected, but younger populations are most at risk. Both adults and children who are food insecure are at higher risk of obesity, obstructive airway disease, diabetes, and hypertension.[95] In children, food insecurity has been associated with higher caries risk;[96] developmental issues (e.g., insecure parental attachment, lower scores on cognitive development); impairments in language and interpersonal skills development; increase in behavioral issues (e.g., self-regulation, self-control, aggressive behavior, anxious/depressed mood); impaired academic performance (e.g., lower math scores, worse reading performance, lower scores on vocabulary and word recognition).[97,98] In adolescents, the major issues were psychosocial issues related to mental health (e.g., anxiety, depression, anti-social behavior, substance use disorders).[97] Some potential effects varied by whether food insecurity was temporary or persistent along with the level of family stress.[98]

Low-income people are subject to the same influences and problems as other Americans (e.g., more sedentary lifestyles, increased portion sizes, ultra- and highly processed foods), but they also face unique challenges in adopting healthful behaviors. Food insecure adults and children are at 50% greater odds of being obese.[99] This may in part be because of disparities in access to purchase health food and shopping behaviors. Those living in low-income communities may not have access to full-service grocery stores and they shop more frequently in stores that have less-healthful options such as convenience/dollar stores.[100] In addition, lower-income neighborhoods provide fewer safe opportunities for physical activity (fewer parks, bike paths, and recreational facilities, unsafe playground equipment, more problems with crime and traffic, and fewer organized sports programs).

Those in food secure households scored slightly higher (49 points) on diet quality than those who were food insecure (45 points).[101] The major differences were food insecure households had lower amounts of fruit, dairy, and protein with larger amounts of refined grains.[101] However, all households need to continue working on improving diet quality consistent with healthy diet patterns in the Dietary Guidelines.

Food insecurity represents a major public health and public policy challenge by causing health problems, increased education costs, and less than optimal productivity. Food and nutrition literacy is an essential aspect of helping food insecure individuals use food resources such as SNAP wisely. In order to educate low-income families, the SNAP Education (SNAP-Ed) was developed in 2002 and is now conducted in collaboration with Extension Food and Nutrition programs at land-grant universities. The educators offer sessions in community sites convenient for the low-income community participants. The education includes healthy eating, food safety, food resource management (meal planning, shopping, and preparation), and physical activity.[102]

Since SNAP benefits are meant to supplement resources for food costs, it is essential for families to have the skills they need to stretch their benefits to minimize the additional food dollars needed to support healthy diet pattern recommended by the Dietary Guidelines and MyPlate website.

The goal of Healthy People 2030 is to increase quality and years of healthy life and to eliminate health disparities; this requires improved food and nutrition security. The objective to eliminate very low food security among children showed little or no detectable change—increasing from 0.59% in 2018 to 0.75% in 2021; the objective to reduce household food insecurity and in doing so reduce hunger showed improvement—decreasing from 11.1% in 2018 to 10.2% in 2021.[103] US federal assistance programs have been discussed earlier in this chapter and in Table 16.2 are resources to address hunger.

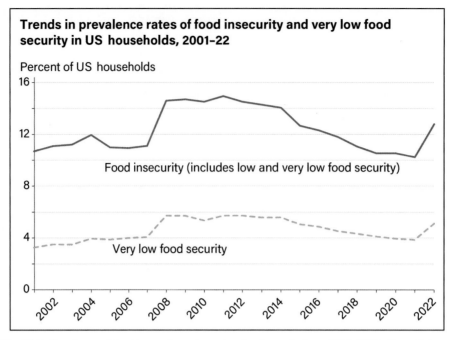

• **Fig. 16.6** Prevalence of food insecurity and very low food security from 1995–2021. (From Coleman-Jensen A, Rabbitt MP, Gregory CA, Singh A. Household Food Security in the United States in 2021, ERR-309, U.S. Department of Agriculture, Economic Research Service; 2022.)

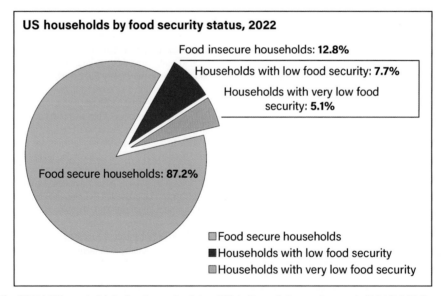

• **Fig. 16.7** US households by food security status, 2021. (From Coleman-Jensen A, Rabbitt MP, Gregory CA, Singh A. Household Food Security in the United States in 2021, ERR-309, U.S. Department of Agriculture, Economic Research Service; 2022.)

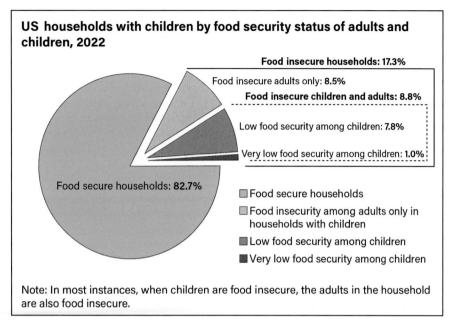

US households with children by food security status of adults and children, 2022

Food insecure households: 17.3%

Food insecure adults only: 8.5%

Food insecure children and adults: 8.8%

Low food security among children: 7.8%

Very low food security among children: 1.0%

Food secure households: 82.7%

- Food secure households
- Food insecurity among adults only in households with children
- Low food security among children
- Very low food security among children

Note: In most instances, when children are food insecure, the adults in the household are also food insecure.

• **Fig. 16.8** US households with children by food security status of adults and children, 2021. Note: In most instances, when children are food insecure, the adults in the household are also food insecure. (From Coleman-Jensen A, Rabbitt MP, Gregory CA, Singh A. Household Food Security in the United States in 2021, ERR-309, U.S. Department of Agriculture, Economic Research Service; 2022.)

◆ CASE APPLICATION FOR THE DENTAL HYGIENIST

A patient reports that he has found a miracle cure for his advanced periodontal disease. He plans to follow a diet and take recommended supplements "to strengthen my gums." This diet eliminates all foods from two food groups from *MyPlate*.

Nutritional Assessment

- Dietary intake, especially which of the food groups are omitted; nutrients most likely to be lacking
- Nutrition knowledge
- Supplements used and dosage
- Economic status
- Where most meals taken; food preparation

Nutritional Diagnosis

Knowledge deficit related to nutritional requirements.

Nutritional Goals

The patient will receive adequate nutrients to maintain oral health status by consuming a well-balanced diet.

Nutritional Implementation

Intervention: Discuss *MyPlate*—different groups, number of servings needed from each group, portion sizes, and nutrients provided from each group.

Rationale: Healthy oral structures depend on a variety of nutrients that can be obtained by following this guideline.

Intervention: Discuss nutrients that are deficient in his proposed diet and why those nutrients are important.

Rationale: When essential nutrients are omitted, the body cannot function effectively and its immune response is compromised.

Intervention: Discuss the importance of obtaining nutrients from foods rather than supplements.

Rationale: Foods are the natural way of obtaining nutrients; when supplements are used, many times they are in proportions that cannot be absorbed or they may interfere with absorption of other nutrients. Other components of food may affect use of the nutrient. In general, most supplements are not as effective as the food itself (see *Health Application 11* in Chapter 11).

Intervention: Discuss specific foods and oral care that would be helpful in preventing further deterioration.

Rationale: Adequate nutrition and oral self-care promote healing and repair of disease tissue. Maintaining a well-balanced diet provides the nutrients needed to support a healthy periodontium and resist disease activity.

Evaluation

The patient will practice effective oral care and consume a well-balanced diet; as a consequence, his periodontal health will improve.

◆ Student Readiness

1. Choose a culture predominant in your area and research the cultural beliefs related to eating patterns.
   - Identify at least one positive aspect about this culture's food pattern.
   - List at least one potential dietary problem for the culture's traditional food pattern and provide some suggestions for altering the diet.
   - Plan a 2-day menu that would meet the *Dietary Guidelines* and *MyPlate* using favorite or traditional foods of the cultural group.
   - Would a patient have any problem following the proposed menu, such as economic hardship or the local availability of special foods?
   - Are there any oral health problems at higher risk in this cultural group?

2. Think of two general statements that apply to all of your family/roommates (e.g., always eat breakfast, never drink milk, etc.). Discuss these statements with a group of your fellow students and see how many actually conform to your statements. Describe some examples of lifelong eating habits learned as a child.

3. State some reasons why people in the United States do not have similar eating patterns.

4. Plan a menu for one day using low-cost healthy foods.

5. A patient wants to know about convenience and fast foods. What would you tell the patient?

6. Study the meats at a grocery store. Categorize the types of meats that contain nitrate preservatives. Look at your own daily intake for three days and evaluate how frequently you are consuming nitrate-containing foods.

7. Some Americans are dependent on commercially prepared frozen foods or purchased foods outside the home. Look at the caloric density of foods consumed in restaurants and the nature of the diseases that relate to obesity and cardiovascular health. What has consumer demand done to change selections offered in commercial food service establishments?

8. Prepare a rough budget showing how your personal funds are expended on a month-to-month basis. Evaluate the percentage of your own personal income that is earmarked for food prepared at home versus food prepared in a restaurant or convenience items purchased in a grocery store. How well do you spend your own food dollar? Make some conclusions about how you could better use your dollar to provide nutrient-dense foods for you and your family.

9. Compare the cost of three foods from a health food store or health food section of a grocery store with the cost of similar items in other sections in the grocery store. Share the pros and cons of choosing the more expensive option.

10. Locate an advertisement online or on social media for a health food product, and list benefits of the product stated in the advertisement. List information about the product that might have been omitted or should be questioned.

11. Compare the cost of three organic foods with the same foods that are not labeled organic. Which would you choose to purchase and why?

12. Discuss current food fads and how they may have adverse effects.

13. What are the warning signs of someone promoting unhealthy or unfounded dietary advice?

14. Discuss the pros and cons of allowing nutritional claims on products.

15. A patient states, "I want to follow the _____ diet because _____ (popular actor) is advertising it." How would you respond?

16. Read a nutrition research article from a reputable journal. Using information provided in this chapter, point out some problems with the validity and applicability of the research. Does the article identify these as problem areas? Summarize the article in one page or less as if it is being presented to a patient.

◆ CASE STUDY

A young couple with three children—ages 3, 5, and 7 years—has been living on unemployment insurance payments for 9 months. The mother expresses concerns about inadequate funds to feed the children. She is worried about their dental health.

1. Prepare a list of social services or federal service agencies in the community that could be contacted to determine potential sources of assistance to support recovery of this couple.
2. What are some nutritional concerns the dental hygienist could address with the patient?
3. What are some foods that are nutrient dense and economical purchases?
4. List some snack foods for the children that are nutritious, economical, and noncariogenic.
5. What methods of food preparation could be suggested to the mother that would preserve the nutritional quality of the food?

References

1. Agency for Healthcare Research and Quality. *2022 National Healthcare Quality and Disparities Report*. AHRQ; 2022. https://www.ahrq.gov/research/findings/nhqrdr/nhqdr22/index.html.
2. Vespa J, Medina L, Armstrong DM. *Demographic Turning Points for the United States: Population Estimates and Projections*. United States Census Bureau; 2020. https://www.census.gov/content/dam/Census/library/publications/2020/demo/p25-1144.pdf.
3. Healthy People 2030, United States Department of Health and Human Services, Office of Disease Prevention and Health Promotion. *Social Determinants of Health*. https://health.gov/healthypeople/objectives-and-data/social-determinants-health
4. United States Department of Agriculture, United States Department of Health and Human Services. *Dietary Guidelines for Americans*. 9th ed. 2020. dietaryguidelines.gov.
5. Ramírez AS, Golash-Boza T, Unger JB, Baezconde-Garbanati L. Questioning the dietary acculturation paradox: a mixed-methods study of the relationship between food and ethnic identity in a group of Mexican-American women. *J Acad Nutr Diet*. 2018;118(3):431–439.
6. Wright KE, Lucero JE, Ferguson JK, et al. The impact that cultural food security has on identity and well-being in the second-generation United States American minority college students. *Food Sec*. 2021;13(3):701–715.
7. Reddy S, Anitha M. Culture and its influence on nutrition and oral health. *Biomed Pharmacology J*. 2015;8(October Spl Edition):613–620.
8. Miller V, Webb P, Cudhea F, et al. Global dietary quality in 185 countries from 1990 to 2018 show wide differences by nation, age, education, and urbanicity. *Nat Food*. 2022;3(9):694–702.
9. Chouraqui JP, Turck D, Briend A, et al. Religious dietary rules and their potential nutritional and health consequences. *Int J Epidemiol*. 2021;50(1):12–26.

10. USDA Economic Research Service. *Summary Findings: Food Price Outlook, 2023 and 2024.* 2023. https://www.ers.usda.gov/data-products/food-price-outlook/summary-findings/

11. USDA Economic Research Service. *Food Prices and Spending.* 2023. https://www.ers.usda.gov/data-products/ag-and-food-statistics-charting-the-essentials/food-prices-and-spending/?topicId=2b168260-a717–4708-a264-cb354e815c67

12. USDA Food and Nutrition Service. *Cost of Food at Home at Three Levels, United States Average, August 2023.* 2023. https://fns-prod.azureedge.us/sites/default/files/resource-files/CostofFoodAug2023LowModLib.pdf

13. Daniel C. Is healthy eating too expensive?: how low-income parents evaluate the cost of food. *Soc Sci Med.* 2020;248:112823.

14. Hartline-Grafton H, Weill J. Replacing the thrifty food plan in order to provide adequate allotments for SNAP beneficiaries. *Food Res Action Cent.* 2012:13. https://frac.org/wp-content/uploads/thrifty_food_plan_2012.pdf.

15. Herforth A, Bai Y, Venkat A, Mahrt K, Ebel A, Masters WA Cost and affordability of healthy diets across and within countries. Background paper for The State of Food Security and Nutrition in the World 2020. FAO Agricultural Development Economics Technical Study No. 2020;9. https://doi.org/10.4060/cb2431en.

16. Vandevijvere S, Pedroni C, De Ridder K, Castetbon K. The cost of diets according to their caloric share of ultraprocessed and minimally processed foods in Belgium. *Nutrients.* 2020;12(9):2787.

17. Carlson A, Frazão E. *Are Healthy Foods Really More Expensive? It Depends on How You Measure the Price.* 2012. http://www.ers.usda.gov/publications/pub-details/?pubid=44679

18. Tiwari A, Aggarwal A, Tang W, Drewnowski A. Cooking at home: a strategy to comply with United States Dietary Guidelines at no extra cost. *Am J Prev Med.* 2017;52(5):616–624.

19. Lin BH, Guthrie J, Smith T. *Dietary Quality by Food Source and Demographics in the United States, 1977–2018.* 2023. http://www.ers.usda.gov/publications/pub-details/?pubid=105955

20. McCullough ML, Chantaprasopsuk S, Islami F, et al. Association of socioeconomic and geographic factors with diet quality in United States adults. *JAMA Netw Open.* 2022;5(6):e2216406.

21. UDSA Food and Nutrition Service. *Thrifty Food Plan, 2021.* USDA; 2021:125. https://www.fns.usda.gov/cnpp/thrifty-food-plan-2021

22. USDA Food and Nutrition Service. *Official USDA Thrifty Food Plan: United States Average.* 2023.

23. Lee S, Choi Y, Jeong HS, Lee J, Sung J. Effect of different cooking methods on the content of vitamins and true retention in selected vegetables. *Food Sci Biotechnol.* 2017;27(2):333–342.

24. Dong L, Qiu CY, Wang RC, et al. Effects of air frying on French fries: The indication role of physicochemical properties on the formation of Maillard hazards, and the changes of starch digestibility. *Front Nutr.* 2022;9:889901.

25. Centers for Disease Control and Prevention. *Estimates of Foodborne Illness in the United States: Estimates of Foodborne Illness.* 2019. https://www.cdc.gov/foodborneburden/index.html

26. USDA Food Safety and Inspection Service. *Foodborne Illness and Disease: Food Safety and Inspection Service.* 2020. http://www.fsis.usda.gov/food-safety/foodborne-illness-and-disease

27. Center for Food Safety and Applied Nutrition. *2019 Food Safety and Nutrition Survey Report.* FDA; 2021. https://www.fda.gov/food/science-research-food/2019-food-safety-and-nutrition-survey-report

28. CDC. *Food Safety: Foods That Can Cause Food Poisoning.* Centers for Disease Control and Prevention; 2023. https://www.cdc.gov/food-safety/foods-linked-illness.html

29. United States Food and Drug Administration, Center for Food Safety and Applied Nutrition. *The New Nutrition Facts Label.* FDA; 2022. https://www.fda.gov/food/nutrition-education-resources-materials/new-nutrition-facts-label.

30. Forde CG, Decker EA. The importance of food processing and eating behavior in promoting healthy and sustainable diets. *Ann Rev Nutr.* 2022;42(1):377–399.

31. Institute of Medicine Committee on Use of Dietary Reference Intakes in Nutrition Labeling. *Overview of food fortification in the United States and Canada. Dietary Reference Intakes: Guiding Principles for Nutrition Labeling and Fortification.* National Academies Press (United States); 2003. https://www.ncbi.nlm.nih.gov/books/NBK208880/.

32. Li L, Pegg RB, Eitenmiller RR, Chun JY, Kerrihard AL. Selected nutrient analyses of fresh, fresh-stored, and frozen fruits and vegetables. *J Food Comp Anal.* 2017;59:8–17.

33. Askari M, Heshmati J, Shahinfar H, Tripathi N, Daneshzad E. Ultra-processed food and the risk of overweight and obesity: a systematic review and *meta*-analysis of observational studies. *Int J Obes.* 2020;44(10):2080–2091.

34. Cascaes AM, Silva NRJD, Fernandez MDS, Bomfim RA, Vaz JDS. Ultra-processed food consumption and dental caries in children and adolescents: a systematic review and *meta*-analysis. *Br J Nutr.* 2023;129(8):1370–1379.

35. Delpino FM, Figueiredo LM, Bielemann RM, et al. Ultra-processed food and risk of type 2 diabetes: a systematic review and *meta*-analysis of longitudinal studies. *Intern J Epidemiol.* 2022;51(4):1120–1141.

36. Bidinotto AB, Martinez-Steele E, Thomson WM, Hugo FN, Hilgert JB. Investigation of direct and indirect association of ultra-processed food intake and periodontitis. *J Periodontol.* 2022;93(4):603–612.

37. Taneri PE, Wehrli F, Roa-Díaz ZM, et al. Association between ultra-processed food intake and all-cause mortality: a systematic review and *meta*-analysis. *Am J Epidemiol.* 2022;191(7):1323–1335.

38. Food and Drug Administration, Center for Food Safety and Applied Nutrition. *Food Irradiation: What You Need to Know.* FDA; 2023. https://www.fda.gov/food/buy-store-serve-safe-food/food-irradiation-what-you-need-know

39. USDA, National Agricultural Statistics Service. *Results From the 2021 Organic Survey.* 2022. https://www.nass.usda.gov/Publications/Highlights/2022/2022_Organic_Highlights.pdf

40. USDA Economic Research Service. *Organic Agriculture.* 2023. https://www.ers.usda.gov/topics/natural-resources-environment/organic-agriculture/

41. Gundala RR, Singh A. What motivates consumers to buy organic foods? Results of an empirical study in the United States. *PLoS One.* 2021;16(9):e0257288.

42. USDA Agricultural Marketing Service. *About the Organic Standards.* https://www.ams.usda.gov/grades-standards/organic-standards

43. USDA. *Conservation and Biological Diversity in Organic Production.* https://www.usda.gov/media/blog/2016/02/29/conservation-and-biological-diversity-organic-production

44. Vigar V, Myers S, Oliver C, Arellano J, Robinson S, Leifert C. A systematic review of organic vs conventional food consumption: is there a measurable benefit on human health? *Nutrients.* 2019;12(1):7.

45. Smith-Spangler C, Brandeau ML, Hunter GE, et al. Are organic foods safer or healthier than conventional alternatives? *Ann Intern Med.* 2012;157(5):348–366.

46. Gómez-Ramos M, del M, Nannou C, Martínez Bueno MJ, et al. Pesticide residues evaluation of organic crops. A critical appraisal. *Food Chem X.* 2020;5:100079.

47. USDA Agricultural Marketing Service. *Pesticide Data Program's databases and annual summaries: Annual Summary, Calendar Year 2021.* 2022. https://www.ams.usda.gov/datasets/pdp/pdpdata

48. Food and Drug Administration. *FDA Announces Transition of Over-the-Counter Medically Important Antimicrobials for Animals to Prescription Status.* FDA; 2023. https://www.fda.gov/animal-veterinary/cvm-updates/fda-announces-transition-over-counter-medically-important-antimicrobials-animals-prescription-status

49. Çakır M, Beatty TKM, Boland MA, Li Q, Park TA, Wang Y. An index number approach to estimating organic price premia at retail. *J Agric Appl Econ Assoc.* 2022;1(1):33–46.

50. Food and Drug Administration. *Menu Labeling Requirements.* FDA; 2023. https://www.fda.gov/food/food-labeling-nutrition/menu-labeling-requirements

51. Alexander E, Rutkow L, Gudzune KA, Cohen JE, McGinty EE. Healthiness of United States chain restaurant meals in 2017. *J Acad Nutr Diet.* 2020;120(8):1359–1367.

52. Pagliai G, Dinu M, Madarena MP, Bonaccio M, Iacoviello L, Sofi F. Consumption of ultra-processed foods and health status: a systematic review and *meta*-analysis. *Br J Nutr.* 2021;125(3):308–318.

53. Chen X, Zhang Z, Yang H, et al. Consumption of ultra-processed foods and health outcomes: a systematic review of epidemiological studies. *Nutr J.* 2020;19:86.

54. Petimar J, Zhang F, Cleveland LP, et al. Estimating the effect of calorie menu labeling on calories purchased in a large restaurant franchise in the southern United States: quasi-experimental study. *BMJ.* 2019;367:l5837.

55. Petimar J, Zhang F, Rimm EB, et al. Changes in the calorie and nutrient content of purchased fast food meals after calorie menu labeling: a natural experiment. *PLoS Med.* 2021;18(7):e1003714.

56. Grummon AH, Petimar J, Soto MJ, et al. Changes in calorie content of menu items at large chain restaurants after implementation of calorie labels. *JAMA Netw Open.* 2021;4(12):e2141353.

57. Food and Drug Administration. *FDA's Approach to the GRAS Provision: A History of Processes.* FDA; 2018. https://www.fda.gov/food/generally-recognized-safe-gras/fdas-approach-gras-provision-history-processes

58. World Health Organization. *Food Additives.* 2022. https://www.who.int/news-room/fact-sheets/detail/food-additives

59. Miller MD, Steinmaus C, Golub MS, et al. Potential impacts of synthetic food dyes on activity and attention in children: a review of the human and animal evidence. *Env Health.* 2022;21(1):1–19.

60. Said Abasse K, Essien EE, Abbas M, et al. Association between dietary nitrate, nitrite intake, and site-specific cancer risk: a systematic review and *meta*-analysis. *Nutrients.* 2022;14(3):666.

61. Ubago-Guisado E, Rodríguez-Barranco M, Ching-López A, et al. Evidence update on the relationship between diet and the most common cancers from the European prospective investigation into cancer and nutrition (EPIC) study: a systematic review. *Nutrients.* 2021;13(10):3582.

62. USDA. *Yearbook of Agriculture: Food and Life.* United States Government Printing Office; 1939. https://www.google.com/books/edition/Food_and_Life/eoVHAQAAMAAJ?hl=en&gbpv=1&dq=More+food+notions+flourish+in+the+United+States+than+in+any+other+civilized+country+on+earth,+and+most+of+them+are+wrong.+They+thrive+in+the+minds+of+the+same+people+who+talk+about+their+operations%3B+and+like+all+mythology,+they+are+a+blend+of+fear,+coincidence,+and+advertising&pg=PA144&printsec=frontcover

63. Tahreem A, Rakha A, Rabail R, et al. Fad diets: facts and fiction. *Front Nutr.* 2022;9:960922.

64. Diekman C, Ryan CD, Oliver TL. Misinformation and disinformation in food science and nutrition: impact on practice. *J Nutr.* 2023;153(1):3–9.

65. Estevan Navarro P, Sospedra I, Perales A, et al. Caffeine health claims on sports supplement labeling. analytical assessment according to EFSA scientific opinion and international evidence and criteria. *Molecules.* 2021;26(7):2095.

66. Autism Science Foundation. *Beware of Non-evidence-Based Treatments.* Autism Science Foundation; 2023. https://autismscience-foundation.org/beware-of-non-evidence-based-treatments/

67. Klein AV, Kiat H. Detox diets for toxin elimination and weight management: a critical review of the evidence. *J Hum Nutr Diet.* 2015;28(6):675–686.

68. National Center for Complementary and Integrative Health. *"Detoxes" and "Cleanses": What You Need To Know.* NCCIH; 2019. https://www.nccih.nih.gov/health/detoxes-and-cleanses-what-you-need-to-know

69. Obert J, Pearlman M, Obert L, Chapin S. Popular weight loss strategies: a review of four weight loss techniques. *Curr Gastroenterol Rep.* 2017;19(12):61.

70. Kardos P, Kun Á, Pléh C, Jordán F. How) should researchers publicize their research papers before peer review? *Scientometrics.* 2023;128(3):2019–2023.

71. Angell M, Kassirer JP. Clinical research – what should the public believe? *N Engl J Med.* 1994;331(3):189–190.

72. Temple NJ. The origins of the obesity epidemic in the USA–lessons for today. *Nutrients.* 2022;14(20):4253.

73. FDA. *Questions and Answers on Dietary Supplements.* FDA; 2022. https://www.fda.gov/food/information-consumers-using-dietary-supplements/questions-and-answers-dietary-supplements

74. Denniss E, Lindberg R, McNaughton SA. Quality and accuracy of online nutrition-related information: a systematic review of content analysis studies. *Public Health Nutr.* 2023;26(7):1345–1357.

75. Siontis KC, Ioannidis JPA. Replication, duplication, and waste in a quarter million systematic reviews and *meta*-analyses. *Circ Cardiovasc Qual Outcomes.* 2018;11(12):e005212.

76. Schuit E, Ioannidis JP. Network *meta*-analyses performed by contracting companies and commissioned by industry. *Syst Rev.* 2016;5(1):198.

77. Toossi S, Jones JW. *The Food and Nutrition Assistance Landscape: Fiscal Year 2022 Annual Report.* USDA Economic Research Service; 2023:34. http://www.ers.usda.gov/publications/pub-details/?pubid=106762.

78. USDA, Supplemental Nutrition Assistance Program. *Addressing Barriers and Challenges–Seniors.* https://www.budget.senate.gov/imo/media/doc/Addressing%20Barriers%20and%20Challenges%20-%20Seniors.pdf

79. Andreyeva T, Tripp AS, Schwartz MB. Dietary quality of Americans by supplemental nutrition assistance program participation status: a systematic review. *Am J Prev Med.* 2015;49(4):594–604.

80. Venkataramani M, Ogunwole SM, Caulfield LE, et al. Maternal, infant, and child health outcomes associated with the special supplemental nutrition program for women, infants, and children: a systematic review. *Ann Intern Med.* 2022;175(10):1411–1422.

81. USDA Economic Research Service. *WIC Program.* 2022. https://www.ers.usda.gov/topics/food-nutrition-assistance/wic-program/

82. USDA Food and Nutrition Service. *Special Supplemental Nutrition Program for Women, Infants, and Children (WIC): Revisions in the WIC Food Packages.* 2022. https://www.govinfo.gov/content/pkg/FR-2022–11–21/pdf/2022–24705.pdf

83. USDA, Food and Nutrition Service. *Indicators of Diet Quality, Nutrition, and Health for Americans by Program Participation Status, 2011–2016: USDA NSLP Report.* 2022. https://www.fns.usda.gov/cn/diet-health-indicators-program-participation-status-2011-2016

84. USDA Food and Nutrition Service. *Nutrition Standards for School Meals.* 2022. https://www.fns.usda.gov/cn/nutrition-standards-school-meals

85. USDA, National Institute of Food and Agriculture. *EFNEP Impact Report 2022.* 2023. http://www.nifa.usda.gov/efnep-impact-report-2022

86. ACL Administration for Community Living. *Nutrition Services.* 2023. http://acl.gov/programs/health-wellness/nutrition-services

87. Feeding America. *Charitable Food Assistance Participation in 2022.* https://www.feedingamerica.org/research/charitable-food-assistance-participation

88. Van Cleve N. Food: facts, fad, and fancy. *Am J Nurs.* 1938;38(3):285–287.

89. Guardia L, Food Research and Action Center, Lacko A. *To End Hunger, We Must End Stigma.* Food Research & Action Center; 2021. https://frac.org/blog/endhungerendstigma

90. USDA Economic Research Service. *Key Statistics & Graphics: Food Security Status of United States Households in 2021.* 2023. https://www.ers.usda.gov/topics/food-nutrition-assistance/food-security-in-the-u-s/key-statistics-graphics/#foodsecure

91. Coleman-Jensen A, Rabbitt MP, Gregory CA, Singh A. *Household Food Security in the United States in 2021.* USDA Economic Research

Service; 2022:51. http://www.ers.usda.gov/publications/pub-details/?pubid=104655.

92. United States Bureau of Labor Statistics. *A Profile of the Working Poor, 2020: BLS Reports.* https://www.bls.gov/opub/reports/working-poor/2020/home.htm

93. Bezuneh M, Yiheyis Z. Household food insecurity, coping strategies, and happiness: the case of two public housing communities. *J Agric Food Syst Community Dev.* 2020;9(3):215–226.

94. Oldroyd L, Eskandari F, Pratt C, Lake AA. The nutritional quality of food parcels provided by food banks and the effectiveness of food banks at reducing food insecurity in developed countries: a mixed-method systematic review. *J Hum Nutr Diet.* 2022;35(6):1202–1229.

95. Nagata JM, Palar K, Gooding HC, Garber AK, Bibbins-Domingo K, Weiser SD. Food insecurity and chronic disease in United States young adults: findings from the national longitudinal study of adolescent to adult health. *J Gen Intern Med.* 2019;34(12):2756–2762.

96. Sabbagh S, Mohammadi-Nasrabadi F, Ravaghi V, et al. Food insecurity and dental caries prevalence in children and adolescents: a systematic review and *meta*-analysis. *Int J Paediatr Dent.* 2023;33(4):346–363.

97. Shankar P, Chung R, Frank D. Association of food insecurity with children's behavioral, emotional, and academic outcomes: a systematic review. *J Dev Behav Pediatr.* 2017;38(1):1–16.

98. Gallegos D, Eivers A, Sondergeld P, Pattinson C. Food insecurity and child development: a state-of-the-art review. *Int J Env Res Public Health.* 2021;18(17):8990.

99. Eskandari F, Lake AA, Rose K, Butler M, O'Malley C. A mixed-method systematic review and *meta*-analysis of the influences of food environments and food insecurity on obesity in high-income countries. *Food Sci Nutr.* 2022;10(11):3689–3723.

100. Drisdelle C, Kestens Y, Hamelin AM, Mercille G. Disparities in access to healthy diets: how food security and food shopping behaviors relate to fruit and vegetable intake. *J Acad Nutr Diet.* 2020;120(11):1847–1858.

101. Gregory CA, Mancino L, Coleman-Jensen A. Food Security and Food Purchase Quality among Low-Income Households: Findings from the National Household Food Acquisition and Purchase Survey (FoodAPS). USDA Economic Research Service; 2019:42. http://www.ers.usda.gov/publications/pub-details/?pubid=93737

102. USDA Economic Research Service. *About SNAP-Ed – Nourishing Communities: Nutrition Education That Works.* https://snap-ed.extension.org/about-snap-ed/

103. USDHHS. Healthy People 2030. *Food Security.* https://health.gov/healthypeople/search?query=food+security

▶ Evolve Resources

Please visit http://evolve.elsevier.com/Mallonee/nutritional for additional practice and study support tools.

17

Effects of Systemic Disease on Nutritional Status and Oral Health

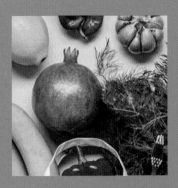

STUDENT LEARNING OUTCOMES

On completion of this chapter, the student will be able to achieve the following learning outcomes:

1. Examine the impact of anorexia, taste/smell disorders, and xerostomia on oral health, evaluate their consequences, and devise tailored interventions for affected patients.
2. Describe the effects of various types of anemia, as well as neutropenia, on nutritional status and oral health and identify nutrition education for patients with anemia.
3. Analyze the impact of gastrointestinal and cardiovascular conditions on oral health and nutrition. Develop a plan for nutrition education of patients with these conditions.
4. Examine the impact of systemic bone and metabolic disorders on oral health and nutritional status, and formulate tailored interventions for affected patients.
5. Evaluate the influence of neuromuscular disorders and cancer on oral health and nutrition, and design suitable interventions for affected patients.
6. Analyze the impact of acquired immunodeficiency and mental health issues on oral health and nutrition, and develop tailored interventions for affected patients.

KEY TERMS

Aneurysm
Anticholinergic
Atherosclerosis
Atrophic glossitis
Binges
Bisphosphonates
Bradykinesia
Chemotherapy
Chemotherapeutic
Dialysate
Epilepsy
Esophagitis

Gastroesophageal reflux disease
Glossodynia
Herpetic ulcerations
Hiatal hernia
Human papillomavirus
Ischemia
Kaposi sarcoma
Leukemia
Leukoplakia
Lipodystrophy
Macroglossia
Mucositis

Necrotizing ulcerative periodontitis
Neoplasia
Neutropenia
Odynophagia
Osteonecrosis
Parkinson's disease
Periapical
Pocketed foods
Purging
Syrup of ipecac
Thrombus

⬡ TEST YOUR NQ

1. **T/F** Anorexia, associated with a chronic disease, can result in an increased susceptibility to infection.
2. **T/F** Antihypertensive, anticholinergic, and antidepressant drugs often cause a decrease in salivary flow.
3. **T/F** Iron supplements should be recommended to a patient who has anemia.
4. **T/F** It is within the scope of practice for a dental hygienist to provide nutritional advice to a patient recently diagnosed with diabetes.
5. **T/F** A patient with a hiatal hernia should be cautioned against eating before a dental appointment to prevent regurgitation while lying in a supine position.
6. **T/F** The health care provider should monitor protein intake closely in a patient with chronic renal failure.
7. **T/F** Kaposi sarcoma is a tumor that occurs frequently in patients with epilepsy.
8. **T/F** Phenytoin (Dilantin) can cause gingival hyperplasia and vitamin deficiencies.
9. **T/F** If a patient has signs/symptoms of an eating disorder, the dental hygienist should not directly ask a patient about having an eating disorder but should casually refer the patient to a health care provider.
10. **T/F** Patients with bulimia generally have low body weight.

As you have already learned, nutritional deficiencies are frequently manifested in the oral, head and neck areas. Oral lesions can be a reflection of, or a marker for, disease elsewhere. The oral cavity cannot be isolated from what is occurring physiologically because oral tissues are nourished by the same blood supply providing oxygen and nutrients to cells throughout the entire body. Oral tissues may reflect changes in nutrient supply or other metabolic alterations. Oral manifestations are a single part of the total systemic state.

Oral problems may develop as a result of disease processes or therapies or by nutritional deficiencies. Subsequent oral issues can cause inadequate intake. Systemic diseases or medications usually prescribed for these conditions may cause alterations in the oral cavity, such as oral lesions, xerostomia, or muscular weakness (Table 17.1). These oral alterations may lead to changes in eating patterns, which frequently have a general debilitating effect on the entire body. For example, food preferences are affected by an individual's ability to chew. Patients with reduced masticatory efficiency usually choose soft foods, which may not provide adequate amounts of essential nutrients. Dentate status, malocclusion, and ill-fitting dentures or partials leading to chewing issues increase risk of malnutrition.[1] The most common nutrients/food groups with lower intake, include fiber, fruits, and vegetables.[2] The body depends on nutrients from foods eaten to regenerate and repair diseased tissues; provisions must be made to provide these nutrients in adequate amounts on a regular basis.

All disease processes result from a combination of factors: the presence of an etiologic agent (e.g., plaque biofilm), the susceptibility or resistance of the host (or activation of immune response), and environmental factors. One of the most important factors in one's ability to combat hostile agents is availability of nutrients acquired from food. Infections can spread rapidly when the immune response is depressed.

Ramifications of a patient's systemic health are important to the dental hygienist because they provide cues to possible oral problems; may change treatment goals, priorities, or scheduling; or may influence dietary recommendations provided to the patient. Thus, the dental hygienist's dietary recommendations should take into consideration the systemic health of a patient and should not contradict dietary instructions provided by the patient's other health care providers. In other words, nutritional advice regarding oral health problems must be provided in the context of the whole patient working with the interprofessional health care team.

More than one-third to 50% of the patients seen in a dental office may not frequently interact with a general health care provider.[3,4] For these individuals and for all patients, dental providers like the dental hygienist are in a key position to assess and detect oral signs and symptoms of systemic health disorders such as prediabetes and diabetes.[5] Clinical observations, radiographic findings, diet screening, and inquiries made while obtaining or updating the health history are used to detect signs and symptoms. They should be the basis for motivating the patient to visit a health care provider. Early diagnosis and management can reduce health care costs.

This chapter presents oral problems frequently caused by systemic health conditions or their treatment because these problems typically affect eating patterns. No attempt is made to cover pathophysiology, and the information given should not be used to diagnose conditions. If the cause of oral signs and symptoms is unknown, refer the patient to a health care provider who can perform a thorough assessment, including diagnostic laboratory evaluation, for accurate diagnosis and treatment.

Effects of Chronic Disease on Intake

Anorexia and Appetite

The term *anorexia nervosa* (AN) refers to a disease associated with a distorted body image, but anorexia also refers to a condition in which a patient has a poor appetite and/or decreased food intake for a variety of reasons. In some situations, it may be unknown whether anorexia is a cause of the illness or an effect of the illness.

The most common causes of anorexia are cancer treatment and aging. During cancer treatment, anorexia may include nausea, swallowing difficulties, depression, and changes in taste sensation.[6] In anorexia of aging, there may be a reduced sensitivity to hunger hormones and increased satiety; reduced gastric motility; decreased salivary secretion and reduced smell and taste; and difficulties shopping and cooking food.[7] All of these result in unintended weight loss which can reach a point where it compromises health leading to a poor prognosis and increased risk for mortality.[6]

Malnutrition and other short-term stresses—such as infection, surgery, and injuries may result in anorexia and depletion of body stores of calories, macronutrients (e.g., protein), and micronutrients (e.g., vitamin C) needed to regenerate and repair cells. In this situation, the body is more susceptible to bacterial or viral invasion.

Management of anorexia is complex and requires an interprofessional health care team. Solely dietary management of anorexia is seldom effective, medications may be needed to increase appetite.[6]

Taste and Smell Disorders

The foods that people choose to eat are modulated by taste (sweet, salty, sour, bitter, and umami), smell, and oral textural perception. Taste and smell dramatically affect appetite and food intake. Chemosensory dysfunction (partial or total loss of smell and taste) has gained a lot of attention due to the issue being one of the symptoms of COVID-19.[8] However, it is common in many disease conditions (e.g., respiratory diseases, neurodegenerative

TABLE 17.1 Oral Problems Associated With Systemic Diseases

Condition	Xerostomia	Taste Alterations	Oral Lesions	Immune Response	Masticatory Efficiency	Delayed Wound Healing	Dysphagia	Sore Tongue	Risk of Bleeding	Dental Caries
Anemias										
Iron-deficiency	X	X	X	X		X		X		
Plummer-Vinson	X	X	X	X		X	X	X		
Megaloblastic		X	X	X				X		
Thalassemia					X					
Aplastic			X						X	
Other Hematologic Diseases										
Polycythemia									X	
Neutropenia			X	X						
Gastrointestinal Problems										
Medications for gastroesophageal reflux	X							X		
Malabsorptive conditions		X	X			X				
Cardiovascular Conditions										
Cardiovascular accidents							X			
Antihypertensive medications	X									
Lipid-lowering medications		X							X	
Skeletal Anomalies										
Systemic bone disturbances					X					
Metabolic Problems										
Diabetes mellitus	X	X		X		X				X
Acromegaly					X					
Hypopituitarism					X					
Cushing's syndrome					X			X		
Hypothyroidism					X					X
Hyperparathyroidism					X					
Renal Disease										
Diminished kidney function			X		X	X			X	
Neuromuscular Problems										
Parkinson's disease	X				X		X			
Developmental disabilities					X		X			
Epilepsy	X									
Neoplasia										
Cancer		X								
Kaposi sarcoma			X							
Leukemia				X						
Acquired Immunodeficiency Syndrome										
AIDS	X		X	X						
Mental Health Problems										
Anorexia nervosa/bulimia			X							X
Medications for mental illness	X									

conditions, and cancer), medications, smoking, and treatment for the conditions to result in chemosensory dysfunction (i.e., disorders of taste and smell).[9–11] Chemosensory dysfunction also increases during the normal aging process and is compounded by a variety of chronic diseases and medications.[9,10,12]

Chemosensory dysfunction significantly affects diet quality with lower intake of total calories, fat, protein, sodium, and potassium.[13] Reactions to loss of taste and smell vary. Strategies to improve dietary intake include making food visually appealing (e.g., a variety of colors, eating environment), avoid cooking foods with unpleasant odors, focus on favorite foods, and add more spices and sauces to foods to offset diminished ability to taste.[14] In addition, it is important to encourage patients to have regular dental visits to identify and manage dental caries and sources of infection which can impart a "bad taste."[15] Oral self-care is also important to keep the mouth and oral appliances free of food debris and plaque biofilm to limit taste alterations and halitosis from these sources.

Xerostomia

Saliva protects hard and soft oral tissues from mechanical, thermal, and chemical irritants in addition to its roles in buffering acids, antimicrobial activity, and remineralization.[16] Medications (e.g., antidepressants, antihistamines, antihypertensives, diuretics, and gastrointestinal drugs), diseases or conditions (e.g., Sjögren's disease, diabetes, Parkinson's disease), and therapies (e.g., radiation) may cause xerostomia.[16,17] Globally the prevalence is 22% and higher in individuals with chronic diseases and taking multiple medications.[18] Hyposalivation is a known risk factor for dental caries and periodontal disease but may also cause taste disturbances, swallowing problems, poor chewing ability, and impact dietary intake.[17]

Xerostomia can affect nutritional status in several ways: (1) chewing is difficult because a bolus cannot be formed without additional moisture; (2) chewing is painful because the mouth is sore; (3) swallowing is difficult because of loss of lubrication from saliva; and (4) food intake may decrease because of changes in taste perception. Individuals with xerostomia may choose softer, easy to chew foods and avoid dry, hard, and crunchy foods. It is important to assess and provide guidance to the patient on healthy options to ensure adequate intake and minimize cariogenic potential. Using gravy and sauces may help with consumption of dry foods. In addition to potential impact on nutrition, regular preventive dental care along with oral self-care education and appropriate use of office and home fluorides is necessary to manage the caries risk associated with xerostomia.[19]

Anemias

Typical symptoms of all the anemias are pallor of the skin, oral mucosa, and conjunctival tissues, along with overall weakness as a result of inadequate oxygen-carrying power of the blood. The occurrence and severity of clinical symptoms depend on the degree of anemia and speed of onset. The type of anemia can be determined only after evaluation of blood tests.

Iron-Deficiency Anemia

Iron-deficiency anemia can be caused by a deficiency of dietary iron, increased blood loss (e.g., gastrointestinal bleeding and menstruation) or decreased absorption (e.g., inflammatory bowel diseases [IBD]).[20] It is likely to occur during periods in which iron requirements are high, such as during infancy or pregnancy. Gradual depletion of iron stores may progress

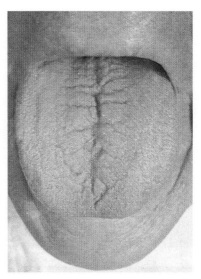

• **Fig. 17.1** Clinical symptoms of iron-deficiency anemia include pallor of the gingiva, mucosa, and tongue. (Courtesy DW Beaven and SE Brooks. From McLaren DS. A *Colour Atlas and Text of Diet-Related Disorders*. 2nd ed. Mosby-Yearbook; 1992.)

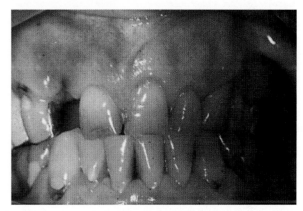

• **Fig. 17.2** Pale gingiva due to anemia. (Courtesy Dr. Edward V. Zegarelli. From Ibsen OAC, Phelan JA. *Oral Pathology for the Dental Hygienist*. 6th ed. Saunders; 2014.)

to iron-deficiency anemia, in which iron levels are inadequate for maintaining hemoglobin levels to provide cellular oxygen. Lethargy and fatigue—in addition to glossitis, aphthous ulcers, and xerostomia associated with iron-deficiency anemia—can lead to changes in appetite and food intake. Clinical symptoms in the oral cavity include gingival and mucosal pallor (Figs. 17.1 and 17.2), angular cheilosis, taste changes, and atrophic glossitis.[21] Atrophic glossitis is described as atrophy of the filiform and fungiform papillae beginning at the tip and lateral borders of the tongue and gradually spreading to the entire dorsum of the tongue.[22] As the papillae gradually shrink in size, bald spots appear, and the tongue becomes smooth, shiny, and red (Fig. 17.3).

Iron-deficiency anemia affects the immune response and places a patient at increased risk for fungal infections, such as candidiasis. After iron supplementation is initiated, the timeline for resolution of oral symptoms and regeneration of filiform papillae depends on the severity of the iron deficiency. Depending on the severity of iron-deficiency anemia, wound healing may be impaired in response to invasive dental treatments, such as tooth extraction, nonsurgical periodontal therapy, and periodontal surgery.

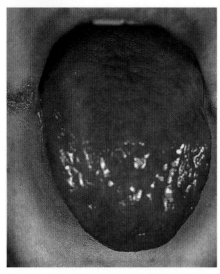

• **Fig. 17.3** Atrophic glossitis. (From Cawson RA, Odell EW. *Cawson's Essentials of Oral Pathology and Oral Medicine.* 8th ed. Churchill Livingstone; 2008.)

🌀 DENTAL CONSIDERATIONS

Assessment
- *Physical:* Burning sensation of the tongue, xerostomia, gingival and mucosal pallor, atrophy of the filiform and fungiform papillae, atrophic glossitis, angular cheilosis, candidiasis.
- *Dietary:* Adequacy of dietary intake, especially red meats, dark-green vegetables, enriched cereals and bread; use of a vitamin-mineral supplement.

Interventions
- Encourage iron-rich foods (see Table 12.12); if principally nonheme sources are consumed at a meal, a source of vitamin C enhances absorption of nonheme iron.
- If the iron supplement causes nausea, encourage the patient to take the supplement with food or discuss the problem with the health care provider rather than discontinuing the supplement.

Evaluation
- Successful outcomes include the patient consuming iron-rich foods and taking the prescribed supplement.

🌀 NUTRITIONAL DIRECTIONS

- If the iron supplement is liquid, dilute with water or juice and drink with a straw to minimize tooth staining.
- Iron stores are replenished very slowly and length of therapy may vary.

Megaloblastic Anemia

Vitamin B$_{12}$ and folic acid are major causes for megaloblastic anemia (a small number of large red blood cells). The vitamin deficiency causes impaired DNA synthesis which inhibits cell division.

Vitamin B$_{12}$ (Cobalamin) Deficiency

Causes of vitamin B$_{12}$ deficiency include inadequate intake, decreased absorption (e.g., loss of intrinsic factor, bariatric surgery, medications), or increased requirements. The body normally stores a 2 to 4 year supply of vitamin B$_{12}$ in the liver.[23] Dietary sources of vitamin B$_{12}$ are animal products including meat, eggs,

and dairy. Vitamin B$_{12}$ deficiency is most common among vegans who consume no animal products.

Anemia due to Vitamin B$_{12}$ deficiency may lead to neurologic damage to the central nervous system so it is important to identify it early. The early diagnostic features include linear or irregular erythema on palatal, buccal, and/or labial mucosa with diffuse "beefy" or bright red patches on the dorsal and ventral borders of the tongue which may progress to atrophic glossitis.[23,24] Symptoms progress to tingling in hands and feet, confusion/cognitive changes, mood changes, smell and taste dysfunction, and balance issues.[25]

Replacement therapy with vitamin B$_{12}$ supplements, nasal spray, or injections are used for treatment and depending on the severity of the symptoms it may take months for improvement. If the central nervous system damage is severe, some symptoms may not be reversed by treatment.

Folic Acid Deficiency

Another type of megaloblastic anemia is caused by folic acid deficiency. Folate is also required for DNA synthesis. Deficiency is frequently associated with decreased intake, increased demand (e.g., pregnancy), malabsorption (e.g., celiac disease), or medications that interfere with folate absorption or metabolism (e.g., phenytoin (Dilantin) or methotrexate).[23] Sources of folic acid include dark green leafy vegetables, fortified breads and cereals, fruits, nuts, eggs, dairy product, and meat.

Adequate folate intake or supplementation in pregnant females is important to reduce the risk for neural tube defects which can include cleft lip and palate in the newborn.[26] Other general symptoms of deficiency are similar to those of vitamin B$_{12}$ deficiency and may include fatigue, headache, heart palpitations, shortness of breath, and gastrointestinal symptoms.[23,27] Oral manifestations of folic acid deficiency anemia include glossitis, atrophy of the papillae, angular cheilitis (Fig. 17.4), and glossodynia (pain in the tongue).[27]

Folate supplementation is necessary because diet alone is inadequate to replace lost stores.[23] Both vitamin B$_{12}$ and folate are closely related and should be evaluated for deficiency and treated. Folate supplementation may produce hematologic improvement within 1 to 2 months.[23]

🌀 DENTAL CONSIDERATIONS

Assessment
- *Physical:* Sex; age; smooth, red, sore, or painful tongue; pale skin and oral mucous membranes; shortness of breath; malabsorption conditions or previous gastrointestinal surgeries.
- *Dietary:* Dietary intake, especially dark-green leafy vegetables, animal products, whole-grain breads, and fortified foods; limit alcohol intake.

Interventions
- If the patient has megaloblastic anemia caused by folate deficiency, encourage rich sources of folate (especially grains fortified with folic acid) along with a supplement meeting the RDA for folate (400 µg; see Table 11.12).
- If the patient is not a vegan, encourage intake of foods from animal sources high in vitamin B$_{12}$ for pernicious anemia. If the patient is a vegan, encourage fortified foods or supplementation. Dietary intake helps reestablish depleted stores.
- Refer the patient to an RDN for guidance on healthy eating patterns to ensure adequate intake of folate and vitamin B$_{12}$ rich foods.

Evaluation
- Desired outcomes include the patient consuming a well-balanced diet and foods high in folate or vitamin B$_{12}$ (as appropriate) and taking supplements to enhance the formation of red blood cells (erythropoiesis).

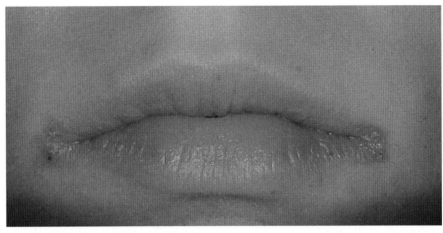

• **Fig. 17.4** Angular cheilitis in folate deficiency anemia. (From Ibsen OAC, Phelan JA. *Oral Pathology for the Dental Hygienist*. 6th ed. Saunders; 2014.)

🔹 NUTRITIONAL DIRECTIONS

- Raw vegetables are a better source of folate than cooked vegetables; heat destroys folate.
- Daily intake of dietary folate is necessary.
- Patients with permanent gastric or ileal damage; malabsorption conditions; or bariatric surgery may need monthly intramuscular or oral vitamin B_{12} supplementation for life.
- Vitamin B_{12} should be obtained from food sources and oral supplementation if indicated. If this is not effective, a B_s injection may be recommended by primary care physician.
- When oral vitamin B_{12} or iron supplements are ordered, take with vitamin C–rich foods to enhance absorption.
- Large doses of folate can negate therapeutic effects of some medications like anticonvulsants; thus consultation with the health care provider is recommended.

Other Hematologic Disorders

Neutropenia

Neutropenia is a diminished number of neutrophils, the most abundant type of white blood cells (WBCs) in the blood and may predispose an immunocompromised patient to life-threatening infections. The risk of infection is directly proportional to etiology, duration, and severity of neutropenia.[28] Neutropenia results from dysfunctional bone marrow: cancer (e.g., leukemia), drugs (e.g., chemotherapeutic agents or antibiotics), radiation therapy, autoimmune disease (e.g., rheumatoid arthritis or systemic lupus erythematosus), bone marrow transplant, nutritional deficiencies (e.g., severe vitamin B_{12}, folate, or copper deficiency), AN, or certain bacterial or viral infections (e.g., human immunodeficiency virus [HIV], malaria, tuberculosis, or Epstein-Barr virus).

The oral cavity is often the first place signs of neutropenia appear and may include aphthous ulcers, mucositis, gingivitis, and viral and fungal infections (e.g., candidiasis).[28] General symptoms may include fever, skin changes, lymphadenopathy, and nail anomalies.[28] As the neutrophil count falls, incidence and severity of infection rise. Oral organisms from the periapical (area around the root apex), and periodontium can disseminate systemically,

causing bacteremias and systemic infection.[29] Mucositis may result in large ulcerative and necrotic lesions with extensive tissue destruction and pain.[29] Mucositis impacts oral self-care and ability to consume food because of the ulcerated lesions and pain.[29] Since poor oral self-care and oral infections may worsen the severity and duration of mucositis, it is essential for the patient at risk for neutropenia to maintain meticulous oral self-care and have regular preventive dental care.[29] When neutropenia is present, invasive dental treatment is usually contraindicated until WBC counts increase. If emergency treatment is indicated, a consultation with the health care provider is necessary to determine if antibiotic prophylaxis is needed.

🔹 DENTAL CONSIDERATIONS

Assessment
- *Physical:* Painful oral mucosal ulcerations (mucositis), candidiasis.
- *Dietary:* Folate and vitamin B_{12} intake.

Interventions
- For neutropenia, encourage foods high in folate (see Table 11.12) and vitamin B_{12} (see Table 11.14) if the patient's intake is questionable.
- Stress the importance of frequent preventive maintenance and meticulous oral self-care.
- Refer the patient to an RDN for nutritional counseling if eating habits are poor.

Evaluation
- Successful outcomes include patient adherence to a diet encompassing a variety of foods, concentrating on iron, vitamin B_{12}, or folate; use of supplementation as recommended by a primary care provider or RDN; and frequent preventive dental care for maintenance of good periodontal health.

🔹 NUTRITIONAL DIRECTIONS

- To ensure adequate iron intake, choose meat, fish, or poultry regularly.
- Choose a vitamin C–rich food with a meal or eat a small amount of meat with each meal to enhance iron absorption.

Gastrointestinal Problems

Gastroesophageal Reflux, Hiatal Hernia, and Esophagitis

Heartburn 30 minutes to 1 hour after eating is the most common symptom of gastroesophageal reflux disease (GERD), a return of gastric contents into the esophagus. GERD has become more prevalent with at least 30% of adults and 10% of children experiencing symptoms at least once per week.[30,31] Risk factors for GERD include lifestyle (e.g., overweight/obesity; excessive alcohol consumption); diet (e.g., trigger foods, acidic foods, coffee, chocolate, fried food and spicy food); eating habits (e.g., large meals particularly before bedtime); neuromuscular conditions (e.g., cerebral palsy); pulmonary conditions (e.g., cystic fibrosis); medications (e.g., calcium channel blockers, nonsteroidal antiinflammatory drugs); hiatal hernia (partial protrusion of the stomach through the diaphragm Fig. 17.5); smoking and secondhand smoke; and pregnancy.[32–35]

Normally, the lower esophageal sphincter prevents gastric acid from refluxing into the esophagus. Acidity from the stomach, alkalinity, pepsin, or bile may damage the esophageal mucosa, and esophagitis (inflammation of the lower esophagus) may result if left untreated. Symptoms include esophageal (e.g., heartburn, regurgitation, Barrett's esophagitis), noncardiac chest pain, laryngeal (e.g., hoarseness, throat pain, throat clearing), pulmonary (e.g., asthma, chronic cough, pulmonary fibrosis), dental (dental erosion, dental caries), ear infections.[30,36] Treatment typically involves medications like proton pump inhibitors along with weight loss for overweight or obese individuals, dietary, and lifestyle changes.[35] The interprofessional team can support the patient in avoiding alcohol, tobacco cessation and avoidance of trigger foods (caffeinated beverages, alcohol, acidic and spicy foods).[35] Other suggestions to help reduce GERD include eating small, frequent meals; eating at least 2 to 3 hours before lying down; and elevating the head of the bed.[35]

Proton pump inhibitors are commonly prescribed for GERD and may interfere with the absorption of vitamin B$_{12}$.[37] Observation for oral signs of vitamin deficiency is appropriate for patients taking these medications.

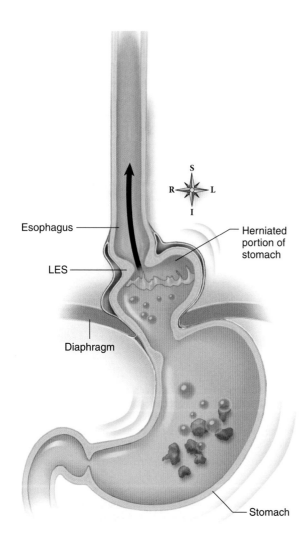

Esophagus

LES

Diaphragm

Herniated portion of stomach

Stomach

• **Fig. 17.5** Hiatal hernia. Note herniated portion of the stomach pushed through the diaphragm. LES, Lower esophageal sphincter. (From *The Human Body in Health & Disease*. 8th ed. 2024.)

🦷 DENTAL CONSIDERATIONS

Assessment
- *Physical:* Type of medications used, heartburn, bitter taste, visual appraisal of weight, enamel erosion, dentin hypersensitivity.
- *Diet:* Adequacy and frequency of intake of trigger foods such as caffeine and alcohol; knowledge of foods that increase reflux or irritate the esophagus.

Interventions
- If weight loss is needed, the dental hygienist can support healthy diet patterns as recommended by the *Dietary Guidelines* and *MyPlate* and refer to an RDN.
- To reduce risk of regurgitation during dental treatment, the patient should be in semisupine position; the patient should not eat for 2 hours before the appointment; and avoid the use of nitrous oxide because it may relax the lower esophageal sphincter.

Evaluation
- The patient plans frequent well-balanced meals, avoiding foods that cause reflux and irritate the esophagus.
- Regular follow up with health care provider for monitoring of GERD management.

🦷 NUTRITIONAL DIRECTIONS

- The effectiveness of avoiding or limiting foods that increase likelihood of reflux to prevent irritation of esophageal tissue varies among patients. General recommendations include limiting caffeine, chocolate, alcohol, mint, and carbonated beverages.
- If citrus fruits and tomato products are avoided or limited, other sources of vitamin C should be selected, including cantaloupe, potatoes, and strawberries.
- Heartburn is not caused by inadequate digestion; digestive enzyme tablets are inappropriate.
- Eat small meals, evenly distributed throughout the day.
- Reduce or eliminate cigarette smoking, which stimulates gastric acid secretion.

Malabsorptive Conditions

Many conditions are associated with malabsorption of nutrients, including IBD (e.g., Crohn's disease, ulcerative colitis); bariatric surgery or small bowel resection; liver disease; pancreatic exocrine insufficiency (e.g., cystic fibrosis, pancreatitis); lactose deficiency; gluten related disorders (e.g., celiac disease, gluten-sensitive enteropathy, tropical sprue), and AIDS.[38] **Gluten** is a protein found mainly in wheat and to a lesser degree in rye, oat, and barley. Different parts of the gastrointestinal tract are affected in these disorders, and manifestations differ from one individual to another with the same condition (see Chapter 3, *Health Application 3*). Malabsorption may occur, affecting many macronutrients (e.g., gluten [protein], fat, and carbohydrates) and micronutrients (e.g., vitamin B_{12}).[38]

General symptoms include chronic diarrhea, bloating, abdominal pain, pallor, poor wound healing, muscle wasting, and unintentional weight loss.[38] Oral problems associated with IBD include swollen, bleeding, erythematous gingiva; diffuse pustular eruptions on the buccal gingiva; aphthous ulcerations (Fig. 17.6); deep oral fissuring; angular cheilitis; taste changes; lichen planus; and cobblestone-like, raised hypertrophic lesions of mucosa (Crohn's disease).[39] Those with IBD also have higher risk for gingivitis, periodontitis, and dental caries.[39] In celiac disease, oral symptoms may include enamel defects and recurrent aphthous ulcers.[40] For individuals with cystic fibrosis, there may be enamel defects however more research is needed to determine if the risk for caries or periodontal disease is higher.[41]

Treatment is dependent on the cause of the malabsorption, avoiding food triggers, and correcting nutrient deficiencies.[38] Different nutritional modalities are required for these conditions and take into account specific nutrient deficiencies identified in the individual. Given the complexities involved, dietary counseling of the patient is outside the scope of the dental hygienist and care requires an interprofessional team. The role of the dental hygienist is to manage and prevent oral disease and support the patient in meeting the recommendations from their interprofessional health care team.[38]

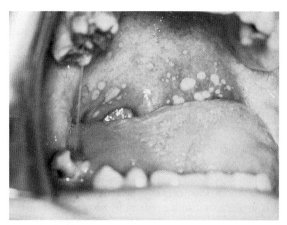

• **Fig. 17.6**   Oral ulcers "due to" ulcerative colitis. (From Ibsen OAC, Phelan JA. *Oral Pathology for the Dental Hygienist*. 6th ed. Saunders; 2014.)

⊙ NUTRITIONAL DIRECTIONS

- Encourage the patient to use a food diary to note symptoms, specific foods, or dietary practices that cause problems.
- Adequate rest and a relaxed, calm day before the dental appointment help to avoid aggravating symptoms.
- Multiple nutrient deficiencies are common and can interfere with effectiveness of the prescribed medication, compromising immune function.

Cardiovascular Conditions

Cardiovascular disease (CVD) encompasses numerous prevalent chronic heart problems, including hypertension, congestive heart failure, myocardial infarction, cerebrovascular accident, and arteriosclerosis. There may be a risk of CVD resulting from systemic exposure to periodontal pathogens.[42,43] Periodontal interventions may reduce systemic inflammation and risk of CVD. However, meta-analyses and evidence-based research have revealed conflicting results regarding the effectiveness of periodontal treatment to prevent or modify the outcomes of CVD, and therefore more research is needed.[44]

In contrast to its many ill effects in other sites of the body, CVD produces few oral effects and usually does not have any oral manifestations that affect food intake. However, medications prescribed for cardiovascular conditions may have oral effects. The dental hygienist should provide support for a healthy dietary pattern based on the *Dietary Guidelines* and *MyPlate* website.

Cerebrovascular Accident

A cerebrovascular accident (also known as a stroke) results if occlusion, or ischemia, occurs in an artery supplying the brain or if hemorrhaging in the brain occurs. Ischemia (inadequate blood flow and lack of oxygen because of constriction or obstruction of arteries) is caused by blockage of one of the arteries in a part of the body (cardiac ischemia, heart muscle). Most strokes are caused by ischemia. An artery may become blocked from atherosclerosis or a thrombus (blood clot). Atherosclerosis is caused by an accumulation of fatty materials (such as cholesterol) on smooth inner walls of arteries (see Fig. 6.3). As this plaque thickens, arteries

⊙ DENTAL CONSIDERATIONS

Assessment
- *Physical:* Edema, anemia, weight loss, abdominal pain, diarrhea, fatigue, swollen and bleeding gingiva, enamel defects, aphthous ulcers, and emotional stress.
- *Dietary:* Iron, folate, vitamin B_{12}, and adequate protein and calories.

Interventions
- Depending on the complexity of the patient's condition, support the patient in following recommendations of their health care team and identify strategies to manage risk for oral disease.
- The use of stress management techniques (e.g., the use of headphones with enjoyable music) during the appointment can prevent aggravating the condition.
- Consult with the interprofessional team to identify dental treatment modifications needed to provide safe dental care (e.g., prophylactic antibiotics).

Evaluation
- Successful outcomes include the patient choosing foods that are well-tolerated and promote weight gain or stability (as needed) and improve quality of life; also, manage oral problems such as aphthous ulcers to minimize their effect on eating.

become progressively narrow and rough, and blood flow carrying oxygen and nutrients may be disrupted. Hemorrhagic strokes may occur as a result of a bleeding aneurysm (weak or thin spot in an arterial wall).

While there are not specific oral lesions associated with stroke, a patient may have poststroke residual issues such as challenges with oral self-care, cognitive impairment, facial paresis, dysphagia, and/or chewing difficulties.[45] Normally, an interprofessional team including a speech-language pathologist, occupational therapist, physical therapist, cardiac team, and RDN will work closely with these patients to return to activities of daily living. However, these residual effects can result in an increased risk for aspiration pneumonia, tooth loss, dental caries, and periodontal disease.[45] Research suggests oral care needs to be incorporated in the early hospital care of stroke patients as well as during rehabilitation, and therefore this is an opportunity for the dental hygienist to be part of the interprofessional collaboration.[45]

Once rehabilitation is complete and the patient returns to the dental office, the dental hygienist's primary role is management of plaque biofilm to reduce risk for aspiration pneumonia and prevent progression of oral disease.[45] Careful attention needs to be made to determine the patient's cognitive and self-care abilities to modify recommendations to support optimal oral self-care. In terms of dietary counseling, the dental hygienist should support the recommendations from the interprofessional team. If the patient continues to experience dysphagia, it will be important to carefully manage water during the dental appointment to minimize the risk for aspiration pneumonia.[45] The patient may be unable to lie in a supine position because of dysphagia and the potential for choking on saliva. Water should be used sparingly, and use of high-speed evacuation may help prevent aspiration. Use of water for rinsing or ultrasonic instrumentation may be contraindicated during dental care.

Neurologic deficits may impact lip force, bite force, oral sensitivity, and chewing making it difficult to form a bolus for swallowing leaving food debris in the mouth.[46] After meals, the mouth should be checked for any pocketed foods (foods retained in the mouth, especially in the vestibule) that should be removed to decrease risk of aspirating the food and developing dental caries.

⬡ NUTRITIONAL DIRECTIONS

- Encourage the patient or caregiver to maintain adequate oral hygiene, particularly because of limited self-cleansing action on the affected side of the oral cavity and risk for aspiration pneumonia.

Hypertension

Hypertension is associated with periodontal disease, although findings are inconsistent about whether periodontal treatment reduces blood pressure, nearly half of studies in a systematic review showed improvement.[47] Patients with diagnosed hypertension or congestive heart failure may have been advised to increase fruit and vegetable consumption, use more low-fat or nonfat dairy products, limit sodium, limit intake of alcohol and caffeine, quit smoking, be physically active, lose weight, and reduce stress (see Chapter 12, *Health Application 12*). The role of the dental hygienist in dietary guidance is supporting recommendations to follow a healthy eating pattern consistent with the *Dietary Guidelines* and. *MyPlate* website and limited added sugars and saturated fat along with sodium.

Antihypertensive medications may include calcium channel blocker diuretics. These medications also negatively affect salivary flow, which causes xerostomia.

Hyperlipidemia

Patients with other types of heart disease involving elevated cholesterol levels or increased risk of atherosclerosis normally have a saturated and total fat restriction. If the individual is overweight or obese, they may also have calorie restrictions (discussed in Chapter 6, *Health Application 6*).

Long-term use of bile acid sequestrants (e.g., cholestyramine and colestipol), prescribed to reduce serum lipids, may cause malabsorption of fat-soluble vitamins (particularly vitamin A and D) and folic acid.[48] Several bile acid sequestrants may cause gastrointestinal disturbances (e.g., nausea, vomiting, abdominal pain) and oral effects such as sour taste and tongue irritation affecting overall food intake.[48]

The dental hygienists should encourage patients to follow the recommended diet and/or a healthy dietary pattern recommended by the *Dietary Guidelines*. For snacks, choose noncariogenic snacks relatively low in fat, such as low-fat or nonfat cheese or skim milk.

⬡ DENTAL CONSIDERATIONS

Assessment
- *Physical:* Slurred speech and inability to communicate effectively; unilateral weakness or paralysis; difficulty chewing and swallowing; loss of oral sensations; lack of tongue control (weak, flabby, and deviates to one side).
- *Dietary:* Chewing and swallowing difficulties, dietary inadequacies.

Interventions
- Monitor the patient's blood pressure at each dental visit.
- If not under the care of a speech language pathologist (SLP) and RDN for dysphagia and swallowing issues are reported, refer to their primary health care provider.
- Carefully review medications and consult with the health care provider before treatment to identify treatment modifications needed.

Evaluation
- Desired outcomes include adequate nourishment using modifications according to the patient's disability, management of plaque biofilm, and oral disease.

⬡ DENTAL CONSIDERATIONS

Assessment
- *Physical:* Medications prescribed, xerostomia, blood pressure.
- *Dietary:* Dietary recommendations, adequacy of food intake.

Interventions
- Because stress is a negative risk factor for most patients with hypertension or heart conditions, minimize stress and consider effects of the disease on the proposed dental treatment. A shortened appointment and use of nitrous oxide may need to be considered.
- Generally, hypertension is often asymptomatic; monitoring blood pressure at each appointment is necessary for early identification and to assess management and safety in providing dental care.
- Refer the patient to the RDN for medical nutrition therapy.

Evaluation
- The patient's blood pressure is within a normal range; the patient takes prescribed medications and follows a healthy dietary pattern in the *Dietary Guidelines* and the *MyPlate* website.

⬡ **NUTRITIONAL DIRECTIONS**

- Salt substitutes are an option to help lower sodium intake. Research shows lower rates of stroke and major CVD events when using a salt substitute as compared to regular salt.[49] However, patients should check with the health care provider or RDN for advice on the use of salt substitutes.
- Another option to help reduce salt use is adding more spices to foods.
- Limiting intake of prepared foods and eating more fresh fruits, vegetables, and whole grains is an easy way to cut down on salt intake. The DASH eating plan is an evidence-based approach to reduce sodium and hypertension.[50] It is one of the eating patterns recommended by the *Dietary Guidelines*.
- Antihypertensive drugs may be responsible for reduced salivary flow. Based on risk assessment, recommend approaches to manage caries risk. This may include nutrition counseling to minimize added sugars and cariogenic foods/beverages; in-office and at-home fluoride therapy; and potentially chlorhexidine 1 week each month along with regular preventive care.[51]
- Calcium channel blockers can cause gingival hyperplasia. Encourage optimal oral self-care.

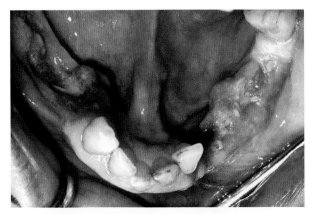

• **Fig. 17.7** Bisphosphonate-associated osteonecrosis of mandibular arch. (From Damm DD, Bouquot JE, Neville BW, et al. *Oral and Maxillofacial Pathology.* 3rd ed. Saunders; 2009.)

Skeletal System

Systemic bone disturbances may initially be detected by the following changes in the maxilla or mandible during an oral examination: (1) significant increase in size or alteration in contour of the maxilla or mandible, (2) alteration in radiographic pattern, (3) mobility of individual teeth without significant periodontal disease, (4) pain or discomfort in the jaw without obvious dental pathology, (5) changes in occlusion of the teeth, or (6) abnormal sequence of deciduous tooth loss or eruption of permanent molars in young patients. These changes may be caused by osteoporosis, metabolic disturbances such as hyperparathyroidism (HPT), or other conditions such as Paget's disease or fibrous dysplasia of bone. Osteoporosis may be the most common bone disease/condition with a global prevalence of nearly 20%.[52] Osteoporosis has implications for maxilla and mandibular bone health and is associated with periodontal disease.[53]

Given the potential to identify and screen for osteoporosis with dental radiographs, particularly with comparison of radiographs over time, dental providers may increasingly be part of referral to a health care provider for initial diagnosis and treatment.[54,55]

Bisphosphonates are medications primarily prescribed for postmenopausal and glucocorticoid-induced osteoporosis and multiple myeloma; intravenous use is sometimes prescribed during chemotherapy for cancer. These drugs decrease bone turnover and inhibit the bone's reparative ability. **Osteonecrosis** (destruction and death of bone tissue due to lack of blood flow to the area) of the jaw after invasive dental procedures is a concern in those using bisphosphonates (Fig. 17.7), however, the risk is very low.[56] Patients at risk for osteonecrosis are those using intravenous bisphosphonates for cancer treatment. Other reasons for osteonecrosis include long duration of use of oral bisphosphonates, preexisting periodontal disease, use of corticosteroids, tobacco use, and comorbid conditions requiring invasive dental procedures (e.g., extractions or dental surgery) or mechanical trauma.[56]

The role of the dental hygienist is to collaborate with the patient in managing periodontal health to minimize infection. In addition, it is important to provide guidance for a healthy eating pattern consistent with the *Dietary Guidelines* and *MyPlate*, and emphasize adequate calcium and vitamin D intake.

⬡ **DENTAL CONSIDERATIONS**

Assessment
- *Physical:* Postmenopausal changes involving bone; osteoporosis/osteopenia.
- *Dietary:* Variety and a well-balanced meal plan.

Interventions
- Encourage consultation with a health care provider to evaluate bone mineral density.
- As a part of the health care team, the dental professional can explain oral concerns related to bisphosphonate use and risk of osteonecrosis of the jaw.
- Preventing and managing oral disease is the primary intervention. If necessary, chlorhexidine rinses, systemic antibiotics, and analgesics may be used for dental treatment.
- Resorption of the edentulous alveolar ridge requires frequent relining of the mandibular denture to avoid oral lesions and ensure the ability to masticate food.
- Provide counseling for tobacco cessation, if necessary (see Chapter 19, *Health Application 19*).

Evaluation
- The patient seeks medical guidance and adheres to prescribed recommendations.

⬡ **NUTRITIONAL DIRECTIONS**

- Encourage adequate intake of calcium and vitamin D rich food sources. Dietary supplementation of calcium and vitamin D should be done in consultation with the health care provider.
- Avoid excessive alcohol consumption.

Metabolic Problems

Diabetes Mellitus

Current evidence supports an interrelationship between diabetes and oral health problems. There is a bidirectional relationship between diabetes and risk of periodontitis.[57,58] Periodontal disease is considered another long-term complication associated with diabetes, along with neuropathy and/or nephropathy. Studies suggest periodontal treatment improves glycemic control and aids in

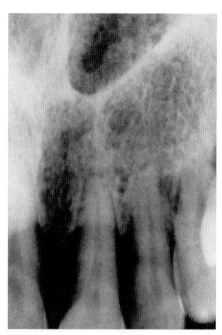

• **Fig. 17.8** Alveolar bone loss in diabetes. (From Ibsen OAC, Phelan JA. *Oral Pathology for the Dental Hygienist.* 6th ed. Saunders; 2014.)

lowering the HbA1c.[59,60] The 2017 classification of periodontal disease also includes diabetes as a risk factor for progression of disease.[61] Poorly controlled diabetes results in more severe periodontal disease and alveolar bone loss contributing to the progression of diabetes (Fig. 17.8).

Patients with poorly controlled or undiagnosed diabetes may have a characteristic fruity-smelling breath (more prevalent in type 1 diabetes), increased thirst, unexplained weight loss, or frequent urination. These symptoms are associated with elevated blood glucose levels. However, patients may be asymptomatic. Diabetes mellitus and nutrition recommendations are discussed in Chapter 7, *Health Application 7.*

Risk of infection is higher in patients with type 1 and type 2 diabetes and the normal healing process is slow.[62] Patients with longstanding, poorly controlled diabetes are at risk of developing oral candidiasis and denture stomatitis (Fig. 17.9), partly due to increased glucose levels in saliva, which provide a substrate for fungal growth.[63] Xerostomia is also prevalent and is partially responsible for altered taste, general tenderness or burning of the mucosa, and carious lesions, all of which may affect nutrient intake. Consultation with the diabetes care provider is necessary to confirm the safety of providing periodontal therapy in the presence of a high HbA1c. However, given treatment may help to lower HbA1c,[59] it may be part of overall management of glycemic control that includes a healthy diet, physical activity, weight loss or maintaining a healthy weight, and medications.

Interventions

- Dental professionals can have a significant, positive effect on the oral and general health of patients with diabetes mellitus.
- Educate patients with diabetes about oral manifestations (e.g., xerostomia) and complications (e.g., periodontitis and oral candidiasis) to promote proper oral health behaviors. Few dental and periodontal changes or mucosal changes are observed in individuals with well-controlled diabetes.
- The office should have a glucometer to check the blood glucose to manage a hypoglycemic event. The patient could bring their own glucometer, but the dental provider needs to know how to use it in case the patient is unable to check their own blood glucose during a hypoglycemic event. Some patients may use a continuous glucose monitoring (CGM) device like Dexcom to provide the glucose values.
- To prevent hypoglycemia during dental treatment, determine, if the patient has a history of hypoglycemia and whether they can identify when their blood glucose is low. Hypoglycemic unawareness often accompanies neuropathy in diabetes and puts the patient at much higher risk for severe hypoglycemia.
- Ensure the patient has eaten regular meals and snacks and taken medications as prescribed.
- The action of insulin and oral diabetes medication tends to peak mid-afternoon and this is often the time for greatest risk of hypoglycemia.
- If hypoglycemia occurs, the patient requires 15 g of a carbohydrate source to bring blood glucose levels to a normal range. If the blood glucose remains below 70 mg/dL after 15 minutes, administer another 15 g of carbohydrate.
- Some oral diabetes medications (e.g., α-glucosidase inhibitor) do not cause hypoglycemia by themselves; however, they are often combined with an oral agent that does. In this scenario, the patient may require a glucose source. Glucose gel is recommended although juice, a regular soft drink, or glucose tablets can also be used.
- When working with individuals who have diabetes, watch for oral signs of poor control including:
  - gingival bleeding when brushing, flossing or probing
  - red, swollen, or tender gingiva
  - oral candidiasis
  - xerostomia
  - suppuration
  - halitosis
  - recession
  - mobile teeth
  - changes in the fit of partial dentures or bridges
  - white or red patches on gingiva, tongue, cheeks, or roof of mouth
- Periodontal infections may need to be managed with systemic antibiotic therapy and topical antimicrobials.[64,65]
- Because of the risk of periodontal disease, meticulous daily oral self-care is imperative in conjunction with regular supportive periodontal therapy for individuals with diabetes.

Evaluation

- The patient's fasting blood glucose levels are normal, and the glycated hemoglobin A1c is less than 7.0%, indicating that the diabetes is well controlled.[66] However, in those at risk for hypoglycemia the A1c goal may be less than 8% so consult with the diabetes provider to confirm the patient's A1c goal.[66]

🔹 DENTAL CONSIDERATIONS

Assessment

- *Physical:* Polyuria, polydipsia, xerostomia, weight loss, weakness, ketosis, or asymptomatic.
- *Dietary:* Polyphagia (increased hunger); adherence to prescribed lifestyle modifications, particularly fruit and vegetable intake.

🔹 NUTRITIONAL DIRECTIONS

- Read labels carefully for sources of added sugars and recommend choosing whole grains. Foods labeled "sugar free" may contain carbohydrates other than sucrose.

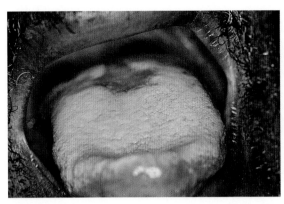

• **Fig. 17.9** Oral candidiasis. (From Swartz MH. *Textbook of Physical Diagnosis: History and Examination.* 7th ed. Saunders: 2014.)

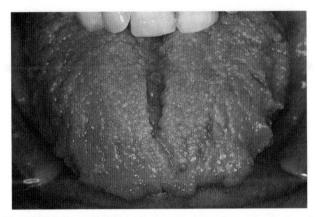

• **Fig. 17.10** In hypothyroidism, the large tongue often protrudes from the mouth, showing indentation on the lateral borders caused by pressure from the teeth. (From Damm DD, Bouquot JE, Neville BW, et al. *Oral and Maxillofacial Pathology.* 3rd ed. Saunders; 2009.)

Hypothyroidism

Hypothyroidism prevalence globally is about 0.2% to 11%.[67] Hypothyroidism may be related to (1) inadequate consumption of iodine, (2) genetic, (3) chronic autoimmune Hashimoto thyroiditis, (4) iatrogenic (e.g., surgical excision or irradiation), (5) thyroid cancer, (6) resistance to thyroid-stimulating hormone, and (7) medications (e.g., lithium, valproate).[67]

An extraoral examination may reveal an enlarged thyroid gland. Intraorally, in children there may be developmental defects of the enamel, delayed eruption, more gingival inflammation, more plaque biofilm, and higher rates of caries.[68] **Macroglossia** (large) tongue, showing indentations on the lateral borders caused by pressure from the teeth (Fig. 17.10) is common in children and adults with hypothyroidism.[69] There may be an association between hypothyroidism and periodontal disease, but more good quality research is needed.[70]

Dietary guidance should include information about the potential for **goitrogens** (chemicals present in broccoli, kale, kohlrabi, cabbage, rutabagas, turnips, cauliflower, Brussels sprouts, horseradish, and soybeans) to inhibit thyroid uptake of iodine and synthesis of thyroid hormones.[71] There is inadequate evidence to determine a safe level of intake of sources of goitrogens so they should be eaten in the context of an overall health dietary pattern. Iodized salt and sources of iodine should also be encouraged.

Hyperparathyroidism

There are three types of HPT with the most common being primary HPT. It is the third most common endocrine disorder after diabetes and hypothyroidism.[72] Primary HPT results from an overactive parathyroid gland(s) and is a disorder of calcium metabolism.[73] Primary hyperthyroidism is seen more often in females. Clinical manifestations result from increased osteoclastic bone resorption, decreasing bone integrity resulting in skeletal deformities and pain.[73] The kidney may also be involved with development of kidney stones and reduced renal function.[73]

Oral symptoms are primarily related to expansion of the maxilla and mandible creating facial swelling/asymmetry which may create malocclusion and make chewing difficult.[72] Pain may be associated with the bone expansion. Tooth mobility or displacement may also occur. Primary HPT may also exacerbate periodontal infection. Loss of the lamina dura is a common radiographic finding in primary HPT.[72] Individuals with HPT are also at higher risk for tooth loss as a result of the effects of the condition on the structure of the maxilla and mandible.[74]

As a result of improved screening of serum calcium levels with routine laboratory tests, most cases of HPT are identified and treated before severe skeletal disease occurs. There are no specific nutrition guidelines for those with HPT so the patient should follow a healthy eating pattern consistent with the *Dietary Guidelines* and *MyPlate* website, but they should get their vitamin D levels evaluated by their primary care provider to determine if supplementation is needed.

Renal Disease

The kidney is the primary organ that eliminates significant amounts of waste products; metabolic and endocrine functions are also affected by kidney disease. Progressive loss of nephrons in the kidney leads to chronic failure. When kidney function diminishes, complications arise as by-products accumulate from protein metabolism, and alterations occur in electrolyte levels and acid–base balance. End-stage renal disease has many causes with the most common being poorly controlled diabetes and hypertension.[75] Patients with end-stage renal disease may have dialysis while awaiting a kidney transplant.

Because of calcium–phosphorus imbalances, renal bone disease is common. The types of bone disease may include: high bone turnover from high hyperparathyroid levels and osteomalacia.[75] Other issues associated with end-stage renal disease is anemia, protein-energy malnutrition, hyperkalemia, and edema (due to inability to excrete water).[75]

The oral cavity reflects many signs of systemic involvement. Platelet abnormalities may result in gingival bleeding and bruising.[76] Anemia is common; thus gingival tissues may be pale in color.[75] Other oral manifestations of chronic renal failure include complaints of a bad taste; malodor from urea buildup; xerostomia from fluid restriction (and use of antihypertensive medications); and oral lesions (e.g., uremic stomatitis, oral hairy leukoplakia [Fig. 17.11]).[76–78] There may also be gingival enlargement secondary to medications like calcium channel blockers and cyclosporine.[78] Those with chronic kidney disease have higher risk for periodontal disease, the more advanced, the higher the risk.[79] Evidence also suggests an increased risk for dental caries.[80]

Nutritional care for these individuals is extremely complex. Dietary restrictions are extensive and include protein, fluid, sodium, and phosphorus. Water soluble vitamins and trace minerals are lost during dialysis in part by removal in the dialysate (material that passes through the membrane during dialysis) so patients can

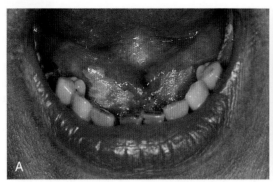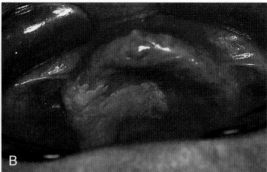

• **Fig. 17.11** (A) Leukoplakia on the floor of the mouth. (B) Leukoplakia on the maxillary alveolar mucosa and palate. (From Ibsen OAC, Phelan JA. *Oral Pathology for the Dental Hygienist.* 6th ed. Saunders; 2014.)

become deficient.[81] Anorexia is often present because of dietary restrictions; poor appetite; depression; gastrointestinal symptoms; difficulty chewing and/or swallowing; difficulty with grocery shopping and cooking; uremia; and bad taste experienced by many patients. High-quality, low protein intake is recommended to reduce nitrogen waste products (urea) and to minimize accumulation in the blood between dialysis treatments. In addition to protein, intake of minerals and electrolytes (e.g., sodium, potassium, and phosphorus) must be adjusted; adequate energy intake must be maintained; and potentially harmful intake of phosphorus, magnesium, aluminum, and some vitamins must be avoided. Fluid intake must be carefully monitored to prevent excess fluid buildup, which has a negative impact on blood pressure. For this reason, nutritional counseling should be left to an RDN who specializes in renal care. These RDNs often have extensive experience with renal patients and have passed an examination to be board certified in renal nutrition.

🔹 DENTAL CONSIDERATIONS

Assessment
- *Physical:* Oral manifestations and deteriorating physical status.
- *Dietary:* Appetite, prescribed diet/diet restrictions, adequacy of oral intake.

Interventions
- Consult the health care provider before treatment because of a bleeding tendency as a result of platelet dysfunction and anticoagulant medication and to determine the necessity for antibiotic prophylaxis to prevent infective endocarditis or infection of the vascular access site for dialysis or both.
- Emphasize the importance of good oral self-care.
- Because of an increased occurrence of oral complications, perform a careful and thorough oral examination to detect problems early.
- Medical care becomes more complicated when systemic conditions (e.g., pneumonia and diabetes) occur secondary to oral infections.
- Because of fluid restrictions for patients on dialysis, minimize water used during treatment. Carefully evaluate the risks and benefits of using ultrasonic and sonic instrumentation due to the water spray generated. If it is used, it is essential to use high-speed evacuation.
- Patients normally require preventive dental care prior to being placed on the transplant waiting list.
- Consult with and refer to an RDN specializing in renal nutrition as needed.
- Dialysis sessions last 3–4 hours and occur at least three times per week. Patients will be tired after their dialysis session so it is best not to schedule dental appointments on the same day.

Evaluation
- The patient is able to describe the relationship between the condition and effects of dietary intake on oral health.

🔹 NUTRITIONAL DIRECTIONS

- Meticulous oral hygiene and frequent recare appointments prevent or reduce oral infections commonly associated with metabolic problems that can lead to difficulties in eating certain foods.
- Antimicrobial mouth rinses are helpful to minimize possible bacterial and fungal infections.

Neuromuscular Problems

Parkinson's Disease

Parkinson's disease is the second most common neurodegenerative disease and is a progressive condition characterized by involuntary muscle tremors; bradykinesia (slowness of movement); muscular weakness; rigidity; a gait with a tendency to lean forward and use rapid, short, steps with reduced arm swing; impaired balance and coordination; and difficulty swallowing (dysphagia), chewing, and speaking (Fig. 17.12).[82,83] Nonmotor characteristics include anosmia (loss of smell), depression, REM sleep disorder, and cognitive decline.[82,83]

Oral effects of Parkinson's disease include xerostomia or sialorrhea (excessive saliva resulting in drooling), burning mouth, and TMD (temporomandibular disorder).[84] While research shows individuals with Parkinson's disease brush and use interdental aids as much as a control group, they report more difficulties performing oral self-care and have higher levels of plaque biofilm.[84] Research also suggests a higher risk for periodontal disease and dental caries.[84] Increased risk for oral disease is likely related to lack of muscular control both orally (affecting chewing and swallowing) and hand control (affecting use of toothbrush, toothpaste, and interdental cleaning).

Treatment consists primarily of managing symptoms of Parkinson's disease. Levodopa is the medication of choice for treatment of early Parkinson's disease motor symptoms.[85] Levodopa has drug–nutrient interactions with protein which reduces effectiveness of the drug.[86]

While chewing and swallowing difficulties may require some changes to form and consistency of food, an overall healthy diet is recommended. The first priority is to correct any malnutrition that may be present. Challenges in managing malnutrition and maintaining body weight may necessitate consultation with an RDN to tailor a diet meeting the patient's needs. However, dental providers

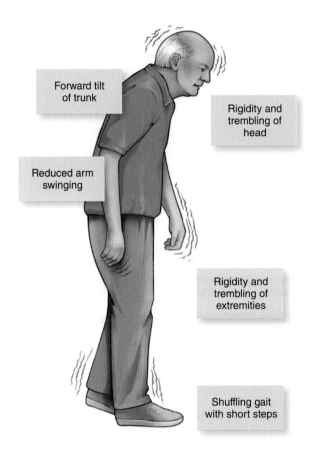

Forward tilt
of trunk

Rigidity and
trembling of
head

Reduced arm
swinging

Rigidity and
trembling of
extremities

Shuffling gait
with short steps

• **Fig. 17.12** Parkinson's disease. The signs include (but are not limited to) rigidity and trembling of the head and extremities, a forward tilt of the trunk, and a shuffling gait with short steps and reduced arm swinging. (From *The Human Body in Health & Disease*. 8th ed. 2024.)

can support the need to choose an overall healthy eating pattern like the Mediterranean Diet that tends to be more plant based.[87,88] Dietary patterns high in fruits, vegetables, legumes, whole grains, nuts, fish, and poultry; low intake of saturated fat; and moderate intake or abstinence of alcohol may protect against Parkinson's disease. However, individuals may need to supplement protein intake to meet their needs.[87] Intake of protein needs to be carefully managed by the health care team and RDN. Physical activity is also important for individuals with Parkinson's disease and has been shown to improve balance, motor function, cognition and sleep.[87]

Children With Special Needs

Many children with special needs have a variety of feeding difficulties which may be related to inadequate food intake, challenges with self-feeding, oral-motor deficits, and behavior issues.[89] These children include those with intellectual disabilities (e.g., Down syndrome), neuromuscular disorders (e.g., cerebral palsy), and neurodevelopmental disorders (e.g., autism spectrum disorder). Neuromuscular conditions like cerebral palsy may impair development of normal feeding reflexes (discussed in Chapter 14) and coordination of these reflexes with respiration. Oral-motor problems may include chewing, biting, lip closure (e.g., lip retraction), tongue movements (e.g., tongue thrust), swallowing, jaw movements (e.g., tonic bite reflex), decreased ability to form a bolus, and drooling (Table 17.2).[90] These conditions put the patient at nutritional risk. These oral-motor problems also impact dental hygiene care. It is essential for the dental hygienist to work with the interprofessional team providing care to the patient. Nutrition care needs to be provided by a knowledgeable nutrition professional working alongside a speech-language pathologist and occupational therapist.

TABLE 17.2	**Feeding Problems in Children With Special Needs**			
Source of Feeding Problems	**Condition**	**Description**	**Feeding Issue**
Jaw movements	Tonic bite reflex or hyperactive bite	Strong jaw closure when teeth or gingiva are stimulated	May bite on feeding utensils and be unable to open jaws
	Jaw thrust	Forceful opening of the jaw to its maximal extent during eating, drinking, attempts to speak, or general excitement	Biting, chewing, and swallowing may be impaired
Tongue movements	Tongue thrust	Forceful and often repetitive protrusion of an often bunched or thick tongue in response to oral stimulation	Food is pushed out of the mouth making feeding difficult
	Tongue retraction	Pulling back the tongue within the oral cavity at presentation of food, spoon, or cup	May be difficult to accept food into the mouth, inability to form a bolus, chew, or swallow
Lips	Lip retraction or inadequate lip closure	Pulling back the lips in a very tight, smile-like pattern at the approach of food, spoon, or cup toward the face	Inability to remove food from a spoon, drink from a cup, or suck liquid from a straw
Sensory processing disorders	Oral sensory hyposensitivity	Decreased oral sensitivity, may not experience pain the same way	Could lead to trauma to soft tissues from bite injuries
	Oral sensory hypersensitivity	Reactions to anything touching the lips or mouth. If not addressed, it progresses to oral defensiveness.	Makes feeding difficult, this occurs frequently when a child has had tube feeding
	Oral defensiveness	A strong adverse reaction to touch. Child may cry, gag, push things away, or turn head away	Limits ability to feed and child may have inadequate intake

Epilepsy

Epilepsy, or psychomotor seizures, in itself does not usually result in any specific oral or feeding problems. However, long-term use of antiepileptic drugs results in loss of bone mineral density.[91] A common antiepileptic medication is phenytoin (Dilantin) and it increases metabolism of vitamins D, K, and folate, which may increase risk for loss of bone mineral density. Other dental considerations associated with phenytoin include increased incidence of infection, delayed healing, gingival hyperplasia (Fig. 17.13), and gingival bleeding. Despite increased need for these nutrients, supplementation of folate or vitamin B$_6$ may decrease bioavailability of phenytoin and it must be carefully monitored by a health care provider. Phenobarbital, which is also used to manage convulsions in epilepsy, may also affect bone health by increasing turnover of vitamins D and K. Overall, individuals with epilepsy should be supported in following a healthy dietary pattern as recommended by the *Dietary Guidelines* and *MyPlate*.

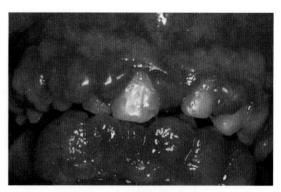

• **Fig. 17.13** Hyperplasia associated with phenytoin use. (Courtesy Barbara D. Altshuler, BSDH, MS, Clinical Assistant Professor, Texas A&M University College of Dentistry, Dallas, TX.)

🔷 DENTAL CONSIDERATIONS

Assessment
- *Physical:* Oral complications related to conditions; medications prescribed; nutrient supplements use; orthostatic hypotension.
- *Dietary:* Adequacy of intake, signs of malnutrition.

Interventions
- Carefully assess oral status.
- To reduce stress and anxiety, keep appointments brief and relaxing.
- Individualize the frequency of preventive oral care based on patient's needs.
- Assess saliva flow and provide tips for preventing xerostomia-associated oral problems (see Chapter 20).
- After supine positioning, have the patient with Parkinson's disease sit upright for at least 2 minutes before standing to avoid orthostatic hypotension.
- Coping strategies for dysphagia, such as massaging the throat before beginning a feeding and reminding the patient to tilt the head forward before swallowing, can help with swallowing problems. However, the challenges can become tedious and taxing for the patient and for health care providers.
- For patients experiencing xerostomia, advise avoidance of alcohol, smoking, and caffeine.
- Encourage a rigorous preventive oral self-care regime tailored to the needs of individuals with neuromuscular problems.
- Schedule appointments at the best time of day for the individual.
- Suggest dental gels, such as fluoride, and dentifrices for individuals with dysphagia rather than mouth rinses that may increase risk of aspiration.
- Refer the patient to the health care provider or RDN if nutrient supplementation is reported. Some nutrients may interfere with absorption of the prescribed medication.
- Suggest adaptations and/or assistive devices so that the patient can maintain independence for teeth or denture cleaning: for example, a mechanical toothbrush, toothbrush handle adaptations, or specialized toothbrushes, such as a Collis curve toothbrush (Fig. 17.14).

Evaluation
- The patient's dental health is maintained, and prescribed medications are taken.

🔷 NUTRITIONAL DIRECTIONS

- Check the fit of a dental prosthesis. An improper fit may impact nutritional status.
- Encourage small, frequent nutrient-dense meals and snacks for patients experiencing anorexia and weight loss. Refer to an RDN.
- Salivary substitutions and topical fluoride treatments may be recommended for patients experiencing xerostomia.
- Antimicrobial rinses are helpful to decrease the chance of bacterial and fungal infections.
- Patients may be at risk for bone loss and osteoporosis so encourage foods high in or fortified with calcium, magnesium, and vitamins D and K.
- Patients taking medications for Parkinson's disease (e.g., levodopa or carbidopa) should take the medication at mealtime for the best absorption and monitor foods high in vitamin B$_6$, protein, and fat, as they may lengthen the time for the medication to show effect or decrease the effectiveness of the medication. Have the patient check with their pharmacist and primary care physician for guidance on the best time to take medications.
- Calcium supplements are not recommended for patients taking phenytoin and phenobarbital unless closely monitored by their primary care physician because large amounts of calcium decrease bioavailability of both the drug and mineral.
- Pyridoxine and folate supplements may alter response of phenytoin and result in increased seizure activity.
- Carbamazepine (Tegretol), another popular anticonvulsant, causes xerostomia, altered taste, and oral sensitivity.

Neoplasia

Neoplasia (abnormal mass of tissue), more frequently referred to as tumors, causes problems not only in the primary site, but also in regional and remote areas. The manifestations at secondary sites away from the primary lesion may be the presenting feature in some cases. The mouth and jaw may be involved in generalized malignant disease.

Anorexia and weight loss along with malnutrition are common symptoms of cancer and cancer therpies.[6] Weight loss is associated with the long-term prognosis for the patient.[6] Anorexia has a complex pathophysiology including the central nervous system and gut hormones that affect hunger and satiety.[6] This is further complicated by cancer and therapies to treat cancer which result in changes of taste and smell.[11]

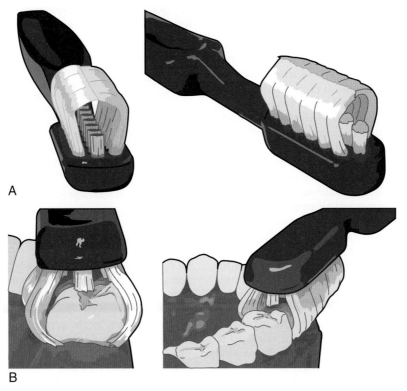

• **Fig. 17.14** (A) Collis curve toothbrush. (B) Use of Collis curve toothbrush.

Oral symptoms or signs (e.g., mucositis) may be secondary to malnutrition, nutrient deficiencies, or the cancer therapy. In addition, the location of the neoplasm itself may be a factor in reduced food intake, especially when the alimentary tract is affected. Intake is reduced in patients with cancer of the oral cavity, pharynx, or esophagus because of odynophagia (pain on swallowing) or dysphagia with about one-third of patients experiencing malnutrition.[92] The National Cancer Institute (NCI) website (https://www.cancer.gov/) provides information about nutrition for patients with cancer and is a good resource. The overarching recommendation is for a healthy eating pattern consistent with the *Dietary Guidelines* and *MyPlate* with referral to an RDN for specialized care in the presence of malnutrition. The NCI provides many strategies for nutrition based on symptoms the patient may experience. For instance, when oral lesions are present, suggestions might include choose nutrient-dense foods that are easy to chew (e.g., scrambled eggs); avoid spicy, salty, citrus, and alcohol; and eat cool or room temperature foods.[93]

Kaposi Sarcoma

Kaposi sarcoma is a highly malignant tumor of blood vessel origin that occurs on the skin and oral mucosa (Fig. 17.15). It is characterized by bluish-red cutaneous nodules, usually on the lower extremities, and occurs frequently in immunocompromised individuals. These lesions appear in many HIV-positive patients. Red-purple macular lesions in the mouth may progress to raised, indurated lesions with central areas of necrosis and ulceration. Lesions can cause obstruction of the esophagus, compromising food intake.

Leukemia

Leukemia is a generalized malignant disease characterized by distorted proliferation and development of WBCs. It is

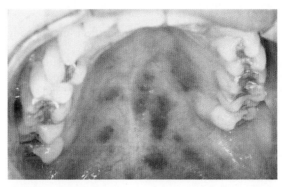

• **Fig. 17.15** Kaposi sarcoma lesions on the hard palate. (From Silverman S Jr. *Color Atlas of Oral Manifestations of AIDS*. 5th ed. Mosby; 1996.)

another neoplastic process with many oral manifestations that detrimentally affect food intake. Several types of leukemia are classified according to the type of WBCs (lymphocytic or myeloid) affected and how quickly it develops and progresses (acute or chronic).

Oral manifestations are some of the first clinical signs of leukemia.[94] The most common oral signs of leukemia are in the gingival tissues followed by alveolar mucosa and hard or soft palate.[94] Gingival tissues may exhibit bleeding, including spontaneous bleeding, and hyperplasia.[94] The mucosa may exhibit ulcers and petechiae.[94] The oral lesions may be the main complaint from patients leading to referral to the health care provider for diagnosis.[94] The dental hygienist can help the patient manage the bacterial load with meticulous oral self-care and some of the same dietary suggestions found in the section on neoplasia would apply to the patient with leukemia. The symptoms the patient experiences will impact diet choices.

Cancer Treatments

Cancer treatment may include surgery, radiation therapy, chemotherapy, biologic therapy, or combinations of these modalities. Chemotherapeutic drugs are used to destroy malignant cells without loss of an excessive number of normal cells. Tumors involving the gastrointestinal tract affect the ability to ingest foods orally or digest and absorb nutrients adequately. Radical surgery in the oropharyngeal area may present problems in chewing and swallowing and alterations in taste sensations.

Radiation therapy significantly affects the alimentary tract. Early transient effects include general loss of appetite, nausea and vomiting, and diarrhea caused by malabsorption secondary to mucosal damage in the gastrointestinal tract. Food intake, particularly energy and protein intake, is affected because of loss of taste sensation, mucositis, xerostomia, difficulty in swallowing,[95] and a burning sensation in the mouth when the larynx or pharynx area is irradiated. The focus of nutrition for those undergoing radiotherapy are adequate calories and protein to prevent weight loss, regain strength, and heal damaged tissues.

Ideally dental care is provided prior to beginning radiotherapy so any teeth with a poor prognosis can be extracted to reduce the risk for osteonecrosis postradiation.[96] Periodontal disease also needs to be treated and managed to reduce the bacterial load. During therapy, patients may need more frequent palliative care to reduce the bacterial load, antimicrobial rinses and fluoride, to manage caries risk, and topical antifungal therapy.[96]

Chemotherapy has more widespread effects on the body than either radiation or surgical treatment. Rapid cell turnover rate in the alimentary tract leads to stomatitis or mucositis, oral ulcerations, and decreased absorptive capacity. Due to the effects of chemotherapy, patients are at risk of malnutrition and should eat a high protein, high calorie nutrient-dense diet. As previously mentioned, the NCI has many resources to help patients manage the effects of chemotherapy and consume a healthy diet to support weight maintenance and healing.

🔷 DENTAL CONSIDERATIONS

Assessment
- *Physical:* Fatigue, periodontal disease caries, adequate weight, weight loss, oral lesions, medications.
- *Dietary:* Maintain high protein, high calorie intake, adequate fluids, food aversions (especially food groups), alterations in taste.

Interventions
- Use of an antimicrobial mouth rinse (i.e., alcohol-free chlorhexidine) may be indicated to reduce inflammation associated with cancer treatment.
- A mechanically altered (Box 19.3) or bland diet (see Chapter 19, Box 19.4) may be recommended as deemed necessary by oral symptoms.
- Discuss the relationship between fermentable carbohydrate intake, effects of xerostomia, plaque biofilm formation, and caries. Caution against eating hard candy containing fermentable carbohydrates to relieve xerostomia.

Evaluation
- A dietary recall reveals adequate nutrients and calories with a minimum of fermentable carbohydrates.

⬡ NUTRITIONAL DIRECTIONS

- Small, frequent meals are appropriate to provide additional calories and to counteract nausea and vomiting.
- Meticulous oral hygiene, frequent recare appointments, and fluoride therapy are essential.
- Adequate food and fluid intake not only improve the physical response to cancer treatment but also create a more positive psychological outlook.
- Avoid foods that are hot, spicy, or acidic (e.g., citrus fruit and juices).
- Avoid alcohol-containing beverages and mouth rinses.
- Commonly used chemotherapeutic agents (bleomycin, cyclophosphamide, and methotrexate) generally cause complications such as stomatitis, nausea, vomiting, diarrhea, and anorexia.

Acquired Immunodeficiency Syndrome

HIV debilitates the body's immune system. Following identification of HIV antibodies in the blood, a positive diagnosis of HIV is made. This retrovirus targets CD4+ T-helper lymphocytes or WBCs that normally function to resist infection. Retroviruses are characterized by the presence of reverse transcriptase, which interferes with production of DNA from RNA. Susceptibility to various opportunistic infections (especially *Pneumocystis carinii*, *Cryptosporidium*, *Candida*, *Mycobacterium*, and herpes simplex) and certain neoplasms (Kaposi sarcoma, non-Hodgkin lymphoma, and oral warts) is increased. These infections can appear in virtually every organ system.

The course of HIV/AIDS is often complicated by wasting of lean body mass, cachexia, opportunistic infections, malignancies, diarrhea, multiple nutrient deficiencies, and particularly protein-energy malnutrition. The cause of malnutrition is multifactorial and may involve inadequate intake, chronic infection, malabsorption, and changes in metabolism.[97] Malnutrition reduces immunity and hastens progression of the disease.[97]

Many oral problems in HIV-positive patients have predictive value for development of AIDS because of their effect on appetite and food intake. Adequate dietary intake maintains nutritional status, improves resistance to opportunistic infections, helps delay progression of disease, and improves quality of life.[97] Good oral health and self-care improves nutritional status by promoting a desirable environment to support adequate food intake.

More than 30 different oral manifestations of HIV disease have been reported since the AIDS epidemic began in the 1980s. Individuals with a compromised immune system should practice preventive measures to avoid bacterial infections evidenced in dental caries and periodontal disease.

Several varieties of oral candidiasis are prevalent in HIV-positive individuals and should be reported to the health care provider. Oral candidiasis produces pain and inhibits production of saliva. Pharyngeal or esophageal lesions of Kaposi sarcoma may cause obstruction, whereas herpetic ulcerations or other ulcerations on the tongue or esophagus can cause difficulty in swallowing. Herpetic ulcerations are painful ulcerations of the oral mucosa with a red center and yellow border. The development of thrush may be attributed to herpes virus, candidiasis, chemotherapy, or drugs such as interferon.

Oral hairy leukoplakia (Fig. 17.16) is found predominantly on the lateral borders of the tongue or occasionally on the buccal or labial mucosa in patients who are HIV positive. The white lesions or filamentous growth do not rub off. HIV-positive patients may have ulcerations that resemble aphthous ulcers with an

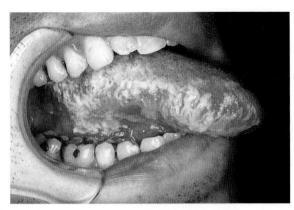

• **Fig. 17.16** Hairy leukoplakia. (From Silverman S Jr. *Color Atlas of Oral Manifestations of AIDS*. 5th ed. Mosby; 1996.)

erythematous margin. These painful ulcers may become extremely large and necrotic; they may persist for several weeks.

With the advent of antiretroviral therapy (ART), HIV-associated wasting is less frequent, particularly in those whose HIV is below the level of detection.[98] However in some patients living with HIV, ART is associated with metabolic diseases such as lipodystrophy (redistribution of fat deposits from peripheral sites like the face to the abdomen and neck), diabetes; and elevated cardiovascular risk.[99] Although prevalence of necrotizing ulcerative periodontitis has decreased since the advent of ART to manage HIV, the literature is conflicting about whether an undetectable viral load and CD4+ count above 200 cells/mm[3] is associated with progression and severity of periodontal disease.[100]

DENTAL CONSIDERATIONS

Assessment
- *Physical:* Weight change, oral infections and malignancies, candidiasis, periodontitis, viral load, CD4+ count, ART and other medications.
- *Dietary:* Implications of oral lesions, adequate dietary intake.

Interventions
- Perform a careful intra- and extraoral examination to identify signs of opportunistic infection.
- Individualize the care plan and treatment for each HIV/AIDS patient.
- Systemic antibiotic therapy may be indicated for infections depending on the level of immunosuppression.
- Oral lesions will affect nutritional status because of discomfort in the mouth. Offer suggestions for palliative care (antimicrobial mouth rinse, antifungal lozenge or mouthwash; pain medication; and nonacidic foods) that will not exacerbate lesions.
- Consultation with the health care provider is necessary to gather information about laboratory values (e.g., platelet count, WBC count, CD4+ count, and viral load), medications, and history of opportunistic infections, and to determine if antibiotic prophylaxis is needed.
- Encourage patient to maintain meticulous oral self-care and regular preventive dental care.
- Side effects of ART include diarrhea, nausea, and vomiting. Frequent vomiting can cause enamel erosion. Preventive dental care and use of topical fluoride therapy at home is essential.

Evaluation
- The patient is meeting goals to manage plaque biofilm and seeking preventive care on the agreed upon schedule. The patient reports following a healthy dietary pattern and is following ART therapy prescribed by the health care provider.

NUTRITIONAL DIRECTIONS

- Support patient in following a healthy dietary pattern consistent with the *Dietary Guidelines* and the *MyPlate* website. Refer any patient with significant weight loss or gain to an RDN for medical nutrition therapy.
- To promote healing and maintenance of oral tissues, encourage adequate nutrient intake.
- To add calories and protein, add protein shakes or smoothies as snacks; use cream instead of milk; add ground meat or poultry or grated cheese to soups, sauces, casseroles, and vegetable dishes; use peanut butter on fruit or crackers; and dip vegetables in sour cream mixes.
- Limit caffeine-containing and alcohol-containing beverages if xerostomia is present.

Mental Health Problems

Eating Disorders

There are three main categories for eating disorders that include AN, bulimia nervosa (BN), and binge eating disorder (BED). AN has the highest mortality rate with 1 in 5 dying from the condition.[101] Commonalities across eating disorders are a severe disturbance in eating behaviors and psychological distress associated with food and eating which impact daily function. They primarily affect young females, but males are also affected.

Diagnosis of AN includes a BMI below $18.5 \, \text{kg/m}^2$, rigid dieting, amenorrhea (for females), and an excessive desire for slimness with a distorted body image (Fig. 17.17). Of the eating disorders, patients with AN are most likely to be severely malnourished. Dental complications (e.g., xerostomia, angular cheilitis, and other mucosal lesions) in advanced stages of malnutrition are generally observed in patients with AN.[102]

BN occurs more frequently than AN. Bulimia is an eating disorder that is not associated with significant weight loss. An individual with bulimia might even be normal weight or slightly overweight and appear healthy. Bulimia is characterized by loss of control over eating resulting in binges (periods of overeating) often followed by purging (a means of counteracting the effects of overindulgence). Conversely, BED is binging on large amounts of food without purging, but the binging is still associated with emotional distress about the binging.

Binges may consist of more than 2000 calories per episode and last 30 minutes to an hour.[103] Binges consist of mostly carbohydrates and those with BN tend to consume more sugar-sweetened beverages.[104] Binges may be planned or spontaneous, but ordinarily are related to depression and/or stress.[103]

Self-induced vomiting is the main method of purging in both AN and BN. Vomiting may be induced by sticking a finger or other object down the throat, applying external pressure to the neck, or drinking syrup of ipecac (emetic drug). Eventually, some individuals with bulimia can vomit by merely contracting their abdominal muscles.

In addition to poor overall health status, nutritional effects of bulimia stem from purging and the method employed for purging. Frequent episodes of self-induced vomiting can cause oral cavity trauma; bruises and lesions on soft tissue in the oral cavity may be observed. Another classic sign of bulimia associated with self-induced vomiting is the presence of abrasions and calluses on dorsal surfaces of fingers and hands secondary to friction of the teeth. Frequent vomiting can cause erosion of tooth enamel (predominantly on the lingual surfaces

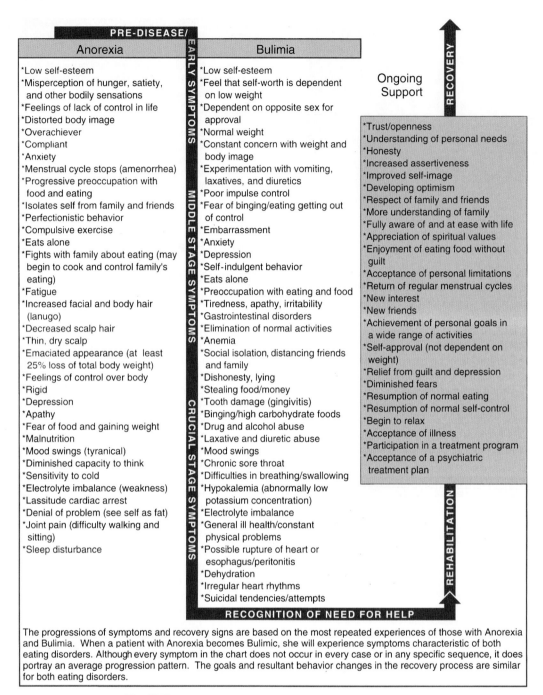

PRE-DISEASE/		
Anorexia	EARLY SYMPTOMS	Bulimia

Anorexia

*Low self-esteem
*Misperception of hunger, satiety, and other bodily sensations
*Feelings of lack of control in life
*Distorted body image
*Overachiever
*Compliant
*Anxiety
*Menstrual cycle stops (amenorrhea)
*Progressive preoccupation with food and eating
*Isolates self from family and friends
*Perfectionistic behavior
*Compulsive exercise
*Eats alone
*Fights with family about eating (may begin to cook and control family's eating)
*Fatigue
*Increased facial and body hair (lanugo)
*Decreased scalp hair
*Thin, dry scalp
*Emaciated appearance (at least 25% loss of total body weight)
*Feelings of control over body
*Rigid
*Depression
*Apathy
*Fear of food and gaining weight
*Malnutrition
*Mood swings (tyranical)
*Diminished capacity to think
*Sensitivity to cold
*Electrolyte imbalance (weakness)
*Lassitude cardiac arrest
*Denial of problem (see self as fat)
*Joint pain (difficulty walking and sitting)
*Sleep disturbance

Bulimia

*Low self-esteem
*Feel that self-worth is dependent on low weight
*Dependent on opposite sex for approval
*Normal weight
*Constant concern with weight and body image
*Experimentation with vomiting, laxatives, and diuretics
*Poor impulse control
*Fear of binging/eating getting out of control
*Embarrassment
*Anxiety
*Depression
*Self-indulgent behavior
*Eats alone
*Preoccupation with eating and food
*Tiredness, apathy, irritability
*Gastrointestinal disorders
*Elimination of normal activities
*Anemia
*Social isolation, distancing friends and family
*Dishonesty, lying
*Stealing food/money
*Tooth damage (gingivitis)
*Binging/high carbohydrate foods
*Drug and alcohol abuse
*Laxative and diuretic abuse
*Mood swings
*Chronic sore throat
*Difficulties in breathing/swallowing
*Hypokalemia (abnormally low potassium concentration)
*Electrolyte imbalance
*General ill health/constant physical problems
*Possible rupture of heart or esophagus/peritonitis
*Dehydration
*Irregular heart rhythms
*Suicidal tendencies/attempts

(vertical labels: EARLY SYMPTOMS, MIDDLE STAGE SYMPTOMS, CRUCIAL STAGE SYMPTOMS)

RECOVERY

Ongoing Support

*Trust/openness
*Understanding of personal needs
*Honesty
*Increased assertiveness
*Improved self-image
*Developing optimism
*Respect of family and friends
*More understanding of family
*Fully aware of and at ease with life
*Appreciation of spiritual values
*Enjoyment of eating food without guilt
*Acceptance of personal limitations
*Return of regular menstrual cycles
*New interest
*New friends
*Achievement of personal goals in a wide range of activities
*Self-approval (not dependent on weight)
*Relief from guilt and depression
*Diminished fears
*Resumption of normal eating
*Resumption of normal self-control
*Begin to relax
*Acceptance of illness
*Participation in a treatment program
*Acceptance of a psychiatric treatment plan

REHABILITATION

RECOGNITION OF NEED FOR HELP

The progressions of symptoms and recovery signs are based on the most repeated experiences of those with Anorexia and Bulimia. When a patient with Anorexia becomes Bulimic, she will experience symptoms characteristic of both eating disorders. Although every symptom in the chart does not occur in every case or in any specific sequence, it does portray an average progression pattern. The goals and resultant behavior changes in the recovery process are similar for both eating disorders.

• **Fig. 17.17** Anorexia nervosa and bulimia: a multidimensional profile.

of the maxillary teeth; Fig. 17.18), dentin hypersensitivity, and enlargement of the parotid glands.[105] Those with eating disorders are five times more likely to have dental erosion (Fig. 17.19) and tend to have diets higher in acidic or carbonated foods/beverages; sweetened foods; and refined carbohydrates.[105] In addition, those with erosion report higher brushing frequency including after vomiting.[105] Signs of malnutrition may also be present and observed during an oral examination (e.g., dry brittle hair, spoon-shaped nails, and cheilosis).

Successful outcomes require comprehensive treatment by an interprofessional team that addresses individual psychosocial, nutritional, and medical problems. The team usually comprises a psychotherapist or psychiatrist, RDN, nurse, social worker, and primary care provider. This interprofessional team of specialties provides effective treatment for the patient and a support system for team members when difficult decisions are necessary or progress seems slow.

Mental Illness

A few of the many different mental illnesses that occur include schizophrenia, depression, and bipolar disorder or mania. Mental health issues are associated with less frequent dental visits, poor oral self-care, higher risk for dental caries, tooth loss,

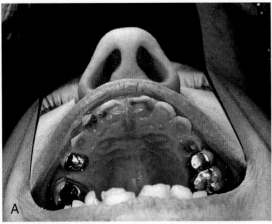
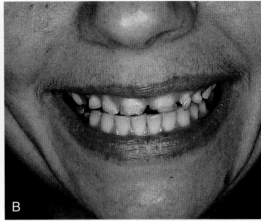

• **Fig. 17.18** (A and B) Enamel erosion caused by bulimia nervosa. (From Ibsen OAC, Phelan JA. *Oral Pathology for the Dental Hygienist*. 6th ed. Saunders; 2014.)

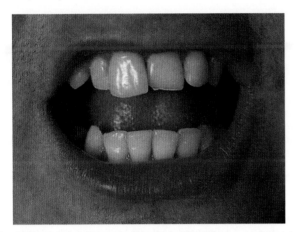

• **Fig. 17.19** Bulimia nervosa. Incisor was capped because of dental caries. Continued vomiting has diminished the size of the surrounding teeth, while prosthesis remains unchanged. (Courtesy Dr. J. Treasure. From McLaren DS. *A Colour Atlas and Text of Diet-Related Disorders*. 2nd ed. Mosby-Yearbook; 1992.)

and bruxism.[106,107] In addition, drugs frequently prescribed to treat the conditions may have side effects that affect oral status. Antipsychotics (e.g., risperidone [Risperdal], olanzapine [Zyprexa], aripiprazole [Abilify]) used to treat schizophrenia frequently cause xerostomia. Anticholinergic properties of tricyclic antidepressants, monoamine oxidase inhibitors, and trazodone used to treat depression also cause xerostomia, increase risk of dental caries, ulcerations, and periodontal disease. Trazodone can also cause an unpleasant taste in the mouth.

DENTAL CONSIDERATIONS

Assessment
- *Physical:* Signs of malnutrition (e.g., thinning hair, cold intolerance, facial hair), fatigue, dehydration, trauma to the soft palate from fingernails or objects used to induce vomiting, location of enamel erosion, parotid enlargement, weight changes.
- *Dietary:* High-carbohydrate diet, very-low-calorie intake or other unusual dietary restrictions or habits, obsession with diet or weight.

Interventions
- Goals of the dental hygiene treatment care plan for patients with psychiatric disorders should be realistic in an effort to maintain oral health and prevent and control oral disease.
- An increased caries rate can be indicative of high-carbohydrate binging, low pH of saliva due to vomiting, and xerostomia. Office and home fluoride therapy should be recommended based on caries risk.
- Discuss specific characteristics observed in the dental assessment with the patient.
- Treatment of an eating disorder involves an interprofessional team of health care professionals, including the dental professional. It is the responsibility of the dental hygienist to recognize the signs and symptoms of a suspected eating disorder, refer patients to a health care provider or a local hospital or eating disorder facility for assessment and treatment, and document the findings and recommendations.
- Chronic use of syrup of ipecac can affect skeletal muscle and cardiac action, which can result in congestive heart failure, arrhythmia, and sudden death.
- Encourage meticulous oral self-care.

Evaluation
- The patient is making realistic changes by protecting the hard and soft tissues, being plaque-free, and being treated by an interprofessional health care team.

NUTRITIONAL DIRECTIONS

- To prevent further damage to teeth, caution the patient against brushing immediately after vomiting; avoid use of hard toothbrushes, abrasive toothpaste, and a "scrubbing" toothbrush method; avoid rinsing with tap water because it reduces the protective effects of saliva; encourage use of a mouth guard during vomiting episodes; rinse with sodium bicarbonate to neutralize the oral environment; and encourage use of daily fluoride and dentinal hypersensitivity products.
- Educate the patient about various ways to relieve xerostomia and strategies for reducing the effect on hard and soft tissues.
- Nutritional advice should be provided to encourage health-centered behaviors rather than discussing calorie values or intake.

◆ **HEALTH APPLICATION 17**

Human Papillomavirus

Human papillomavirus (HPV) is a common sexually transmitted infection with a prevalence of 40% in the United States.[108] HPV is a risk factor for oral cancer (Box 17.1). However, there are more than 200 different types of HPV and most do not progress to disease. In the United States, the most common HPV-associated cancer is oropharyngeal cancer.[109] HPV strains are numbered; HPV-16 and HPV-18 have been identified as subtypes associated with risk factors for oral squamous cell carcinomas.

HPV-positive oropharyngeal cancer account for nearly 20,000 cases annually with males most affected.[110] More disturbing is the fact that the 5 years survival rate after diagnosis is only 68% and mortality is almost three times higher for males.[110] These lesions can be recognized during an intraoral examination; however, HPV lesions vary in form (Fig. 17.20). Dental professionals are well-positioned to refer patients with lesions identified during an intra- and extraoral examination to the health care provider. HPV can be present and communicable even when lesions are not present. Salivary diagnostic testing is available to detect the presence of HPV. Currently, two

HPV vaccines have received FDA approval for protection against HPV-16 and HPV-18. The vaccine requires two doses and can start at age 9 years.[111] Children starting the series on or after age 15 years will need three doses of the vaccine.[111] HPV vaccination is not currently recommended for those over 26 years of age.[111] Treatment regimens for cancer (surgery, chemotherapy, and/or radiation) vary according to the cancer site and stage. The treatments cause or exacerbate symptoms such as anorexia, alterations or loss of taste, xerostomia, mucositis, nausea, and vomiting, all of which have an impact on eating. Before, during, and after treatment, patients with oral cancer often experience complications related to these symptoms. Malnutrition, a frequent complication, has serious implications on the outcome and response to treatment as previously discussed.

As the association between HPV and oral cancer strengthens, early detection and education is the emerging responsibility of dental professionals. Communicating the message on this sensitive topic may require additional training.

• BOX 17.1   Evidence-Based Risk Factors for Oral, Pharyngeal, and Laryngeal Cancers

- Human papillomavirus infection
- Tobacco use
- Chewing betel quid containing betel leaf, areca nut, and lime (areca nut is the carcinogenic agent)
- Tobacco and alcohol use

Data from National Cancer Institute. *Oral Cavity, Oropharynx, Hypopharynx, & Larynx Cancer Prevention (PDQ)-Health Professional Version.* 2023. https://www.cancer.gov/types/head-and-neck/hp/oral-prevention-pdq.

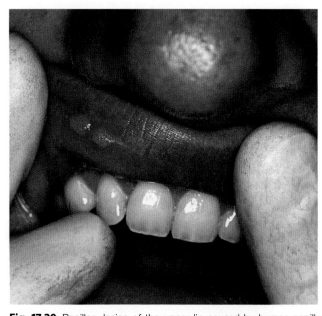

• **Fig. 17.20** Papillary lesion of the upper lip caused by human papillomavirus in a patient with human immunodeficiency virus infection. (From Ibsen OAC, Phelan JA. *Oral Pathology for the Dental Hygienist.* 6th ed. Saunders; 2014.)

◆ **CASE APPLICATION FOR THE DENTAL HYGIENIST**

Janie, a 17-year-old cheerleader in high school, came in for her 6-month recare appointment. She complained, "my teeth seem to be wearing down," and "I'm getting holes in my front teeth." Further questioning indicated frequent vomiting to control her weight because "everyone does it," she said.

Nutritional Assessment
- Weight changes
- Oral assessment
- Food, nutrient, and calorie intake
- Awareness of the relationship between health and nutritional intake
- Dietary habits

Nutritional Diagnosis
Consumption of large amounts of high-carbohydrate, low-nutrient foods in a short time, several times a week, followed by regurgitation.

Nutritional Goals
Patient will limit fermentable carbohydrates to reduce the incidence of decay.

Nutritional Implementation
Intervention: Conduct an oral examination to note if any of the oral manifestations are present: trauma to the soft palate, erythematous pharyngeal area, enamel erosion, angular cheilosis, salivary gland enlargement, and xerostomia.

Rationale: These self-inflicted oral complications can indicate to the dental professional the need to investigate further the possibility of an eating disorder in a patient who denies the problem.

Intervention: Discuss effects of frequent vomiting on the oral cavity and appropriate methods to prevent further damage to soft tissues and teeth.

Rationale: Avoidance of brushing immediately after purging and daily using fluoride along with desensitizing agents to decrease further problems in the oral cavity.

Intervention: Become the dental liaison in the interprofessional health care team for this patient.

Rationale: Because of complicated issues involved with an eating disorder, an interprofessional healthcare team is required to treat patients. The dental hygienist plays a crucial role in overall care of these patients.

◆ CASE APPLICATION FOR THE DENTAL HYGIENIST—CONT'D

Intervention: Discuss specific foods that help to prevent further deterioration of the teeth.

Rationale: Adequate nutrition is essential to support a healthy periodontium and prevent destructive dental activities. Frequent intake of simple carbohydrate foods is a factor in caries risk.

Evaluation

The patient is actively seeking treatment for her eating disorder. She plans to achieve small goals as she works toward improving intake of all nutrients and decreasing episodes of binging and purging to improve her oral hygiene status.

◆ Student Readiness

1. List ways to make a low-sodium diet more appealing. Using favorite foods, create a low-sodium diet for yourself for day.
2. Describe several oral manifestations seen in various systemic diseases causing oral pain, making eating difficult and less enjoyable.
3. Identify strategies for a patient who is experiencing (1) nausea and vomiting, (2) bitter or metallic taste in the mouth, (3) chewing and swallowing difficulties, (4) stomatitis, and (5) xerostomia.
4. What factors contribute to anorexia in a patient with HIV/AIDS?
5. What are some cancer treatments, and what oral problems can result from these therapies?
6. Choose a systemic disease from this chapter. Search for a recent (within the past 3 years) systematic review and/or meta-analysis using the name of the disease, oral health, and nutrition as the key terms. Review the article and determine the outcomes. Present the outcomes to others in the course. Consider further research and write an article on the disease to submit to a dental hygiene journal for publication or present a poster at a dental hygiene association meeting.

◆ CASE STUDY

A new patient is seen in the office with complaints of recurrent aphthous ulcers. These ulcers make it very difficult for him to eat, and he has lost about 8 lb. During an oral examination, candidiasis, hairy leukoplakia, and a flat, bluish, nonsymptomatic lesion on the palate, indicative of Kaposi sarcoma, are noted. HIV/AIDS may be a possible diagnosis.

1. What additional information would you like to obtain from this patient?
2. Would this patient benefit from nutrition information given by the dental hygienist? If so, on what areas should the dental hygienist concentrate?
3. What dietary modifications and dental care instructions would you provide to this patient?
4. Create a list of helpful additional resources, mobile apps, and agencies for this patient.

References

1. Hussein S, Kantawalla RF, Dickie S, Suarez-Durall P, Enciso R, Mulligan R. Association of oral health and mini nutritional assessment in older adults: a systematic review with *meta*-analyses. *J Prosthodont Res.* 2022;66(2):208–220.
2. Moynihan P, Varghese R. Impact of wearing dentures on dietary intake, nutritional status, and eating: a systematic review. *JDR Clin Transl Res.* 2022;7(4):334–351.
3. Strauss SM, Alfano MC, Shelley D, Fulmer T. Identifying unaddressed systemic health conditions at dental visits: patients who visited dental practices but not general health care providers in 2008. *Am J Public Health.* 2012;102(2):253–255.
4. Chandrupatla SG, Ramachandra R, Dantala S, Pushpanjali K, Tavares M. Importance and potential of dentists in identifying patients at high risk of diabetes. *Curr Diabetes Rev.* 2019;15(1):67–73.
5. Estrich CG, Araujo MWB, Lipman RD. Prediabetes and diabetes screening in dental care settings: NHANES 2013 to 2016. *JDR Clin Trans Res.* 2019;4(1):76–85.
6. Hariyanto TI, Kurniawan A. Appetite problem in cancer patients: Pathophysiology, diagnosis, and treatment. *Cancer Treat Res Commun.* 2021;27:100336.
7. Cox NJ, Ibrahim K, Sayer AA, Robinson SM, Roberts HC. Assessment and treatment of the anorexia of aging: a systematic review. *Nutrients.* 2019;11(1):144.
8. De Luca P, Di Stadio A, Colacurcio V, et al. Long COVID, audio-vestibular symptoms and persistent chemosensory dysfunction: a systematic review of the current evidence. *Acta Otorhinolaryngol Ital.* 2022;42(Suppl. 1):S87–S93.
9. Doty RL, Hawkes CH. Chemosensory dysfunction in neurodegenerative diseases. *Handb Clin Neurol.* 2019;164:325–360.
10. Schiffman SS. Influence of medications on taste and smell. *World J Otorhinolaryngol Head Neck Surg.* 2018;4(1):84–91.
11. Spotten LE, Corish CA, Lorton CM, et al. Subjective and objective taste and smell changes in cancer. *Ann Oncol.* 2017;28(5):969–984.
12. Hoffman HJ, Rawal S, Li CM, Duffy VB. New chemosensory component in the United States National Health and Nutrition Examination Survey (NHANES): first-year results for measured olfactory dysfunction. *Rev Endocr Metab Disord.* 2016;17(2):221–240.
13. Roxbury CR, Bernstein IA, Lin SY, Rowan NR. Association between chemosensory dysfunction and diet quality in United States adults. *Am J Rhinol Allergy.* 2022;36(1):47–56.
14. Høier ATZB, Chaaban N, Andersen BV. Possibilities for maintaining appetite in recovering COVID-19 patients. *Foods.* 2021;10(2):464.
15. Thomas DC, Chablani D, Parekh S, Pichammal RC, Shanmugasundaram K, Pitchumani PK. Dysgeusia. *J Am Dent Assoc.* 2022;153(3):251–264.
16. Pedersen AML, Sørensen CE, Proctor GB, Carpenter GH, Ekström J. Salivary secretion in health and disease. *J Oral Rehabil.* 2018;45(9):730–746.
17. Fornari CB, Bergonci D, Stein CB, Agostini BA, Rigo L. Prevalence of xerostomia and its association with systemic diseases and medications in the elderly: a cross-sectional study. *Sao Paulo Med J.* 2021;139(4):380–387.
18. Agostini BA, Cericato GO, Silveira ERda, et al. How common is dry mouth? Systematic review and *meta*-regression analysis of prevalence estimates. *Braz Dent J.* 2018;29(6):606–618.
19. Barbe AG. Medication-induced xerostomia and hyposalivation in the elderly: culprits, complications, and management. *Drugs Aging.* 2018;35(10):877–885.
20. Kumar A, Sharma E, Marley A, Samaan MA, Brookes MJ. Iron deficiency anaemia: pathophysiology, assessment, practical management. *BMJ Open Gastroenterol.* 2022;9(1):e000759.

21. Napeñas JJ, Brennan MT, Elad S. Oral manifestations of systemic diseases. *Dermatologic Clinics*. 2020;38(4):495–505.

22. Chiang CP, Chang JYF, Wang YP, Wu YH, Wu YC, Sun A. Atrophic glossitis: Etiology, serum autoantibodies, anemia, hematinic deficiencies, hyperhomocysteinemia, and management. *J Formos Med Assoc*. 2020;119(4):774–780.

23. Hariz A, Bhattacharya PT. *Megaloblastic anemia*. StatPearls. StatPearls Publishing; 2023. http://www.ncbi.nlm.nih.gov/books/NBK537254/.

24. Zhou P, Hua H, Yan Z, Zheng L, Liu X. Diagnostic value of oral "beefy red" patch in vitamin B12 deficiency. *TCRM*. 2018;14:1391–1397.

25. National Heart, Lung, and Blood Institute. *Vitamin B12–Deficiency Anemia*. 2022. https://www.nhlbi.nih.gov/health/anemia/vitamin-b12-deficiency-anemia

26. Viswanathan M, Urrutia RP, Hudson KN, Middleton JC, Kahwati LC. Folic acid supplementation to prevent neural tube defects: updated evidence report and systematic review for the United States Preventive Services Task Force. *JAMA*. 2023;330(5):460–466.

27. Office of Dietary Supplements. *Folate: Fact Sheet for Health Professionals*. https://ods.od.nih.gov/factsheets/Folate-Health Professional/

28. Connelly JA, Walkovich K. Diagnosis and therapeutic decision-making for the neutropenic patient. *Hematol Am Soc Hematol Educ Program*. 2021;2021(1):492–503.

29. Zecha JAEM, Raber-Durlacher JE, Laheij AMGA, et al. The impact of the oral cavity in febrile neutropenia and infectious complications in patients treated with myelosuppressive chemotherapy. *Support Care Cancer*. 2019;27(10):3667–3679.

30. Yadlapati R, Gyawali CP, Pandolfino JE Consensus Conference Participants. AGA clinical practice update on the personalized approach to the evaluation and management of GERD: expert review. Clin Gastroenterol Hepatol. 2022;20(5):984–994.e1

31. Singendonk M, Goudswaard E, Langendam M, et al. Prevalence of gastroesophageal reflux disease symptoms in infants and children: a systematic review. *J Pediatr Gastroenterol Nutr*. 2019;68(6):811–817.

32. National Institute of Diabetes and Digestive and Kidney Diseases. *Symptoms & Causes of GER & GERD in Children*. National Institute of Diabetes and Digestive and Kidney Diseases; 2020. https://www.niddk.nih.gov/health-information/digestive-diseases/acid-reflux-ger-gerd-children/symptoms-causes

33. National Institute of Diabetes and Digestive and Kidney Diseases. *Symptoms & Causes of GER & GERD*. 2020. https://www.niddk.nih.gov/health-information/digestive-diseases/acid-reflux-ger-gerd-adults/symptoms-causes

34. Fox M, Gyawali CP. Dietary factors involved in GERD management. *Best Pract Res Clin Gastroenterol*. 2023;62–63. 101826.

35. Katz PO, Dunbar KB, Schnoll-Sussman FH, Greer KB, Yadlapati R, Spechler SJ. ACG clinical guideline for the diagnosis and management of gastroesophageal reflux disease. *Am J Gastroenterol*. 2022;117(1):27.

36. Chen JW, Vela MF, Peterson KA, Carlson DA. AGA clinical practice update on the diagnosis and management of extraesophageal gastroesophageal reflux disease: expert review. *Clin Gastroenterol Hepatol*. 2023;21(6):1414–1421.e3.

37. Wynn R.L., Meiller T.F., Crossley H.L. *Omeprazole*. Vol. 28. Lexicomp, Inc.; 2023. https://online-lexi-com

38. Zuvarox T, Belletieri C. *Malabsorption syndromes*. In: StatPearls. StatPearls Publishing; 2023. http://www.ncbi.nlm.nih.gov/books/NBK553106/.

39. Lauritano D, Boccalari E, Di Stasio D, et al. Prevalence of oral lesions and correlation with intestinal symptoms of inflammatory bowel disease: a systematic review. *Diagnostics*. 2019;9(3):77.

40. Alsadat FA, Alamoudi NM, El-Housseiny AA, Felemban OM, Dardeer FM, Saadah OI. Oral and dental manifestations of celiac disease in children: a case-control study. *BMC Oral Health*. 2021;21(1):669.

41. Pawlaczyk-Kamieńska T, Borysewicz-Lewicka M, Śniatała R, Batura-Gabryel H, Cofta S. Dental and periodontal manifestations in patients with cystic fibrosis – a systematic review. *J Cyst Fibros*. 2019;18(6):762–771.

42. Larvin H, Kang J, Aggarwal VR, Pavitt S, Wu J. Risk of incident cardiovascular disease in people with periodontal disease: a systematic review and *meta*-analysis. *Clin Exp Dent Res*. 2021;7(1):109–122.

43. Sanz M, Marco Del Castillo A, Jepsen S, et al. Periodontitis and cardiovascular diseases: consensus report. *J Clin Periodontol*. 2020;47(3):268–288.

44. Ye Z, Cao Y, Miao C, et al. Periodontal therapy for primary or secondary prevention of cardiovascular disease in people with periodontitis. *Cochrane Database Syst Rev*. 2022;10(10):CD009197.

45. Cardoso AF, Ribeiro LE, Santos T, et al. Oral hygiene in patients with stroke: a best practice implementation project protocol. *Nurs Rep*. 2023;13(1):148–156.

46. Schimmel M, Ono T, Lam OLT, Müller F. Oro-facial impairment in stroke patients. *J Oral Rehabil*. 2017;44(4):313–326.

47. Muñoz Aguilera E, Suvan J, Buti J, et al. Periodontitis is associated with hypertension: a systematic review and *meta*-analysis. *Cardiovasc Res*. 2020;116(1):28–39.

48. Wynn RL, Meiller TF, Crossley HL *Cholestramine Resin*. Vol. 28. Lexicomp, Inc.; 2023. https://online-lexi-com

49. Neal B, Wu Y, Feng X, et al. Effect of salt substitution on cardiovascular events and death. *N Engl J Med*. 2021;385(12):1067–1077.

50. Jeong SY, Wee CC, Kovell LC, et al. Effects of diet on 10-year atherosclerotic cardiovascular disease risk (from the DASH trial). *Am J Cardiol*. 2023;187:10–17.

51. Featherstone JDB, Crystal YO, Alston P, et al. Evidence-based caries management for all ages-practical guidelines. *Front Oral Health*. 2021;2:14.

52. Xiao Pl, Cui Ay, Hsu Cj, et al. Global, regional prevalence, and risk factors of osteoporosis according to the World Health Organization diagnostic criteria: a systematic review and *meta*-analysis. *Osteoporos Int*. 2022;33(10):2137–2153.

53. Peng J, Chen J, Liu Y, Lyu J, Zhang B. Association between periodontitis and osteoporosis in United States adults from the National Health and Nutrition Examination Survey: a cross-sectional analysis. *BMC Oral Health*. 2023;23(1):254.

54. Yeung AWK, Mozos I. The innovative and sustainable use of dental panoramic radiographs for the detection of osteoporosis. *Int J Environ Res Public Health*. 2020;17(7):2449.

55. Mupparapu M, Akintoye SO. Application of panoramic radiography in the detection of osteopenia and osteoporosis-current state of the art. *Curr Osteoporos Rep*. 2023;21(4):354–359.

56. Ruggiero SL, Dodson TB, Aghaloo T, Carlson, Eric R, Ward, Brent B, Kademani D. American Association of Oral and Maxillofacial Surgeons position paper on medication-related osteonecrosis of the jaw—2022 update. *J Oral Maxillofac Surg*. 2022;80(5):920–943.

57. Stöhr J, Barbaresko J, Neuenschwander M, Schlesinger S. Bidirectional association between periodontal disease and diabetes mellitus: a systematic review and *meta*-analysis of cohort studies. *Sci Rep*. 2021;11(1):13686.

58. Wu CZ, Yuan YH, Liu HH, et al. Epidemiologic relationship between periodontitis and type 2 diabetes mellitus. *BMC Oral Health*. 2020;20(1):204.

59. Baeza M, Morales A, Cisterna C, et al. Effect of periodontal treatment in patients with periodontitis and diabetes: systematic review and *meta*-analysis. *J Appl Oral Sci*. 2020;28:e20190248.

60. Simpson TC, Clarkson JE, Worthington HV, et al. Treatment of periodontitis for glycaemic control in people with diabetes mellitus. *Cochrane Database Syst Rev*. 2022;4(4):CD004714.

61. Tonetti MS, Greenwell H, Kornman KS. Staging and grading of periodontitis: framework and proposal of a new classification and case definition. *J Periodontol*. 2018;89(S1):S159–S172.

62. Carey IM, Critchley JA, DeWilde S, Harris T, Hosking FJ, Cook DG. Risk of infection in Type 1 and Type 2 diabetes compared with the general population: a matched cohort study. *Diabetes Care*. 2018;41(3):513–521.

63. Martorano-Fernandes L, Dornelas-Figueira LM, Marcello-Machado RM, et al. Oral candidiasis and denture stomatitis in diabetic patients: systematic review and *meta*-analysis. *Braz Oral Res*. 2020;34:e113.

64. Mugri MH. Efficacy of systemic amoxicillin-metronidazole in periodontitis patients with diabetes mellitus: a systematic review of randomized clinical trials. *Medicina (Kaunas)*. 2022;58(11):1605.

65. Alshehri M, Alshail F, Alshehri FA. Effect of scaling and root planing with and without adjunctive use of an essential-oil-based oral rinse in the treatment of periodontal inflammation in type-2 diabetic patients. *J Investig Clin Dent*. 2017;8(1).

66. ElSayed NA, Aleppo G, Aroda VR, et al. 6. Glycemic targets: standards of care in diabetes—2023. *Diabetes Care*. 2023;46(Supplement_1):S97–S110.

67. Taylor PN, Albrecht D, Scholz A, et al. Global epidemiology of hyperthyroidism and hypothyroidism. *Nat Rev Endocrinol*. 2018;14(5):301–316.

68. Venkatesh Babu NS, Patel PB. Oral health status of children suffering from thyroid disorders. *J Indian Soc Pedod Prev Dent*. 2016;34(2):139–144.

69. Patil N, Rehman A, Jialal I. *Hypothyroidism*. StatPearls. StatPearls Publishing; 2023. http://www.ncbi.nlm.nih.gov/books/NBK519536/.

70. Aldulaijan HA, Cohen RE, Stellrecht EM, Levine MJ, Yerke LM. Relationship between hypothyroidism and periodontitis: a scoping review. *Clin Exp Dent Res*. 2020;6(1):147–157.

71. Babiker A, Alawi A, Al Atawi M, Al Alwan I. The role of micronutrients in thyroid dysfunction. *Sudan J Paediatr*. 2020;20(1):13–19.

72. Palla B, Burian E, Fliefel R, Otto S. Systematic review of oral manifestations related to hyperparathyroidism. *Clin Oral Investig*. 2018;22(1):1–27.

73. Bilezikian JP, Bandeira L, Khan A, Cusano NE. Hyperparathyroidism. *Lancet*. 2018;391(10116):168–178.

74. Lexomboon D, Tägt M, Nilsson I-L, Buhlin K, Häbel H, Sandborgh-Englund G. Effects of primary hyperparathyroidism on oral health. A longitudinal register-based study. *Oral Dis*. 2023;29(7):2954–2961.

75. Hashmi MF, Benjamin O, Lappin SL. *End-stage renal disease*. StatPearls. StatPearls Publishing; 2023. http://www.ncbi.nlm.nih.gov/books/NBK499861/.

76. Hande A, Jidewar N, Gadge R. Oral manifestations in patients with renal diseases. *J Datta Meghe Institute Med Sci Univ*. 2020;15(2):238.

77. Dembowska E, Jaroń A, Gabrysz-Trybek E, Bladowska J, Trybek G. Oral mucosa status in patients with end-stage chronic kidney disease undergoing hemodialysis. *Int J Environ Res Public Health*. 2023;20(1):835.

78. Proctor R, Kumar N, Stein A, Moles D, Porter S. Oral and dental aspects of chronic renal failure. *J Dent Res*. 2005;84(3):199–208.

79. Serni L, Caroti L, Barbato L, et al. Association between chronic kidney disease and periodontitis. A systematic review and *meta*-analysis. *Oral Dis*. 2023;29(1):40–50.

80. Kreher D, Ernst BLV, Ziebolz D, et al. Prevalence of dental caries in patients on renal replacement therapy—a systematic review. *J Clin Med*. 2023;12(4):1507.

81. Bévier A, Novel-Catin E, Blond E, et al. Water-soluble vitamins and trace elements losses during on-line hemodiafiltration. *Nutrients*. 2022;14(17):3454.

82. Simon DK, Tanner CM, Brundin P. Parkinson disease epidemiology, pathology, genetics, and pathophysiology. *Clin Geriatr Med*. 2020;36(1):1–12.

83. National Institute on Aging. *Parkinson's Disease: Causes, Symptoms, and Treatments*. National Institute on Aging. https://www.nia.nih.gov/health/parkinsons-disease

84. Verhoeff MC, Eikenboom D, Koutris M, et al. Parkinson's disease and oral health: a systematic review. *Arch Oral Biol*. 2023;151:105712.

85. Pringsheim T, Day GS, Smith DB, et al. Dopaminergic therapy for motor symptoms in early Parkinson disease practice guideline summary: a report of the AAN Guideline Subcommittee. *Neurology*. 2021;97(20):942–957.

86. Agnieszka W, Paweł P, Małgorzata K. How to optimize the effectiveness and safety of Parkinson's disease therapy? – a systematic review of drugs interactions with food and dietary supplements. *Curr Neuropharmacol*. 2022;20(7):1427–1447.

87. Lister T. Nutrition and lifestyle interventions for managing Parkinson's disease: a narrative review. *JMD*. 2020;13(2):97–104.

88. Bianchi VE, Rizzi L, Somaa F. The role of nutrition on Parkinson's disease: a systematic review. *Nutr Neurosci*. 2023;26(7):605–628.

89. Manikandan B, Gloria JK, Samuel R, Russell PS. Feeding difficulties among children with special needs: a cross-sectional study from India. *OTJR*. 2022;43(4):592–599.

90. Min K-C, Seo S-M, Woo H-S. Effect of oral motor facilitation technique on oral motor and feeding skills in children with cerebral palsy : a case study. *BMC Pediatr*. 2022;22(1):626.

91. Griepp DW, Kim DJ, Ganz M, et al. The effects of antiepileptic drugs on bone health: a systematic review. *Epilepsy Res*. 2021;173:106619.

92. Bao X, Liu F, Lin J, et al. Nutritional assessment and prognosis of oral cancer patients: a large-scale prospective study. *BMC Cancer*. 2020;20(1):146.

93. National Cancer Institute. *Nutrition in Cancer Care (PDQ)—Health Professional Version*. 2023. https://www.cancer.gov/about-cancer/treatment/side-effects/appetite-loss/nutrition-hp-pdq

94. Quispe RA, Aguiar EM, de Oliveira CT, Neves ACX, Santos PSdaS. Oral manifestations of leukemia as part of early diagnosis. *Hematol Transfus Cell Ther*. 2022;44(3):392–401.

95. Conigliaro T, Boyce LM, Lopez CA, Tonorezos ES. Food intake during cancer therapy: a systematic review. *Am J Clin Oncol*. 2020;43(11):813–819.

96. Kawashita Y, Soutome S, Umeda M, Saito T. Oral management strategies for radiotherapy of head and neck cancer. *Jpn Dent Sci Rev*. 2020;56(1):62–67.

97. Rezazadeh L, Ostadrahimi A, Tutunchi H, Naemi Kermanshahi M, Pourmoradian S. Nutrition interventions to address nutritional problems in HIV-positive patients: translating knowledge into practice. *J Health Popul Nutr*. 2023;42:94.

98. Mavarani L, Albayrak-Rena S, Potthoff A, et al. Changes in body mass index, weight, and waist-to-hip ratio over five years in HIV-positive individuals in the HIV Heart Aging Study compared to the general population. *Infection*. 2023;51(4):1081–1091.

99. Lagathu C, Béréziat V, Gorwood J, et al. Metabolic complications affecting adipose tissue, lipid and glucose metabolism associated with HIV antiretroviral treatment. *Expert Opin Drug Saf*. 2019;18(9):829–840.

100. Gonclaves LS, Goncalves BML, Fontes TV. Periodontal disease in HIV-infected adults in the HAART era: clinical, immunological, and microbiological aspects. *Arch Oral Biol*. 2013;58(10):1385–1396.

101. Qian J, Wu Y, Liu F, et al. An update on the prevalence of eating disorders in the general population: a systematic review and *meta*-analysis. *Eat Weight Disord*. 2022;27(2):415–428.

102. Cuadrado-Ríos S, Huamán-Garaicoa F, Cruz-Moreira K. Anorexia and bulimia nervosa in the practice of the paediatric dentist. *Eur Eat Disord Rev*. 2023;31(1):9–23.

103. Mourilhe C, Moraes CEde, Veiga Gda, et al. An evaluation of binge eating characteristics in individuals with eating disorders: a systematic review and *meta*-analysis. *Appetite*. 2021;162:105176.

104. Moraes CEF de, Antunes MML, Mourilhe C, Sichieri R, Hay P, Appolinario JC. Food consumption during binge eating episodes in binge eating spectrum conditions from a representative sample of a Brazilian metropolitan city. *Nutrients*. 2023;15(7):1573.

105. Lin JA, Woods ER, Bern EM. Common and emergent oral and gastrointestinal manifestations of eating disorders. *Gastroenterol Hepatol*. 2021;17(4):157–167.

106. Tiwari T, Kelly A, Randall CL, Tranby E, Franstve-Hawley J. Association between mental health and oral health status and care utilization. *Front Oral Health*. 2022;2:732882.

107. Kisely S, Sawyer E, Siskind D, Lalloo R. The oral health of people with anxiety and depressive disorders - a systematic review and *meta*-analysis. *J Affect Disord*. 2016;200:119–132.

108. Lewis RM, Laprise JF, Gargano JW, et al. Estimated prevalence and incidence of disease-associated HPV types among 15–59-year-olds in the United States. *Sex Transm Dis*. 2021;48(4):273–277.

109. Liao CI, Francoeur AA, Kapp DS, Caesar MAP, Huh WK, Chan JK. Trends in human papillomavirus-associated cancers, demographic characteristics, and vaccinations in the United States, 2001–2017. *JAMA Netw Open*. 2022;5(3):e222530.

110. Gribb JP, Wheelock JH, Park ES. Human papilloma virus (HPV) and the current state of oropharyngeal cancer prevention and treatment. *Dela J Public Health*. 2023;9(1):26–28.

111. CDC. *Human Papillomavirus (HPV) Vaccine*. Centers for Disease Control and Prevention; 2023. https://www.cdc.gov/hpv/parents/vaccine-for-hpv.html

▶ Evolve Resources

Please visit http://evolve.elsevier.com/Mallonee/nutritional for additional practice and study support tools.

18

Nutritional Aspects of Dental Caries: Causes, Prevention, and Treatment

STUDENT LEARNING OBJECTIVES

On completion of this chapter, the student will be able to achieve the following learning outcomes:

1. Explain the role that each of the following plays in the caries process: tooth, saliva, food, and plaque biofilm.
2. Discuss the following related to cariogenic foods, as well as cariostatic and noncariogenic properties of food:
   - List cariogenic food and beverages.
   - List examples of fermentable carbohydrates potentially increasing risk to dental health.

- Identify foods that stimulate salivary flow.
- Suggest food and beverage choices and their timing to reduce the cariogenicity of a patient's diet.
- Describe characteristics of foods having noncariogenic or cariostatic properties.
3. Provide nutrition education to a patient at risk for dental caries.

KEY TERMS

Acidogenic
Caries Management by Risk Assessment
   (CaMBRA)
Casein

Macrodontia
Noncariogenic
Silver diamine fluoride (SDF)

⬙ TEST YOUR NQ

1. **T/F** Cariogenic carbohydrates are the only reason for the development of carious lesions.
2. **T/F** Nutrients have a role in the composition and structure of teeth during development.
3. **T/F** Bicarbonates, phosphates, and proteins in saliva dilute and neutralize plaque acids in the mouth.
4. **T/F** Sucrose, fructose, glucose, and maltose have equal potential to cause dental caries.
5. **T/F** Most sugar alcohols—including sorbitol, mannitol, and xylitol—are cariogenic.

6. **T/F** For a tooth to demineralize, the plaque pH needs to be 6 or higher as a result of consuming cariogenic foods.
7. **T/F** The total quantity of sugar is of greatest importance when assessing the patient's diet.
8. **T/F** A fermentable carbohydrate consumed with a meal is less cariogenic than the same food consumed as a snack.
9. **T/F** The revised Recommended Dietary Allowances provide helpful nutrition information for patients trying to reduce dental caries.
10. **T/F** Providing patients with information about the caries process leads to desirable dietary and oral behavior changes.

Nutritional status and oral health have a strong interrelationship. Countless research studies have shown the importance of diet in the development, maintenance, and repair of hard and soft oral tissues. Dental caries is an oral infectious disease that is multifactorial, transmissible, and of bacterial origin (Fig. 18.1).

Diet and nutrients play a role in dental caries. Some foods exert a cariogenic effect, whereas others are cariostatic or anticariogenic and offer protection to reduce caries. Nutrients also have topical and systemic effects, which can be primary or secondary factors in the development of dental caries. However, many factors must be considered if the situation is to be defined as cariogenic. A list of cariogenic foods would be misleading because no food is cariogenic in all situations.

The primary oral health goal of *Healthy People 2030* is to improve oral health by increasing access to oral health care,

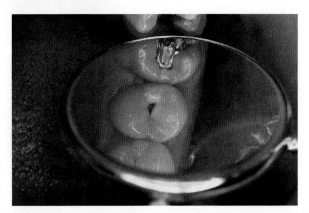

• **Fig. 18.1** Dental caries. (Reproduced with permission from Iannucci JM, Howerton LJ. *Dental Radiography: Principles and Techniques*. 5th ed. St. Louis, MO: Elsevier; 2017.)

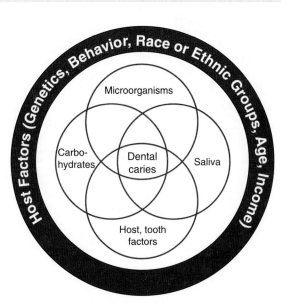

• **Fig. 18.2** Major factors that interact in the dental caries process.

including preventive services.[1] There is a focus on reducing the proportion of adults and adolescents with active or untreated tooth decay. Additionally, there is an effort to reduce consumption of added sugars by people aged 2 years and over.[1]

Even with advancements in the quality of digital radiography, emerging technology for early detection of caries, improved restorative materials, multiple fluoride options, application of sealants, frequent dental care appointments, dental health education, and improved access to care, dental caries remain the most common chronic childhood disease. Although a remarkable reduction in caries has been observed in school-age children since the 1970s, certain racial, ethnic, and lower-income population groups continue to be problematic. Data for *Healthy People 2030* from the National Survey of Children's Health estimated that 68.7% of low-income children and adolescents received preventive dental services in 2020–21.[1] Dental visits in the past year among low-income adults were 36.3%.[2] Barriers to dental care include cost; lack of dental insurance, public programs, or providers for underserved groups; fear of dentistry; difficulties in accessing services; or oral health literacy.

Major Factors in the Dental Caries Process

No single factor is responsible for formation of a carious lesion (Fig. 18.2). A combination of factors is involved, including a susceptible host or tooth surface, a sufficient quantity of cariogenic microorganisms in the mouth, the presence of fermentable carbohydrates, and a particular composition or flow of saliva. All of these must be present simultaneously for an adequate time to allow decay to occur.

Tooth Structure

Increasing resistance of the tooth against demineralization begins in the preeruptive phase. An adequate intake of nutrients during growth and development of enamel and dentin is essential. The most influential nutrients include calcium; phosphorus; vitamins A, C, and D; fluoride; and protein. Indirectly, some fermentable carbohydrates play a role in the formation of caries before tooth eruption. Consider a child who snacks on cookies, candy, or ice cream throughout the day and is not hungry for meat, vegetables, fruit, and dairy such as milk that may be offered at mealtime. A child's diet high in low-nutrient (or calorie-dense) carbohydrates

may be deficient in required nutrients for optimal growth and development of the dentition. Other factors, such as genetic or metabolic disturbances, can be responsible for poor tooth formation. Dental anomalies include **macrodontia** (abnormally large teeth) and enamel hypoplasia.

After the tooth erupts, the depth of the natural anatomic pits and fissures and the position of the teeth are relevant factors in the development of dental caries. Deep pits and fissures increase susceptibility for dental caries because of the potential for plaque biofilm and food entrapment. Overlapping and crowding of teeth also offer areas for these materials to collect and ferment, compounded by difficulty keeping these areas clean.

Host Factors

Food selection, dietary patterns, oral hygiene habits, genetics, race or ethnicity, age, and income are factors that determine susceptibility to caries.

Saliva

Availability of essential nutrients during the development of salivary glands, which begins during the fourth week in utero, has a significant impact on the amount of saliva and its composition. Of particular importance are vitamin A, iron, and protein, which have a role in normal growth, development, and secretion of saliva.

The protection provided by an adequate salivary flow and buffering capacity of saliva ultimately reduces the destructive capabilities of fermentable carbohydrates on teeth. This fact is recognized in patients with xerostomia, who are at high risk for development of caries because of decreased salivary production.

Saliva provides protection against caries in several ways. First, saliva acts as a buffer by neutralizing much of the acid produced by plaque biofilm as a result of carbohydrate metabolism. Second, normal saliva contains bicarbonate, phosphate, and protein, which dilute and neutralize acids to maintain a neutral oral pH, which is around 7. After an acidic drink is consumed, the pH of the oral cavity is rapidly normalized by the components of saliva. However, if the frequency or duration of the acidic drink is extended, it becomes more difficult for saliva to buffer the continuous supply of acid and it loses its caries protection.

Particularly important to the prevention of dental caries is the flow of saliva. An adequate salivary flow enables rapid transport of foods from the mouth, decreasing the length of time harmful bacteria and food particles are able to attach to teeth and cause caries to develop. Consumption of citrus fruits (e.g., 100% orange juice and lemons or fresh lemon juice) promotes saliva formation by means of their citric acid content; however, intake needs to be monitored because of the potential to cause enamel erosion.

Because saliva is saturated with calcium, phosphate, and fluoride ions, the potential for remineralization (restoration of damaged enamel) and resistance to enamel dissolution exists. Finally, antimicrobial elements in saliva, such as immunoglobulin A, either interfere with adherence of bacteria or compete with bacteria to attach to the tooth surface. An alkaline saliva offers protection, whereas an acidic saliva increases susceptibility to caries.

Plaque Biofilm and Its Bacterial Components

Plaque biofilm is a complex environment of bacteria, polysaccharides, proteins, and lipids. Plaque biofilm forms a local barrier on enamel and may interfere with demineralization. However, acids produced in plaque biofilm have harmful properties that offset the benefit of its barrier effect.

Composition of plaque biofilm is altered as it matures, and is strongly influenced by diet. As a by-product of the metabolism of sucrose and glucose, bacteria produce acids that lower the pH, resulting in a more favorable environment for the development of certain bacteria, such as *Streptococcus mutans*. *S. mutans*, a gram-positive, anaerobic, spherical bacterium, is widely implicated in initiation of dental caries. Other microorganisms, such as bacteria from other mutans streptococci and the *Lactobacillus* species, are capable of fermenting carbohydrates. They also thrive in an acidic environment.

When a carbohydrate has been ingested, its metabolism by salivary amylase begins within 2 to 3 minutes and can persist for hours. The metabolic products are acetic, butyric, formic, lactic, and propionic acids. Concentration of the acids escalates as carbohydrate intake continues, whereas the pH of the plaque decreases. Demineralization of enamel occurs when the "critical pH" of 5.5 is reached. Incipient demineralization of cementum and dentin can occur with a pH of 6.7; this is a real concern for areas of gingival recession. In addition, demineralization is faster on root surfaces than on enamel because dentin contains less mineral content. In interproximal areas or in deep pits and fissures, the pH can decrease to four and remain at that pH for an hour. The pH of acids produced by bacteria in plaque biofilm is eventually neutralized after elimination of cariogenic foods as saliva exerts its protective action.

● DENTAL CONSIDERATIONS

- Evaluate the patient for deep pits and fissures, amount of plaque biofilm in the oral cavity, and composition and flow of saliva. Encourage use of sealants in deep pits and fissures of young patients to prevent plaque biofilm accumulation.
- Silver diamine fluoride (SDF) is a noninvasive and easily applied fluoride modality for caries management. The effectiveness of SDF can be a promising strategy for populations at risk for dental decay.

Educating the patient and parents/caregivers on black staining of the arrested lesion is essential. Further studies are indicated to determine a minimum concentration of SDF that is safe and effective.[3]
- Recommend a combination of fluoride sources for patients at high risk for caries. Fluoride in plaque biofilm and saliva inhibits demineralization and enhances remineralization of tooth surfaces.
- For patients with a high caries rate, the use of chlorhexidine or other antimicrobial agents may be beneficial due to their ability to disorganize dental biofilm. Educate the patient that this practice can suppress harmful plaque and organisms. Counsel the patient regarding the potential of chlorhexidine staining teeth. The research regarding the use of chlorhexidine for inhibiting caries formation is inconclusive.[4–6]
- Encourage meticulous oral hygiene habits, including regular recare visits.
- Caution parents to avoid sharing utensils with children, a practice allowing transfer of the cariogenic microorganism *S. mutans*.

● NUTRITIONAL DIRECTIONS

- Eating a variety of sources from the food groups in moderation ensures adequate nutrient intake. Encouraging healthy eating habits is a factor in growth, development, and maintenance of teeth; prevention of dental caries; and general wellness.
- Firm, fibrous foods (such as raw fruits and vegetables), sugar free chewing gum, sour foods, and citrus fruits stimulate salivary flow. An increase in the flow rate has a positive impact on resistance of teeth to caries. However, sour foods and citrus foods should be consumed in moderation. due to increased acidity

Cariogenic Foods

Cariogenic foods and beverages are fermentable carbohydrates that can be metabolized by oral bacteria and reduce salivary pH below 5.5 (Fig. 18.3). As previously discussed, fermentable carbohydrates are a factor in the development of demineralization and dental caries. The average daily consumption from added sugars among 2- to 18-year-olds has declined over the last two decades but is still above the *Dietary Guidelines* recommendation of less than 10% of energy per day.[7] The major sources of added sugars are sugar-sweetened beverages (e.g., soft drinks, fruit drinks, sport and energy drinks and sweetened coffee/tea drinks).[8] A reported 63% of adults aged 18 and older in the United States reported drinking sugar-sweetened beverages once daily or more.[9] Other sources of added sugars include desserts and sweet snacks (e.g., ice cream and frozen dairy desserts, cakes, pies, cookies, brownies, doughnuts, sweet rolls and pastries), coffee, tea, and candy.[8] Nondiet sports and energy drinks are fast-growing sugar-sweetened beverage choices. Almost one in four US adults consumes sports and energy drinks at least one time per week.[10] A 16-oz bottle of a regular sports drink contains 21 g of added sugars, a 16-oz can of energy drink contains 54 g, and 12-oz sugar-sweetened soda may contain as much as 39 g of sugar.[10,11]

The small size of sugar molecules allows salivary amylase to split the molecules into components that can be easily metabolized by plaque bacteria. Sucrose is not the only culprit; other monosaccharides and disaccharides—such as fructose, glucose, and maltose—all produce similar amounts of substrate for metabolism by plaque bacteria to produce acid. Sucrose is used to produce glucans, facilitating the adherence of bacteria, such as *S. mutans*, to the dental pellicle. Glucose and other carbohydrates are also used to

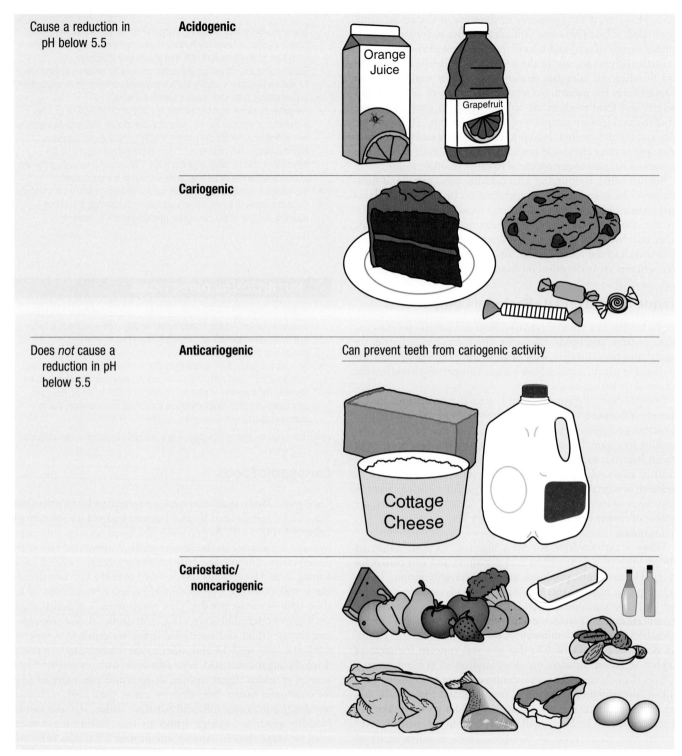

Cause a reduction in
pH below 5.5

Acidogenic

Cariogenic

Does *not* cause a
reduction in pH
below 5.5

Anticariogenic   Can prevent teeth from cariogenic activity

**Cariostatic/
noncariogenic**

• **Fig. 18.3** Cariogenicity of foods and beverages.

produce extracellular polysaccharides. Therefore, diets containing glucose, and the disaccharides can increase plaque biofilm mass and facilitate its retention and colonization. "Natural sugars"—such as honey (fructose and glucose), molasses (sucrose and invert sugar), and brown sugar (sugar and molasses)—have cariogenic potential similar to sucrose. Box 18.1 lists examples of fermentable carbohydrates potentially increasing risk to dental health.

Polysaccharides—starchy foods such as rice, potatoes, and corn—are less cariogenic than monosaccharides and disaccharides. Physical and chemical properties of starches are very different from the properties of simple carbohydrates, and render complex carbohydrates less damaging to enamel. These unique properties prevent starch from providing a readily available energy source for cariogenic microflora, and it is less likely to produce

• BOX 18.1 **Foods That Can Cause the pH of Plaque Biofilm to Fall Below 5.5**

- Alcohol
- Bananas
- Beans, baked
- White bread
- Candy
- Cereals, non–presweetened, ready-to-eat
- Cereals, presweetened, ready-to-eat
- Chips
- Cookies
- Crackers
- Dill pickles
- Doughnuts, plain
- Energy drinks
- Flavored coffees and teas
- Fruit, dried
- Fruit drinks
- Fruit smoothies
- Gelatin, flavored
- Sugar-sweetened hard candy
- Honey
- Ice cream
- Jams and jellies
- Marshmallows
- Nondairy creamers
- Oatmeal, instant cooked
- Pasta
- Peanut butter
- Pretzels
- Rice, instant and/or cooked
- Sauerkraut
- Snack cakes
- Soft drinks, regular and diet
- Sports drinks
- Tomato juice
- Flavored yogurts

caries than mono- or disaccharides. In contrast to sucrose, the large number of glucose units needed to form a starch, make it almost insoluble. Because starch must be hydrolyzed (split into smaller glucose units) before acid can be produced, the time a starch is in the mouth is usually not long enough to be completely metabolized if oral self-care is completed promptly. Normal saliva flow readily neutralizes any acids produced by polysaccharides.

When starches and simple carbohydrates are combined (as in pastries or sugar-coated cereals), their potential to produce caries is equal to or greater than that of sucrose. Also, processed starches, as found in instant oatmeal, are often more fermentable than their non-processed counterparts because of partial hydrolysis or diminution of particle size. The cariogenic activity is also related to the form of starch.

Fresh fruit is another food group of low cariogenicity because of its low percentage of carbohydrate and high percentage of water. Firm fruits such as apples play a protective role by stimulating saliva flow. The high concentration of fructose found in juices is potentially a source of substrate for plaque bacteria that may influence caries risk. This is shown in early childhood caries, which occurs in children given unlimited amounts of fruit juice and other fermentable carbohydrate beverages. Citric fruits and juices are acidogenic and can reduce the salivary pH to less than 5.5. The sticky nature of dried fruit (e.g., raisins) also increases risk of decay.

Cariostatic/Noncariogenic Properties of Food

Cariostatic or noncariogenic foods and beverages do not cause a reduction in salivary pH below 5.5 (see Fig. 18.3).

Nonnutritive Sweeteners

Aspartame, saccharin, sucralose, neotame, and acesulfame are a few examples of nonnutritive sweeteners. These sweeteners are not metabolized by microorganisms and do not promote dental caries. Foods made from these sweeteners are generally higher in cost, and therefore may not be feasible for low-income patients. Other

components of foods using these substitutes, such as raisins, may offset the benefits of using nonnutritive sweeteners to prevent dental caries.

Protein and Fat

Protein and fat are two nutrient classes that may be considered cariostatic because they do not lower plaque pH. Generally, protein may contribute to buffering effects of saliva. Consuming foods with fat and protein following a fermentable carbohydrate may increase plaque pH.[12] Meat, seafood, poultry, eggs, nuts, seeds, margarine, and oils are examples of potentially cariostatic foods.

Anticariogenic Properties of Food

Anticariogenic foods or beverages do not cause a reduction in pH below 5.5 and may protect teeth from cariogenic activity (see Fig. 18.3).

Sugar Alcohols

Some food components can protect teeth by decreasing demineralization, enhancing remineralization, or increasing salivary flow, even in the presence of a fermentable carbohydrate. Sugar alcohols, such as mannitol and sorbitol, are often used as substitute sweeteners. They are viable alternatives to sugar because of their sweet taste but have the added benefit of being noncariogenic, a carbohydrate that does not increase salivary pH (see Table 4.1 in Chapter 4 and Fig. 18.3). Sugar alcohols ferment more slowly in the mouth than monosaccharides and disaccharides; buffering effects of saliva competently neutralize destructive acids produced by plaque bacteria.

Another sugar alcohol, xylitol, is found naturally in plants and is equal to or sweeter than sucrose. Xylitol may be classified as anticariogenic because oral flora may not contain enzymes to ferment it, and metabolizing microorganisms, such as *S. mutans*, are inhibited. Salivary pH does not drop below 5.5. Chewing gums, mints, and candies containing xylitol may inhibit enamel demineralization.[13] This inhibitory effect is enhanced by increased salivary flow, increased oral clearance, and greater buffering capabilities. Compounded by increased mastication, the outcome can be remineralization of incipient decay.

The US Food and Drug Administration (FDA) recognizes sugar alcohols to be xylitol, sorbitol, mannitol, maltitol, isomalt, lactitol, hydrogenated starch hydrolysates, hydrogenated glucose syrups, and erythritol, or a combination of these. On food labels, products containing any of these sugar alcohols can state, "…the noncariogenic carbohydrate sweetener present in the food "does not promote," "may reduce the risk of," "useful [or is useful] in not promoting," or "expressly [or is expressly] for not promoting" dental caries."[14] The dental professional uses this information to educate the patient when choosing products containing sugar alcohols.

Phosphorus and Calcium

Phosphorus and calcium also provide qualities protecting against caries. Dispersion of these minerals throughout plaque biofilm may provide a buffering effect, increasing plaque pH. Ultimately, this action curtails demineralization of enamel.

Protein, especially the principal protein in milk, casein, and the minerals phosphorus and calcium are all ingredients of other anticariogenic—or even cariostatic—foods, such as cheese and milk. Despite the fact that lactose is cariogenic (although the least cariogenic of all mono-, di- and polysaccharides), these other elements in milk and dairy products decrease risk of dental caries. Cheese, produced from milk, contains several anticariogenic properties and has the potential to reduce demineralization (or enhance remineralization) of tooth enamel.

An increase of salivary flow occurs when chewing hard cheeses. This increased salivary flow provides a neutral environment and increases clearance of carbohydrates. Following the *MyPlate* website recommendation for the milk and milk products group (using low-fat dairy products) is prudent advice for a dental patient. Eating these foods as snacks or at the end of a meal can provide anticariogenic effects.

Other Foods With Protective Factors

A constituent in chocolate, known as the cocoa factor, has shown anticariogenic properties. The classic Vipeholm study compared the caries rate of individuals consuming chocolate with the rate for individuals consuming other types of "nonchocolate" candies under similar circumstances. The results indicated a slightly lower caries incidence in individuals consuming chocolate.[15]

Glycyrrhiza, the active ingredient in licorice, can also be considered anticariogenic due to the potential to reduce *S. mutans* in saliva.[16] However, glycyrrhiza contraindicated with some antihypertensive medications, has a staining capability, and can cause sodium retention and increased blood pressure.[17] Grapefruit and other fruits containing citric acid can stimulate saliva production. However, they are generally considered acidogenic because of their ability to lower salivary pH and increase caries risk. Emerging research indicates probiotics have properties that may interrupt caries formation.[18] Probiotics specific to oral health are live bacteria that are beneficial to the host (for more information see Chapter 3).

◈ DENTAL CONSIDERATIONS

- Educate patients about the caries process, and how to prevent demineralization of enamel, including the role that diet plays in initiation and progression of decay. Use terms that are appropriate and understandable for the patient.
- The dental hygienist should know which foods and situations have the potential to be cariogenic, create awareness of the potential harm, and offer suggestions for appropriate consumption of sweetened foods or alternative choices for sugar-containing foods (Box 18.1).
- Use of a variety of fluoride modalities, products containing appropriate levels of xylitol, and application of sealants increases protection of the tooth.
- Consider using an antimicrobial agent to control existing plaque biofilm, reduce the number of *S. mutans*, and prevent the formation of new plaque biofilm.
- Educate the patient regarding sports and energy drinks. Although these beverages are promoted to support intense physical activity since they contain electrolytes, vitamins, and minerals, remind patients that excessive consumption can lead to dental decay and in most cases are unnecessary.
- Exercise caution in recommending high-fat foods for their potential anticariogenic properties to patients with chronic diseases such as heart disease or diabetes mellitus because of their deleterious effects on these conditions.

◈ NUTRITIONAL DIRECTIONS

- Using the *Dietary Guidelines* and *MyPlate* website, evaluate the patient's diet for adequate nutritional intake and frequency of fermentable carbohydrate consumption.
- Substitute nonnutritive sweeteners for sucrose, if practical, use a high-intensity sweetener. Provide several options to sweeten coffee and tea instead of table sugar, especially if the beverage is consumed between meals. Include the patient in the conversation to determine if they are open to using a nonnutritive sweetener in place of table sugar.
- "Natural sugars," such as honey and molasses, are as cariogenic as refined carbohydrates.
- Encourage the consumption of healthy beverages, such as water, reduced fat milk. Limit consumption of vegetable and 100% fruit juices to 4–6 oz daily.
- Food sources of probiotics include yogurt, kefir, buttermilk, tempeh, and miso.
- Energy drinks may contain vitamins and minerals, but the main ingredients are added sugars and stimulants (e.g., caffeine and guarana). The amount of caffeine varies widely among drinks but can be as high as 500 mg of caffeine per can, which is comparable to approximately 14 cans of caffeinated soda. The consumption of energy drinks has been associated with insomnia, nervousness, and headache and can lead to tachycardia, seizures, and cardiac arrest.[10]
- Excessive intake of beverages or other products containing caffeine because of the potential interaction with certain drugs (e.g., bronchodilators, antibacterials, and antipsychotics).[10]
- Frequent use of medications containing fermentable carbohydrates, including antacids and cough drops are cariogenic.
- Increased use of products containing sugar alcohols (e.g., chewing gum, hard candy, dentifrices, and some medications) can cause gastrointestinal distress.
- Although sorbitol and mannitol ferment slowly in the mouth, which allows saliva to neutralize the acids produced, frequent use can potentially cause caries. This occurs especially in a patient with xerostomia using these products for relief of symptoms.
- Xylitol-containing chewing gums may inhibit growth of microorganisms, thereby reducing caries rate. Use of these gums after eating is recommended when proper oral care cannot be completed.
- High-sugar foods are generally high in fat as well. *MyPlate* website recommends that intake of high-sugar and high-fat foods should be limited.
- The *Dietary Guidelines* and *MyPlate* website recommend no more than 10% of total calories be from added sugar. The National Academy of Medicine (formerly the Institute of Medicine) recommends that added sugars should not exceed 25% of the total calories.[19]
- Popular sugar-sweetened beverages include sodas, fruit drinks, sports drinks, energy drinks, chocolate milk, and many vitamin waters.
- Compare labels; some low-fat or nonfat foods that compensate for flavor by increasing sugar or sodium content (e.g., frozen dairy products).
- Because physical properties of milk are comparable to saliva, increasing low-fat milk intake as a saliva substitute may also offer protection against caries for a patient experiencing xerostomia.
- Encourage proper oral hygiene techniques to avoid complications associated with exposure to natural sugars (lactose in milk) and added sugars (some fruit juices).

Other Factors Influencing Cariogenicity

The amount and type of carbohydrates are not the only determinants of food intake that influence caries prevalence and severity. Other considerations include retentiveness of the carbohydrate, duration for which teeth remain exposed, sequence in which a

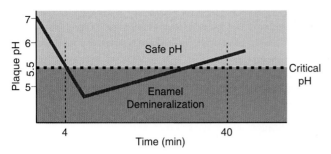

• **Fig. 18.4** Stephan curve: time involvement of carbohydrate consumption and enamel demineralization.

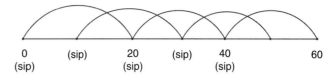

Minutes of acid exposure per sip of soda

• **Fig. 18.5** The increased consumption of soft drinks and sports drinks results in an enhanced caries risk. Although oral clearance is rapid, consuming such drinks over an extended time creates a cariogenic environment. If only soda is consumed, each sip results in at least 20 min of acid exposure. In this example, the patient took a sip at approximately 10-min intervals and finished the drink in 5 sips for a total of 60 min of acid exposure.

carbohydrate is consumed, and whether food is eaten with a meal or as a snack. Some foods thought to have low cariogenic potential (e.g., cornflakes, crackers, or potato chips) may be more acidogenic than simple-carbohydrate foods because of their retentiveness in embrasures, pits, and fissures. Preventive practices, such as regular recare appointments, appropriate oral hygiene practices, sealants, xylitol, and fluoride use, should also be considered when discussing cariogenicity.

Physical Form

How quickly a cariogenic food is cleared from the mouth is a factor related to caries development. Ingestion of hard candy results in prolonged exposure. A sticky and retentive carbohydrate (e.g., chewy fruit snacks) remains in contact with the enamel surface for a longer period than sweetened fluids. Slow oral clearance of fermentable carbohydrate means longer exposure of the tooth to acid attack.

Fermentable carbohydrates that are chewy, such as caramels, adhere to teeth. However, the additional mastication required to process these foods stimulates saliva flow, making them less retentive and less damaging than dry, sticky foods, such as pretzels. Caramels are higher in sucrose than pretzels, supporting the concept of quantity of fermentable carbohydrates having a limited impact.

Frequency of Intake

Closely related to the physical form of a food in caries potential is frequency of fermentable carbohydrate intake. Longer periods of oral exposure to a fermentable carbohydrate lead to a greater risk of demineralization and less opportunity for teeth to remineralize. In comparing two individuals who eat equal amounts of fermentable carbohydrates, the one who eats more frequently throughout the day has the greatest potential for decay. With each exposure, a decrease in pH begins within 2 to 3 minutes; at a pH of 5.5 or less (the critical pH), enamel decalcification occurs. Within 40 minutes, the pH has increased to its initial value. The classic Stephan curve shows the pH changes of dental plaque after rinsing with a sugar solution (Fig. 18.4). Using a similar scenario, if a person eats a candy bar within a 5-minute period, the teeth would be exposed to a critical pH that lasts for approximately 40 minutes before the pH returns to the original level. If another person eats the same candy bar in five bites, but only takes a bite every hour, the total acid exposure would be approximately 200 minutes (5 bites × 40 minutes = 200 minutes of acid exposure).

Frequent consumption of soft drinks, sports drinks, energy drinks, and flavored coffees and teas compounded with a decline in dairy products can also influence caries risk and erosion despite the rapid oral clearance of these beverages (Fig. 18.5). The pH of diet and regular soft drinks, bottled iced teas, and sports drinks ranges from 2.5 to 3.5. Although these drinks are popular snacks, low-fat dairy products, water, and limited consumption of 100% fruit juice are preferable beverage alternatives. The American Academy of Pediatrics recommends infants under 6 months be fed only breast milk or an infant formula; avoid fruit juice before 1 year of age. Limit fruit juice to 4 oz/day for children 1 to 6 years old and 8 oz/day for children 7 to 18 years old.[20]

Timing and Sequence in a Meal

Another consideration is whether the cariogenic food is eaten with meals or snacks. Participants in the Vipeholm study who ate foods high in sugar between meals in addition to mealtime had a significantly higher decay rate than participants who consumed these foods at mealtime only.[15] Despite these results, recommendations to eliminate snacks are not always realistic. Children cannot eat enough food in three meals to get all the nutrients they need, and snacks are warranted. Foods chosen for snacks should produce little or no acid (Box 18.2), and oral self-care should follow a snack.

The location of an acidogenic food within a meal presents another consideration for caries potential. Drinking coffee with sugar after a meal has been determined to lower plaque pH, whereas consuming cheese after a fermentable carbohydrate within a meal prevents the decrease of plaque pH that would occur if this fermentable carbohydrate were eaten alone. Cariogenic foods create less risk of enamel demineralization if paired or followed by a noncariogenic or cariostatic food.

🦷 DENTAL CONSIDERATIONS

- Review diet history for patterns of fermentable carbohydrate consumption, frequency, form, and time consumed.
- Further questioning can reveal dietary habits the patient failed to recognize as being relevant to oral health.
- Fermentable carbohydrates alone do not cause dental decay. It is one factor in the decay process.

• BOX 18.2 Noncariogenic Foods

- Cheeses[a]
  - American
  - Blue cheese
  - Brie
  - Cheddar
  - Cheese spread
  - Cream cheese
  - Gouda
  - Monterey jack
  - Mozzarella
  - Swiss
- Yogurt[b]
- Nuts
- Chewing gum with xylitol
- Cocoa products
- Protein food sources[c]
  - Meat
  - Seafood
  - Poultry
  - Eggs
- Fat food sources[c]
  - Margarine
  - Butter
  - Oils

[a]These natural cheeses are high in fat. Reduced-fat or low-fat cheeses can be recommended.
[b]Encourage use of low-fat or skim versions, sugar free or plain.
[c]Follow *MyPlate* website and *Dietary Guidelines* for serving sizes and low-fat choices, and preparation methods.
Adapted from American Dental Association. *Diet and Dental Health.* https://www.mouthhealthy.org/en/all-topics-a-z/diet-and-dental-health. American Dental Association. *Nutrition: What You Eat Affects Your Teeth.* https://www.mouthhealthy.org/en/nutrition/food-tips.

• BOX 18.3 Populations That Would Benefit From Diet Education to Reduce Caries Risk

Early Childhood Caries
- Parents before pregnancy
- Parents during pregnancy
- Parents of young children

Lifecycle Stages
Adolescents
Older Adults

Root Caries and Xerostomia
- Periodontal patients
- Chronic disease states, for example, diabetes mellitus, chronic renal disease
- Polypharmacy
- Radiation therapy
- Gingival recession

Habits or Conditions
- Special needs individuals with oral sensitivity, restrictive eating behaviors, challenging oral health behaviors, etc.
- Frequent use of hard candy or chewing gum, cough drops, chewing tobacco, medication containing a fermentable carbohydrate source
- Frequent consumption of sports or energy drinks
- Frequent vomiting (e.g., bulimia)
- Poor oral hygiene
- Patients with orthodontic appliances
- Patients with dexterity challenges

Dental Issues
- Intake of low-fluoridation or nonfluoridated water
- Unsealed deep pits and fissures
- Family history of high caries risk
- Levels of cariogenic bacteria

NUTRITIONAL DIRECTIONS

- Consume fermentable carbohydrates at mealtimes (when possible) to allow other foods to neutralize acids in saliva.
- Foods that require chewing (e.g., sugar-free chewing gum, raw fruits, and vegetables) help increase salivary flow. This aids in providing additional buffering effects and accelerated removal of retentive foods.
- Noncariogenic snacks include raw fruits and vegetables, low-fat cheese, skim milk, low-fat yogurt, peanuts, popcorn, seeds, pizza, and tacos.
- Cariogenic snacks before bedtime should be omitted or followed by careful oral hygiene. Salivary flow is reduced when sleeping; clearance of plaque biofilm acids is limited. Uninterrupted acid production for 2 hours can be harmful.
- Consume fermentable carbohydrates within a meal, or eat a noncariogenic food last.
- Carbohydrate foods that are retentive (e.g., graham crackers or potato chips) are retained in the mouth longer, creating a greater potential for decay.
- Use products made with a nonnutritive sweetener, such as aspartame or sucralose in moderation (two to three products per day). Some patients may not tolerate large amounts of aspartame or other nonnutritive sweetener, or choose not to use them. Choose alternative noncariogenic food items and practice oral self-care.
- Limit purchasing soft drinks, and sports and energy drinks in large, resealable containers in an effort to decrease the frequency and duration of consumption.
- Athletes require fluid for hydration. In most events, lasting less than 4 hours, water is the preferred source of hydration rather than high-carbohydrate sports drinks.

Dental Hygiene Care Plan

Providing nutrition education is an essential component of the preventive program. Although all patients benefit from nutrition education, certain populations (Box 18.3) require special attention by the dental hygienist. As mentioned, the quantity of fermentable carbohydrates consumed is of concern, especially nutritionally. However, the form of the carbohydrate, how often it is consumed, and whether it is eaten with meals or snacks are more important for oral health than the amount consumed.

Assessment

When a dental nutrition care plan is necessary, many factors must be considered. Anthropometric measures (i.e., height and weight), clinical signs, dental and dietary assessment, health and dental history, and laboratory data (if applicable) are addressed in Chapter 21. In addition, an assessment takes into account a patient's learning style, literacy level, cultural heritage, and socioeconomic status. Caries Management by Risk Assessment (CaMBRA) is a popular tool used by dental professionals to identify risk of caries and to determine preventive and therapeutic goals for both children and adult patients.

The first step is to identify disease indicators (e.g., low income), caries risk factors (e.g., frequent snacks), and caries protective factors (e.g., use of products with xylitol) along with the clinical evaluation (e.g., number of existing restorations). Note that the age 6-to-adult form includes identification of medications associated with xerostomia while the 0-to-6-years form highlights acid exposure associated with childhood caries, such as the availability of bottles or sippy cups between meals or in the bed. The second step is to create and implement a treatment plan of action based on the risk outcome. The risk form can be used as a pedagogical tool by the dental professional to educate the patient. Risk factors are color coded for ease in explanation. For example, green designates *low risk*. A risk score can be obtained and compared to future risk forms. Detailed instructions on use of the form and educating patients are available on the American Dental Association website. Accompanying patient education material and sources are also provided.

Gathering information about the quality of the patient's meal pattern and eating habits is an important step in assessing the cariogenic potential of a diet. A food diary (Fig. 18.6), which provides food data for one day, can be obtained through an interview by the dental hygienist, or the patient can be asked to return the completed form at a recare appointment. This practical assessment tool is helpful in determining adequacy of the overall diet and habits related to carbohydrate intake. Fig. 18.7 shows a second example of a food diary.

Using *MyPlate* website as a guide, the dental hygienist can review adequacy of food intake with participation of the patient. Actively involving the patient in as many steps as possible enhances motivation and adherence. Ask the patient to highlight all fermentable carbohydrates on the food diary (see Figs. 18.6 and 18.7). Review the food diary and discuss any oversights with the patient as needed. Classify each fermentable carbohydrate as cariogenic or noncariogenic to assess caries potential (Fig. 18.8). This classification requires identifying the carbohydrate according to its form, frequency of consumption, and the time when it was eaten. More than two hours of acid exposure in one day is generally considered high.

Goals

When all the facts are gathered, help the patient develop realistic goals. These goals need to be flexible to meet the patient's needs, preferences, and lifestyle. Achievement of long-term goals is possible only if the patient is able and motivated to make behavioral changes, such as altering choices of cariogenic snacks or limiting frequency of cariogenic foods.

Education

Providing current information about detrimental dietary habits is instrumental in determining appropriate goals. Education alone does not guarantee behavioral change. For example, a patient

Food Diary Day ————				
Time	Place	Food Eaten	Amount Eaten	How Prepared
Example: 6:00 A.M.	Kitchen	Orange juice Whole wheat bread Diet margarine Egg	½ c 2 slices 1 tsp 1	Unsweetened Toasted Tub Fried in oil

Instructions:
1. List EVERYTHING you eat or drink on 3 consecutive, typical days.
2. Use 2 weekdays and 1 weekend day.
3. Include extras such as chewing gum, sugar and cream in coffee, or mustard on a sandwich.

• **Fig. 18.6** Food diary. Typically used for 1 to 7 days. (A customizable version is available on Evolve.)

Daily Food and Activity Diary

	Monday	Tuesday	Wednesday	Thursday	Friday	Saturday	Sunday
Breakfast							
Lunch							
Dinner							
Activity							

GOALS: DIET   **PHYSICAL ACTIVITY**

          BEHAVIOR

• **Fig. 18.7** Another example of a food diary. (From United States Department of Health and Human Services. National Heart, Lung and Blood Institute. https://www.nhlbi.nih.gov/health/educational/lose_wt/eat/diary.pdf.)

Carbohydrate Intake Analysis Worksheet

Fermentable CHO	Cariogenic?	Reason	Period of Exposure to Enamel
Banana and coffee with sugar	Yes	2 carbohydrates eaten at the same time; banana is retentive.	40 minutes
Pizza and regular soda (consumed together)	No	If soda is consumed with meal, carbohydrates in pizza (crust, sauce) and soda will be neutralized by fat and protein of other components of pizza.	0 minutes
Pizza and regular soda (consumed separately)	Yes	If consumption of soda is continued after the meal, there are no components to neutralize the carbohydrates in the soda.	20 minutes

TOTAL EXPOSURE TIME: _____

• **Fig. 18.8** Example of a carbohydrate intake analysis. (A customizable version is available on Evolve.)

may recite the process of decay and list components responsible for caries development, but if several areas of decay are evident at each 6-month recare visit, behavioral change has not occurred. Individualize dietary advice based on the patient's lifestyle, rather than requesting a change in lifestyle to accommodate recommendations. The patient's assessment and goals are the basis for any recommendations. The dental professional should attempt to dispel myths, redirect inappropriate habits, and provide new thoughts.

◆ **HEALTH APPLICATION 18**

Genetically Modified Foods

Genetically modified organisms (GMOs) consist of taking genetic material (DNA) from one plant, animal, or microorganism and inserting it into the permanent genetic code of another. This technology is also referred to as "genetic engineering" and "biotechnology."

The first genetically modified (GM) food, introduced in the mid-1990s, was herbicide-resistant soybeans. Currently, more than 85% of corn, soybeans, cotton, and sugar beets in the United States are genetically engineered. Additionally, other GM plants include quinoa, canola (rapeseed), rice, potatoes, and bananas. While the United States is the leading producer of GM foods, developing countries are planting GM crops at a more rapid rate than rich countries. Currently, GM foods are mostly plants, but foods derived from GM microorganisms or GM animals may become available in the near future. Very few fresh fruits and vegetables are GM, but highly processed foods, such as vegetable oils or breakfast cereals, most likely contain some percentage of GM ingredients.

GM plants are modified in the laboratory and marketed because of a perceived advantage either to the farmer or consumer, such as lower price, improved durability, or nutritional value. The purposes of genetic engineering are to (1) speed growth, (2) resist disease, (3) repel insects, (4) withstand harsh growing conditions, and (5) improve nutritional quality. The world faces serious problems in feeding 9 billion people by 2050. Agriculture production must be increased and ecosystem services maintained at a time when conditions for growing crops are predicted to worsen in many parts of the world.[21]

Malnutrition in developing countries is a consequence of a dearth of certain vitamins in staple foods, losses during crop processing, and overreliance on a single primary food source. Golden Rice is a GM rice that provides vitamin A. The beta-carotene in this rice is effectively converted to vitamin A and can be used to improve the vitamin A status of young children in developing countries.[22]

Insect resistance is accomplished by incorporating the gene for a toxin from the bacterium *Bacillus thuringiensis*. This toxin, used as a conventional insecticide in agriculture, is safe for human consumption. Viral resistance makes plants less susceptible to diseases caused by viruses, resulting in higher crop production.[23] The potential for GM seeds to result in bigger yields should lead to lower prices.

Altering the genetic makeup of plants and animals has been very controversial with concerns from many experts about the long-term effects on humans and the environment. Some of the concerns voiced include the potential for GM foods to cause (1) organ damage, (2) disrupt endocrine functions, (3) decrease fertility, (4) increase allergies, (5) increase pesticide resistance, (6) accelerate aging, and (7) promote immune system disorders. Indeed, no studies have tracked the long-term effect that GMOs may have on humans.

The main issues widely debated are the potential for GM foods to provoke allergic reaction, gene transfer, and cross-contamination. In response to the allegation that GM crops may increase allergenicity, foods that are considered highly allergenic are highly discouraged in producing GM products. When foods are digested and absorbed, a possibility exists that the genes can transfer through the digestive system, increasing antibiotic resistance and pesticide residues in the body. The World Health Organization indicates that the probability of transfer occurring is low, but using technology without antibiotic-resistant genes has been encouraged by an expert World Health Organization panel.[24,25] Some are fearful that modified plants or animals may have genetic changes that are unexpected and harmful. Some are concerned that the protein that was intended to be created during the manufacturing process may be different than what is actually created. Any minor error in a DNA sequence could cause various unintended effects and health issues.

A few of the concerns are legitimate. Whereas GM technology was supposed to decrease the need for pesticides to fight weeds and insects, herbicides in the production of two GM crops (soybeans and corn) have actually increased.[26] Resistant weeds have become a major problem for farmers using GM seeds. Genes from GM plants have cross-pollinated into conventional crops or related wild species as well as mixing with crops derived from conventional seeds with those grown using GM crops. This occurred when traces of maize approved for animals appeared in maize products produced for human consumption in the United States.[24,25]

The United States and Canada modified existing regulatory statutes to control GM foods. In the United States, three different government agencies have jurisdiction of GM foods. The US Environmental Protection Agency (EPA) evaluates GM plants for environmental safety. The US Department of Agriculture evaluates whether the plant is safe to grow; they are concerned with potential hazards of the plant itself. They ensure that the function of the introduced gene is known and the gene does not cause plant disease. The FDA evaluates whether the plant is safe to eat. The FDA has no control over the production of corn, but they regulate a box of cornflakes because it is a food product. To the FDA, GM foods are substantially equivalent to unmodified, "natural" foods, and are not subject to FDA regulations. Companies who create new GM foods are not required to consult the FDA nor are they required to follow any recommendations made by the FDA.

GM foods currently available have passed risk assessments and are not likely to present risks for human health. Conversely, there is little scientific data tracking the long-term effects that GMOs may have on humans, and the information available does not ensure complete safety. It is possible that GM foods may cause unexpected health consequences that will not be evident for years. Furthermore, it is impossible to design a long-term safety test in humans. Each new GM food should be assessed on an individual basis before being allowed on the market. General statements regarding the safety of all GM foods are inappropriate.

Most Americans would prefer that GM foods be labeled. Very low concentrations of GMOs in foods often cannot be detected. Proponents of labeling genetically engineered foods feel that consumers have a right to know where products come from when they are making food purchases. If all GM foods and food products are to be labeled, Congress must enact sweeping changes in the existing food labeling policy and establish acceptable limits of GM contamination in non-GM products. Labeling is mandatory in the European Union. Organic foods do not contain GM products.

There are many challenges for GM products in the areas of safety testing, regulation, international policy, and food labeling. This technology has enormous potential benefits, but caution is needed to avoid causing unintended harm to human health and the environment.

◆ CASE APPLICATION FOR THE DENTAL HYGIENIST

At his 6-month recare visit, John S. presented with six new areas of decay: one occlusal area (class I carious lesion), two proximal surfaces of posterior teeth (class II), and three proximal surfaces of anterior teeth (class III). There is bleeding on probing, suggesting active periodontal disease. John admits that his busy schedule prevents him from flossing his teeth. He stopped smoking and replaced it with chewing gum and hard candy since his last appointment. When asked about work, John states he takes antacids to settle his stomach because of the added pressures of his job.

Nutritional Assessment
- Food, nutrient, and caloric intake
- Frequency of eating between meals
- Eating habits
- Motivation level
- Knowledge level

Nutritional Diagnosis

Altered nutrition: frequent intake of chewing gum, hard candy, and antacids at various intervals throughout the day compounded by an increased plaque index, a measure of the quantity and location of plaque biofilm.

Nutritional Goals

The patient will improve his overall nutrient intake and make substitutions or modify the habits increasing his caries risk.

Nutritional Implementation

Intervention: Provide a food diary (see Figs. 18.8 and 18.9) with an explanation for its use and instructions emphasizing the importance of listing everything put into his mouth.
Rationale: The food record provides additional information about John's intake and reveals habits that he may have neglected to mention, thinking they were not relevant to his dental needs.
Intervention: Review the food record with John to identify health aspects and aspects needing revision. Allow John to make the necessary changes.
Rationale: The probability of a patient adhering to a recommended regimen is enhanced when the patient is actively involved in the decision-making process. The dental hygienist can suggest possible solutions and direct misguided changes. The patient ultimately makes required changes.

Intervention: Explain the caries process, and factors involved.
Rationale: Understanding the total picture of his particular dental status can be motivating for John and may help him make needed changes.
Intervention: Stress that not only the quantity of fermentable carbohydrates in his diet, but also spacing, duration, frequency, and form of intake lead to caries. Use the Carbohydrate Intake Analysis Worksheet (see Fig. 18.10) as an educational tool to enhance the explanation.
Rationale: Each time the patient consumes a fermentable carbohydrate, even if it is a small mint, he is decreasing the plaque pH to an acidic level for 40 minutes. By consuming sugar-containing mints six times throughout the day, the acid produced by plaque bacteria may be present for 4 hours.
Intervention: Educate John about the cariogenic potential of sugar-containing antacids and discuss options to avoid or reduce use of antacids. Another option may be to use sugar-free antacids, although his condition should be evaluated by his health care provider if it persists.
Rationale: Sugar-containing antacids contain simple carbohydrates and have cariogenic potential. Antacids are high in sodium and can interfere with absorption of many nutrients. Suggestions to decrease use of antacids include consuming small, frequent meals; eating slowly; avoiding excessive amounts of caffeine products and alcohol; and reducing stress. Referral to the health care provider is necessary for persistent heartburn to ensure diagnosis and management of gastroesophageal reflux, which may increase the risk for caries and dental erosion and esophageal cancer.
Intervention: Praise John for his ability to quit smoking (see Chapter 19, *Health Application 19*).
Rationale: Smoking is a very difficult habit to break; many who stop smoking will start again, especially in stressful situations.
Intervention: Recommend fluoride treatments in the office and at home; sealants, if applicable; an antimicrobial rinse; and optimum oral self-care practices.
Rationale: Omitting the carbohydrate source is not the only factor involved in the caries process. In John's situation, protecting susceptible tooth surfaces and removing plaque biofilm also help eliminate the potential for caries.

Evaluation

The patient returns for his 6-month recare appointment, caries free with a reduction in gingival bleeding. He is still not smoking and uses a chewing gum and mints with xylitol. He has begun an exercise program, which is helping to relieve his stress, and he has decreased the use of antacids.

◆ Student Readiness

1. Explain the role of firm, fibrous foods in protecting the tooth against caries.
2. List several noncariogenic substitutions for fermentable carbohydrate snacks.
3. What are the different roles that carbohydrates, protein, and fat play in the decay process?
4. Identify at least four nutritional foods contraindicated for a caries-active patient.
5. Complete a 1- to 3-day food diary (see Figs. 18.8 and 18.9). Assess for nutrient adequacy, comparing it with *MyPlate* website. Highlight the fermentable carbohydrates.
6. Based on the food diary from Question 5, complete the example Carbohydrate Intake Analysis worksheet (see Fig. 18.10). Determine your cariogenic behaviors and the number of minutes of acid production. Based on this intake record, create a realistic and appropriate meal pattern. Discuss the rationale for modifications and substitutions.
7. Compare the pH, grams of sugar, and milligrams of caffeine for an 8-oz serving of 100% apple juice, skim milk, an energy drink, a sports drink, soda, a fruit drink, and water. Provide a conclusion based on your findings.

◆ CASE STUDY

Carol is a 42-year-old married high school graduate with three teenage children. She is a homemaker and does all the cooking and grocery shopping. Each member of Carol's family continues to have new areas of decay at each recare visit. The dental hygienist decides to have Carol write down her food consumption from the previous day while waiting for her appointment. Her food record showed the following details:

Breakfast: skipped
Morning snack: glazed doughnut, coffee with cream and sugar
Lunch: grilled cheese sandwich, taco chips, gelatin salad with fruit and whipped cream, coffee with cream and sugar
Afternoon snack: candy bar and two or three homemade cookies throughout the afternoon
Dinner: meat loaf, fried potatoes, buttered carrots, roll with margarine
Evening snack: chocolate chip ice cream

1. What other information needs to be obtained before starting to educate the patient?
2. What dental information does Carol need to have?
3. What dietary recommendations should a dental hygienist suggest? What are some specific substitutions and modifications that can be made?
4. Approximately how many minutes of acid production occurred on the enamel surfaces this day?

CASE STUDY

As a new mother, Barbara wanted to take precautionary measures to prevent her daughter from having rampant dental decay, like the neighborhood children. She breastfed the infant until 9 months of age and refused to allow any sugar-containing foods, including ice cream. The daughter was frequently observed carrying a box of crackers and her sippy cup around the house. By age 3 years, she has six carious lesions.

1. When should nutrition education have first been initiated for Barbara? Explain.
2. Describe the procedure that a dental professional would take to educate Barbara.
3. What suggestions would you recommend to Barbara?

References

1. National Center for Health Statistics. Chapter 32: Oral conditions. *Healthy People 2030 Midcourse Review*. 2016. https://www.cdc.gov/nchs/data/hpdata2020/HP2020MCR-C32-OH.pdf.
2. National Center for Health Statistics. *Health, United States, 2020–2021: Table Dental Visits in the Past Year Among Adults Aged 18 and Over, by Selected Characteristics: United States, Selected Years 1997–2019*. 2021. https://www.cdc.gov/nchs/hus/data-finder.htm.
3. Wakhloo T, Reddy SG, Sharma SK, et al. Silver diamine fluoride vs atraumatic restorative treatment in pediatric dental caries management: a systematic review and *meta*-analysis. *J Int Soc Prev Community Dent*. 2021;11(4):367–375.
4. Figuero E, Nobrega DF, Garcia-Gargallo M, et al. Mechanical and chemical plaque control in the simultaneous management of gingivitis and caries: a systematic review. *J Clin Periodontol*. 2017;44(suppl 18):S116–S134.
5. Takenaka S, Ohsumi T, Noiri Y. Evidence-based strategy for dental biofilms: current evidence of mouthwashes on dental biofilm and gingivitis. *Jpn Dent Sci Rev*. 2019;55(1):33–40.
6. Tran K, Butcher R. *Chlorhexidine for Oral Care: A Review of Clinical Effectiveness and Guidelines*. Canadian Agency for Drugs and Technologies in Health; 2019. Available from: https://www.ncbi.nlm.nih.gov/books/NBK541430/.
7. Ricciuto L, Fulgoni VL, Gaine PC, Scott MO, DiFrancesco L. Trends in added sugars intake and sources among United States children, adolescents, and teens using NHANES 2001–2018. *J Nutr*. 2022;152(2):568–578.
8. United States Department of Agriculture and United States Department of Health and Human Services. *Dietary Guidelines for Americans, 2020–2025*. 9th ed. December 2020.
9. Chevinsky JR, Lee SH, Blanck HM, Park S. Prevalence of self-reported intake of sugar-sweetened beverages among United States adults in 50 states and the District of Columbia, 2010 and 2015. *Prev Chronic Dis*. 2021;18:200434.
10. Park S, Onufrak S, Blanck HM, et al. Characteristics associated with consumption of sports and energy drinks among United States adults: National Health Interview Survey, 2010. *J Acad Nutr Diet*. 2013;113(1):112–119.
11. Field AE, Sonneville KR, Falbe J, et al. Association of sports drinks with weight gain among adolescents and young adults. *Obes (Silver Spring, Md)*. 2014;22(10):2238–2243.
12. Tenelanda-López D, Valdivia-Moral P, Castro-Sánchez M. Eating habits and their relationship to oral health. *Nutrients*. 2020;12(9):2619. https://doi.org/10.3390/nu12092619.
13. ALHumaid J, Bamashmous M. *Meta*-analysis on the effectiveness of xylitol in caries prevention. *J Int Soc Prev Community Dent*. 2022;12(2):133–138.
14. Food and Drug Administration. Code of Federal Regulations Title 21, Volume 2: Food labeling, specific requirements for health claims. In: *Health Claims: Dietary Noncariogenic Carbohydrate Sweeteners and Dental Caries*. https://www.ecfr.gov/current/title-21/chapter-I/subchapter-B/part-101/subpart-E/section-101.80; https://www.accessdata.fda.gov/scripts/cdrh/cfdocs/cfcfr/cfrsearch.cfm?fr=101.80.
15. Gustaffson BE, Quensel CE, Lanke LS, et al. The Vipeholm dental caries study: the effect of different levels of carbohydrate intake on caries activity in 436 individuals observed for 5 years. *Acta Odontol Scand*. 1954;11:232–364.
16. Kim YR, Nam SH. A randomized, double-blind, placebo-controlled clinical trial of a mouthwash containing *Glycyrrhiza uralensis* extract for preventing dental caries. *Int J Env Res Public Health*. 2021;19(1):242. https://doi.org/10.3390/ijerph19010242.
17. Kwon YJ, Son DH, Chung TH, Lee YJ. A review of the pharmacological efficacy and safety of licorice root from corroborative clinical trial findings. *J Med Food*. 2020;23(1):12–20. https://doi.org/10.1089/jmf.2019.4459.
18. Shi J, Wang Q, Ruan G, et al. Efficacy of probiotics against dental caries in children: a systematic review and *meta*-analysis. *Crit Rev Food Sci Nutr*. 2022:1–18.
19. National Academies of Sciences, Engineering, and Medicine; Health and Medicine Division; Food and Nutrition Board; Committee on the Dietary Reference Intakes for Energy. *Dietary Reference Intakes for Energy*. National Academies Press (United States); 2023. https://www.ncbi.nlm.nih.gov/books/NBK588659/ https://doi.org/10.17226/26818.
20. Hayman MB, Abrams SA, Section on Gastroenterology, Hepatology and Nutrition and Committee on Nutrition Fruit juice in infants, children, and adolescents: current recommendations. *Pediatrics*. 2017;139(6):e20170967.
21. Raybould A, Poppy GM. Commercializing genetically modified crops under EU regulations: objectives and barriers. *GM Crop Food*. 2012;3(1):9–20.
22. De Steur H, Demont M, Gellynck X, et al. The social and economic impact of biofortification through genetic modification. *Curr Opin Biotechnol*. 2017;44:161–168.
23. Wani SH, Choudhary M, Barmukh R, et al. Molecular mechanisms, genetic mapping, and genome editing for insect pest resistance in field crops. *Theor Appl Genet*. 2022;135(11):3875–3895.
24. United States Food and Drug Administration. *How GMOs Are Regulated in the United States*. https://www.fda.gov/food/agricultural-biotechnology/how-gmos-are-regulated-united-states.
25. National Library of Medicine. Medline Plus. *Genetically Engineered Foods*. https://medlineplus.gov/ency/article/002432.htm.
26. Perry ED, Ciliberto F, Hennessy DA, et al. Genetically engineered crops and pesticide use in United States maize and soybeans. *Sci Adv*. 2016;2:e1600850.

▶ Evolve Resources

Please visit http://evolve.elsevier.com/Mallonee/nutritional for additional practice and study support tools.

19

Nutritional Aspects of Gingivitis and Periodontal Disease

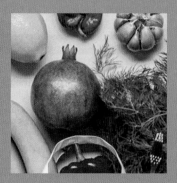

STUDENT LEARNING OUTCOMES

On completion of this chapter, the student will be able to achieve the following student learning outcomes:

1. Describe the role that nutrition plays in periodontal health and disease for a patient.
2. List the effects of food consistency and composition in periodontal disease.
3. Describe nutritional factors associated with gingivitis and periodontitis.
4. Discuss the following related to periodontal surgery and necrotizing periodontal disease:

- Discuss components of nutritional education for a periodontal patient.
- List major differences between full liquid, mechanically altered, bland, and regular diets.
- Discuss nutrient deficiencies and oral health issues related to necrotizing periodontal disease.

KEY TERMS

Clinical attachment loss	Full liquid diet	Purulent exudate
Fibrotic	Mechanically altered diet	Suppuration

TEST YOUR NQ

1. **T/F** Vitamin-mineral supplementation beyond recommended levels is ineffective in controlling or preventing periodontal disease.
2. **T/F** Firm, fibrous foods physically remove plaque biofilm from the gingiva and tooth surface.
3. **T/F** A deficiency of vitamin C causes gingivitis.
4. **T/F** A bland, soft diet is commonly prescribed for a patient with necrotizing ulcerative gingivitis (NUG)/necrotizing ulcerative periodontitis (NUP).
5. **T/F** An appropriate instruction to a patient after periodontal surgery is, "Eat whatever foods you can manage."
6. **T/F** An individual with uncontrolled diabetes should be referred to a registered dietitian nutritionist for nutrition counseling if the diet

needs to be modified because of oral discomfort, such as with NUG/NUP or after a periodontal procedure.
7. **T/F** Whole milk and milkshakes mixed with an instant breakfast mix are acceptable on a full liquid diet.
8. **T/F** A mechanically altered diet is similar to a regular diet except in consistency and texture.
9. **T/F** It is acceptable for a dental hygienist to recommend an instant breakfast drink or liquid supplement to a periodontal patient who is temporarily following a full liquid diet.
10. **T/F** The dental hygienist should complete the nutritional assessment and provide nutritional education immediately after periodontal surgery.

Gingivitis is characterized by inflammation; swelling, changes in contour or consistency; presence of plaque biofilm or calculus or both; no evidence of attachment loss or radiographic bone loss; and bleeding on probing is between 10% and 30% (Fig. 19.1A).[1] Gingivitis is often reversible with appropriate oral self-care techniques to remove biofilm. Gingivitis can progress to periodontal disease.

Periodontal disease is a chronic, inflammatory, and infectious disease (see Fig. 19.1B). It is the result of a loss of connective tissue and alveolar bone. Common findings are gingival bleeding, inflammation, attachment loss, **suppuration** (formation or discharge of pus), tooth mobility, and furcation involvement.[2] Two targets for *Healthy People 2030* are (1) to reduce the prevalence of

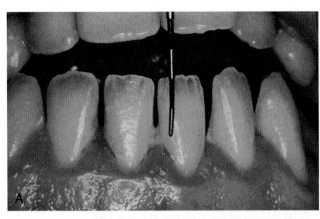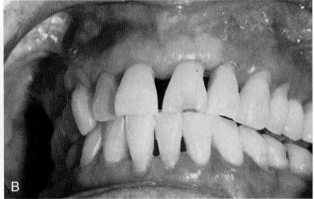

• **Fig. 19.1** (A) Gingivitis. (B) Periodontal disease. (A, From Perry DA, Beemsterboer P, Essex G. *Periodontology for the Dental Hygienist*. 4th ed. Saunders Elsevier; 2014. B, Courtesy Barbara D. Altshuler, BSDH, MS, Clinical Assistant Professor, Caruth School of Dental Hygiene, The Texas A&M University System, Baylor College of Dentistry, Dallas, TX.)

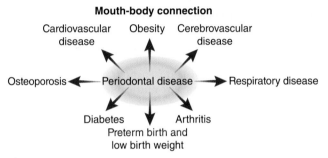

• **Fig. 19.2** The possible connections between periodontal disease and other systemic diseases or conditions.

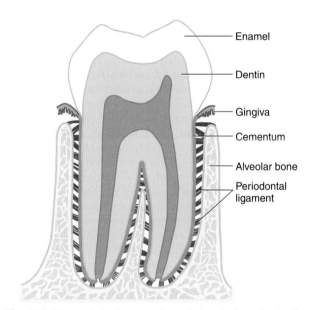

• **Fig. 19.3** The periodontium consists of the gingiva, alveolar bone, cementum, and periodontal ligament. (From Fehrenbach MJ, Popowics T. *Illustrated Dental Embryology, Histology, and Anatomy*. 4th ed. Saunders Elsevier; 2016.)

moderate and severe periodontitis from nearly 44.5% to 39.3% in people aged 45 to 74 years and (2) to reduce the prevalence of tooth loss from 8.9% to 5.4%.[3]

The inflammatory process of gingivitis and periodontal disease is affected by the host's immune response—the body's ability to protect itself from destructive periodontal pathogens and infection. Nutritional deficiencies, which may occur from adolescence through adulthood, can modify the body's response to periodontal disease. Bacteria associated with periodontal disease may increase the risk of systemic diseases or conditions such as cardiovascular disease, stroke, premature births, respiratory infections, and uncontrolled diabetes (Fig. 19.2).[4,5]

The involvement of nutrition in periodontal disease is not as clear as it is for dental caries. Predisposing, etiologic, and contributing factors of periodontal disease are diverse; however, the primary initiating agent is plaque biofilm accumulation around teeth and gingiva. Nutrient deficiencies, excesses, or imbalances do not initiate periodontal disease, and megadoses of vitamin-mineral supplements do not cure or prevent periodontal disease. Indirectly, nutritional status may alter development, resistance, or repair of the periodontium (Fig. 19.3), which ultimately affects severity and extent of the disease.[6] In addition, a patient's health, medications, and food choices influence the properties of plaque biofilm and saliva. The buffering and antimicrobial effects of saliva are significant factors in periodontal disease. A change in composition or amount of saliva can influence development and maturation of plaque biofilm (see discussion of xerostomia in Chapter 20).

Physical Effects of Food on Periodontal Health

Food Composition

The classes of macronutrients and micronutrients that have physiologic roles in growth, maintenance, and repair include carbohydrates, proteins, fats, vitamins, minerals, and water. At least 50 nutrients are provided by food, most of which are required for a healthy periodontium. An imbalance of one or more nutrients can be a factor in the disruption of tissue integrity and immune response. Consuming adequate amounts of each is the ultimate goal.

Normal growth and development of periodontal and oral mucosal tissues depend on sufficient intake of vitamin A (salivary glands, epithelial tissue), vitamin C (collagen, connective

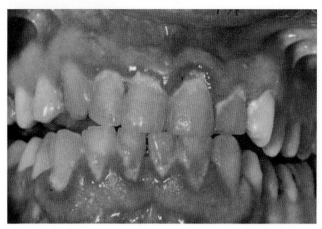

• **Fig. 19.4** Gingivitis-related malnutrition. (From Perry DA, Beemsterboer P, Essex G. *Periodontology for the Dental Hygienist*. 4th ed. Saunders Elsevier; 2014.)

• **BOX 19.1**   **Nutritional Involvement in Periodontal Disease**

A patient's dietary intake plays a role in periodontal health, directly and indirectly affecting:
• Growth and development, maintenance, and repair of the periodontium
• Amount and type of supragingival plaque biofilm
• Inflammation and immune response for optimal healing
• Amount and type of saliva
• Host resistance to decrease the susceptibility to infection

tissue), and vitamin B complex (epithelial and connective tissue). Calcification of the alveolus and cementum requires amino acids, calcium, phosphorus, vitamin D, and magnesium. Maintenance of oral tissues and integrity of the host's immune and repair responses requires sufficient amounts of vitamins A, C, D, and E; proteins; carbohydrates; fiber; calcium; iron; zinc; folic acid; and omega-3 fatty acids. Higher caloric ranges also are indicated for increased metabolic needs for individuals with periodontal disease (Refer to Chapters 4–12 for more descriptive information on the effects of specific nutrients on the periodontium.)[7–9] Note the inflammation, bulbous tissue, edema, and suppuration in Fig. 19.4 depicting gingivitis-related malnutrition.

Supragingival plaque biofilm adhesion and formation is influenced by frequent dietary consumption of monosaccharides (e.g., glucose) and disaccharides, particularly sucrose.[10] Subgingival plaque biofilm seems to be protected from local effects of sugars.

Nutritional intervention needs to be a component of the dental hygiene care plan for periodontal disease because poor nutrition affects the entire body, having an adverse effect on the periodontium. In combination with local irritating factors, such as plaque biofilm or tobacco use, systemic factors can increase risk or severity of periodontal disease of a patient but is not solely responsible for periodontal disease.[6] A nutrition assessment by the dental hygienist can reveal dietary deficiencies that should be corrected for optimal healing. Referral to a registered dietitian nutritionist (RDN) may be indicated, particularly for compromised patients requiring medical nutrition therapy, such as patients with uncontrolled diabetes.

Food Consistency

Another factor affecting periodontal health is the texture of food. Chewing firm, coarse, and fibrous foods, such as raw fruits and vegetables, increases the chewing (or oral processing) time and stimulates salivary flow.[11] The increase in saliva enhances oral clearance of food, thereby reducing oral pH and risk for caries.[12,13] However, plaque biofilm is not physically removed by eating firm textured foods. Soft, sticky foods with fermentable carbohydrates increase retention of food, which enhances dental biofilm growth.[14]

Nutritional Considerations for Periodontal Patients

Increased nutrients and energy are required by periodontal patients experiencing stress, tissue catabolism, or infection. A thorough assessment of the periodontal patient, as described in Chapter 21, provides valuable data needed to formulate a nutrition plan.

A medical and social history can indicate whether a patient is at risk of nutrient deficiencies because of alcohol use disorder, eating disorders, or other chronic disease (e.g., inflammatory bowel disease). These patients would benefit from medical nutrition therapy by an RDN to normalize nutrient levels before treatment.

Dietary education using *MyPlate* website and the *Dietary Guidelines* of all periodontal patients by the dental hygienist facilitates tissue repair and wound healing, improves resistance to infection, and reduces the number and severity of complications. In particular, the Mediterranean diet and DASH dietary patterns have been shown to result in lower risk for periodontal disease.[15] These dietary patterns include less red meat with more fruit, vegetable, nuts, and whole grain intake (fiber) and are healthy options for most patients. Optimally, good nutritional status results in a shorter recovery time and a more rapid return to health (Box 19.1).

Gingivitis

Gingivitis is an inflammatory process beginning in the interdental papillae and advancing to the attached gingiva. The color of the gingiva varies from slight redness to a darker reddish blue. The gingiva bleeds easily and is either edematous and spongy, or **fibrotic** (formation of fibrous tissue of the gingiva owing to chronic inflammation). The stippling of the gingiva disappears, and probing depths may increase without loss of attachment. Gingivitis is associated with a large accumulation of plaque biofilm and calculus on teeth (Fig. 19.5), which is exacerbated by frequent exposure to fermentable carbohydrates and retentive foods.

Gingival disease may be nonplaque (or biofilm) induced or plaque induced. Nonplaque induced gingivitis may be related to infectious agents (e.g., viral and fungal), immune conditions, reactive processes, neoplasms, trauma, vitamin deficiency (scurvy), and gingival pigmentation.[16]

Of the possible etiologies, the primary nutrition related cause of nonplaque induced gingivitis is scurvy, however, it is rarely seen in the United States. Scurvy's clinical features include: hemorrhage, bluish red gingiva, a widened periodontal ligament, and tooth mobility. Correcting the vitamin C deficiency through appropriate food choices, and sometimes supplementation, improves symptoms of scurvy. Inadequate levels of vitamin C has also been associated with progression of periodontitis, however, it is unclear

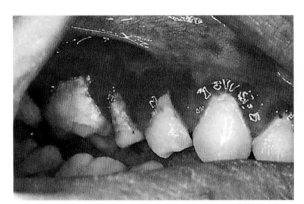

• **Fig. 19.5** Gingivitis, with heavy calculus present. (From Darby ML, Walsh MM. *Dental Hygiene: Theory and Practice.* 4th ed. Saunders Elsevier; 2015.)

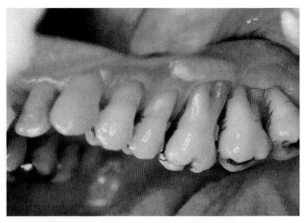

• **Fig. 19.6** Clinical attachment loss. (From Perry DA, Beemsterboer P, Essex G. *Periodontology for the Dental Hygienist.* 4th ed. Saunders Elsevier; 2014.)

if supplementation improves periodontal status.[17,18] Therefore, it is essential that dental hygienists assess and encourage adequate intake of good sources for vitamin C to maintain adequate levels.

A lack of nutrients does not cause gingival inflammation but may be a predisposing factor by disrupting the process of tissue repair. Adequate nutrients can hasten healing and repair processes. Controlling or modifying the etiologic factors can reverse clinical characteristics. Nutritional interventions for varying severities of gingivitis are the same as those for promoting overall health by encouraging adequate intake of all food groups and analyzing fermentable carbohydrate intake to determine potentially damaging habits that intensify the gingivitis.

Periodontitis

Periodontitis is an inflammatory disease characterized by progressive **clinical attachment loss** (Fig. 19.6).[19] Severity of the gingival inflammation, bleeding, gingival recession, bone loss (Fig. 19.7), tooth mobility, and periodontal pocket formation varies according to duration of disease and the host factors such as smoking and diabetes. It can be localized or generalized with **purulent exudate** or drainage of fluids from the gingival sulcus.

Initiation and progression of periodontitis do not occur unless plaque biofilm is present. As with gingivitis, certain types of food (e.g., soft, retentive, or fermentable carbohydrate) can enhance food retention providing a source of nutrients for growth of microorganisms in plaque biofilm. In addition to retentive carbohydrates, dietary carbohydrates provide a nutrient source for bacterial growth in the early stages of biofilm development.[20] Then anaerobic organisms in periodontal disease are less dependent on dietary carbohydrates and more interdependent on other organisms for nutrients for growth.[20]

Systemically, nutritional status affects the immune response in periodontal disease. Adequate Vitamin D intake appears to have a role in limiting inflammation, bleeding, and is associated with less severe periodontal disease.[21] Low calcium levels have also been associated with higher risk for periodontal disease.[7] This suggests the importance of counseling patients on the need to consume dairy products and check with their primary care provider about assessing vitamin D levels to ensure the patient is not deficient. As noted previously in the chapter, inadequate vitamin C intake may increase risk for periodontal disease.[6,17,18] A recent systematic review found intake of omega-3 fatty acids, green/oolong tea, polyphenols, and flavonoids as adjunctive therapy had a beneficial effect on pocket depth and bleeding after non-surgical periodontal therapy.[22] Probiotics along with non-surgical periodontal therapy have also been shown to improve plaque and gingival index; pocket depth; attachment level; bleeding on probing, and levels of subgingival microorganisms.[23] Given average intake of vegetables, fruits, dairy, whole grains, and seafood are below recommended levels in adults,[24] dental hygienists are in an ideal position to educate and encourage patients to follow the healthy dietary patterns in *MyPlate* website and the *Dietary Guidelines* to provide these nutrients.

🦷 DENTAL CONSIDERATIONS

Assessment
- *Physical:* Gingival tissue is red to reddish blue, or pink if fibrotic; interdental papillae are often bulbous; spontaneous bleeding on probing; the gingival margin is coronal to the cementoenamel junction; periodontal condition may be asymptomatic.
- *Dietary:* Adequate nutrient and calorie intake; frequency and amount of alcohol consumption.

Intervention
- Educate the patient that tissue damage associated with gingivitis is reversible.
- Encourage tailored oral self-care regimens.
- Provide oral prophylaxis, including biofilm and endotoxin debridement.

Evaluation
- Satisfactory response to therapy, resulting in healthy tissue; patient is able to demonstrate adequate oral hygiene techniques; adequate dietary intake.

🦷 NUTRITIONAL DIRECTIONS

- Optimal nutrient intake impacts the growth, development, maintenance, and repair of the periodontium throughout the life cycle.
- Encourage nutrient-dense foods that are not retentive. Soft foods are followed by appropriate oral hygiene.
- Encourage a variety of foods, including foods and beverages rich in vitamin C. Use the *Dietary Guidelines* and *MyPlate* website as a guide.
- Poor nutrient intake is not the sole reason for periodontal disease. It is one risk factor that can affect the severity and extent of the disease.

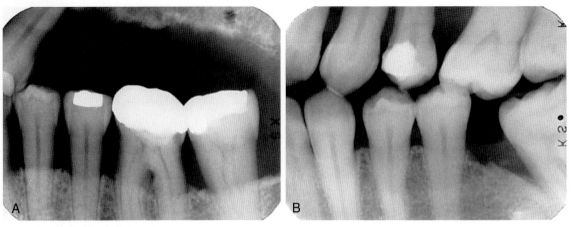

• **Fig. 19.7** Horizontal (A) and vertical (B) bone loss. (From Iannucci JM, Howerton LJ. *Dental Radiography: Principles and Techniques*. 4th ed. Saunders Elsevier; 2012.)

Periodontal Surgery

Preoperative

If periodontal surgery is indicated, the body's immunologic competency is important for optimal healing and preventing or minimizing infections. The dental hygienist should conduct a preliminary assessment of the patient for adequate nutrient reserves before the dental procedure. If the recommendations of the *Dietary Guidelines* and *MyPlate* website are met, the patient's dietary intake is considered adequate for most healthy individuals. Generally, minor periodontal surgical procedures on a healthy patient with an adequate intake do not require special dietary modification. Surgery on a medically complex patient, particularly for those who may be inadequately nourished or malnourished, may require attention to nutrition prior to surgery. An elective surgery may need to be postponed for 1 or 2 weeks to allow improvement in nutritional status. A medically compromised patient is best served by an RDN who can appropriately assess and determine energy and other nutrient requirements.

Before surgery, the patient should be given a tailored meal plan listing nutrient-dense, fortified and enriched foods and beverages to consume during the recovery period. Milk and 100% fruit juices contain more nutrients than soft drinks, even if caloric value is similar. The dental hygienist should consider the extent of the surgery, its potential discomfort, and the patient's ability to eat after the periodontal procedure, and encourage food choices that avoid tissue trauma. The patient's food preferences and dislikes are other factors to be taken into consideration.

Postoperative

Because of blood loss, increased catabolism, tissue regeneration, and host defense activities after periodontal surgery, adequate nutrient intake is required. Meeting the requirements for calories, proteins, vitamins, minerals, and decaffeinated fluids (8–10 glasses a day) may enhance recovery.

Dietary intake can be influenced by complications of anorexia, nausea, dysphagia, and oral discomfort. The texture of foods depends on extent of the surgery and symptoms of the patient. A full liquid diet may be required the first 1 to 3 days (Box 19.2). Recommendation of a nutritional supplement drink as part of the full liquid diet may be warranted after surgery to improve periodontal healing.[25] Many high-protein supplement drinks are available over the counter for patients. For medically complex patients such as those with diabetes, coordinate efforts with an RDN to ensure the patient is getting the proper nutritional guidance to maintain glycemic control.

A full liquid diet provides food in a liquid form for patients who are unable to chew. It should consist of high-protein, high-calorie fluids and semisolid foods to promote optimal healing. Fluids can be drunk from a cup. A full liquid diet is used only temporarily because nutrient and caloric value is usually inadequate. Any special diet modifications (e.g., low sodium, low fat) and patient preferences should be considered.

A periodontal dressing may be used to cover and protect the surgical site; shield the tissue from irritation; help control postoperative bleeding, edema, and infection; and prevent accumulation of food debris and bacteria. Cool liquids and foods for the first 24 hours may be appealing and aid in minimizing swelling. Discourage smoking and using straws because sucking pressure could dislodge a blood clot. The full liquid diet can progress to a mechanically altered diet when tolerated. A mechanically altered diet (Box 19.3) consists of a regular diet altered in consistency and texture by whipping, blending, grinding, chopping, or mashing foods for ease in mastication when chewing is compromised. Foods are generally moist. Depending on the surgery performed, it may be necessary to avoid seeds and nuts. The mechanically altered diet is recommended for 3 to 7 days until the patient can tolerate regular foods. Consuming small, frequent meals (e.g., six small feedings one-half the size of a regular meal) may provide adequate intake and is easier for the patient. Bland foods (Box 19.4) may be necessary to avoid irritating sensitive tissue. A high-protein liquid nutritional supplement may be recommended depending on the patient's ability to consume the mechanically altered diet to ensure adequate nutrients to support recovery.

🦷 DENTAL CONSIDERATIONS

Assessment

• *Physical:* Pale-pink to purplish-red gingival tissue (firm to spongy); interdental papillae may not fill the interdental spaces; bleeding on probing and suppuration may occur; probing depths of 4 mm or more; tooth mobility, furcation involvement, and pain may be present.
• *Dietary:* Adequacy of dietary and fluid intake; avoidance of alcohol; use of vitamin-mineral supplements.

DENTAL CONSIDERATIONS—CONT'D

Interventions

- Oral prophylaxis to debride and reduce plaque biofilm, and thus reduce infectious microorganisms.
- The periodontist or dentist may recommend an antimicrobial such as chlorhexidine mouth rinse to aid healing.
- Instruct the patient to avoid hard, sticky, and brittle foods and to follow the guidelines for a mechanically altered diet for 1 to 2 days.
- Encourage appropriate techniques for optimal oral self-care.
- Provide smoking-cessation counseling, if needed (see *Health Application 19* at the end of this chapter).
- Collaborate with the diabetes care provider to maintain glycemic control during healing.
- Identify and recommend modification of open margins, overhangs, inadequate restorations.
- Recommend or provide fluoride therapy for desensitization, if needed.

Evaluation

- Absence of inflammation and other signs of periodontal issues, such as pain and ulcerations; adherence to an adequate diet; avoiding alcohol and smoking; maintaining regular recare appointments with a healthy periodontal clinical assessment.

NUTRITIONAL DIRECTIONS

- Postsurgical patients may require a full liquid or mechanically altered diet until the patient can chew comfortably.
- To meet energy and nutrient needs, postsurgical patients typically require small, frequent meals and nutrient-dense foods and beverages.
- A patient receiving medical nutrition therapy, such as for diabetes, may need a referral to an RDN.
- Discuss with the patient how alcohol misuse may contribute to periodontal issues because of enhanced bleeding tendencies and a propensity toward malnutrition.
- There is emerging evidence that probiotics may inhibit growth of plaque biofilm and bacteria associated with periodontal disease (see Table 20.1 in Chapter 20). Probiotics vary in means of administration, including foods, tablets, chewing gums, and lozenges. Probiotics are live microorganisms differing in strains and strengths; therefore, selecting the correct strain for a specific oral issue is essential and complex (see Chapter 3). Other considerations for selecting a probiotic include mode and time of administration; health of the patient; and retention and exposure times in the oral cavity. Further rigorous research is needed in this area.[26–28]

• BOX 19.2   Full Liquid Diet: Oral Surgery

Purpose

To provide a high-protein, high-calorie liquid diet to promote healing in cleft lip and cleft palate repair, oral surgery (when chewing is difficult), or mouth irritations when solid foods are not tolerated.

Adequacy

This diet meets the Dietary Reference Intakes for energy, carbohydrates, protein, fat, calcium, and vitamin C for children and adults. It may be inadequate in all other nutrients. Nutritional adequacy can be improved by the addition of a commercial nutritional supplement. For prolonged use, a multivitamin-mineral supplement should be considered.

Description

All foods are liquid or semisolid at room temperature. All foods are of a consistency that can be drunk from a cup without a spoon or straw.

Guidelines

This is a transitional diet: it should be followed by the mechanically altered diet to a regular diet. Oral nutritional supplements are recommended after 48 hours. Refer to an RDN or a health care provider if the patient requires longer time on this diet. A multivitamin-mineral supplement may be needed. Six small meals are recommended.

Sample Menu for Full Liquid Diet for Oral Surgery Patients

Breakfast	Snack	Lunch	Snack	Dinner
½ cup apple juice	8 oz malted milk	½ cup cranberry juice	½ cup ice cream with chocolate syrup	½ cup grape juice½ cup gelatin
8 oz smoothie made with yogurt and fruit		8 oz strained cream of pea soup with pureed ham		
1 cup cream of wheat cereal with butter		12 oz milkshake mixed with instant breakfast powder		8 oz tomato soup made with milk and additional milk powder
1 cup whole milk		8 oz whole milk		8 oz vanilla yogurt
		½ cup custard		1 cup eggnog
				½ cup of pudding

Approximate Nutrient Composition for Sample Full Liquid Diet for Oral Surgery Patients

Calories, 2649
Carbohydrate, 345 g
Protein, 102 g
Fat, 100 g
Cholesterol, 484 mg
Dietary fiber, 13 g

Sodium, 3622 mg
Potassium, 5191 mg
Calcium, 3019 mg
Iron, 18 mg
Vitamin A, 2086 µg RAE (retinol activity equivalents)
Vitamin C, 113 mg

From Texas Academy of Nutrition and Dietetics. *Texas Academy of Nutrition and Dietetics MNT Manual.* 2013.

• BOX 19.3 Mechanically Altered Diet

Purpose

To provide a well-balanced diet, soft in texture and consistency, for patients with chewing difficulties due to poor or missing dentition, oral surgery, or radiation of the head and neck area, which may make the mouth sore.

Adequacy

If a variety of foods is selected, the diet meets the Dietary Reference Intakes for nutrients for most adults.

Description

1. The diet consists of a regular diet with alterations in consistency and texture.
2. Foods are generally tender—finely chopped, ground, or pureed—although very soft whole foods may be eaten as tolerated.
3. Patient tolerance to food texture and consistency may vary; modifications should be made accordingly.

Mechanically Altered Diet Food List

Food	Allowed	Avoid
Soup	Broth or creamed soups made with allowed foods, or strained	Soup with large pieces of food or whole meats or crunchy vegetables
Meat and meat substitutes	Any chopped or ground meat or poultry, very tender, baked, broiled, creamed or stewed whole meat, fish, or poultry; bacon, cheese, and cottage cheese; eggs; smooth peanut butter; soft dried beans and peas; boiled, creamed, poached, scrambled, souffléd eggs; soft casseroles	Whole cuts of meat; fried meat, fish, poultry and eggs; hot dogs and other meat in casings; crunchy peanut butter; pizza with thick, tough crust
Potato and substitutes	Any white or sweet potatoes, mashed, baked, creamed, scalloped, or boiled; macaroni, noodles, rice, pasta	Fried potatoes, potato chips, potato skins; whole grain or brown rice
Vegetables	Vegetable juice; any well-cooked, soft vegetable without seeds or skins; peeled raw tomatoes	Corn and other raw vegetables, unless tolerated
Bread	Any enriched or whole grain breads, soft rolls, doughnuts, pancakes, crackers, and biscuits	Hard, crusty bread; bread containing nuts or dried fruit; bagels; taco shells; popcorn
Cereals	Cooked cereals, cereals that require minimal chewing	Cereals containing nuts, coconut, dried fruit; shredded wheat cereal; granola; cereals that remain crunchy in milk
Fats	Any	None
Fruits	Any fruit juice; all canned or cooked fruit, soft fresh fruit	All other raw fruits and fruits with skins, dried fruits
Milk	Any	None
Desserts	Any except those to "avoid"	Desserts containing coconut, nuts, dried fruits; fried, tough, or chewy items
Beverages	Any	None
Miscellaneous	Honey, iodized salt, sugar, sugar substitutes, syrup, jelly, ketchup, mustard, pepper, herbs, ground spices, cream sauces and gravies, chocolate, vinegar, lemon juice, cranberry sauce	Whole spices, pickles, popcorn, nuts, coconut

Sample Menu for Mechanically Altered Diet

Breakfast
½ cup orange juice
1 cup oatmeal with brown sugar
1 slice whole-wheat toast
1 tsp margarine
1 cup skim milk

Lunch
3 oz ground beef
½ cup mashed potatoes with gravy
½ cup well-cooked green beans
2 slices peeled tomato
1 ripe banana
1 whole-wheat bun
1 tsp mayonnaise
½ cup ice cream
1 cup skim milk

Dinner
3 oz broiled salmon
1 medium baked potato (no peel)
½ cup well-cooked broccoli
1 slice whole-wheat bread
1 tsp margarine
1 small brownie without nuts
1 cup chocolate skim milk
½ cup vegetable juice

Snack
1 tbsp smooth peanut butter
3 squares graham crackers
½ cup apple juice

Approximate Nutrient Composition for Mechanically Altered Diet

Calories, 1898
Carbohydrate, 287 g
Protein, 154 g
Fat, 60 g
Cholesterol, 307 mg
Dietary fiber, 26 g

Sodium, 3114 mg
Potassium, 5700 mg
Calcium, 1587 mg
Iron, 16 mg
Vitamin A, 1199 µg RAE (retinol activity equivalents)
Vitamin C, 186 mg

Adapted from Texas Academy of Nutrition and Dietetics. *Texas Academy of Nutrition and Dietetics MNT Manual.* 2013.

• BOX 19.4 **Bland Diet**

Purpose

To provide a temporary well-balanced diet for dental patients with ulcerations.

Foods and Fluids to Avoid
- Caffeine-containing beverages (coffee, tea, cola, cocoa)
- Alcohol
- Peppermint
- Chocolate
- Black and red pepper
- Chili pepper
- Chili powder
- Acidic foods
- Citrus fruits

  Intolerance to these and other foods varies. Foods that cause discomfort should be avoided.

Necrotizing Periodontal Diseases

Necrotizing gingivitis (NG) and necrotizing periodontitis (NP) are classified as acute periodontal diseases with a low prevalence.[29] The primary etiology is an immunocompromised host with secondary factors that include bacteria (e.g., spirochetes); systemic immunocompromised conditions (e.g., diabetes or human immunodeficiency virus/AIDS); local factors (e.g., smoking, poor oral hygiene); psychological stress and inadequate sleep; and systemic factors (e.g., malnutrition and alcohol).[29] NG is characterized by necrosis of interdental papillae; pseudomembrane formation; gingival bleeding; halitosis, adenopathy and/or fever; and pain (Fig. 19.8). Common complaints include a burning mouth and anorexia.[29]

Malnutrition is a contributing factor to NG because of the association with lowered host resistance. While it is important for the patient with necrotizing periodontal disease to consume an overall healthy dietary pattern following *MyPlate* website and the *Dietary Guidelines*, the necrotic tissues and pain may limit the ability to consume adequate food.

Begin by obtaining the patient's health, dental, and social histories as the first step in nutritional management, followed by an extraoral and intraoral examination. In addition, a 24-hour food recall (see Chapter 18, Figs. 18.7 and 18.8) provides important insights into dietary practices and potential nutrient deficiencies. A 3- to 7-day food record may help provide a more accurate picture of food intake. Information gathered provides valuable clues regarding nutritional factors needing to be altered or eliminated. Dietary information allows the dental hygienist to make recommendations suited to the patient's eating patterns with consideration of the patient's food preferences and habits as well as financial resources. Maintaining food intake as closely as possible to the regular eating pattern while encouraging a healthy dietary pattern based on *MyPlate* website may result in greater compliance.

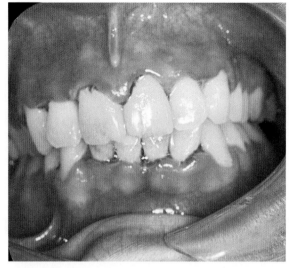

• **Fig. 19.8** Necrotizing gingivitis. (Reproduced with permission from Ibsen OAC, Phelan JA. *Oral Pathology for the Dental Hygienist.* 6th ed. St. Louis, MO: Saunders Elsevier; 2014.)

The severity of NG/NP will impact initial dietary recommendations. The goal is to provide adequate nutrients and calories, avoid alcohol, and consume noncaffeinated fluids to maintain hydration. Based on the food record, liquid nutritional supplement and a multivitamin with mineral supplement may be suggested to ensure nutrient and caloric adequacy during acute periods of the disease.

Lip and tongue ulcers, extremely painful inflamed gingival tissue, and possibly initial removal of calculus may warrant a full liquid diet for 1 to 3 days (see Box 19.2). As tolerated, the patient progresses to a mechanically altered diet (see Box 19.3). A patient's tolerance to consistency varies; the dental hygienist needs to tailor the dietary information to the patient. A patient with necrosis and ulcerations may need to eliminate nuts and seeds that can lodge in the ulcer and cause further discomfort. Encourage fluids with meals to make chewing foods easier.

Provide examples of acceptable bland and soothing foods (e.g., gelatin, puddings), while recommending avoidance of spicy and acidic foods (e.g., citrus fruits and tomatoes), that can irritate the oral mucosa (see Box 19.4). Frequent small meals are beneficial for a patient who is having difficulty eating; choosing a variety of foods according to *MyPlate* website and the *Dietary Guidelines* healthy diet patterns is important. Additional protein intake (in the form of yogurt, cheese or reduced fat milk) can be effective in meeting the increased needs related to fever and infection. Adequate decaffeinated fluid intake is essential. A regular diet should be resumed as soon as the patient is able to consume foods of normal consistency and texture. Recurrence of NG is possible, and preventive guidelines should be emphasized. Each episode of NG increases the risk of progression to NP.[29] If the patient continues to be immunocompromised, there is a greater risk of progression of NP so the patient's oral health needs careful monitoring.[29]

DENTAL CONSIDERATIONS

Assessment
- *Physical:* Inflamed and hemorrhagic gingivae; interdental papillae necrosis with cratering; pseudomembrane (grayish sloughing of the marginal gingivae); halitosis; pain; fever; malaise.
- *Dietary:* Adequate nutrient, calorie, and fluid intake; amount and frequency of alcohol consumption.

Interventions
- Explain extrinsic and intrinsic etiologic factors associated with the type and severity of periodontal disease the patient is experiencing.
- Treatment includes debridement with local anesthesia, pain control, and possibly antibiotics.

(Continued)

◆ DENTAL CONSIDERATIONS—CONT'D

- Educate the patient on appropriate oral self-care procedures and recommend use of non–alcohol-containing antimicrobial mouth rinses.
- Explain how fermentable carbohydrates enhance plaque biofilm formation by providing substrates for bacterial growth and biofilm maturation. Also, explain how soft, retentive foods cling to the tooth, allowing adherence of plaque biofilm.
- When nutrient requirements are increased because of a periodontal condition and therapeutic treatment is needed, a multivitamin supplement may be recommended. Care should be taken to ensure that the nutrients in the supplement do not exceed 100% of the RDA unless recommended by an RDN.

- Many foods on a full liquid diet are milk based. Consider the needs of a patient who is lactose intolerant. A referral to an RDN may be needed.
- Ask the patient about any allergies to antibiotics.

Evaluation

- The patient improves nutritional adequacy of foods chosen; limits or avoids smoking and alcohol consumption; oral hygiene improves with each visit; and clinical signs and symptoms of necrotizing periodontal diseases improve.

◆ NUTRITIONAL DIRECTIONS

- Initially, a liquid diet may be needed; advancement to a mechanically altered diet is followed by a regular diet, depending on the patient's tolerance and comfort.
- Liquid nutrition supplements may be needed. The patient should check the label for the grams of added sugars to choose those with less sugar.

- Cooler-temperature foods are more soothing when ulcerations are present in the oral cavity.

◆ HEALTH APPLICATION 19

Tobacco Cessation

Throughout this text, there are multiple references to the impact of smoking on health, including a negative influence on nutrient absorption. This health application focuses on one of the essential roles of dental professionals: implementing tobacco cessation protocols for dental patients.

Approximately 47.1 million US adults use any tobacco product, with the most common being cigarettes 12.8% and e-cigarettes (3.7%).[30] Current tobacco use was more prevalent in individuals living in rural areas, who were non-Hispanic white.[30] Tobacco use is associated with cancer, coronary heart disease, stroke, respiratory diseases, and diabetes.[31,32] In the oral cavity, tobacco and nicotine products increase the risk of periodontal disease, oral cancers, leukoplakia, hairy tongue, delayed healing, dental implant failure, loss of taste and smell, malodor, and extrinsic staining.[33,34] All forms of tobacco have health consequences (Box 19.5).

The addictive ingredient of tobacco is nicotine. Nicotine is a stimulant that increases the heart rate and blood pressure.[35] Because of the addictive nature of tobacco, an individual may attempt to quit on multiple occasions, requiring repeated intervention. Furthermore, global exposure to secondhand smoke results in 1.2 million deaths annually. In adults, secondhand smoke is associated with ischemic heart disease, stroke, chronic obstructive pulmonary disease (COPD), and lung cancer.[36] In children, secondhand smoke is linked to asthma, ear infections, low birthweight, lower respiratory tract infections, and sudden infant death syndrome (SIDS).[36] In addition, early childhood caries has been associated with secondhand (or passive) smoking.[37,38] An evidence-based and frequently used protocol to assist with tobacco cessation is the Five A's Approach: Ask, Advise, Assess, Assist, and Arrange.[39] *Ask* involves identifying and documenting tobacco use at every visit. Tobacco (nicotine) use should be a part of every health history. Fig. 19.9 provides an example of a tobacco use assessment form available for use with patients. The dental hygienist should determine if the patient is a current user, former user, or they never used tobacco, as well as the form, frequency, and duration of tobacco (nicotine) use. Box 19.6 provides questions to aid the dental professional in starting and continuing this essential conversation.

Advise advocates for all tobacco users to quit. The dental hygienist must send a clear message about health risks at every appointment. It can be as simple as providing basic information about tobacco use. The message should be clear, nonjudgmental and tailored to the patient. A helpful statement may be, "I cannot see what tobacco is doing to your heart, lungs, brain, and other organs, but I would like to show you some changes in your mouth." This opens opportunities to educate the patient on the importance of oral self-examinations in order to recognize abnormal situations.

Assess will focus on patients who report any type of tobacco (nicotine) use. The dental hygienist will assess the patient's willingness to quit. The response of the patient will determine the next step. Fig. 19.10 provides a flow chart on the process, including direction for when a patient is ready or not ready to quit.

Assist is determined by the patient's willingness to quit. Whatever the response, the dental hygienist will provide information on the benefits of tobacco cessation. For those who are ready to quit, the dental hygienist will *elicit* information to enhance their motivation to quit; *provide* education (e.g., establish quit date), information on the available pharmacotherapy (Box 19.7); and refer the patient to support services. Popular resources include quitlines, online programs, cell phone apps, pamphlets, or local smoking-cessation programs. The final step within *Assist* is to *elicit* again by asking the patient to commit to an initial step in the action plan.

Arrange is the final step, in which the dental professional will establish a follow-up contact (e.g., phone call, email, text), provide encouragement, answer questions, review information, and modify the plan as needed.

During the tobacco cessation process, the dental hygienist should encourage and praise the patient.

All states have tobacco quitlines available with a toll-free number 1-800-QUIT NOW. It is a free cessation service staffed by counselors trained to help quit smoking by coaching, self-help kits, cessation information, and referrals to local programs. The coaching is on an individual basis and anonymous. The National Cancer Institute provides help through chat at 877–448–7848 in English and Spanish. Smokefree.gov (http://www.smokefree.gov/) provides a number of resources to help with tobacco cessation.

Except in the presence of contraindications, pharmacotherapy can be an effective support for nicotine addiction when going through smoking cessation (see Box 19.7). Medication can minimize the discomfort of nicotine withdrawal. A combination of tobacco cessation methods increases the likelihood for success.

Dental professionals are well-situated to provide tobacco education and promote abstinence or cessation. It is the responsibility and ethical obligation of all dental professionals to intervene and educate patients.

• BOX 19.5   Tobacco Products

- Regular cigarettes
- Low-tar (light) cigarettes
- Smokeless tobacco
  - Spitless tobacco products
  - Moist snuff
  - Sticks
  - Orbs
  - Strips

- Cigars
- Pipes
- Electronic cigarettes
- Imported tobacco products
  - Hookah
  - Flavored tobacco

Tobacco Use Assessment Form

Name _____

Date _____

1.   Do you use tobacco in any form?   ☐ Yes   ☐ No

1A.   If no, have you ever used tobacco in the past?   ☐ Yes   ☐ No

How long did you use tobacco?   _____ years _____ months

How long ago did you stop?   _____ years _____ months

If you are not currently a tobacco user, no other questions should be answered. Thank you for completing this form.

Questions 2-10 are for current tobacco users only.

2.   If you smoke, what type? (Check)   How many? (Number)
     ☐ Cigarettes   _____ Cigarettes per day
     ☐ Cigars   _____ Cigars per day
     ☐ Pipe   _____ Bowls per day

3.   If you chew/use snuff, what type? How much?
     ☐ Snuff   _____ Days a can lasts
     ☐ Chewing   _____ Pouches per week
     ☐ Other (describe) _____
     Amount _____ per _____
3A. How long do you keep a chew in your mouth?
     _____minutes

4.   How many days of the week do you use tobacco?
     7   6   5   4   3   2   1

5.   How soon after you wake up do you first use tobacco?
     ☐ within 30 minutes   ☐ more than 30 minutes

6.   Does the person closest to you use tobacco?
     ☐ Yes   ☐ No

7.   How interested are you in stopping your use of tobacco?
     ☐ not at all   ☐ a little ☐ somewhat ☐ yes ☐ very much

8.   Have you tried to stop using tobacco before?   ☐ Yes   ☐ No

8A. How long ago was your last attempt to quit?
     _____ years _____ months

9.   Have you discussed stopping with another physician, dentist,
     or dental hygienist?   ☐ Yes   ☐ No

10. If you decided to stop using tobacco completely during the next two
     weeks, how confident are you that you would succeed?
     ☐ not at all   ☐ a little ☐ somewhat ☐ very confident

Thank you for completing this form

Client Tobacco Use Assessment Form

Contact Record

Date client contacted	Client asked Y/N	Advice given Y/N	Assist describe service

• **Fig. 19.9** Tobacco use assessment form. (Adapted from the United States Department of Health and Human Services. *Tobacco Effects in the Mouth, National Institutes of Health Publication No. 94–3330.* U.S. Government Printing Office; 1992.)

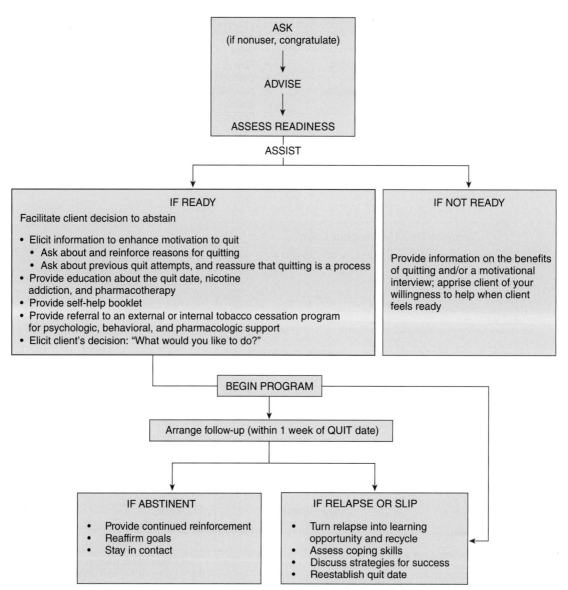

ASK
(if nonuser, congratulate)

↓

ADVISE

↓

ASSESS READINESS

ASSIST

IF READY

Facilitate client decision to abstain

- Elicit information to enhance motivation to quit
  - Ask about and reinforce reasons for quitting
  - Ask about previous quit attempts, and reassure that quitting is a process
- Provide education about the quit date, nicotine addiction, and pharmacotherapy
- Provide self-help booklet
- Provide referral to an external or internal tobacco cessation program for psychologic, behavioral, and pharmacologic support
- Elicit client's decision: "What would you like to do?"

IF NOT READY

Provide information on the benefits of quitting and/or a motivational interview; apprise client of your willingness to help when client feels ready

BEGIN PROGRAM

Arrange follow-up (within 1 week of QUIT date)

IF ABSTINENT

- Provide continued reinforcement
- Reaffirm goals
- Stay in contact

IF RELAPSE OR SLIP

- Turn relapse into learning opportunity and recycle
- Assess coping skills
- Discuss strategies for success
- Reestablish quit date

• **Fig. 19.10** Tobacco intervention flow chart. (Reproduced with permission from Darby ML, Walsh MM. *Dental Hygiene: Theory and Practice.* 4th ed. St. Louis, MO: Saunders Elsevier; 2015.)

• **BOX 19.6** **Questions for Tobacco Cessation**

- Do you use any tobacco or nicotine products?
- Have you ever used tobacco or nicotine in the past?
- How much do you smoke or vape?
- What forms of tobacco do you use?
- How many cigarettes or vape cartridges do you smoke each day?
- Why do you continue to smoke?
- How soon after you wake up do you smoke your first cigarette?
- Do others in your household smoke?
- Do you smoke inside your home or car?
- Do you want to quit smoking?
- Tell me about your last quit attempt(s).
  Did you use a smoking-cessation medication?
  Did you receive any professional support?

• **BOX 19.7** **Pharmacotherapy for Tobacco Cessation**

- Nicotine Replacement
  Gum
  Lozenges
  Patch
  Nasal spray
  Inhaler
- Nonnicotine Replacement
  Bupropion
  Clonidine
  Nortriptyline
  Varenicline
- Combination Therapy

◆ CASE APPLICATION FOR THE DENTAL HYGIENIST

Jenny is a 20-year-old college student. It has been 9 months since her last recare visit because of her busy school-and-work schedule. She continues to smoke despite the dental hygienist's encouragement to quit. An oral examination exhibits inflamed gingiva bleeding on touch and a grayish pseudomembrane covering the marginal gingiva. The dental hygienist also notices an unusual odor from the patient's mouth. A 24-hour dietary recall is as follows:

7:30 a.m.: large coffee with cream and sugar; pastry
10:00 a.m.: 12 oz cola; potato chips
2:30 p.m.: 3 slices pizza; 12 oz cola
7:30 p.m.: 12 oz can of ravioli; 8 oz milk
11:30 p.m.: hot chocolate; 8 sandwich cookies

Nutritional Assessment

- Food, nutrient, caloric intake
- Eating habits
- Social history
- Motivation level
- Knowledge level

Nutritional Diagnosis

Identify the patient's irregular eating patterns; choices of high-calorie, low nutrient-dense foods; stress from school and work; and smoking.

Nutritional Goals

Jenny will attempt to discontinue smoking or avoid smoking during periods of acute inflammation. With the help of the dental hygienist, she will review her busy schedule and prioritize events to incorporate a variety of foods, including some choices that are quickly prepared or healthier options from vending machines.

Nutritional Implementation

Intervention: Question Jenny further on the level of oral discomfort she is experiencing. Determine whether a relationship exists between oral health and food choices. Depending on her response, a full liquid diet may initially be suggested, followed by a mechanically altered diet within 1 to 3 days, as tolerated.

Rationale: Oral conditions can interfere with chewing or swallowing. Jenny might be eating too little or omitting foods too painful to eat. Consequently, she may be experiencing a deteriorating nutritional status, which is negatively affecting her oral status. Altering the consistency of her diet can increase nutrient intake by minimizing the task of chewing and swallowing. Every patient's oral situation is unique and tolerance levels vary greatly. The dental hygienist should listen closely to Jenny's response to individualize recommendations to meet her needs.

Intervention: Encourage Jenny to eat a variety of foods, making choices as similar to her normal eating patterns as possible.

Rationale: Systemic factors, such as nutrient deficiencies, influence inflammatory response of the gingiva. The dental hygienist should explain the role of nutrients in maintaining a healthy periodontium, suggesting food choices that vary only slightly from Jenny's regular food intake to enhance compliance. Essential education tools include *MyPlate* website and *Dietary Guidelines*. Temporary use of a multivitamin supplement may be recommended.

Intervention: Identify the frequency and form of fermentable carbohydrates in Jenny's diet, along with soft and sticky foods.

Rationale: Foods and drinks—such as coffee with sugar, pastries, potato chips, and cookies—influence formation of plaque. With Jenny's cooperation, practical and realistic modifications can be established in her diet, which are compatible with the demands of her busy lifestyle. The dental hygienist should discuss use of dairy products (e.g., cheese on pizza and hot chocolate) in her diet.

Intervention: Continue efforts to eliminate smoking. Evaluate Jenny's readiness to quit tobacco use. Refer her to the National Network of Smoking Cessation quitlines at 1-800-QUIT-NOW or http://www.smokefree.gov.

Rationale: Smoking may promote plaque biofilm accumulation and inhibit the healing process. Heat, staining, and smoke from cigarettes can lead to unfavorable gingival changes. Evidence suggests that quitlines are convenient, effective, and preferred by smokers.[40]

Intervention: During an oral examination, note any areas of ulceration.

Rationale: Depending on the patient's tolerance, a bland diet may be recommended because discomfort may be experienced from highly seasoned or acidic foods. Nuts, popcorn hulls, and seeds are avoided because they can become lodged in an ulcerated area and hence become painful. Finally, cooler-temperature foods are more soothing.

Evaluation

The patient comes to each of her recare appointments, with improvement in oral health noted each time. At a 1-month reevaluation appointment, Jenny is (1) consuming a regular diet including a variety of foods; (2) eating fermentable carbohydrates only with meals; (3) choosing firm, fibrous foods more frequently; and (4) attending a smoking-cessation program. She is also able to verbalize reasons for these lifestyle changes.

◆ Student Readiness

1. List at least four factors detrimentally affecting nutritional status in a periodontally involved patient. Why is it important to concentrate on nutrient intake?
2. Discuss the difference between a mechanically altered and a full liquid diet. What dental situations benefit from use of each of these diets?
3. Describe a periodontal situation in which small, frequent meals should be recommended. Explain the rationale to a patient.
4. What dietary strategies can be offered to a patient experiencing oral discomfort?
5. Conduct an Internet search for "supplements for periodontal disease" or "supplements for periodontal health." Choose one or two supplements identified to treat or prevent periodontal disease. Based on your knowledge of nutrition, dietary supplements, and periodontal disease, provide a rationale for suggesting or not suggesting the supplement(s).
6. If you are not in a "Tobacco-Free" work or school environment, investigate how you can begin this process. Find several tobacco-free policies at other schools of similar size to present to faculty or an administrator, or speak directly with the owner of your work place. One person or a small group can make an impact.

◆ CASE STUDY

A 43-year-old man comes to his recare appointment complaining of "sore and bleeding gums, especially after brushing." He is a busy executive and entertains his clients frequently. Consequently, he dines out often and averages two to three alcoholic drinks each day. His medical history is uneventful—no medications or health alerts. An oral examination reveals bleeding on probing with pocket depths generalized at 4 to 6 mm with moderate gingival inflammation.

The dental hygienist asks him to recall everything he has eaten on the previous day. His food consumption is high in fat, calories, and sodium because of heavy reliance on dining out. His diet also lacks variety and is low in nutrient value.

1. List several secondary factors precipitating the periodontal problem. What changes in his lifestyle could be suggested?
2. From the limited information presented, what additional data can the dental hygienist gather to help him modify his diet?
3. What vitamins and minerals might be inadequate or deficient, that could cause progression of his periodontal condition?
4. What diet should be suggested? What is the rationale? Provide a realistic menu for one day on the recommended diet.

References

1. Trombelli L, Farina R, Silva CO, Tatakis DN. Plaque-induced gingivitis: case definition and diagnostic considerations. *J Periodontol.* 2018;89(S1):S46–S73.
2. Tonetti MS, Greenwell H, Kornman KS. Staging and grading of periodontitis: framework and proposal of a new classification and case definition. *J Periodontol.* 2018;89(S1):S159–S172.
3. USDHHS, Office of Disease Prevention and Health Promotion. *Healthy People 2030.* https://health.gov/healthypeople
4. Hajishengallis G. Interconnection of periodontal disease and comorbidities: evidence, mechanisms, and implications. *Periodontol 2000.* 2022;89(1):9–18.
5. Jepsen S, Caton JG, Albandar JM, et al. Periodontal manifestations of systemic diseases and developmental and acquired conditions: consensus report of workgroup 3 of the 2017 World Workshop on the Classification of Periodontal and Peri-Implant Diseases and Conditions. *J Periodontol.* 2018;89(Suppl 1):S237–S248.
6. Chapple ILC, Bouchard P, Cagetti MG, et al. Interaction of lifestyle, behaviour or systemic diseases with dental caries and periodontal diseases: consensus report of group 2 of the joint EFP/ORCA workshop on the boundaries between caries and periodontal diseases. *J Clin Periodontol.* 2017;44(Suppl 18):S39–S51.
7. Varela-López A, Giampieri F, Bullón P, Battino M, Quiles JL. A systematic review on the implication of minerals in the onset, severity and treatment of periodontal disease. *Mol Basel Switz.* 2016;21(9):1183.
8. Dommisch H, Kuzmanova D, Jönsson D, Grant M, Chapple I. Effect of micronutrient malnutrition on periodontal disease and periodontal therapy. *Periodontol 2000.* 2018;78(1):129–153.
9. Saleh MHA, Decker A, Tattan M, et al. Supplement consumption and periodontal health: an exploratory survey using the BigMouth repository. *Medicina.* 2023;59(5):919.
10. Marsh PD, Zaura E. Dental biofilm: ecological interactions in health and disease. *J Clin Periodontol.* 2017;44(S18):S12–S22.
11. Choy JYM, Goh AT, Chatonidi G, et al. Impact of food texture modifications on oral processing behaviour, bolus properties and postprandial glucose responses. *Curr Res Food Sci.* 2021;4:891–899.
12. Lynge Pedersen AM, Belstrøm D. The role of natural salivary defences in maintaining a healthy oral microbiota. *J Dent.* 2019;80(Suppl 1):S3–S12.
13. Dawes C, Pedersen AML, Villa A, et al. The functions of human saliva: a review sponsored by the World Workshop on Oral Medicine VI. *Arch Oral Biol.* 2015;60(6):863–874.
14. Halvorsrud K, Lewney J, Craig D, Moynihan PJ. Effects of starch on oral health: systematic review to inform WHO guideline. *J Dent Res.* 2019;98(1):46–53.
15. Altun E, Walther C, Borof K, et al. Association between dietary pattern and periodontitis—a cross-sectional study. *Nutrients.* 2021;13(11):4167.
16. Holmstrup P, Plemons J, Meyle J. Non–plaque-induced gingival diseases. *J Periodontol.* 2018;89(S1):S28–S45.
17. Tada A, Miura H. The relationship between vitamin C and periodontal diseases: a systematic review. *Int J Env Res Public Health.* 2019;16(14):2472.
18. Li W, Song J, Chen Z. The association between dietary vitamin C intake and periodontitis: result from the NHANES (2009–2014). *BMC Oral Health.* 2022;22:390.
19. Papapanou PN, Sanz M, Buduneli N, et al. Periodontitis: consensus report of workgroup 2 of the 2017 World Workshop on the Classification of Periodontal and Peri-Implant Diseases and Conditions. *J Periodontol.* 2018;89(S1):S173–S182.
20. Sanz M, Beighton D, Curtis MA, et al. Role of microbial biofilms in the maintenance of oral health and in the development of dental caries and periodontal diseases. Consensus report of group 1 of the Joint EFP/ORCA workshop on the boundaries between caries and periodontal disease. *J Clin Periodontol.* 2017;44(S18):S5–S11.
21. Lu EMC. The role of vitamin D in periodontal health and disease. *J Periodontal Res.* 2023;58(2):213–224.
22. Woelber JP, Reichenbächer K, Groß T, Vach K, Ratka-Krüger P, Bartha V. Dietary and nutraceutical interventions as an adjunct to non-surgical periodontal therapy—a systematic review. *Nutrients.* 2023;15(6):1538.
23. Li J, Zhao G, Zhang HM, Zhu FF. Probiotic adjuvant treatment in combination with scaling and root planing in chronic periodontitis: a systematic review and *meta*-analysis. *Benef Microbes.* 2023;14(2):95–107.
24. U.S. Department of Agriculture, U.S. Department of Health and Human Services. *Dietary Guidelines for Americans.* 9th ed. 2020. dietaryguidelines.gov.
25. Lee J, Park JC, Jung UW, et al. Improvement in periodontal healing after periodontal surgery supported by nutritional supplement drinks. *J Periodontal Implant Sci.* 2014;44(3):109–117. https://doi.org/10.5051/jpis.2014.44.3.109.
26. Gheisary Z, Mahmood R, Harri Shivanantham A, et al. The clinical, microbiological, and immunological effects of probiotic supplementation on prevention and treatment of periodontal diseases: a systematic review and *meta*-analysis. *Nutrients.* 2022;14(5):1036.
27. Hill C, Guarner F, Reid G, et al. The International Scientific Association for Probiotics and Prebiotics consensus statement on the scope and appropriate use of the term probiotic. *Nat Rev Gastroenterol Hepatol.* 2014;11(8):506–514.
28. Martin-Cabezas R, Davideau JL, Tenenbaum H, Huck O. Clinical efficacy of probiotics as an adjunctive therapy to non-surgical periodontal treatment of chronic periodontitis: a systematic review and *meta*-analysis. *J Clin Periodontol.* 2016;43(6):520–530.
29. Herrera D, Retamal-Valdes B, Alonso B, Feres M. Acute periodontal lesions (periodontal abscesses and necrotizing periodontal diseases) and *endo*-periodontal lesions. *J Periodontol.* 2018;89(S1):S85–S102.
30. Cornelius ME. Tobacco product use among adults—United States, 2020. *MMWR Morb Mortal Wkly Rep.* 2022;71:398–30511. https://doi.org/10.15585/mmwr.mm7111a1.
31. Hajat C, Stein E, Ramstrom L, Shantikumar S, Polosa R. The health impact of smokeless tobacco products: a systematic review. *Harm Reduct J.* 2021;18(1):123.
32. Centers for Disease Control and Prevention. *Health Effects of Smoking—Smoking-Related Illnesses.* Centers for Disease Control and Prevention; 2022. https://www.cdc.gov/tobacco/campaign/tips/diseases/index.html
33. Leite FRM, Nascimento GG, Scheutz F, López R. Effect of smoking on periodontitis: a systematic review and *meta*-regression. *Am J Prev Med.* 2018;54(6):831–841.

34. Abbott AJ, Reibel YG, Arnett MC, Marka N, Drake MA. Oral and systemic health implications of electronic cigarette usage as compared to conventional tobacco cigarettes: a review of the literature. *J Dent Hyg*. 2023;97(4):21–35.

35. Le Foll B, Piper ME, Fowler CD, et al. Tobacco and nicotine use. *Nat Rev Dis Primer*. 2022;8(1):1–16.

36. Carreras G, Lugo A, Gallus S, et al. Burden of disease attributable to second-hand smoke exposure: a systematic review. *Prev Med*. 2019;129:105833.

37. Lam PPY, Chua H, Ekambaram M, Lo ECM, Yiu CKY. Risk predictors of early childhood caries increment--a systematic review and *meta*-analysis. *J Evid-Based Dent Pract*. 2022;22(3):101732.

38. Chaffee BW, Urata J, Couch ET, Silverstein S. Dental professionals' engagement in tobacco, electronic cigarette, and cannabis patient counseling. *JDR Clin Transl Res*. 2020;5(2):133–145.

39. Fiore MC, Jaen CR, Baker TB. *Treating Tobacco Use and Dependence: 2008 Update*. US Department of Health and Human Services; 2008.

40. United States Public Health Service Office of the Surgeon General, National Center for Chronic Disease Prevention and Health Promotion (United States) Office on Smoking and Health. *Smoking Cessation: A Report of the Surgeon General*. US Department of Health and Human Services; 2020. http://www.ncbi.nlm.nih.gov/books/NBK555591/.

▶ Evolve Resources

Please visit http://evolve.elsevier.com/Mallonee/nutritional for additional practice and study support tools.

20

Nutritional Aspects of Alterations in the Oral Cavity

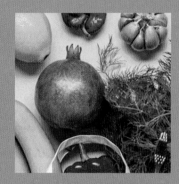

STUDENT LEARNING OBJECTIVES

On completion of this chapter, the student will be able to achieve the following learning outcomes:

1. Describe the common signs and symptoms of xerostomia. Also, synthesize appropriate dietary and oral hygiene recommendations for a patient with orthodontics, xerostomia, root caries, or dentin hypersensitivity.
2. Discuss normal dentition, and identify *Dietary Guidelines* appropriate for a patient undergoing oral surgery and a patient with a new denture, before and after insertion.
3. Describe the common signs and symptoms of glossitis. Also, synthesize appropriate dietary and oral hygiene recommendations for a patient with a loss of alveolar bone, glossitis, or temporomandibular disorder.

KEY TERMS

Abrasion
Benign migratory glossitis
Crepitus

Dentin hypersensitivity
Erosion
Functional food

Lichen planus
Temporomandibular disorder
Tinnitus

TEST YOUR NQ

1. **T/F** While charting for dental caries, the dental hygienist notes several root surface caries and documents xerostomia as the cause. This is a correct assessment.
2. **T/F** Xerostomia is a consequence of the aging process.
3. **T/F** Xerostomia can be a contributing factor to malnutrition in an older patient.
4. **T/F** Root caries are frequently seen in adolescents.
5. **T/F** The primary component of alveolar bone is compact cortical bone.
6. **T/F** Glossitis can be a symptom of a nutrient deficiency.
7. **T/F** Masticatory efficiency, or chewing, is a factor in providing a well-structured alveolar process.
8. **T/F** A relationship exists between nutritional status of a patient and tooth mobility, missing teeth, and denture performance.
9. **T/F** High-fiber, nutrient-dense foods are recommended for the first few days after insertion of new dentures to promote healing and prevent loss of alveolar bone.
10. **T/F** To maintain a normal serum calcium level, calcium is obtained from the alveolar process when the patient is in negative calcium balance.

Instructing patients to follow the *Dietary Guidelines* and utilize guidance for healthy eating patterns using *MyPlate* website is practical nutrition advice for optimum general and oral health. Various oral conditions can interfere with food intake and influence a patient's nutritional status. These situations require modifications of eating patterns based on individual needs. The oral health team can serve as a valuable member of an interprofessional team in provision of care for complicated cases, such as patients with renal disease. Management of oral manifestations that may result from a chronic condition and palliative care should be the primary focus of the oral health teams. Dietary advice should be provided to a patient by a Registered Dietitian or physician.

Orthodontics

Orthodontic treatment presents unique nutritional implications. Risk of decalcification, erosion, gingival inflammation, alveolar bone loss, and decline of the periodontal ligament are concerns that may compromise orthodontic outcomes and long-term oral health. Optimal nutrient intake is a factor that can minimize these negative oral health situations. The treatment time varies widely and is dependent on the complexity of the situation and patient compliance. The level of comfort and duration of discomfort also vary, with common complaints of pain localized to the teeth, soft tissues, and tongue, particularly in the first days after placement or adjustment. Pain can last from 1 day to 2 weeks.[1] These symptoms impact food choices, quantity of foods, and food preparation. Eating foods that require biting and chewing may be difficult.

Irregular meal patterns, frequent consumption of acidic beverages and snack habits typical of many adolescents create an additional challenge during orthodontic treatment. Health and science courses at school provide adolescents with sufficient knowledge to make better choices, but this information may not be applied. Choosing snacks or meals from vending machines, convenience stores, or fast food restaurants is commonplace. Fortunately, many schools are opting to have nutrient-dense snacks or meals for purchase. In addition, fast food restaurants and convenience stores are offering progressively more nutrient-dense options to consumers.

🦷 DENTAL CONSIDERATIONS

Assessment
- *Physical:* Gingival inflammation, dental caries, decalcification of teeth, soft tissue lesions from sharp appliances, erosion, root resorption, and accumulation of food debris around brackets.
- *Dietary:* Frequency and times fermentable carbohydrates are consumed, form of food chosen.

Interventions
- Individualize nutrition education to motivate adolescents to improve their eating and oral hygiene habits. For any plan to succeed, the adolescent must be willing to change.
- After initial placement, adjustments or repairs in orthodontic care may require a full liquid or mechanically altered (see Chapter 19) diet for 1 to 2 days.
- Emphasize the importance of oral self-care, daily fluoride use, and possibly an alcohol-free antimicrobial rinse.
- Because fermentable carbohydrates are a factor in demineralization and plaque biofilm formation, conduct a dietary analysis using a 3- to 7-day food diary (see Chapter 18). Based on this assessment, counsel the orthodontic patient, including recommendations to modify the frequency of consuming fermentable/refined carbohydrates.
- Remind the patient that appliances can be damaged with sticky, hard, or firm foods, or chewing ice.
- Soft tissue trauma caused by sharp appliances can lead to discomfort and avoidance of certain foods. Warm saltwater rinses (8 oz water with 1 tsp salt) and utility wax (to cover the offending surface of the appliance) provide comfort until the situation can be resolved.

Evaluation
- The patient has demonstrated acceptable plaque biofilm control abilities; soft tissues are free of trauma; the patient is choosing a variety of foods based on *MyPlate* website.

🦷 NUTRITIONAL DIRECTIONS

- Although a mechanically altered diet allows for ease of chewing and is less painful, it consists of soft, sticky, and retentive foods that can adhere around the brackets, contributing to plaque biofilm formation. Consequently, this diet can result in gingival inflammation and increased caries risk. Encourage and educate the patient regarding an optimal oral self-care regimen.
- Commonly chosen soft foods include mashed potatoes, rice, pasta, bananas, soups, cheese, and boiled vegetables.[1]

- Liquids such as milkshakes or smoothies may also be well-tolerated. Since these drinks are fermentable carbohydrates, highlight the need for optimal oral self-care.
- Foods such as carrots and apples should not be avoided but rather cut into small pieces.
- Corn on the cob, apples, carrots, meat dishes, nuts, chewing gum, chewy candy, and crackers are foods commonly identified as difficult to consume with orthodontic bands.[1]
- Soft drinks, energy drinks, specialized coffee drinks, and sports drinks, often contain fermentable carbohydrates along with citric or phosphoric acid and should be avoided to minimize enamel decalcification and erosion.
- Adequate nutritional intake is indispensable for the maintenance and repair of "hard and soft tissue" and to withstand the stresses of tooth movement.
- Foods with a low nutrient value and fermentable carbohydrates minimize success of orthodontic treatment and increase the risk of oral complications.

Xerostomia

Good oral health depends on adequate salivary flow. Common factors contributing to xerostomia are listed in Box 20.1. Because xerostomia is most commonly characterized by diminished or absent salivary flow or a change in the viscosity of saliva, xerostomia has a negative impact on oral tissues and dietary intake (Fig. 20.1). Chapter 3 provides some basic information about the functions of saliva and xerostomia.

• BOX 20.1   Factors Contributing to Xerostomia

Medications
- Analgesics
- Antianxiety agents
- Anticholinergics
- Anticonvulsants
- Antidepressants
- Antihistamines
- Antihypertensives
- Antiinflammatories
- Antiobesity agents
- Anti-Parkinson agents
- Antipsychotics
- Bronchodilators
- Decongestants
- Diuretics
- Gastrointestinal agents
- Narcotics

Other Considerations
- Antineoplastic therapy (chemotherapy and radiation)
- Autoimmune diseases (Sjögren's syndrome)
- Poorly controlled diabetes
- Uncontrolled hypertension
- Stress and depression
- Use of medical or recreational cannabis
- Significant nutrient deficiency (e.g., vitamins A and C, protein)
- Liquid diets, due to lack of mastication
- Dehydration
- Excessive use of alcohol or tobacco
- Consumption of excess caffeine or spicy food

Adapted from American Dental Association. *Xerostomia (Dry Mouth)*. https://www.ada.org/en/resources/research/science-and-research-institute/oral-health-topics/xerostomia.

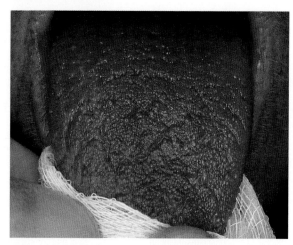

• **Fig. 20.1** Appearance of mouth of patient with xerostomia. (From Ibsen OAC, Phelan JA. *Oral Pathology for the Dental Hygienist*. 6th ed. Elsevier; 2014.)

The dental professional should determine from the medical history the patient's risk for xerostomia. An estimated 22% of the global population experiences some level of xerostomia.[2] Salivary flow does not significantly decrease as a result of aging. Adults most frequently experience xerostomia in relation to taking multiple medications (see Box 20.1). Xerostomia can also be a result of one or more chronic diseases, such as Sjögren's syndrome (Fig. 20.2). Xerostomia results in various oral complications compromising a patient's nutrient intake (Box 20.2). Overall, the goals for a patient with xerostomia are to protect the oral cavity from the destructive effects of xerostomia, treat existing conditions, and provide relief from the dryness to improve the quality of the diet and quality of life. The dental professional should be able to recognize and provide suggestions for patients experiencing xerostomia.

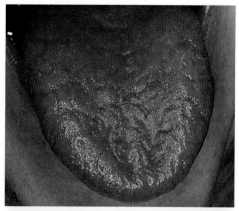
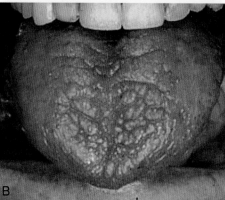

• **Fig. 20.2** Appearance of mouth of patient with Sjögren's syndrome causing xerostomia. (A) Sjögren's syndrome with severe xerostomia and a lack of papillae on the dorsal tongue. (B) In severe cases, a cobblestone appearance of the tongue may be seen. (From Ibsen OAC, Peters SM. *Oral Pathology for the Dental Hygienist: With General Pathology Introductions*. 8th ed. Elsevier; 2023.)

🦷 DENTAL CONSIDERATIONS

Assessment

- *Physical:* Dry mouth; dysgeusia; burning sensation of the tongue or oral mucous membranes; dry and crusty mucosa; difficulty in swallowing and speaking (see Box 20.2); medications (see Box 20.1); antineoplastic therapy (chemotherapy and radiation); systemic diseases (diabetes, Sjögren's syndrome, acquired immune deficiency syndrome); stress and depression; dehydration; and weight loss.
- *Dietary:* Inadequate intake of vitamins A and C, fluid, fiber, potassium, vitamin B$_6$, iron, calcium, zinc, and protein; taste changes; lack of interest in eating; and poor appetite.

Interventions

- If the patient complains of oral dryness, the dental hygienist can place a mouth mirror or tongue blade on the oral mucosa and watch for stickiness on removal. Milking the major salivary glands (submandibular, sublingual, and parotid) to observe the amount of saliva produced is another assessment option.
- After a thorough oral examination of the patient with oral dryness, a sialometry test can be performed. Saliva flow tests take approximately 10 to 15 minutes and provide fast results of not only the flow but also consistency, pH, and quantity of saliva. A low salivary rate with this type of test may raise suspicion and indicate systemic disease. A more invasive procedure, scintigraphy, is a diagnostic test performed in the hospital to observe salivary function. Examples include tumors, cysts, salivary stones, duct blockage, and trauma.
- Because burning mouth syndrome cannot be identified clinically, listen to the patient's symptoms. Patients may compare the burning sensation to consumption of hot peppers, typically complaining of having an intense burning sensation on the anterior two-thirds of the tongue or oral mucous membranes. This is commonly associated with taste changes and xerostomia.

- Discomfort with a removable appliance may occur because of the tongue sticking to the prosthesis, an inability to retain the appliance properly, and gingival lesions created by an improperly fitting denture.
- A complete assessment allows the dental professional to formulate appropriate intervention strategies for xerostomia.
- Each patient's situation is unique; thus oral therapy must be individualized.
- Educate the patient about techniques and procedures to relieve symptoms of xerostomia effective in minimizing oral discomfort and related conditions, especially increased dental caries.
- More than 500 over-the-counter and prescription medications indicate xerostomia to be a possible side effect.[3] Because drugs are a common cause of xerostomia, review the patient's medications to identify any drugs associated with xerostomia (see Box 20.1). The patient may want to discuss an alternative medication or a reduction in dosage with the health care provider. If the medication cannot be changed or the dosage cannot be reduced, provide alternative options for maintaining oral health.
- Schedule frequent recare appointments to monitor the oral cavity.
- Discuss the importance of excellent daily oral hygiene.
- Advise fluoride therapy to reduce the risk of caries.
- Pilocarpine or cevimeline may be prescribed by the health care provider for relief from xerostomia.[4]
- After assessing food intake, note any changes in appetite affecting overall dietary adequacy resulting in weight changes.
- Malic acid may counteract the harmful effects of drug-induced xerostomia on enamel.[4]

Evaluation

- The patient uses oral hygiene and dietary interventions to relieve xerostomia.

◈ NUTRITIONAL DIRECTIONS

- Use products formulated to relieve xerostomia (e.g., sprays or oral rinses).
- Use unflavored or mildly flavored oral hygiene products that have a neutral pH.
- Use lip balm to help keep lips moist.
- Consume fluids with meals and between meals; frequent sips of fluids between bites facilitate chewing and swallowing.
- Use a humidifier to maintain the humidity in the air.
- Choose nutrient-dense, soft, moist foods (e.g., macaroni and cheese, cottage cheese, or applesauce).
- Use gravies and sauces to moisten dry foods (e.g., roast beef).
- Choose foods principally made with a nonnutritive sweetener or sugar alcohols (e.g., gum, hard candy, lozenges, or popsicles), especially between meals.

- Avoid or limit foods that are dry (e.g., saltines), crumbly (e.g., whole-wheat muffins), sticky (e.g., peanut butter), and spicy (e.g., salsa or chili peppers); alcohol; commercial mouthwashes containing alcohol; tobacco; and caffeine.
- Suck on ice chips between meals.
- Carry a water bottle during the day.
- Enhance appetite by presenting foods in interesting, appealing, and appetizing ways. Suggestions to improve the appearance and appeal of food can involve colorful combinations of foods. Imagine the lack of appeal of a plate with cauliflower, mashed potatoes, and baked white fish compared with a colorful plate of baked salmon, steamed broccoli, and a baked yam.

• BOX 20.2   Consequences of Xerostomia Influencing Nutrient Intake

- Increased rate of caries (root, cervical or incisal/cuspal tips)
- Secondary oral candidiasis
- Enlargement of salivary glands secondary to sialadenitis
- Inability to keep mouth moist
- Sticky or tacky saliva
- Absence of salivary pooling
- Difficulty in chewing and swallowing
- Burning or sensitive oral mucosa
- Dry, crusty, smooth, or shiny mucosa
- Low tolerance to spicy and acidic foods
- Ulcerations
- Food sticking to hard palate or tongue
- Painful tongue—atrophied, fissured, inflamed, edematous, burning sensation
- Angular cheilosis—cracking or burning at the corners of the mouth
- Altered or lack of taste—lack of interest in eating, possible unintentional weight loss
- Difficulty wearing dentures
- Dentin hypersensitivity—hot, cold, sweet, touch
- Dry throat—difficulty with swallowing

Adapted from American Dental Association. *Xerostomia (Dry Mouth)*. https://www.ada.org/en/resources/research/science-and-research-institute/oral-health-topics/xerostomia.

Root Caries and Dentin Hypersensitivity

Because the population of older adults who have retained their teeth is increasing, root caries are increasingly common. New carious lesions in adults are typically located on the root, below the cementoenamel junction, in areas of gingival recession. The area around the cementoenamel junction is particularly susceptible because it often has an anatomically thin layer of enamel. The cementum, which is thinner and contains fewer minerals than enamel, is also more susceptible. Demineralization of cementum can occur at a pH of 6.7 or less. Adequate removal of plaque biofilm from exposed root surfaces is very difficult because of root morphology allowing bacteria and cariogenic material to accumulate, thus increasing caries risk. Xerostomia frequently compounds the risk for root caries because of limited buffering and dilution capacity of decreased amounts of saliva along with poor oral clearance. Also, prevalence of root caries is increased when carbohydrates are consumed frequently.

In addition to root caries, other problems often associated with gingival recession are abrasion and erosion of enamel and cementum. **Erosion** is the permanent depletion of tooth surfaces due to the action of an external or internal chemical substance (Fig. 20.3). Erosion is the major cause of hypersensitivity and often occurs as a consequence of exposure to acids such as those found in food and beverages (extrinsic) and acid from gastroesophageal reflux or excessive vomiting (intrinsic). **Abrasion** is the permanent depletion of tooth surfaces as a result of pathologic tooth wear, such as toothbrush abrasion (Fig. 20.4). Erosion and abrasion produce dentin exposure, which can lead to dentin hypersensitivity. **Dentin hypersensitivity** is an extremely painful feeling resulting from a stimulus to the exposed dentin.

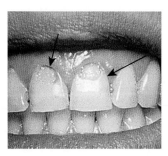

• **Fig. 20.3** Erosion (*arrows*) caused by frequently sucking on lemons. (Reproduced with permission from Darby ML, Walsh MM. *Dental Hygiene: Theory and Practice*. 4th ed. St. Louis, MO: Saunders Elsevier; 2015.)

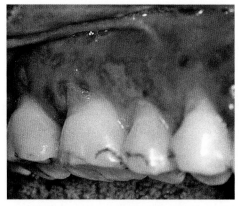

• **Fig. 20.4** Toothbrush abrasion. (Reproduced with permission from Newman MG, Takei HH, Klokkevold PR, Carranza FA: *Carranza's Clinical Periodontology*. 12th ed. St. Louis, MO: Saunders Elsevier; 2014.)

⬡ **DENTAL CONSIDERATIONS**

Assessment

- *Physical:* Gingival recession, oral infections, a narrow region of attached gingiva, toothbrush abrasion, use of fluoridated water, oral hygiene status, and xerostomia.
- *Dietary:* Diet history and carbohydrate analysis, frequency of eating, use of sugar-sweetened medications (cough syrup or lozenges), or intake of hard candy.

Interventions

- Patients complaining of a sudden, sharp pain in areas where dentin is exposed and recession exists, may be experiencing dentin hypersensitivity.
- Onset of dentin hypersensitivity is often related to temperature, primarily cold, or touch.
- Recommend 3-month recare visits, meticulous oral hygiene, topical fluoride treatments at home, and fluoridated water. Self-applied fluoride gels reduce enamel solubility and oral bacteria. Desensitizing toothpastes and mouth rinses may also be beneficial.[5]
- For patients with areas of hypersensitivity, recommend the following: (1) brushing before consuming acidic foods to neutralize the pH of saliva; (2) using a straw for acidic drinks; (3) decreasing frequency of intake or following with a chewing gum containing xylitol or a noncariogenic food (e.g., cheese or milk); or (4) avoiding foods causing discomfort (e.g., hot coffee or iced beverages).
- Avoid brushing immediately after consuming acidic foods and beverages to minimize erosion. Wait at least 40 minutes to brush or a minimum of 20 minutes.
- Recommend using soft-bristled toothbrushes.
- Saliva is one of the best protective measures for the demineralization effects of erosion by neutralizing the acid. Tips to increase saliva flow should be recommended.

Evaluation

- The patient is free of pain, can eat comfortably, has avoided controllable risk factors, and has incorporated appropriate oral hygiene procedures into a home care regimen.

⬡ **NUTRITIONAL DIRECTIONS**

- Minimize the acidic attacks on teeth. Consumption of carbonated beverages (regular and diet), sports drinks, energy drinks, pickled products, wine, citrus products (e.g., grapefruit and orange juice), and ciders, is acidic and should be minimized because it can contribute to erosion.
- Because dairy products, especially cheddar cheese, are cariostatic, their consumption with or without cariogenic foods can decrease the risk of caries.

Dentition Status

Over the decades, a steady reduction in tooth loss has occurred. However, approximately 13% of individuals older than age 65 years still incur loss of all natural teeth.[5,6] Although many mistakenly believe that tooth loss is a normal element of aging, education level and race/ethnicity of the patient are the strongest determinants of tooth loss.[7] Smoking status has also been identified as a variable. Although complete dentition is not required for adequate nutrient intake, loss of teeth or supporting periodontium and/or an improperly fitting prosthesis are frequently associated with poor food selection and limited chewing ability. Compromised nutritional intake may be a result of tooth loss, tooth mobility, edentulous status, and discomfort from removable appliances.

Malnutrition or inability to comply with nutritional recommendations may result from declining dentition status.

A patient with complete dentures, less than 20 functioning teeth, or few pairs of opposing teeth has lower nutrient intake than a patient with adequate dentition[8] The patient's masticatory efficiency and biting force increasingly decline with each tooth lost. The number of teeth and presence of advanced mobility determine food choices. Well-fitting dentures and/or implants may improve quality of the diet; with loss of chewing ability, however, the patient may choose predominantly soft foods with less variety.[9] Because of the number of variables that can have an impact on nutrient intake, it is imperative for the dental professional to provide personalized nutrition education for patients who are edentulous, wear a dental prosthesis, or have missing or compromised teeth. It is also essential for dental professionals to work collaboratively with and educate registered dietitian nutritionists (RDNs) and physicians to assess patients at risk of malnutrition due to their dentate status.

⬡ **DENTAL CONSIDERATIONS**

Assessment

- *Physical:* Masticatory efficiency, biting force, number of teeth and location, and fit of dentures.
- *Dietary:* Adequacy of calories and nutrients, especially protein; fiber; vitamins A, B_{12}, and C, folic acid; iron, magnesium, zinc; and fluids; interest in foods.

Interventions

- Most tooth loss is a result of caries or periodontal disease. Tooth loss can be prevented with education, early diagnosis, and regular preventive care. For a dental health educator, it is important to educate the patient, community, and other health care providers regarding prevention and recognition of signs and symptoms of oral disease.
- Nutrient deficiencies frequently interfere with maintenance and repair of oral soft and hard tissues.
- During the appointment preceding placement of a new denture, educate the patient about the initial days of adaptation so that appropriate foods can be made available for the adjustment period.
- Swallowing foods may initially present a challenge to a new denture wearer because a full upper denture interferes with the ability to determine the location of food in the mouth. Days 1 and 2 of placement may necessitate a full liquid diet (see Chapter 19) to allow the patient to master swallowing with the new prosthesis before having to deal with chewing or biting firmer-textured foods.
- A high-protein liquid nutrition supplement may be necessary to meet caloric and nutrient needs to promote healing from extractions or sore spots or both.
- Encourage intake of dairy products fortified with vitamin D to slow the rate of bone loss.
- During the next 2 to 3 days the patient should advance to a mechanically altered diet as tolerated (see Chapter 19), which slowly introduces foods that require limited mastication.
- Discuss the possible decline in taste, a limited ability to identify texture and temperature of foods, and challenges in forming a bolus with food (mass of food) to be swallowed, for patients with a complete set of dentures.
- As sore spots heal, the patient should add firmer-textured foods. This process is essential for masticatory efficiency and stability of the denture and to enhance the patient's nutritional status and increase fiber intake.
- Examine the denture for fit. An appointment to reline or make new dentures may be needed. Explain the significance of a properly fitting denture to the patient, including its relationship to a poor-quality diet.

⬥ DENTAL CONSIDERATIONS—CONT'D

- Patients with a compromised dentition status frequently have inadequate intake of whole grains, fruits, vegetables, and proteins.
- Chewy, hard, or fibrous foods are often avoided because of low masticatory performance.
- Ensure adequate nutrient intake by encouraging a variety of food and beverages based on *MyPlate* website and *Dietary Guidelines*.

Evaluation

- The patient is choosing a variety of foods from each of the *MyPlate* website groups and understands the importance of a complete and functioning dentition to overall general health.

⬥ **NUTRITIONAL DIRECTIONS**

- Fortified foods may improve nutrient intake.
- Cut food into small pieces.
- Peel and chop fruits and vegetables; cooked fruits and vegetables may be better tolerated.
- Chew food well and longer.
- Evenly distribute food on both sides of the mouth.
- Chew in a straight up-and-down motion rather than a rotary motion and avoid biting with anterior teeth.
- Avoid foods such as chewing gum, sticky foods (e.g., caramels), berries with seeds, and nuts.

Oral and Maxillofacial Surgery

Oral and maxillofacial surgeries include extractions, orthognathic surgery (to correct conditions of the jaw and face), dental implants, and maxillomandibular fixation. The dental hygienist is a vital part of the dental team providing comprehensive treatment to a patient for optimal outcomes.

The role of the dental hygienist includes obtaining an assessment of the nutritional needs for patients before a surgical procedure to cope better with the postsurgical demands and to minimize complications. The patient must have an adequate nutrient and fluid intake to meet the stress of surgery (e.g., blood loss and catabolism), provide for optimal healing, and increase resistance to infection, which shortens the recovery period. Patients who are malnourished as a result of various chronic diseases and conditions—such as anorexia nervosa, chemotherapy, or alcohol abuse—are at increased risk because they are likely to be immunosuppressed. A compromised immune response may compound the severity of complications. These patients should be referred to an RDN for medical nutrition therapy before the procedure. Based on a nutrition assessment and consideration of the procedure, recommendations can be developed to help the patient plan and purchase appropriate food for the recovery period. Postoperative recommendations should also be addressed by the dental professional.

⬥ **DENTAL CONSIDERATIONS**

Assessment

- *Physical:* Oral dysfunction that affects speech, mastication, or swallowing; medical history.
- *Dietary:* Dietary intake, including decaffeinated fluids.

Interventions

- When general anesthesia is used for the surgical procedure, the stomach should be empty at the time of the operation to avoid aspirating vomitus.
- If the patient loses weight unintentionally, healing seems delayed, history of bisphosphonate use exists, or overall health declines, the patient should be referred to a health care provider or RDN.
- Recommendations for oral surgery such as extractions include reminding the patient to avoid alcohol and smoking, avoid sipping through a straw, drink adequate decaffeinated fluids, and refrain from brushing during the first 24 hours to avoid a dry socket.
- Emphasize meeting the recommendations of *MyPlate* website. The key factor for optimal healing during the recovery process is adequate intake of calories, carbohydrates, proteins, fats, vitamins, minerals, and fluids.
- Provide written instructions to reinforce postsurgical nutritional needs.
- Depending on severity of the operative procedure, the patient may tolerate solid foods after surgery. If not, the dental hygienist can suggest a full liquid diet (see Chapter 19) for 1 to 2 days with progression to a mechanically altered diet (see Chapter 19, Box 19.3) and then to a regular diet when tolerated.
- Suggest nutrient-dense, enriched and fortified foods and fluids that the patient enjoys.
- Because nutrient requirements increase after surgery, patients may find it difficult to consume adequate amounts of food. To increase protein and calories, suggest a high-protein liquid nutritional supplement or add milk powder to milk, milkshakes, soups, yogurt, or pudding. A multivitamin with minerals may be necessary.

Evaluation

- The patient is able to verbalize the problem and discuss ways to continue maintaining a healthy oral cavity and an adequate nutrient intake.

⬥ **NUTRITIONAL DIRECTIONS**

- Cold foods may be soothing to the oral cavity postoperatively.
- Frequent small meals with nutrient-dense foods help meet nutrient needs.

Loss of Alveolar Bone

Several factors, including poor calcium intake over a lifetime, create a physiologic negative calcium balance. To maintain a normal serum calcium level, the body obtains calcium from other internal sources. The calcium from spongy cancellous bone, the primary component of the alveolar process, can readily be absorbed. The status of the alveolus, which may undergo resorption before other bones, may be an early indicator of osteoporosis. When osteoporotic change in the alveolus is detected, the dental professional should refer the patient to a health care provider for further evaluation. Progressive loss of the alveolar ridge leads to tooth loss.

After tooth extractions, accelerated atrophy of alveolar bone occurs (within months). A reduction in masticatory efficiency, as occurs in individuals with dentures, also increases resorption, loss of bone mass, or alveolar osteoporosis. The mandible has greater resorption than the maxilla. As the alveolar ridge reduces in height and volume, it becomes increasingly difficult to fit dentures properly, and relined or new dentures are necessary. Management of osteoporosis is discussed in *Health Application 9* in Chapter 9.

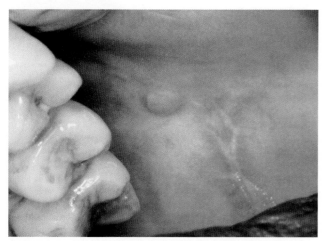

• **Fig. 20.5** Mild lichen planus on the buccal mucosa. The patient was prescribed a mouthwash and pain subsided within 24 h. (Courtesy Amy L. Sullivan, University of Mississippi Medical Center, Jackson, MS.)

Glossitis

A chronic inflammation of the tongue, or glossitis, is very painful. Glossitis may be caused by bacteria, fungus, virus, or disease, and unknown causes. Nutrient deficiency (e.g., B vitamins) or an allergic reaction to food or drugs can result in glossitis. Additionally, psychological stress can be related to psychogenic glossitis. There are many forms of glossitis. One of the most common forms of glossitis is "geographic tongue" or **benign migratory glossitis**. Clinically, benign migratory glossitis appears as multiple reddish flat areas with a loss of filiform papillae on the dorsum of the tongue. The dental hygienist may also identify and document a grooved or fissured tongue as part of the intraoral examination.[10] Although usually asymptomatic, having a patient avoid dietary triggers such as hot, spicy, or acidic foods is recommended. Dental professionals should also closely examine the oral cavity for any signs of lichen planus, considering a potential link.[10]

Lichen planus is a chronic inflammatory disease with an itchy rash found most often in the mouth. It is associated with various systemic diseases, such as hypertension and diabetes.[11,12] A mouthwash consisting of Maalox, Benadryl, and dexamethasone (Decadron)—or similar variations—is another commonly prescribed treatment for pain and irritation in patients with glossitis, lichen planus, and benign migratory glossitis (Fig. 20.5). Ultimately, more options for pain control provide a better quality of life for the patient. Once pain is controlled, patients can continue with normal eating, consuming a balanced diet based on the *Dietary Guidelines.*

Glossitis typically appears reddish with a slight to total atrophy of the filiform and fungiform papillae on the dorsum of the tongue. Depending on the degree of atrophy, the tongue inevitably appears shiny, smooth, and red (see Chapter 11). The atrophy can be localized or generalized. The tongue size can shrink because of dehydration or become enlarged (macroglossia) as a result of edema. A thorough assessment determines the extent and cause of glossitis.

With benign migratory glossitis, an assessment of the tongue might reveal erythematous or atrophic patches surrounded by a yellow-white border, often changing pattern or appearance. These erythematous patches may extend onto the buccal mucosa

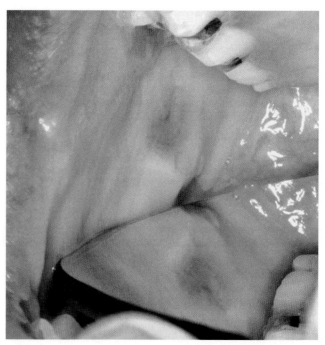

• **Fig. 20.6** The irritation on the buccal mucosa appeared after eating acidic and spicy foods. (Courtesy Amy L. Sullivan, University of Mississippi Medical Center, Jackson, MS.)

(Fig. 20.6). When patients engage in the previously mentioned triggers (spicy foods), antihistamine or corticosteroid rinses may be suggested.[13] In those cases in which lichen planus is also observed, an assessment might reveal whitish plaques on the dorsal part of the tongue and even the buccal mucosa.

🦷 DENTAL CONSIDERATIONS

Assessment
- *Physical:* Burning sensation, pain, or tenderness of the tongue; atrophy of papillae on the dorsum of the tongue; tongue size (microglossia or macroglossia); appearance of the tongue (e.g., shiny, smooth, red); diminished, altered, or lost taste sensation; change in the alveolus.
- *Dietary:* Nutritional status.

Intervention
- Macroglossia is commonly observed in individuals who are edentulous.
- Individualize dietary instructions with the goal of improving nutritional quality of the diet.
- Suggest enhancing the taste and appearance of foods on the plate.

Evaluation
- The patient is developing or maintaining healthful eating and exercise patterns and behaviors and has met with the health care provider for further evaluation.

📋 NUTRITIONAL DIRECTIONS

- Choose soft, nutrient-dense, enriched, and fortified foods (e.g., tuna salad, cream soups, cottage cheese).
- Liquid nutrition supplements, such as instant breakfast, may help provide adequate nutrients.

Temporomandibular Disorder

When a patient complains of orofacial pain, frequent headaches, impaired mandibular movement, or **tinnitus** (ringing in the ears), and the extraoral examination reveals clicking, **crepitus** (crackling or crunching sound), and popping of the temporomandibular joint, the diagnosis can be **temporomandibular** **disorder**. Clenching, grinding, stress, malocclusion, injury, and bone abnormalities are common conditions that result in temporomandibular disorder. Limited jaw opening and associated discomfort can inhibit intake. Recommendations may include avoiding gum chewing and foods that require significant chewing, such as caramels, taffy, and bagels. A mechanically altered diet (see Chapter 19) may also be warranted.

◆ HEALTH APPLICATION 20

Functional Nutrition

"Functional" implies that the food has value in providing some type of health benefits beyond basic nutrition and may function to optimize health by reducing or minimizing the risk of certain diseases and other health conditions. Functional foods are found in virtually all food categories and can include conventional foods and fortified, enriched, or enhanced foods with potentially beneficial effects on health when consumed as a part of a varied diet. The term functional foods has no legal meaning in the United States. In fact, the Academy of Nutrition and Dietetics, the International Food Information Council, Institute of Food Technologists, the European Commission, Health Canada, European Commission, and the Japanese Ministry of Health, Labour, and Welfare all define functional foods slightly differently.

Foods have always been known to provide therapeutic benefits. Thus all foods, because they provide nutritive value, are functional to some extent. After determining the role for essential elements (e.g., protein, carbohydrates, vitamins) of foods in deficiency diseases, scientists began to recognize physiologically active components in plant and animal products that can reduce risk for various chronic diseases or otherwise provide desirable physiologic effects. Implying that some foods are "good" and others are "bad" leads to misinformed food choices. Dietary supplements are not foods. Some food components—not the traditional nutrients of carbohydrate, proteins, fats, vitamins, and minerals—may provide positive health benefits. Foods containing these components are defined as functional foods. Beneficial nutrients in functional foods may be naturally present, or may be added during manufacturing.[14] According to the Academy of Nutrition and Dietetics, functional foods include minimally processed, whole foods along with fortified, enriched or enhanced foods.[15,16]

The scientifically sound approach to labeling and marketing a functional food is through the use of US Food and Drug Administration (FDA)–approved health claims as outlined by the Nutrition Labeling and Education Act (1990) discussed in Chapter 1. Under the Nutrition Labeling and Education Act, a health claim can be authorized by the FDA with the consensus of qualified experts acknowledging that scientific studies support the validity of the relationship described in that claim. Scientific agreement requires consistent findings from well-designed clinical and epidemiologic studies and expert opinions from independent scientists. Strong evidence supports some of the claims, but there is only weak evidence for others. When research confirms links between food components and health, the FDA permits additional health claims

Health-related statements or claims allowed on labels include[17]:
- nutrient content claims that indicate a specific nutrient at a certain level
- structure and function claims that describe the effect of dietary components on the normal structure or function of the body
- dietary guidance claims in reference to health benefits of broad categories of foods or diets, not a disease-or health-related condition
- qualified health claims that convey a relationship between components in the diet and reduced risk of disease

Examples of functional foods include natural components of fruits and vegetables, milk, fortified or enhanced foods, and even some foods previously thought of as unhealthy, such as chocolate and red wine. More than a dozen classes of biologically active plant chemicals are known as phytochemicals and antioxidants (Table 20.1). These natural components found in vegetables such as cabbage, carrots, broccoli, and tomatoes may reduce the risk of cancer. Foods that have been fortified to enhance the level of a specific food component include products such as calcium-fortified orange juice, fiber-supplemented snack bars, or folate-enriched cereals. Oat products reduce serum cholesterol, reducing risk of coronary heart disease. Food products are constantly being developed with beneficial components, such as cholesterol-lowering margarine and products with soy protein.

Frequently, the press reports about a perfectly legitimate scientific study or a firm will begin marketing a functional food on the basis of "emerging evidence." Conversely, consumers worry that new technological developments may influence the safety of the food. For instance, many prefer natural additives as opposed to synthetics. Lack of nutritional knowledge may limit the acceptance of functional foods. However, people should not automatically assume that consuming functional foods will necessarily improve their health. Adding a food containing a particular nutrient does not mean that the nutrient will always have the desired effect.

Research regarding how foods or food components and dietary supplements may promote health and reduce chronic disease is providing a steady stream of new information. Dietary recommendations from established scientific authorities are slow in coming because of the need for a strong, consensus-based body of evidence before changing dietary advice for the public. Increasing intake of selected foods may not be wise without considering potential negative consequences and thinking whether or not these specific elements are needed. Factors such as overall nutritional value and calorie intake of an individual's diet, and the claims on package labels backed up by sound scientific evidence, should be considered before routinely encouraging or choosing these foods. When evaluating functional foods, safe levels of intake must be considered. In many cases, optimal levels of nutrients and other physiologically active components in the foods have yet to be determined.

A person who does not have cardiovascular disease or an elevated cholesterol level would not benefit from using sterol-enhanced products. The vitamins in vitamin-enhanced drinks are probably well-absorbed, but the vitamins may not be the ones deficient in the diet and most of these products have more sugar than a regular soda. Many of these products indicate improvement of athletic performance, conditioning, recovery from fatigue after exercise, and avoidance of injury. Some of these claims may be valid. However, these foods should be used only when scientific evidence clearly supports the claim and when the physiologic changes caused by the functional ingredient are understood. The best way a consumer can evaluate the effectiveness of a food product is by trying it for several weeks to observe for benefits.

Functional foods are an important part of wellness because they offer potential for consumers to optimize their health through diet, but they are not "magic bullets" or a universal panacea for poor health habits. Functional foods are not a substitute for a well-balanced diet and regular physical activity within the framework of a healthy lifestyle. Consumers will probably continue to choose functional foods that they enjoy eating, they are familiar with, and the foods readily accessible to them. When referring to functional foods, the important thing is that what *is* eaten may be more important to health than what is *not* eaten. The best advice is to discuss appropriate intake of functional foods and strategies for achieving dietary intake goals in the context of a healthful diet based on the *Dietary Guidelines* and *MyPlate* website to optimize health and potentially decrease the risk of chronic diseases.

TABLE 20.1 Examples of Functional Components

Class/Component	Source[a]	Potential Benefit
Carotenoids		
Beta carotene	Carrots, pumpkin, sweet potato, cantaloupe, spinach, tomatoes	Neutralizes free radicals that may damage cells; bolsters cellular antioxidant defenses; can be made into vitamin A in the body
Lutein, zeaxanthin	Kale, collard, spinach, corn, eggs, citrus fruits, asparagus, carrots, broccoli	Supports maintenance of eye health
Lycopene	Tomatoes and processed tomato products (more effective after heating), watermelon, red/pink grapefruit	Supports maintenance of prostate health
Dietary (Functional and Total) Fiber		
Insoluble fiber	Wheat bran, corn bran, fruit skins	Supports maintenance of digestive health; may reduce risk of some types of cancer
Beta glucan[b]	Oat bran, oatmeal, oat flour, barley, rye	May reduce risk of CVD
Soluble fiber[b]	Psyllium seed husk, peas, beans, apples, citrus fruit	May reduce risk of CVD and some types of cancer
Whole grains[b]	Cereal grains, whole-wheat bread, oatmeal, brown rice	May reduce risk of CVD and some types of cancer; may contribute to maintenance of healthy blood glucose levels
Fatty Acids		
MUFAs[b]	Tree nuts, olive oil, canola oil	May reduce risk of CVD
PUFAs—omega-3 fatty acids—delta-ALA	Walnuts, flaxseeds, flaxseed oil	Support maintenance of heart and eye health; supports maintenance of mental function
PUFAs—omega-3 fatty acids—DHA/EPA	Salmon, tuna, marine, other fish oils	May reduce risk of CVD; contributes to maintenance of eye health and mental function
CLA	Beef and lamb; some cheese	Supports maintenance of desirable body composition and immune health
Flavonoids		
Anthocyanins—cyanidin, delphinidin, malvidin	Berries, cherries, red grapes	Bolster cellular antioxidant defenses; supports maintenance of healthy brain function
Flavonols—catechins, epicatechins, epigallocatechin	Tea, cocoa, chocolate, apples, grapes	Support maintenance of heart health
Procyanidins and proanthocyanidins	Cranberries, cocoa, apples, strawberries, grapes, red wine, peanuts, cinnamon, tea, chocolate	Support maintenance of urinary tract health and heart health
Flavanones—hesperetin, naringin	Citrus fruits	Neutralize free radicals that may damage cells; bolster cellular antioxidant defenses
Flavonols—quercetin, kaempferol, isorhamnetin, myricetin	Onions, apples, tea, broccoli	Neutralize free radicals that may damage cells; bolster cellular antioxidant defenses
Isothiocyanates		
Sulforaphane	Cauliflower, broccoli, brussels sprouts, cabbage, kale, horseradish	May enhance detoxification of undesirable compounds; bolster cellular antioxidant defenses
Minerals		
Calcium[b]	Sardines, spinach, yogurt, low-fat dairy products, fortified foods and beverages	May reduce the risk of osteoporosis
Magnesium	Spinach, pumpkin seeds, whole-grain breads and cereals, halibut, almonds, brazil nuts, beans	Supports maintenance of normal muscle and nerve function, immune health, and bone health
Potassium[b]	Potatoes, low-fat dairy products, whole-grain breads and cereals, citrus juices, beans, banana, leafy greens	May reduce risk of high blood pressure and stroke in combination with a low sodium diet
Selenium	Fish, red meat, whole grains, garlic, liver, eggs	Neutralizes free radicals that may damage cells; supports maintenance of immune and prostate health

TABLE
20.1

TABLE 20.1   Examples of Functional Components—Cont'd

Class/Component	Source[a]	Potential Benefit
Phenolic Acids		
Caffeic acid, ferulic acid	Apples, pears, citrus fruits, some vegetables, whole grains, coffee	Bolster cellular antioxidant defenses; support maintenance of eye and heart health
Plant Stanols/Sterols		
Free stanols/sterols[b]	Corn, soy, wheat, fortified foods and beverages	May reduce risk of CVD
Stanol/sterol esters[b]	Stanol ester dietary supplements, fortified foods and beverages, including table spreads	May reduce risk of CVD
Polyols		
Sugar alcohols[b]—xylitol, sorbitol, mannitol, lactitol	Some chewing gums and other food applications	May reduce risk of dental caries
Prebiotics		
Inulin, FOS, polydextrose	Whole grains, onions, some fruits, garlic, honey, leeks, fortified foods and beverages	Supports maintenance of digestive health; supports calcium absorption
Probiotics		
Yeast, *Lactobacilli*, *Bifidobacteria*, other specific strains of beneficial bacteria	Certain yogurts and other cultured dairy and nondairy products	Support maintenance of digestive and immune health; benefits are strain specific
Phytoestrogens		
Isoflavones—daidzein, genistein	Soybeans and soy-based foods	Support maintenance of bone and immune health, and healthy brain function; for females, support menopausal health
Lignans	Flaxseeds, rye, some vegetables, seeds and nuts, lentils, triticale, broccoli, cauliflower, carrots	Support maintenance of heart and immune health
Soy Protein		
Soy protein	Soybeans and soy-based foods like milk, yogurt, cheese and tofu	May reduce risk of CVD
Sulfides/Thiols		
Diallyl sulfide, allyl methyl trisulfide	Garlic, onions, leeks, scallions	May enhance detoxification of undesirable compounds; support maintenance of heart, immune and digestive health
Dithiolethiones	Cruciferous vegetables	May enhance detoxification of undesirable compounds; support maintenance of healthy immune function
Vitamins		
A[c]	Organ meats, milk, eggs, carrots, sweet potato, spinach	Supports maintenance of eye, immune and bone health; contributes to cell integrity
Thiamin (vitamin B_1)	Lentils, peas, brown or enriched white rice, pistachios, certain fortified breakfast cereals	Supports maintenance of mental function; helps regulate metabolism
Riboflavin (vitamin B_2)	Lean meats, eggs, green leafy vegetables, dairy products, certain fortified breakfast cereals	Supports cell growth; helps regulate metabolism
Niacin (vitamin B_3)	Dairy products, poultry, fish, nuts, eggs, certain fortified breakfast cereals	Supports cell growth; helps regulate metabolism
Pantothenic acid (vitamin B_5)	Sweet potato, organ meats, lobster, soybeans, lentils, certain fortified breakfast cereals	Helps regulate metabolism and hormone synthesis

[a]Examples are not an all-inclusive list.
[b]US Food and Drug Administration–approved health claim for component.
[c]Preformed vitamin A is found in foods that come from animals. Provitamin A carotenoids are found in many dark colored fruits and vegetables and are a major source of vitamin A for vegetarians.
ALA, Aminolevulinic acid; *CVD*, cardiovascular disease; *CLA*, conjugated linoleic acid; *DHA*, docosahexaenoic acid; *EPA*, eicosapentaenoic acid; *FOS*, fructo-oligosaccharides; *MUFAs*, monounsaturated fatty acids; *PUFAs*, polyunsaturated fatty acids.
Data from International Food Information Council Foundation. *Functional Foods.* 2009. https://foodinsight.org/wp-content/uploads/2009/10/FINAL-IFIC-Fndtn-Functional-Foods-Backgrounder-with-Tips-and-changes-03-11-09.pdf.

◆ CASE APPLICATION FOR THE DENTAL HYGIENIST

Mrs. Owen is a 73-year-old patient with a complete dentition in the maxillary arch and a removable mandibular partial denture. The mandibular canines and incisors are present, all of which have periodontal involvement with 3 to 5 mm of gingival recession. Root caries are present on the mandibular right and left canine. Examination reveals dry, cracked lips; a lack of salivary pool; and an ill-fitting mandibular prosthesis. The medical history reveals high blood pressure and a 10-year history of antihypertensive drug use. Mrs. Owen complains of difficulty in swallowing dry food, xerostomia, and taste alterations.

While obtaining a 24-hour food recall, the dental hygienist realizes that Mrs. Owen has lost interest in food. She states, "I just don't feel like eating. Food doesn't taste good, and I don't like cooking for myself." If she eats breakfast, she typically has orange juice and a doughnut; for lunch, she has canned soup; and before bedtime, part of a frozen dinner. A jar of hard candy sits in her living room from which she often takes a piece throughout the day, and she is constantly drinking soda for relief of xerostomia.

Nutritional Assessment
- Food intake for possible nutrient deficiencies
- Oral factors affecting motivation to eat
- Social and medical factors affecting nutrient intake
- Knowledge and motivation level
- Financial status

Nutritional Diagnosis
Several factors are involved with Mrs. Owen's poor nutrient intake: xerostomia; root caries; an ill-fitting prosthesis; frequent intake of hard candy; lack of variety in food; choice of soft, low nutrient-dense foods; and social isolation.

Nutritional Goals
Mrs. Owen has agreed to improve her overall nutritional status gradually by replacing soft, low nutrient-dense foods with high-fiber foods and using sugar-free candies and soda to prevent root caries.

Nutritional Implementation
Intervention: Increase intake of calcium-rich foods, such as low-fat milk, yogurt, and cheese.
Rationale: Adequate calcium and vitamin D intakes help to protect the alveolar bone from resorption.
Intervention: Provide education on xerostomia and its effects on the oral cavity and dietary process.
Rationale: An understanding of the cause and effect of xerostomia can help Mrs. Owen make necessary changes.
Intervention: Limit the intake of commercially prepared frozen meals and other processed foods high in sodium. Suggest that she could prepare several meals and freeze them in individual portion sizes when she feels like cooking.
Rationale: An occasional frozen meal is quick and effortless and a better choice than not eating. However, it is expensive and generally needs to be supplemented with other foods for adequate nutrients. Because many foods are high in sodium, an important factor for Mrs. Owen's hypertension, remind her to read labels and to purchase ones that contain less than 500 mg of sodium per serving.
Intervention: Suggest (1) frequent sips of a nutritious beverage (e.g., milk or juices) or a noncariogenic fluid (e.g., water) throughout the day; (2) use of products designed for patients with xerostomia, such as Bioténe or Oral Balance; (3) foods containing nonnutritive sweeteners or sugar alcohols (e.g., products containing xylitol); and (4) foods that stimulate saliva flow, such as citrus, tart, or sour foods (e.g., sugar-free lemon drops). Remind the patient of gastrointestinal distress associated with excessive consumption of products containing sugar alcohols.
Rationale: High-nutrient or noncariogenic fluids keep the mouth moist to relieve xerostomia. Products containing xylitol consumed after a meal can deter demineralization and promote remineralization. Citrus, tart, or sour foods and chewing gum stimulate saliva flow.
Intervention: Emphasize the importance of practicing proper oral hygiene techniques and explain the caries and periodontal disease process.
Rationale: Because dentition status is related to nutritional status, Mrs. Owen would benefit from retaining each natural tooth as long as possible. Xerostomia is also a contributing factor to root caries; however, plaque biofilm must be present for xerostomia to play a role in caries development. Proper daily oral hygiene care would improve her oral status and prevent further complications.
Intervention: Apply topical fluoride in the office, and instruct the patient on self-applied home fluoride treatments.
Rationale: Topical fluoride application reduces caries risk by disrupting destructive bacteria from metabolizing fermentable carbohydrates. Application of fluoride is based on caries risk, not age.
Intervention: Instruct the patient to use a daily antimicrobial rinse for 2 weeks after each treatment.
Rationale: Antimicrobial agents are used as an adjunct to other strategies for caries reduction. Antimicrobial agents effectively control plaque biofilm formation and maturation.
Intervention: Avoid dry, spicy, and some acidic foods. Avoid alcohol, caffeine, and tobacco as well.
Rationale: These choices can worsen xerostomia or irritate the mucosa.
Intervention: Encourage involvement with a local senior group and provide information for food assistance programs for older adults, such as Meals on Wheels.
Rationale: An older adult who lives alone may experience a decreased appetite and lack motivation to prepare appropriate meals. Socializing with others during meals enhances the enjoyment of eating.

Evaluation
Mrs. Owen's mandibular partial denture has been adjusted. The nutrition goals established with the dental hygienist are gradually being met. She has substituted a few pieces of sugar-free candy for hard sugar-containing candy. She prepares more meals, and has joined the community senior citizen center. She recently began using home fluoride treatments, completed the antimicrobial rinse, and now remains caries free. She appears to be a much happier individual at present.

◆ Student Readiness

1. To understand what a patient with xerostomia experiences, eat several saltine crackers with no fluid, and note the dryness of the oral cavity. Imagine this situation indefinitely and its impact on a patient's food intake. Now, try a product designed to relieve xerostomia to understand its effect before recommending it to a patient.

2. Discuss at least two changes in the oral cavity that can change a patient's taste sensation. What recommendations can a dental hygienist provide?

3. Prepare an educational program for interdisciplinary health care professionals on recognizing changes in the oral cavity affecting nutrient intake and, ultimately, general health. List at least three health care professionals who would benefit from this knowledge.

References

1. Al Jawad FA, Cunningham SJ, Croft N, et al. A qualitative study of the early effects of fixed orthodontic treatment on dietary intake and behavior in adolescent patients. *Eur J Orthod*. 2011;34:432–436.
2. Agostini BA, Cericato GO, Silveira ERD, et al. How common is dry mouth? Systematic review and meta-regression analysis of prevalence estimates. *Braz Dent J*. 2018;29(6):606–618.
3. Mark AM. Is your mouth always dry? *J Am Dent Assoc*. 2020;151(12):972.
4. Molina A, Garcia-Gargallo M, Montero E, et al. Clinical efficacy of desensitizing mouthwashes for the control of dentin hypersensitivity and root sensitivity: a systematic review and meta-analysis. *Int J Dent Hyg*. 2017;15:84–94.
5. Fleming E, Afful J, Griffin SO. *Centers for Disease Control and Prevention Prevalence of tooth loss among older adults: United States 2015-2018. NCHS Data Brief, No 368*. National Center for Health Statistics; 2020. https://www.cdc.gov/nchs/data/databriefs/db368-h.pdf.
6. Borg-Bartolo R, Roccuzzo A, Molinero-Mourelle P, et al. Global prevalence of edentulism and dental caries in middle-aged and elderly persons: a systematic review and meta-analysis. *J Dent*. 2022;127:104335.
7. Kim JK, Baker LA, Seirawan H, et al. Prevalence of oral health problems in US adults, NHANES 1999-2004: exploring differences by age, education, and race/ethnicity. *Spec Care Dentist*. 2012;32(6):234–241.
8. Factors. Associated with tooth loss in general population of Bialystok, Poland. *Int J Environ Res Public Health*. 2022;19(4):2369.
9. Saarela RKT, Lindroos E, Soini H, et al. Dentition, nutritional status and adequacy of dietary intake among older residents in assisted living facilities. *Gerodontology*. 2016;33:225–232.
10. Scariot R, Bastista TBD, Olandoski M, et al. Host and clinical aspects in patients with benign migratory glossitis. *Arch Oral Biol*. 2017;73:259–268.
11. Mozaffari HR, Sharifi R, Sadeghi M. Prevalence of oral lichen planus in diabetes mellitus: a meta-analysis study. *Acta Inform Med*. 2016;24(6):390–393.
12. Sun Y, Chen D, Deng X, et al. Prevalence of oral lichen planus in patients with diabetes mellitus: a cross-sectional study. *Oral Dis*. 2022. https://doi.org/10.1111/odi.14323.
13. Sandhu S, Klein BA, Al-Hadlaq M, et al. Oral lichen planus: comparative efficacy and treatment costs-a systematic review. *BMC Oral Health*. 2022;22(1):161.
14. International Food Information Council. *Functional Foods: Superheroes for Health*. FoodInsight.org; 2023.
15. Crowe KM, Francis C. Position of the Academy of Nutrition and Dietetics: functional foods. *J Acad Nutr Diet*. 2013;113(8):1096–1103.
16. Ellis E. *Functional Foods*. 2022. https://www.eatright.org/health/wellness/healthful-habits/functional-foods.
17. U.S. Food and Drug Administration. *Label Claims for Conventional Foods and Dietary Supplements*. https://www.fda.gov/food/food-labeling-nutrition/label-claims-conventional-foods-and-dietary-supplements.

▶ Evolve Resources

Please visit http://evolve.elsevier.com/Mallonee/nutritional for additional practice and study support tools.

21

Nutritional Assessment and Education for Dental Patients

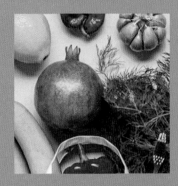

STUDENT LEARNING OUTCOMES

On completion of this chapter, the student will be able to achieve the following learning outcomes:

1. Discuss the importance of a thorough health, social, and dental history in relation to assessment of nutritional status.
2. Explain the types of methods to obtain diet history and determine situations in which each may be used effectively: 24-hour recall, food frequency questionnaire, food diary/food record.
3. Discuss the following related to dietary treatment plans and nutrition education sessions:
   * Formulate a dietary treatment plan for a dental problem influenced by nutrition.

* Identify steps and considerations in implementing a dietary treatment plan.
* Assimilate the steps of a nutrition education session.
* Discuss motivational interviewing techniques that can be incorporated when providing nutrition education in relation to oral health in the clinical setting.
4. Practice several communication skills that the dental professional should employ when educating a patient.

KEY TERMS

Anthropometry
Diet history

Food frequency questionnaire
Motivational interviewing

24-Hour recall

TEST YOUR NQ

1. **T/F** When health and dental histories have been reviewed, the dental professional has adequate information to begin nutrition education with the patient.
2. **T/F** A clinical oral examination is a very sensitive tool for identifying nutritional deficiencies.
3. **T/F** Using food models helps the patient to learn how to determine portion sizes quickly and accurately.
4. **T/F** When providing nutrition education, the dental professional should suggest minimal changes to the patient's usual intake and reinforce positive practices.
5. **T/F** Results of dietary discussion sessions do not need to be documented or communicated with other dental staff members.
6. **T/F** Providing a standardized low-carbohydrate menu is sufficient for most patients with a high caries rate.

7. **T/F** The dental professional should highlight all foods on the food diary that may contribute to increasing the risk for caries.
8. **T/F** After the nutrition education session, the patient should have enough information and motivation to make the necessary changes.
9. **T/F** "What type of snacks do you eat?" is an example of an open-ended question.
10. **T/F** Listening involves interpreting the words spoken, the manner in which they are said, and nonverbal actions directly observed.
11. **T/F** In motivational interviewing, inappropriate behaviors are discussed and a course of treatment is presented.
12. **T/F** It is better to elicit a patient's motivation and thoughts than to present the dental professional's opinions.

Health is a multidimensional and interprofessional concept, encompassing the interaction of many elements. Dissemination of information to a patient does not guarantee that the patient will establish healthier patterns. For example, millions of people start or continue smoking despite documented health risks. To facilitate positive changes toward a desired health behavior, the health care educator must tailor the message to meet the patient's needs, practices, habits, attitudes, beliefs, and values.

The relationship between nutrition and the oral cavity has already been established in this book. As you have learned, signs of a nutrient deficiency, excess, or imbalance can be detectable in the mouth. Conversely, integrity of the oral cavity is a factor in nutrient intake. Nutrition education should be patient centered, should emphasize prevention, and provide evidence-based information. Through the dental hygiene process of care (assessment, diagnosis, planning, implementation, and evaluation), the dental hygienist is ideally situated to address nutritional status as it relates to oral health.[1] The position of the Academy of Nutrition and Dietetics states, "The Academy supports the integration of oral health with nutrition services, education, and research. Collaboration between dietetics and oral health care professionals is recommended for oral health promotion and disease prevention and intervention."[2] Nutrition is essential for general health and dental health. The American Dental Hygienists' Association *Standards for Clinical Dental Hygiene Practice* state that one of the dental hygienist's responsibilities is assessment of nutrition history and dietary practices with integration of nutrition counseling into comprehensive dental hygiene care.[1] Poor eating habits are widespread among Americans; nutrition education as a primary source of prevention to reduce oral disease risk is indicated for most patients. When the instruction requires more than general nutrition information for improved oral health, or involves complex medical nutrition therapy, a referral to the health care provider or registered dietitian nutritionist (RDN) is necessary.

A nutrition assessment involves compiling and comparing information about the patient from various sources to provide meaningful evaluation and effective education. Providing nutritional information without a complete assessment is inappropriate. All steps in the assessment require critical thinking by the dental professional. The evaluation tools to be discussed in this chapter include health, social, and dental histories; clinical evaluations; dietary intake evaluation; and biochemical analysis.

Patient Assessment

For effective education, a comprehensive picture of the patient is essential. The most effective technique for gathering a medical, social, and dental history for the dental professional is to gather this information during the assessment phase of the patient's appointment.

If information gathered is incomplete, it hinders the development of a treatment plan to adequately address a patient's most immediate needs. Consider this scenario: a patient with rampant caries is told to substitute sugar-free candy for mints. The patient agrees to try this until she discovers that sugar-free mints cost more money and are unrealistic with her limited income. The patient is unaware of other acceptable alternatives and continues with the mints. Thus the information essential for making appropriate recommendations for the patient was overlooked. Another example: a dental hygienist recommends a fluoride supplement to a young patient who drinks only bottled water containing fluoride, without assessing all fluoride sources being consumed. Fluoride supplements in addition to regular consumption of bottled water with fluoride could potentially lead to fluorosis; this highlights the importance of a thorough assessment.

Health History

The health history is designed to identify health-related considerations and side effects from medications putting a patient at nutritional risk. The presence of some medical conditions could affect nutritional status by interfering with a patient's ability to chew, digest, absorb, metabolize, or excrete nutrients. Medications (over-the-counter and prescription), herbs, and supplements have numerous side effects and interactions altering eating behaviors or affecting nutritional status or both. A patient taking an antihypertensive medication may experience drug-induced xerostomia and its consequent dental complications.[3] Changes in taste and appetite, increased risk of dental problems, gastrointestinal distress, nausea or vomiting, and xerostomia are just a few drug-induced side effects. Many medications also have drug–nutrient interactions (e.g., prednisone), which may influence nutrient needs.[4]

By reviewing the health history and clarifying statements with the patient, the clinician can discover additional health-related information. Patients may not report valuable information because they (1) perceive it as irrelevant for dental professionals, (2) have forgotten it, (3) are confused by the question, or (4) are apprehensive about their visit to the dental office. Patients frequently neglect to disclose the use of oral contraceptives, antiobesity drugs, or dietary supplements, which can have several dental and nutritional implications[5] A few minutes of further questioning by the dental professional can save hours of time and effort spent trying to treat the complications. A thorough health history provides the dental professional with a strong foundation for developing a plan for dietary education. In addition, a blood pressure measurement for all patients and a blood glucose level of patients with diabetes can be obtained to augment the assessment.

Social History

A social history identifies factors influencing food intake. Personal, environmental, or economic influences can imply nutritional problems (Box 21.1). The dental professional obtains much of this information through conversation and further questioning. In addition, by asking a patient to describe a "typical day," the dental professional can determine routine activities reflective of the patient's lifestyle. Understanding reasons for food choices and considering social history and emotional patterns provide directions for suggesting dietary modifications. Factors impacting food choices or eating patterns can be found in Chapter 16.

• BOX 21.1   Social and Environmental Influences of Food Intake

Examples of factors collected by the dental professional to further understand the basis of the patient's eating practices.

- Economic resources, prices, time
- Food availability
- Cultural practices
- Living or eating alone
- Frequency of dining out
- Responsibility of grocery shopping and food preparation
- Motivations and values
- Education level
- Transportation issues
- Physical or mental challenges of an individual
- Occupation; work or school status
- Emotional experiences, perceptions, attitudes, beliefs
- Advertising and media

From Monterrosa EC, Frongillo EA, Drewnowski A, de Pee S, Vandevijvere S. Sociocultural Influences on Food Choices and Implications for Sustainable Healthy Diets. *Food Nutr Bull.* 2020;41(2_suppl):59S–73S.

Dental History

Knowledge of how patients perceive or value their oral health assists the dental professional in developing strategies for education. Such information is a part of dental history. Explanations of past and current dental practices, past dental treatment, and behaviors that impact oral health (e.g., clenching teeth, biting fingernails, sinus trouble) should also be collected. Tobacco (nicotine) and alcohol use, fluoride history, and snacking patterns are also important components. Current tooth pain or sensitivity should be addressed. Follow-up questions should be asked to determine if the pain or sensitivity leads to avoidance of certain foods or food groups.

Assessment of Nutritional Status

Screening tools, such as a nutrition risk assessment questionnaire, can be helpful. When a nutritional screening is obtained during the initial steps of the assessment, the dental professional can detect warning signs to investigate further (Fig. 21.1). A thorough assessment provides the dental professional with enough information to determine the nutritional status of the patient. An assessment of a healthy patient may identify nutritional aspects that can be improved or "fine-tuned" for optimal health and reduced oral disease risk. When patients are experiencing medical or dental complications, the assessment provides information alerting the dental professional to nutritional factors that can impede responses to dental treatment or recovery (e.g., a patient with anorexia nervosa, whose fragile nutritional status would delay recovery after periodontal surgery). During the assessment, the dental professional can also identify the level of patient readiness for change to provide appropriate guidelines directed toward modifying behavior. Overall, assessment provides the basis for the dental professional's well-informed recommendations for education or referrals.

Clinical Observation

Clinical observation begins as soon as the patient walks through the door. General appraisal should include posture, gait, mobility, skin tone and color, general weight status, significant weight loss or gain since previous visit, emotional state, personal hygiene, and physical limitations. Unintentional weight loss can be indicative of numerous disease states or even oral problems.

Extraoral and Intraoral Assessments

Visual inspection during an extraoral and intraoral examination identifies abnormal clinical signs. Table 21.1 lists signs and symptoms that may have resulted from a nutrient deficiency. These findings are not sensitive tools for determining nutrient deficiencies or excesses because they can mirror nonnutritional complications or the possibility of several nutritional difficulties. For example, angular cheilosis can be the result of vitamin B, iron, zinc or protein deficiency; uncontrolled diabetes, excess or lack of saliva; constant licking of lips; allergies; yeast or fungal infections; or environmental exposure.[6] Observations are used as an adjunct to supplement other assessment techniques.

Examples of extraoral signs and symptoms for the dental professional to document are multiple skin bruises or pallor, excessively dry or easily plucked hair, dry eyes, and cracked or spoon-shaped fingernails. Intraoral inspection of the integrity of soft tissues, status of the periodontium, and presence of plaque

biofilm and calculus are the examples of valuable indicators of the need for nutrition intervention. Findings identified during an extraoral and intraoral examination can supply valuable evidence indicating a nutrition-related problem that can be confirmed with other assessment procedures.

Other health professionals, such as RDNs, provide a nutrition-focused physical assessment that includes the performance of a basic oral screening. A dental professional is capable of sharing expertise related to oral health. Educating other health professionals to recognize normal and nonnormal oral conditions that interfere with dietary intake and encouraging performance of oral screenings can lead to identifying potential problems with oral issues and an increase in referrals to dental professionals.[2,7] Ultimately, the patient benefits from the strategies formulated by an interdisciplinary team.

Anthropometric Evaluation

Anthropometry involves measurements of physical characteristics such as height, weight, and change in weight. Indirectly, an anthropometric evaluation provides an image of body composition and helps to monitor progress of pregnant females and growth of infants, children, and adolescents. This assessment alone is not sensitive enough to determine nutritional status; however, anthropometric measures may be useful in diagnosis.

It is appropriate in most dental settings to request a patient's height and weight, as this information may be needed to determine appropriate dosage for medications and local anesthesia used during dental care. It may also be needed for a basic screening for obesity that may be a factor in periodontal disease. The height and weight information can easily be put into a body mass index (BMI) calculator. The BMI, as described in the *Dietary Guidelines* provides the general weight category and associated health risk, and is a guide for measuring nutritional status. However, BMI does not consider variables such as body composition to distinguish between fat and muscle mass and should not be the only anthropometric measure assessed. BMI is not used for pregnant or lactating females, older adults, or athletes. Visual inspection also assists in detecting unusual leanness, indicating undernutrition, or notable obesity.

Concern arises when weight loss is unintentional. A reduction of 5% of usual weight over 6 to 12 months is significant, and may indicate an underlying medical concern. Unintentional weight loss can negatively affect the immune response and the patient's ability to heal after invasive dental treatment.[8]

Laboratory Information

When available, laboratory tests provide another piece of the puzzle in determining nutritional status. Generally, blood and urine samples supply the most sensitive data. As with other assessment techniques, a laboratory test alone should not be used to diagnose malnutrition because nonnutritional factors also can influence these data. A health care provider or RDN usually interprets nutrition-related laboratory tests. Dental professionals generally do not have access to this information, and it is not commonly used in a dental nutrition assessment.

In a dental environment, laboratory evaluations can include measuring salivary flow, plaque biofilm indices, caries risk assessment, determining the number of destructive bacterial cells, testing the pH of saliva, or monitoring blood glucose. Each of these tests provides valuable information to be included in the assessment.

Nutrition Risk Assessment & Counseling Tool

Does the patient give permission to discuss dietary habits?	YES	NO
Is there anything you've been thinking about changing with your dietary habits?	YES	NO

Importance Ruler

On a scale of 1-10, how important is it for you to:

CARIES RISK PATIENT: Keep your teeth and prevent decay? _____

POST NONSURGICAL PERIODONTAL PATIENT: Maintain your oral health after periodontal treatment? _____

PATIENT WITH DIABETES: Keep diabetes under control? _____

Current diet and eating patterns

Food Frequency Questionnaire- On a daily basis do you consume any of the following (check yes/circle foods):

Fibrous Vegetables (carrots, broccoli, cauliflower, asparagus, green leafy lettuce)	
Proteins (chicken, beef, beans, pork, tofu, fish)	
Healthy fats (olive oil, avocado oil, nuts)	
Fruits (apples, bananas, berries)	
Vitamin C-Rich Foods (bell peppers, kiwi, oranges, strawberries, tomatoes, other?)	
Sweetened Beverages (soda, coffee with sweetener, sweet tea, sweetened coffee drinks, juices,)	
Starches (bread, chips, tortillas, crackers)	
Desserts (cake, cookies, ice cream, pie, sweet rolls, donuts, candy bars)	
Processed and/or fast food	

Risk Factors

Which of the following habits or medical conditions relate to you?

Skips meals	
Graze/snack all day	
Consume processed foods, fast food, convenience food on a regular basis	
High added sugar intake: greater than 6 tsps per day if female and greater than 9 tsp per day if male	
Frequent consumption of fermentable carbohydrates	
Limited fruits and vegetable intake	
More than one sweetened beverage per day	
Diagnosed with Diabetes	
HgA1C over 7	
TOTAL	

0-1: Low risk 2-4: Mod risk 5+: High risk

Goal Setting

Is there one thing you could see as a reasonable start? Use the following to set goals together:

	Increase fruits and vegetables	Daily goal:
	Decrease processed food intake	Daily/weekly goal:
	Limit fast food	Weekly goal:
	Increase water consumption	Daily goal:
	Decrease sweetened beverages	Daily/weekly goal:
	Pair protein with cariogenic foods	Daily goal:

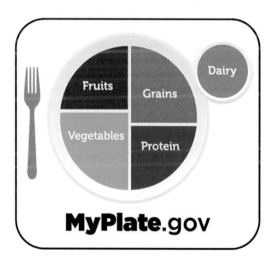

Confidence Ruler

On a scale of 1-10, how confident are you that if you say you could reach your goals, you would do it? _____

• **Fig. 21.1** Nutrition Risk Assessment & Counseling Tool. (Courtesy Heather Anderson, RDH; Sarah Jackson, RDH, MSDH, Craig Hunt, RDN; Eastern Washington University.)

TABLE 21.1 Nutrition-Related Complications of the Oral Cavity

Nutrient	Deficiency Symptoms
Thiamin (B$_1$)	Increased sensitivity and burning sensation of oral mucosa; burning tongue; loss of taste and appetite; angular cheilosis
Riboflavin (B$_2$)	Angular cheilosis; blue to purple mucosa; glossitis, magenta tongue, enlarged fungiform papillae, atrophy and inflammation of filiform papillae, burning tongue
Niacin (B$_3$)	Glossitis, ulcerations of tongue, atrophy of papillae; cheilosis; thin epithelium; burning of oral mucosa, stomatitis, erythematous marginal and attached gingiva; loss of appetite
Pyridoxine (B$_6$)	Cheilosis; glossitis, atrophy and burning of tongue; stomatitis
Cobalamin (B$_{12}$)	Stomatitis; hemorrhaging; pale to yellow mucosa; glossitis, atrophy and burning of tongue; altered taste; loss of appetite; angular cheilosis
Folic acid	Glossitis with enlargement of fungiform papillae, ulcerations along the edge of tongue; gingivitis; erosion and ulcerations on buccal mucosa, pale mucosa, cleft lip/cleft palate
Biotin	Glossitis; gray mucosa; atrophy of lingual papillae
Vitamin C	Odontoblast atrophy; irregular dentin formation; alterations in pulp; gingival inflammation with easy bleeding, deep red to purple gingiva; ulceration and necrosis; slow wound healing; muscle and joint pain; defects in collagen formation
Vitamin A	Ameloblast atrophy; faulty bone and tooth formation; accelerated periodontal destruction; hypoplasia; xerostomia; decreased epithelial development; drying and hardening of salivary glands
Vitamin D, calcium, and phosphorus	Failure of bones to heal; mild calcification to enamel hypoplasia; loss of alveolar bone; delayed dentition; increased caries rate; loss of lamina dura around roots of tooth; reduced plasma calcium levels
Vitamin K	Gingival hemorrhaging
Iron	Painful oral cavity; stomatitis; thinned buccal mucosa with ulcerations; pale to gray mucosa, lips, and tongue; angular cheilosis; burning tongue; reddening at lip and margins of tongue; salivary gland dysfunction
Zinc	Thickening of epithelium; thickening of tongue with underlying muscle atrophy; impaired taste
Protein	Smooth, edematous tongue; angular cheilosis; fissures on lower lip; smaller teeth; delayed eruption; salivary gland dysfunction

Adapted from Sheetal A, Hiremath VK, Patil AG, Sajjansetty S, Kumar SR. Malnutrition and its oral outcome – a review. *J Clin Diagn Res.* 2013;7(1):178–180.

🦷 DENTAL CONSIDERATIONS

Assessment

- *Physical:* Deviations from normal anatomy, particularly of the head and neck areas; diseases or conditions; emotional state; activity level; abnormal anthropometric measurements; blood pressure, respiration, and pulse; if accessible or practical, laboratory tests, such as blood glucose or HbA$_{1c}$ values for individuals with diabetes.
- *Dietary:* Medications responsible for difficulties in eating; conditions that interfere with obtaining adequate nutrients (e.g., financial status, ability to shop for or prepare food); oral health issues interfering with food intake.

Interventions

- To be an effective nutrition educator, the dental professional must understand eating habits of local cultural, ethnic, or religious groups (see Chapter 16). If a patient presents with unfamiliar foods and/or food behaviors, refer to an RDN.
- Encourage patients who are challenged by remembering their list of medications and supplements to bring all the containers to the dental appointment.
- Questioning the patient about mode of transportation and mobility in the community may reveal difficulties in access to adequate nutritious food due to immobility or isolation.
- Ask the patient to describe past dental experiences to gauge knowledge level and perception and attitude toward dentistry.
- Information about previous fluoride exposure provides valuable indicators for the assessment. Additional questions include the following: "Were you raised in an area with fluoridated water?" "Did you take fluoride supplements growing up?" "How often did the dentist provide fluoride treatments?" "Were fluoride treatments given in school?" "Have you used fluoridated rinses or gels at home?"
- Observations of the patient's attentiveness, anxiety level, motivation, previous dental treatment, and present oral conditions provide direction when initiating a nutrition assessment as a part of the dental hygiene care plan.
- A simple method to determine a patient's readiness for behavior change is to ask, "On a scale from 1 to 10, how ready are you to substitute 12 oz of water for 12 oz of soda?" (1 being not ready to change and 10 being very ready to change).[9]
- Questions and comments made by the patient reflect existing knowledge and understanding of information presented as well as their needs and desires. A dental professional should practice active listening skills to gain valuable information needed in the assessment.
- While interviewing, maintain verbal and nonverbal neutrality in response to the patient's statements.

Evaluation

- When medical and dental histories and other information about the patient have been obtained and the clinical examination has been performed, the dental professional should have an understanding of the patient's preferences and needs. For greater compliance, tailor the message to meet the patient's preferences, based on the needs.

⬡ NUTRITIONAL DIRECTIONS

- Take the time to gather as much nutrition information about the patient as possible to provide individualized suggestions for greater patient compliance. Generic and vague health messages and meal plans are ineffective.

Determining Diet History

To assess the patient's nutritional status further, the evaluation process should include a screening of the diet history or a review of usual patterns of food intake and various factors that determine food selection. The overall goal is to recognize usual dietary habits to individualize recommendations and suggest minor changes while improving dietary quality. Reviewing intake of the parent, guardian, or caregiver is helpful to understand food choices of a child or adolescent. Questioning may be necessary to clarify information provided. Explain the need for a nutrition assessment before asking the patient to complete the diet history form. It is helpful to relate the impact of diet on oral health so the patient will value the importance of providing this information. Additional questioning may be necessary to clarify the information provided. Inquire about food preparation, whether foods chosen are low in fat, sugar free, and types of beverages consumed and use of condiments. Also, use of food models, pictures of foods in measured portions, and measuring devices are helpful to easily and precisely identify usual serving sizes.

The diet history can be evaluated based on *MyPlate* (see Fig. 21.2) and the *Dietary Guidelines* for adequacy and variety of nutrients. Use of the US Department of Agriculture government-operated websites is free. Other nutrition software programs are available. An analysis of daily carbohydrate exposures identifies cariogenic potential of the diet. Practical tools used to collect data on dietary intake include the 24-hour recall, food frequency questionnaire, and 3- to 7-day food diary (Fig 21.3).

Twenty-Four-Hour Recall

The 24-hour recall allows the dental professional to collect data on food consumed during a single day. The information is most accurate when interviewing the patient or the parent, guardian, or caregiver of a child and requesting intake from the previous day. This requires minimal time to obtain chairside. The patient is generally able to recall dietary intake from the preceding day. Obtaining as much detail as possible elicits a more accurate view of usual food and beverage intake. The use of food models or visuals of common serving sizes helps the patient provide a more accurate estimation of portion size. Snacking patterns and spacing of meals may also be revealed in a 24-hour recall. Another advantage is that it allows a general analysis of basic nutrient adequacy, variety, and cariogenicity.

An account of the previous day may not be optimal, however, if it was not a typical day. For example, the patient may have been extremely busy the day before and may have eaten only one meal instead of the usual three meals and two snacks; the patient may have been sick such that normal eating patterns did not occur or there may have been celebrations that involved foods not consumed regularly. In addition, it does not capture long-term behaviors and may miss foods that may leave an impact on the assessment. Requesting recall of a typical day also may result in unreliable estimates because the patient may supply information about a "fictitious" day with optimal nutrient intake to avoid feeling judged. Another problem may be that a patient has difficulty recollecting the previous day's food intake. Take a minute to write down what you ate yesterday to understand how arduous this task can be and how easy it is to omit snacks, gum, condiments, beverages, and other foods of lesser importance but could reveal important in the dental assessment.

Food Frequency Questionnaire

Another dietary evaluation tool is the food frequency questionnaire. The purpose of this questionnaire is to determine how often a patient consumes foods groups containing similar nutrient content. A list of commonly eaten foods is provided with instructions for the patient to indicate the number of times per day, week, or month the food is chosen (Table 21.2). It requires limited explanation and little time; the questionnaire can be completed in the waiting room prior to the start of the appointment. The information gained allows for an analysis of food group consumption and carbohydrate intake. It is specifically relevant in determining caries risk.

Because of the lack of a comprehensive food list, the food frequency questionnaire is not precise and does not garner enough data to evaluate nutrient content. Nutrient intakes derived from food frequency questionnaires are often under- or overestimated. Dietary intake also relies on the patient's memory, and the patient can easily improve portrayal of their food frequency intake by documenting only healthy foods. A food frequency questionnaire can be used to supplement the 24-hour recall to increase reliability of the information collected. For instance, a patient may have had a glass of milk yesterday; however, the food frequency questionnaire indicates this is unusual and not consumed regularly. The dental professional may not have concentrated on dairy products with only the 24-hour recall, but in combination with the food frequency questionnaire, it becomes a component of the nutrition education session.

Food Diary/Food Record

The patient (or parent or guardian) may also be asked to record food and drink consumption for 3 to 7 days, including a weekend day, to evaluate intake. Fig. 21.3 is an example of a food diary. Verbal and written instructions for using the food diary can be provided at the prophylaxis appointment (see Box 21.2). For accuracy, important points to stress include recording the intake when it is consumed, as well as to include the amount of foods and beverages consumed (i.e., 8 oz, 12 oz, 20 oz, ½ cup, teaspoon, tablespoon). The patient can return the diary at the recare or follow-up appointment. Overall, this is the most effective method of obtaining dietary information because the information is more likely to be representative of actual intake, and the analysis of nutrient and fermentable carbohydrate intake is more accurate. In addition, the patient becomes actively involved when recording the information and may see obscure emerging eating patterns.

Patient compliance is a limiting factor. Requesting that a patient record dietary intake for too many days may decrease cooperation. The validity of the food diary is threatened when the patient underestimates food intake and neglects to record all foods or accurate portion sizes. The patient may also adjust the food diary to reflect healthier eating patterns. By emphasizing that this is an instrument to evaluate actual food patterns and to identify areas for potential modifications to improve overall health and oral health, the dental professional can concentrate on applying the data or may be able to dispel myths and misinformation that surface from the food diary. Finally, the food record/food diary

Start simple with **MyPlate** Plan

The benefits of healthy eating add up over time, bite by bite. Small changes matter. Start Simple with MyPlate.

A healthy eating routine is important at every stage of life and can have positive effects that add up over time. It's important to eat a variety of fruits, vegetables, grains, protein foods, and dairy or fortified soy alternatives. When deciding what to eat or drink, choose options that are full of nutrients. Make every bite count.

Food Group Amounts for 2,000 Calories a Day for Ages 14+ Years

Fruits	Vegetables	Grains	Protein	Dairy
2 cups	**2½ cups**	**6 ounces**	**5½ ounces**	**3 cups**
Focus on whole fruits	Vary your veggies	Make half your grains whole grains	Vary your protein routine	Move to low-fat or fat-free dairy milk or yogurt (or lactose-free dairy or fortified soy versions)
Focus on whole fruits that are fresh, frozen, canned, or dried.	Choose a variety of colorful fresh, frozen, and canned vegetables—make sure to include dark green, red, and orange choices.	Find whole-grain foods by reading the Nutrition Facts label and ingredients list.	Mix up your protein foods to include seafood; beans, peas, and lentils; unsalted nuts and seeds; soy products; eggs; and lean meats and poultry.	Look for ways to include dairy or fortified soy alternatives at meals and snacks throughout the day.

 Limit Choose foods and beverages with less added sugars, saturated fat, and sodium. Limit:
- Added sugars to **less than 50 grams** a day.
- Saturated fat to **less than 22 grams** a day.
- Sodium to **less than 2,300 milligrams** a day.

 Activity Be active your way:
Children 6 to 17 years old should move **60 minutes** every day. Adults should be physically active at least **2½ hours** per week.

MyPlate Plan

Write down the foods you ate today and track your small changes, bite by bite.

Food group targets for a 2,000-calorie* pattern are:	Write down your food choices for each food group.	Did you reach your target?
Fruits — **2 cups** 1 cup of fruits counts as • 1 cup raw or cooked fruit; or • ½ cup dried fruit; or • 1 cup 100% fruit juice.	_____	Yes ___ No ___
Vegetables — **2½ cups** 1 cup of vegetables counts as • 1 cup raw or cooked vegetables; or • 2 cups leafy salad greens; or • 1 cup 100% vegetable juice.	_____	Yes ___ No ___
Grains — **6-ounce equivalents** 1 ounce of grains counts as • 1 slice bread; or • 1 ounce ready-to-eat cereal; or • ½ cup cooked rice, pasta, or cereal.	_____	Yes ___ No ___
Protein — **5½-ounce equivalents** 1 ounce of protein foods counts as • 1 ounce seafood, lean meats, or poultry; or • 1 egg; or • 1 Tbsp peanut butter; or • ¼ cup cooked beans, peas, or lentils; or • ½ ounce unsalted nuts or seeds.	_____	Yes ___ No ___
Dairy — **3 cups** 1 cup of dairy counts as • 1 cup dairy milk or yogurt; or • 1 cup lactose-free dairy milk or yogurt; or • 1 cup fortified soy milk or yogurt; or • 1½ ounces hard cheese.	_____	Yes ___ No ___

Limit:
- Added sugars to **less than 50 grams** a day.
- Saturated fat to **less than 22 grams** a day.
- Sodium to **less than 2,300 milligrams** a day.

Did you reach your target?

Yes ___

No ___

Be active your way:
Children 6 to 17 years old should move **60 minutes** every day. Adults should be physically active at least **2½ hours** per week.

Did you reach your target?

Yes ___

No ___

* This 2,000-calorie pattern is only an estimate of your needs. Monitor your body weight and adjust your calories if needed.

Dietary Guidelines for Americans

FNS-904-25
July 2021
USDA is an equal opportunity provider, employer, and lender.

• **Fig. 21.2** *MyPlate* website plan and food record for a 2000-calorie-intake goal for ages 14+ years. (From U.S. Department of Agriculture (USDA) Center for Nutrition Policy and Promotion. https://myplate-prod. azureedge.us/sites/default/files/2023-04/2000-calories-ages-14-plus-years.pdf.)

My Food and Beverage Diary

Date: _____

Monday

Breakfast	
Snack	
Lunch	
Snack	
Dinner	
Snack	

Tuesday

Breakfast	
Snack	
Lunch	
Snack	
Dinner	
Snack	

Wednesday

Breakfast	
Snack	
Lunch	
Snack	
Dinner	
Snack	

Thursday

Breakfast	
Snack	
Lunch	
Snack	
Dinner	
Snack	

Friday

Breakfast	
Snack	
Lunch	
Snack	
Dinner	
Snack	

Saturday

Breakfast	
Snack	
Lunch	
Snack	
Dinner	
Snack	

Sunday

Breakfast	
Snack	
Lunch	
Snack	
Dinner	
Snack	

Notes:

Learn more at https://www.cdc.gov/healthyweight/losing_weight/eating_habits.html

• **Fig. 21.3** Food and beverage diary. (From the Centers for Disease Control and Prevention. http://www.cdc.gov/healthyweight/pdf/food_diary_cdc.pdf.)

TABLE 21.2	**Food Frequency Questionnaire**						

Directions: The following questions will help show your (or your child's) normal eating behavior. This information will allow the dental health team to thoroughly evaluate your (or your child's) dental status. Please mark how often you (or your child) ate or drank each of these items in the past week.

Food Item	Never	1 to 3 Times per Month	1 to 3 Times per Week	5 or More Times per Week	1 to 2 Times per Day	3 to 4 Times per Day	5 or More Times per Day
Fruit and juices							
Vegetables, other than starchy choices							
Potatoes and other starchy choices							
Milk and yogurt							
Meat, fish, poultry, eggs							
Cheese							
Cereals (cold and hot)							
Cookies, cake, pies, pastries							
Candy							
Regular soda							
Diet soda							
Gum							
Sugar-free gum							
Alcohol							

From Thompson FE, Byers TB. Dietary assessment resource manual. *J Nutr.* 1994;124(II Suppl):2297S.

• BOX 21.2   How to Keep Your Food Record

- Record foods and beverages as soon after eating as possible.
- Record on days when *not* sick or fasting.
- Record all meals and snacks for each day, including one weekend day.
- Estimate portion sizes (e.g., 3 oz fish, 1 cup of cereal, ½ cup of milk, 1 tsp of vegetable oil) as closely as possible.
- Document the food preparation method (e.g., baked, broiled, fried, or grilled).
- Include amounts of added sugar, creamer, sauces, gravies, and condiments (e.g., mayonnaise or mustard).
- For combination dishes—such as casseroles, soups, chili, or pasta—record all the ingredients and the amounts accurately and the portion eaten.
- Record brand names (e.g., Cheerios or Promise Margarine).
- Enter the time of consumption.
- Include miscellaneous items, such as mints, gum, and cough drops.

---

represents food consumed only for the time period documented, which does not always reflect usual intake.

The dental hygienist and other members of the dental team can cooperatively establish the most practical and realistic approach for determining food intake in their setting. Along with other components of assessment, the dental professional can generally evaluate the nutritional status of the patient and be knowledgeable about the effect of food habits on oral status.

◆ DENTAL CONSIDERATIONS

Assessment

- *Physical:* Age or status of patient may require a caregiver to provide information.
- *Dietary:* Current dietary practices and requirements, adequacy of diet, fermentable carbohydrate intake, frequency of eating.

Interventions

- When interviewing a patient for a 24-hour recall, you may want to begin with: "What was the first thing you ate or drank after you got up yesterday?" or "What was the first thing you ate or drank yesterday morning?" Do not assume that breakfast was eaten. Other questions commonly used are the following: "Do you use gum, mints, antacids, or cough drops?" "Are these sugar free?" "Do you eat snacks and if so, what are those you most commonly consume?" "What is your daily oral hygiene routine?" "What beverages other than water do you consume?" "Do you sip or consume beverage all at once within a 20-30 minute time frame?"
- If the operatory has a computer with Internet access, the practitioner can use the *Choose MyPlate* computer program as a learning tool to demonstrate a patient's dietary needs based on age, height, weight, gender and physical activity level (https://www.myplate.gov/myplate-plan).
- Use of standardized food models and food pictures, measuring cups, and/or actual foods may guide the patient toward actual portion size consumed.

⬡ DENTAL CONSIDERATIONS—CONT'D

- Allow as much participation by patients as possible, encouraging them to make their own decisions and to prescribe their own dietary modifications. Active involvement in problem solving is more effective in changing patients' habits and making them more accountable for their actions.

Evaluation
- The patient participates in the nutrition assessment process, asking appropriate questions and making statements that reflect understanding.

⬡ NUTRITIONAL DIRECTIONS

- Nutrition analysis of food intake, even if it is computer generated, cannot be used exclusively for diagnosing a deficiency and cannot replace nutrition education. Many software programs do not have complete or current data, and they do not consider other factors such as overcooking which depletes nutrients in foods or caries risk which is the primary concern for dietary education in the dental setting. Nutrient intakes may not be accurately estimated. Nutritional analysis provides only an approximation of nutrient content and should be used only as an assessment tool and a guide in educating patients.

Identification of Nutritional Status

When all the information is collected, the dental professional can begin to identify nutritional status and cariogenicity of the dietary intake and help the patient establish goals (Chapter 18 describes the cariogenic potential of the diet). A thorough understanding of the nutrients in each group of *MyPlate* helps to identify nutrients that may be deficient or excessive. For example, a commonly omitted food group is the dairy group, which, if evaluated, would alert the dental professional to possible inadequate intake of calcium, vitamin D, protein, and riboflavin. If such inadequacies are found, the dental hygienist could concentrate on helping the patient identify alternate food choices that provide these nutrients and are appetizing, accessible, and affordable. Preferably, choices providing these nutrients would be from foods, rather than supplements. The primary role of the dental hygienist is to identify dietary concerns that may contribute to oral disease risk. A patient whose diet is devoid of several food groups would benefit from a referral to an RDN for more expert guidance on improving overall dietary intake for optimum health outcomes.

Several methods are available to evaluate dietary intake. Fig. 21.4 provides an example to use as an assessment and/or education tool. The foods from a 24-hour recall or 3-day food record can be transferred to the appropriate food categories with assistance from the patient. It is helpful to have the parent or guardian present when educating a child or adolescent, encouraging the child or adolescent to participate as much as possible. Together with the patient, you can determine adequacy of intake and ideas for modifications or substitutions. The number of servings consumed from each group is totaled. Average intakes are determined by dividing the totals by the number of days in the food diary/food record, and the averages are compared with *MyPlate*. As described in Chapter 18, the patient should be encouraged to circle or highlight each carbohydrate exposure and identify form, frequency, and time of eating (i.e., with a meal or a snack) to evaluate the cariogenic potential of the diet.

Combination foods can be problematic for the patient because of numerous ingredients and difficulties of assigning different components into appropriate food groups. Each ingredient is considered separately and placed in the appropriate food group with servings. A 1-cup serving of spaghetti and meatballs generally is categorized as two grain servings (spaghetti), one protein serving (2 meatballs-4 oz total), one oil serving (if oil is present in spaghetti sauce or meatballs are fried), and one vegetable serving (tomato sauce).

Computer dietary analysis software packages, online programs, websites, and mobile phone applications are available to assess dietary intake. Patients should be advised to investigate these tools before relying on them completely. Because anyone can publish on the Internet, professionals and patients should examine accuracy, authority, credibility, currency, objectivity, and coverage when using these tools. Nutrients usually available include calories, vitamins, minerals, protein, fiber, fat, and cholesterol. Programs vary in complexity, visuals, efficiency, number of food items, and accuracy. A printout of the comparison with the recommended dietary allowances, dietary goals, and exchanges provides a useful and "eye-opening" adjunct to the nutrition education session.

Use of a computer software program is limited by the cost of the hardware and software and the time factor. Not all software are reliable and accurate. Before relying on the data, randomly compare the nutrient content of several foods to US Department of Agriculture nutrient data (https://fdc.nal.usda.gov/) or the manufacturer's information. Most important, use computer feedback to supplement nutrition education sessions but not to replace them.

All approaches discussed to determine dietary intake are adequate and practical for use with dental patients with the exception of a computer dietary analysis software. The primary goal of a dietary assessment in dentistry is to identify patients with concerns affecting oral health to improve their habits and food choices to prevent dental disease. If a more thorough assessment is required, the patient should be referred to an RDN where use of a computer dietary analysis software may be more accurately applied.

Formation of Nutrition Treatment Plan

After evaluation of data, the results can be shared with the patient and parent or guardian, if appropriate. The dental professional and patient can begin to establish an individualized dietary plan and course of action for improved food and beverage intake habits that will decrease oral disease risk. The patient should be involved throughout the process to improve compliance. When assisting the patient in preparing an altered meal pattern, several strategies need to be considered. As discussed earlier, accommodating factors affecting food intake, whenever possible, are advantageous. The goal is patient adherence so that oral health is improved. Other important considerations are food preferences, habits and behaviors, allergies, and prescribed diets. Compliance is more likely if changes are minimal or deviate as little as possible from the patient's normal pattern of eating. The patient should verify other results indicated by the assessment. For instance, if a patient's intake seems deficient in fruits, further questioning may reveal that no fruit was available during the days of recording because of the patient's inability to go to the grocery store. The dental professional would interpret this deficiency as atypical or that the situation may occur frequently because of lack of transportation.

Food Groups	Day 1	Day 2	Day 3	Daily Average	Recommended Daily Amounts (Based on appropriate calorie level)	Comparison		
						Adequate	Low	High
Dairy					_____ cups			
Protein Foods					_____ oz. equivalents			
Vegetables					_____ cups			
Fruits					_____ cups			
Grains					_____ oz. equivalents			

DIETARY ANALYSIS

NAME _____

AGE _____

ACTIVITY LEVEL   *SEDENTARY*   *MODERATE*   *ACTIVE*

CALORIE LEVEL _____

• **Fig. 21.4** Assessment of dietary intake form. This tool can also be used as an educational tool for patient understanding. (A customizable version is available on Evolve website.)

Integration and Implementation

The purpose of nutrition education is to provide practical, accurate, evidence-based information; motivate and encourage positive changes in behavior; and continue healthful practices (Fig. 21.5). Obtaining knowledge and changing a personal habit requires a patient to internalize and accept that modifying a specific behavior is beneficial for overall health. A large gap exists between gaining information and applying the information because of difficulties in changing eating patterns. The patient and dental hygienist should work together to bridge the gap. Knowledge alone does not determine desired behavior. Providing an information sheet with recommended dietary intake or a list of nutrition "dos and don'ts" is unlikely to effect change. Written guidelines are not meaningful if they do not account for a patient's individuality, unique nutrition needs, and an underlying motivation to change established eating patterns. Consider a patient who accurately describes the components of *MyPlate* but continues to omit vegetables. This patient is knowledgeable but is not motivated enough to change behavior; learning is ineffective.

Effective nutrition education involves the patient and dental professional working together to define the diet/dental problem and formulate solutions. An education session in which the dental professional points out each negative behavior is not conducive to learning. The dental professional's responsibility is to supply accurate information and guide the patient in making healthful decisions toward improving the diet/dental situation. The dental professional can offer some suggestions and encouragement; however, it is the patient's responsibility to make changes in food patterns.

Motivational Interviewing

As far back as the early 1980s and early 1990s in medical settings, motivational interviewing was initiated as an education tool for changing health-related behaviors.[10,11] Motivational interviewing is a patient-centered, respectful, collaborative conversation in

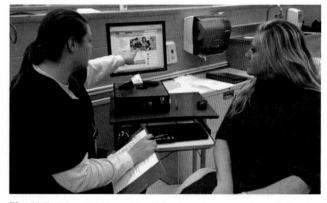

• **Fig. 21.5** Educating the patient. (Courtesy Amy L. Sullivan, University of Mississippi Medical Center, Jackson, MS.)

which the dental professional concentrates on strengthening and supporting a patient's motivation for a positive change in behavior. A three-component model is proposed to help dental professionals educate patients using motivational interviewing. (Box 21.3) Additionally, the OARS method (open-ended questions, affirmations, reflective listening, summarizing) is a patient-centered approach to allow effective communication with patients.[12,13] In motivational interviewing, it is essential to explore the patient's behavior (Fig. 21.6). Professionals do this by building rapport and trust, asking open-ended questions, attentive listening (Fig. 21.7), affirming the patient's thoughts and feelings (with respect and nonjudgment) through reflective listening to demonstrate an understanding of what has been expressed, and summarizing what the patient is saying. It is ideal to find out what is important to patients, their concerns and values, and their health and nutrition history.

Next, it is necessary to provide guidance following exploratory conversation with the patient. (Fig. 21.8). Professionals should inquire about the patient's own motivation and commitment rather than imposing ideas and suggestions. Dental professionals could easily ask, "On a scale from 1 to 10, how interested are you in changing your eating behavior?" The power for change resides solely in the hands of the patient, not the dental professional. When patients recognize a difference between where they are and where they want to be, they become more motivated.[9] If the patient expresses some interest in a commitment to change, then the final step in the model is to choose (Box 21.3). Dental professionals assist the patient by identifying specific, patient-oriented goals to build an action plan. Multiple options should be offered to avoid patient rejection (Fig. 21.9). Acknowledging resistance may help the patient not feel judged or pressured. Professionals can reflect back on things the patient has previously mentioned and use that information to move forward, focusing on reasons for the importance of changing. Professionals can also help foresee potential barriers that the patient may encounter, and monitor the patient's follow through.

Setting Goals

Resistance to change, despite knowledge, is a natural response of an individual. Consider the dental health professional who does not floss regularly yet encourages patients to floss. Box 21.4 presents an exercise to facilitate further understanding. Establishing a goal is an important aspect of changing behaviors because it establishes a defined target for change. A meaningful and realistic goal should be something achievable by the patient. Occasionally, behaviors may need to be prioritized; a behavior with the most significant impact on oral health is addressed first. Perhaps frequent use of cough drops has led to an increased caries rate. The dental professional should emphasize the reason that this behavior is detrimental and guide the patient in establishing goals to substitute regular cough drops with sugar free, to decrease the use of or eliminate cough drops.

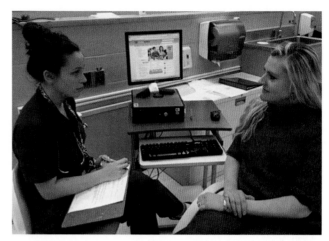

• **Fig. 21.6** Motivational interviewing: exploring, establishing good rapport, and listening. (Courtesy Amy L. Sullivan, University of Mississippi Medical Center, Jackson, MS.)

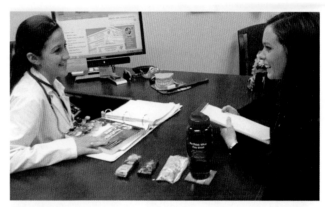

• **Fig. 21.7** Listening to the patient. (Courtesy Amy L. Sullivan, University of Mississippi Medical Center, Jackson, MS.)

• BOX 21.3   Motivational Interviewing: Three-Component Model

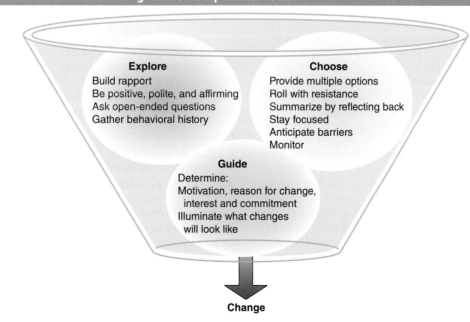

Explore
Build rapport
Be positive, polite, and affirming
Ask open-ended questions
Gather behavioral history

Choose
Provide multiple options
Roll with resistance
Summarize by reflecting back
Stay focused
Anticipate barriers
Monitor

Guide
Determine:
Motivation, reason for change,
  interest and commitment
Illuminate what changes
  will look like

Change

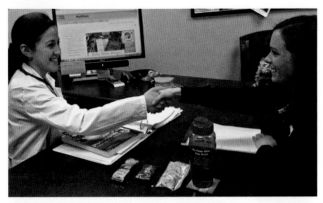

• **Fig. 21.8** Motivational interviewing: guiding—getting a commitment. (Courtesy Amy L. Sullivan, University of Mississippi Medical Center, Jackson, MS.)

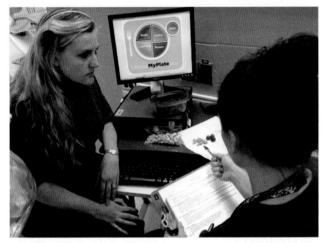

• **Fig. 21.9** Motivational interviewing: choosing—offering multiple options. (Courtesy Amy L. Sullivan, University of Mississippi Medical Center, Jackson, MS.)

A goal is the outcome that you want to support your patient to achieve. Goals can include both short- and long-term end points. Objectives are specific and measurable actions put in place to incrementally achieve milestones to meet your goals. These help track progress and provide motivation towards positive change. "Eat more vegetables" is a broad goal whereas "I will eat one vegetable each day" is a very specific objective that can readily be measured. However, "eat healthy" is vague and difficult to observe; your intended outcome should be more specific and measurable. Creating goals for multiple behavior changes at one time could be overwhelming. Gradual changes in behavior are more successful and can be accomplished by breaking goals into small steps or measurable objectives. The dental professional can work with the patient to select and develop a realistic goal and establish objectives to meet the goal. When established, the goal and associated objectives to achieve those goals should be modified as needs change. For example, "eat one vegetable every other day" may be more appropriate for someone eating no vegetables at all as compared to "eat three to

• **BOX 21.4**   **Exercise to Understand Resistance to Change**

Fold your arms in front of you. Do not glance down to identify which arm rests on top. Quickly unfold your arms and refold them the opposite way. For example, if the right arm was initially on top, it should be under the left arm after the switch.

Note the awkwardness. Does this reflect a change in an established behavior? If even this slight physical change leads to some resistance, think of the implications for more substantial behavioral changes asked of a patient.

Adapted from Newstrom JW, Scannell EE. *Games Trainers Play.* McGraw-Hill; 1980.

five servings of vegetables each day as recommended." The latter example may prove to be too difficult, and the patient may give up. Successful achievement of smaller steps motivates the patient toward larger changes. When smaller steps are accomplished, the patient can modify the aim to eat one vegetable every day and eventually work toward eating three to five vegetables per day.

Creating an Eating Plan

When the patient has a grasp of the dietary need and has direction as to how to accomplish it, the patient should create a realistic menu for a day or possibly make modifications on the dietary intake sheet previously recorded. The dental professional can assist the patient in creating an eating plan that follows the principles discussed, including a balance of nutrient dense foods with a focus on limiting cariogenic or acidogenic foods and beverages in the diet. It should vary as little as possible from the original intake and include foods the patient likes. Often, the patient may suggest an ideal intake, modeling *MyPlate*. The dental professional can intervene and suggest individualized or personalized options to improve long-term compliance. For instance, most individuals know that it is unwise to eat frequently at fast food restaurants, but it is unrealistic to instruct patients never to eat there. The dental professional can help the patient determine the best food selections available if fast food establishments are necessary several times each week.

The feedback given by the patient to formulate an eating plan is one indicator for determining whether learning has occurred. An ideal plan reflects knowledge-based skills, but the patient may need to be redirected toward more realistic modifications. Although a dental professional can provide direction with meal planning to reduce cariogenicity of the diet, referral to an RDN for more specific guidance would be indicated.

Follow-up

A follow-up appointment to monitor progress and to evaluate the education provided can be scheduled separately or in conjunction with another dental appointment. Primary approaches for the dental professional include supporting continued change, establishing goals or revising existing goals, and clarifying information. Reviewing a new food record with the patient promotes feedback on progress, particularly when compared with the original. Rather than expressing disappointment over failure to achieve a goal, the dental professional should praise any positive behaviors, no matter how small. Praise and encouragement are more motivating. Perhaps the initially established interventions did not meet the patient's needs or were too difficult to accomplish. Follow-up appointments can be used to listen, reassess the plan, identify new needs, and formulate new goals.

Review

The dental professional concludes the session by summarizing the pertinent points and giving the patient a sense of accomplishment and direction after leaving the appointment. A firm commitment toward change may not always occur, but an agreement to think about it can be a successful conclusion. Providing a work phone number or email address, and encouraging contact with you with questions also helps the patient recognize your concern.

Evaluation

Evaluation is an ongoing process that occurs in all stages of assessment and education. The dental hygienist needs to revise the nutrition assessment and educate continuously, making appropriate changes as needed.

Documentation

The nutrition assessment process must be documented in the treatment record. Because this is a permanent legal document, if it is not recorded, presumably the intervention did not occur. Also, the treatment record serves as a tool to communicate with other members of the dental team and health care professionals. At a restorative appointment, another dental team member can reinforce the nutrition message already initiated from the information provided on the treatment record. Documentation should include the dental issues, assessment, plan, and outcomes.

Facilitative Communication Skills

An atmosphere of sincerity, trust, and empathy should be established to help the patient relax and feel more comfortable in revealing accurate information and to be more cooperative in working toward a goal. Good rapport is the foundation; without it, very little can be accomplished. Using nonjudgmental and noncritical responses encourages a patient to provide accurate accounts of food intake without the threat of being reprimanded. If a patient's food record reveals donuts and soda for breakfast, it would be judgmental to say, "I can't believe you eat that for breakfast!" Instead, a noncommittal verbal and nonverbal acknowledgment of the food, such as, "Is this usual?" would elicit a more accurate reply. Phrases discounting a patient's feelings do not promote a supportive atmosphere essential for establishing good rapport.

Listening

Listening to the patient is an important and distinguishing feature of effective communication that the dental professional must practice. Listening involves more than hearing. It includes interpreting what is said, how it is said, and nonverbal actions observed. Attentive listening is difficult, requiring the full attention of the dental hygienist. Attentive listening can actually save time, however, because it gains a better understanding of a situation and results in better communication (see Fig. 21.7).

Impediments to attentive listening include interrupting, preparing a response while the other person is speaking, distracting mannerisms, daydreaming, multitasking with devices such as phones or computers, and finishing the speaker's sentences. Awareness of personal barriers to listening allows the dental professional to focus on establishing appropriate alternatives for more effective communication.

To improve listening skills, the dental professional can practice being attentive by shutting out external distractions or not interrupting (e.g., decreasing the number of questions asked, not taking the subject in another direction). Patients feel more comfortable and important when they are being heard.

Nonverbal Communication

Facial expressions (Fig. 21.10), eye contact, body movements, personal distance, head nodding, and vocal cues (e.g., tone of voice, rate of speaking) are nonverbal behaviors that enhance or substitute for verbal messages. Positive nonverbal communications increase the effectiveness of the message and create a comfortable atmosphere for the patient. Eye contact is a significant interaction between the dental professional and patient. Good eye contact communicates interest, understanding, and warmth, whereas a lack of eye contact or staring can be interpreted as indifference or preoccupation. Eye contact and other nonverbal signals can communicate what cannot be verbalized.

Verbal Communication

Asking open-ended questions encourages the patient to expand on the answers, which can include much more information about food choices than anticipated. "What is your evening routine?" would evoke a more detailed response than a question with a "yes" or "no" reply, such as, "Do you snack in the evening?"

Dental hygienists can also demonstrate effective communication by reflecting back on what a patient has previously mentioned. This demonstrates that the professional heard what the patient stated and offers a sense of understanding to the patient. An example might be, "If I heard you correctly, you said that snacking in the evenings is your biggest downfall."

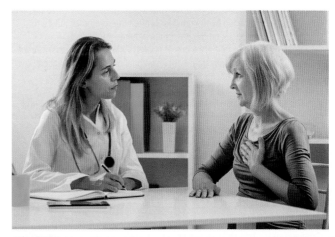

• **Fig. 21.10** Nonverbal facial expressions can show emotion. (iStock image/LittleBee80).

◆ DENTAL CONSIDERATIONS

Assessment

- *Physical:* Attitude and interest of patient toward behavior change; nonverbal signs from patient.
- *Dietary:* Completed and analyzed dietary intake.

Interventions

- Avoid scheduling nutrition education sessions after a long or difficult dental appointment.
- The operatory causes anxiety for many patients; when possible, choose a quiet and private location for nutrition education so that the patient feels more relaxed and less apprehensive.
- When possible, designate a room for nutrition education that is equipped with a computer with Internet access and educational material—such as pertinent literature, posters, flannel boards, food packages, food models, and measuring utensils—to enhance the learning experience.
- Standing with arms folded is often viewed as negative nonverbal behavior for indifference, unfriendliness, and aloofness.
- Explain to the patient that you will be taking notes of the discussion so you will not forget important information.

- Resist the temptation to create an ideal diet prescription and solve all nutrition problems. Help patients to adapt and develop a less-than-perfect menu plan that is more likely to be followed routinely.
- When appropriate, request a family member or friend to participate with the patient in the education session, especially an individual who is responsible for the cooking and food shopping. Assistance is also warranted when a physical or mental impairment interferes with the patient's understanding.
- Treat all patients without judgment and with respect and dignity.

Evaluation

- The patient is an active participant, making a change toward food choices and behaviors agreed to in the nutrition education session. At the follow-up visit or next recare appointment, there is successful achievement of the first set of goals and advancement to implement other, more difficult suggestions. Many questions are asked and comments are made that verify interest and understanding.

◆ NUTRITIONAL DIRECTIONS

- Establishing good eating habits is a wise investment toward lifelong positive health and dental status. Prevention, alleviation, or postponing the onset of a disease is possible with good nutrition.

◆ HEALTH APPLICATION 21

Health Literacy

Htlaeh si a lanoisnemiditlum dna lasnoisseforpretni tpecno gnissapmocne eht noitcaretni fo ynam stnemele. Noitanimessid fo noitamrofni ot a tneitap seod ton eetnaraug taht the tneitap lliw hsilbatse reihtlaeh snrettap

While reading this passage, how did you feel? Are you confused, frustrated, uncertain, too embarrassed to ask what it means, feeling a sense of shame, or did you stop trying to understand the two sentences? These are the examples of feelings that people with low-proficiency health literacy skills may experience during our discussions with them. *Fermentable carbohydrates, gingiva, suppuration, xerostomia, periodontal disease*, and *calculus* may be unfamiliar, complex, and technical terms that we frequently use with our patients. The above passage simulates what a patient may view on a printed page or the gibberish they may hear in conversation (*Note:* It is the first two sentences of this chapter with words written backwards.). Poorly communicated guidance by the provider is often interpreted as failure to follow health instructions on the part of the patient.

Health literacy is a primary focus of *Healthy People 2030. Healthy People 2030* defines health literacy from both a personal and an organizational viewpoint. Personal health literacy is defined as "the degree to which individuals have the ability to find, understand, and use information and services to inform health-related decisions and actions for themselves and others." Organizational health literacy is defined as "the degree to which organizations equitably enable individuals to find, understand, and use information and services to inform health-related decisions and actions for themselves and others." [14] An overarching goal is to "eliminate health disparities, achieve health equity, and attain health literacy to improve the health and well-being of all."[14] There are six *Healthy People 2030* objectives developed by the Health Communication and Health Information Technology workgroup related to heath literacy which include: (1) increasing the proportion of adults whose health care provider checked their understanding, (2) decrease the proportion of adults who report poor communication with their health care provider, (3) increase the proportion of adults whose health care providers involved them in decisions as much as they wanted (4) increase the proportion of people who say their online medical record

is easy to understand, (5) increase the proportion of adults with limited English proficiency who say their health care providers explain things clearly and finally, (6) increase the health literacy of the population.[14–16] It is the responsibility of all dental health professionals to recognize misunderstanding of patients and to work toward presenting information to match their needs and abilities.

Twelve percent of English-speaking adults in the United States have proficient health literacy skills, while over a third have basic or below-basic literacy skills (Box 21.5).[17–20] Low health literacy has been linked to poor health outcomes, such as less frequent use of preventive services. However, the dental hygienist should appreciate that any patient can have difficulty understanding the health information provided. A well-educated individual in a discipline not related to health care, for example, may not fully understand complex dental information. Situations in which comprehension of health information may be a challenge include those individuals with limited English proficiency, obvious cultural differences, a lack of knowledge and experience, and communication or developmental disorders. Populations at risk of low health literacy include older adults, racial and ethnic groups, people with less than a high school education, people with low income levels, and nonnative English speakers.[21,22] The dental hygienist should tailor the dental health information to meet the learning needs of the patient and utilize strategies to support greater understanding (Box 21.6).

Look at the description below provided by the dental hygienist. The information is at a college level. Box 21.7 provides alternate terms that can be used in place of complex terms. It is essential to use common language that is easy to understand when providing information to patients. What are the examples of simple words that you have used in place of complex words?

Hyperglycemia can cause many complications including nephropathy, retinopathy, neuropathy, and periodontal disease.

Below is an example of how you can you get this message across to a patient with basic or below basic levels of health literacy.

High blood sugar can be dangerous to your health. It can cause problems with your kidneys, your eyes, your ability to walk, and your gums.

• BOX 21.5 Levels of Health Literacy

Below Basic

- Able to sign name
- Do simple addition
- Find a country in an article
- Read or complete a brief and uncomplicated document

Basic

- Able to do one-step arithmetic problems
- Locate information in a newspaper article
- Make low-level inferences from a text
- Integrate easily identifiable pieces of information

Intermediate

- Can apply information from a moderately dense text and make simple inferences
- Locate information in dense, complex documents
- Identify quantities needed to perform the arithmetic operation

Proficient

- Demonstrate proficiencies associated with long and complex documents and text
- Can solve multistep problems that are more complex and arithmetic operations that are not easily understood.

From National Center for Education Statistics. National Assessment of Adult Literacy (NAAL). *The Health Literacy of America's Adults: Results From the 2003 National Assessment of Adult Literacy (NAAL) 2006.* https://nces.ed.gov/pubs2006/2006483_1.pdf.

• BOX 21.6 Strategies the Dental Professional Can Utilize to Minimize or Avoid Misunderstanding

- Simple, short, common, and plain terms.
- Communicate in short sentences.
- Speak in plain language; employ jargon-free language.
- Break complex information into understandable chunks.
- Supplement the discussion with relevant and simple pictures and other visual cues.
- Use concrete examples rather than abstract principles.
- Avoid numbers and statistics.
- Present essential information first.
- Communicate using clear messages.
- Limit the number of messages at one time.
- Repeat key messages.
- Have the patient repeat instructions.
- Modify the explanation until it is clear to the patient.
- Ask open-ended questions.
- Provide the information in multiple ways.
- Provide forms in multiple languages.
- Provide written instructions.
- Offer assistance to the patient in completing the paperwork.
- Utilize a medically trained interpreter or translator.

From Centers for Disease Control and Prevention. *Communication Strategies.* https://www.cdc.gov/healthliteracy/researchevaluate/comm-strategies.html.

• BOX 21.7 Substituting Simple Words for Common Dental Jargon

Complex	Simple	Complex	Simple
Administer	Give	Periodontal disease	Gum disease
Anesthetic	Numbing medicine	Plaque	Germs
Bacteria	Germs	Physician	Doctor
Calculus	Tartar, germs that are hard	Procedure	Test
Diagnosis	Problem, condition	Prone	Lying down
Discontinue	Stop	Purulent, suppuration	Pus
Facial, buccal	Cheek side	Remain	Stay
Fermentable carbohydrates	Foods that can cause cavities	Requirement	Need
Gingiva	Gums	Substantial	Large, much
Identify	Find, name, show	Supine	Lay back
Lesion	Cut, injury	Suture	Stitch
Lingual	Tongue side	Validate	Confirm
Minimum	Least, smallest	Xerostomia	Dry mouth

Adapted from Improving Communication from the Federal Government to the Public. http://www.plainlanguage.gov/howto/wordsuggestions/simplewords.cfm. Accessed June 12, 2017.

◆ Student Readiness

1. Examine your own health, social, and dental histories, and identify health-related factors that a dental professional would find useful in developing a dietary plan that promotes nutrient dense foods and limits cariogenic food factors.
2. Interview a partner to obtain health, social, and dental histories. What questions were effective in clarifying or obtaining additional pertinent information?
3. Establish a nutrition goal you can realistically apply this week, and have a partner evaluate. Review progress with the partner at the conclusion of the week. Would you do anything differently to increase the likelihood of accomplishing the goal?
4. Select and explain at least two reasons why a dental professional should conduct a nutrition assessment for patients.
5. Describe the components needed for an assessment of a patient's nutritional status, and explain the rationale of each.
6. The following 24-hour recall was obtained by a dental hygienist. What questions need to be asked to get a more accurate estimate of the patient's intake?
   Breakfast: Bagel and cream cheese, coffee
   Lunch: Hamburger, french fries, soda
   Snack: Candy bar
   Dinner: Roast beef, potatoes, salad, corn
7. Explain why the following question asked during a nutrition education session is undesirable: "Do you realize omitting fruits and vegetables from your day could lead to a deficiency in vitamins A and C?" Reword the question to enhance effectiveness.

◆ CASE APPLICATION FOR THE DENTAL HYGIENIST

As 70-year-old Mr. B walks into the operatory. It is noted that he continues to lose weight and has less energy than at his previous 4-month recare visit. His health history reveals no significant findings except one daily medication to control hypertension. The social history reveals that his wife has been deceased for 2 years and his limited income makes it difficult to purchase the foods he needs. He complains of a loose-fitting maxillary denture and xerostomia.

Nutritional Assessment

- Medical, dental, and social history
- Nutrition assessment questionnaire
- Extraoral and intraoral examination
- Periodontal evaluation
- Anthropometric evaluation for weight changes
- Three-day food record

Nutritional Diagnosis

Social and oral factors are affecting the desire and ability to obtain adequate nutrition.

Nutritional Goals

The patient will seek support from referral to community senior food programs (See Chapter 16, Table 16.3) and begin to improve his calorie intake by eating a variety of nutrient dense foods.

Nutritional Implementation

Intervention: Ask open-ended questions pertaining to his late wife.
Rationale: Weight change can stem from lack of transportation and education. Mr. B's late wife may have done all the shopping (primary driver) and cooking previously. Educating Mr. B on finding transportation or educating him on what foods should be included in a meal may be appropriate.
Intervention: Examine the oral cavity for any deviation from normal and the fit of the maxillary denture.
Rationale: Ill-fitting dentures can be a result of weight loss, which can be responsible for creating sore spots. The presence of oral infections can decrease the ability and desire to eat, ultimately affecting nutritional status. Identifying such areas can allow for treatment and education on prevention.

Intervention: Provide instruction for completing a 3-day food record.
Rationale: This component completes the assessment process. Determining typical eating habits and patterns and the variety of foods gives direction to the nutrition education. Look for the predominant use of soft foods, highly salted foods, convenience foods, and fermentable carbohydrates; variety; low calories; and number of meals daily.
Intervention: Educate Mr. B regarding basic information about nutrient needs and the relationship between diet, oral health and overall health status.
Rationale: Depression over a spouse's death and dining alone are two factors decreasing an older individual's desire to eat. Referral to a congregate senior meal site may provide support and companionship needed to improve his desire to eat.
Intervention: Explain to Mr. B that frequent consumption of acid-containing beverages (e.g., sodas, citrus juices) can put him at high risk for caries. Due to his xerostomia, the lack of saliva may contribute to a more cariogenic environment, especially if food clearance is slowed and his remaining teeth have gingival recession.
Rationale: Patients with xerostomia have limited cleansing and buffering capabilities because of reduced quantities of saliva. Even foods generally noncariogenic when saliva flow is adequate, can be detrimental when saliva flow is diminished. Suggest rinsing with water to dilute the effects of citrus juices or to remove foods higher in fermentable carbohydrates (e.g., rinsing away remnants of crackers or pretzels).
Intervention: Provide positive feedback on any changes, even small ones, that Mr. B makes.
Rationale: An older adult may be more resistant to modifications in well-established habits. Small goals are more realistic. Allow him to make the goals based on the information presented to him. Recognize any change as a sign of effort. A follow-up on his progress is important to establish new goals or modify goals as necessary.

Evaluation

At a return visit, Mr. B's new 24-hour recall reveals adequate calorie intake and improvement in variety of food choices. He has slowly begun to gain back some of his weight. He has sought the support of various local senior citizen groups. His denture has been repaired, and he presents a healthy oral cavity.

◆ CASE STUDY

The dental hygienist has reviewed Jim S's medical, dental, and social histories at the prophylaxis appointment, indicating no significant changes. Jim presents with observable weight gain since the last 6-month recare appointment and three new areas of dental caries. He has no idea why the areas of decay occurred. A 3-day food diary is explained, and a nutrition education session is established following his restorative treatment. At the restorative appointment, the patient forgot to bring his complete food diary. The dental hygienist attributed this to a lack of interest. A 24-hour recall is obtained, and the session is conducted in the operatory.

1. Prioritize the diet and dental information that Jim S needs.
2. Explain why and how a nutrition education session could be beneficial to Jim.
3. What questions should be asked before and during the session to gain additional information?
4. State several reasons why the education session may not be effective to motivate behavior change. How could these situations be modified to enhance motivation?

References

1. American Dental Hygienists' Association (ADHA). *Standards for Clinical Dental Hygiene Practice.* ADHA; 2016. https://www.adha.org/wp-content/uploads/2023/03/2016-Revised-Standards-for-Clinical-Dental-Hygiene-Practice-1.pdf.
2. Touger-Decker R, Mobley C. Position of the Academy of Nutrition and Dietetics: oral health and nutrition. *J Acad Nutr Diet.* 2013;113(5):693–701.
3. Ramírez Martínez-Acitores L, Hernández Ruiz de Azcárate F, Casañas E, Serrano J, Hernández G, López-Pintor RM. Xerostomia and salivary flow in patients taking antihypertensive drugs. *Int J Environ Res Public Health.* 2020;17(7):2478.
4. Bhupathiraju SN, Hu F. *Nutrient Drug Interactions.* https://www.merckmanuals.com/professional/nutritional-disorders/nutrition-general-considerations/nutrient-drug-interactions.
5. Guzman JR, Paterniti DA, Liu Y, Tarn DM. Factors related to disclosure and nondisclosure of dietary supplements in primary care, integrative medicine, and naturopathic medicine. *J Fam Med Dis Prev.* 2019;5(4). https://doi.org/10.23937/2469-5793/1510109.

6. Federico JR, Basehore BM, Zito PM. *Angular chelitis. StatPearls.* StatPearls Publishing; 2023.

7. Mallonee LF, Boyd LD, Stegeman CA. Practice paper of the Academy of Nutrition and Dietetics: oral health and nutrition. *J Acad Nutr Diet.* 2014;114(6):958.

8. Mayo Clinic. *Unexplained Weight Loss.* https://www.mayoclinic.org/symptoms/unexplained-weight-loss/basics/when-to-see-doctor/sym-20050700.

9. Chapman-Novakofski K, Rios LKD. Education and counseling: behavioral change. In: Morrow K, Raymond JL, eds. *Krause and Mahan's Food and the Nutrition Care Process.* 16th ed. Elsevier; 2023.

10. Miller WR. Motivational interviewing with problem drinkers. *Behav Psychother.* 1983;11:147–172.

11. Rollnick S, Heather N, Bell A. Negotiating behaviour change in medical settings: the development of brief motivational interviewing. *J Ment Health.* 1992;1(1):25–37.

12. Arnett M, Gwozdek A. Motivational interviewing for dental hygienists. *Dimens Dent Hyg.* 2017:54–57.

13. Gillam DG, Yusuf H. Brief motivational interviewing in dental practice. *Dent J (Basel).* 2019;7(2):51.

14. Office of Disease Prevention and Health Promotion. Health literacy in Healthy People 2030. In: *Healthy People 2030.* U.S. Department of Health and Human Services. https://health.gov/healthypeople/priority-areas/health-literacy-healthy-people-2030.

15. Office of Disease Prevention and Health Promotion. Health communication. In: *Healthy People 2030.* U.S. Department of Health and Human Services. https://health.gov/healthypeople/objectives-and-data/browse-objectives/health-communication.

16. Office of Disease Prevention and Health Promotion. Health information technology (IT). In: *Healthy People 2030.* U.S. Department of Health and Human Services. https://health.gov/healthypeople/objectives-and-data/browse-objectives/health-it.

17. National Assessment of Adult Literacy. *Demographics.* http://nces.ed.gov/naal/kf_demographics.asp#3.

18. U.S. Department of Health and Human Services. Office of the Surgeon General. *Health literacy Reports and Publications.* https://www.hhs.gov/surgeongeneral/reports-and-publications/health-literacy/index.html.

19. International Education Statistics (IES). National Center for Education Statistics (NCES). *Program for the International Assessment of Adult Competencies.* https://nces.ed.gov/surveys/piaac/.

20. National Center for Education Statistics. *Highlights of the 2017 U.S PIAAC Results Web Report (NCES 2020-777).* U.S. Department of Education. Institute of Education Sciences, National Center for Education Statistics. https://nces.ed.gov/surveys/piaac/national_results.asp.

21. American Medical Association. Health literacy: report of the Council on Scientific Affairs. Ad Hoc Committee on Health Literacy for the Council on Scientific Affairs, American Medical Association. *JAMA.* 1999;281:552–557. 1.

22. Shahid R, Shoker M, Chu LM, et al. Impact of low health literacy on patients' health outcomes: a multicenter cohort study. *BMC Health Serv Res.* 2022;22:1148. https://doi.org/10.1186/s12913-022-08527-9.

▶ Evolve Resources

Please visit http://evolve.elsevier.com/Mallonee/nutritional for additional practice and study support tools.

Glossary

abrasion permanent depletion of tooth surfaces as a result of pathologic tooth wear, such as toothbrush abrasion.

Acceptable Macronutrient Distribution Ranges (AMDRs) a part of the latest dietary reference intakes (DRIs); established for the macronutrients (fat, carbohydrate, protein, and two polyunsaturated fats) to ensure sufficient intakes of essential nutrients while reducing risk of chronic diseases.

accessory organs organs, such as salivary glands, liver, gallbladder, and pancreas, that provide secretions essential for the digestive process.

achlorhydria absence of hydrochloric acid in the stomach, a condition that occurs primarily in older patients.

acidogenic foods and beverages that cause a reduction of salivary pH to less than 5.5.

active site the region of an enzyme that selectively binds a substrate and contains the amino acids that directly participate in the chemical transformation converting a substrate into a product.

active transport absorption within the gastrointestinal tract from a region of lower concentration to one of a higher concentration; requires a carrier and cellular energy.

added sugars sugars added to foods during processing or at the table.

adenosine triphosphate (ATP) main form of energy used by the cells.

adequate intake (AI) average amount of a nutrient that seems to maintain a defined nutritional state; derived from mean nutrient intakes by groups of healthy people.

adipose tissue body fat.

aerobic lives and grows in the presence of oxygen.

age-related macular degeneration (AMD) deterioration in the central area of the retina (back of the eye) in which lesions lead to loss of central vision.

aldosterone hormone secreted by the adrenal cortex that signals the kidney to retain sodium and water, and excrete potassium and hydrogen ions; ultimately causes edema and high blood pressure.

alopecia hair loss.

α-linolenic acid organic compound found in many vegetable oils.

alternative medicine use of medical and health care systems that are not considered part of conventional Western medicine.

alveolar bone the bone of the maxillae and mandible that contains the sockets for the teeth.

alveolar process crest of the maxilla and mandible.

ameloblasts tall columnar epithelial cells in the inner layer of the enamel; enamel-forming cells.

amenorrhea absence of menses.

amino acids basic building blocks or monomer units for proteins.

amorphous having no definite form.

amphiphilic compound with molecules with a water-soluble group attached to a water-insoluble grouping.

amylase an enzyme that begins the process of digesting dietary carbohydrates.

anabolism use of absorbed nutrients to build or synthesize more complex compounds.

anencephaly absence of a major portion of the brain and skull.

aneurysm bulge or ballooning in the wall of an artery. When an aneurysm becomes too large, it may burst and cause dangerous bleeding or death.

anhydrous contains no water, a hydrophobic or "water-fearing" substance.

anion ion carrying a negative charge as a result of an accumulation of electrons.

anorexia lack or loss of appetite.

anosmia loss of smell.

anthropometric measurements of physical characteristics, such as height, weight, and change in weight.

anticariogenic foods and beverages that may reduce the risk of caries by preventing plaque from recognizing a cariogenic food.

anticholinergic medication used to block parasympathetic nerve impulses.

anticoagulant drug or substance that delays or prevents the clotting of blood (e.g., heparin).

antidiuretic hormone (ADH) hormone released by the pituitary gland to act on the kidneys that control urine output.

antigenic having the properties of an antigen (substance that comes in contact with target cells, inducing an immune response or sensitivity).

antioxidant synthetic or natural substance that prevents or delays the damaging effects of a reactive substance seeking an electron.

apatite calcium phosphate complex that forms crystalline salts within the matrix of bone and teeth.

appetite external factors that influence people to seek and eat food even when not hungry.

ariboflavinosis symptoms associated with riboflavin deficiency (angular cheilitis, glossitis, dermatitis, and anemia).

ataxia gait disorder characterized by uncoordinated muscle movements.

atherosclerosis degenerative disease caused by progressive accumulation of fatty materials on smooth inner walls of the arteries of the heart, narrowing the arteries and disrupting blood flow.

atrophic gastritis chronic stomach inflammation with atrophy of the mucous membrane and glands, resulting in diminished hydrochloric acid production.

atrophic gingivitis condition characterized by redness, pain, and wasting of the gingival tissue owing to local and systemic causes.

atrophic glossitis atrophy of the filiform and fungiform papillae beginning at the tip and lateral borders of the tongue and gradually spreading to the entire dorsum of the tongue.

avoidant/restrictive food intake disorder (ARFID) a condition in children who have difficulty eating; body image is not a characteristic of this eating disorder classification.

autoimmune disorder condition in which the body produces antibodies against one's own tissues (e.g., celiac disease).

avidin biotin-binding glycoprotein substance present in raw egg white.

baby bottle tooth decay (BBTD) see early childhood caries.

bariatric surgery surgical procedure that promotes weight loss by restricting food intake or interrupting the digestive process to prevent absorption of some kilocalories and nutrients.

basal energy expenditure person's total calorie requirement.

basal metabolic rate energy required for involuntary physiological functions to maintain life, including respiration, circulation, and maintenance of muscle tone and body temperature.

benign migratory glossitis "geographic tongue"; multiple reddish flat areas with a loss of filiform papillae on the dorsum of the tongue, which may also be grooved or fissured.

beriberi dietary deficiency of thiamin characterized by neuropathy, diarrhea, weight loss, fatigue, and poor memory.

bile emulsifier that helps in digestion of fats.

binges periods of overeating.

bioactive a substance that has an effect on a living organism; in nutrition, bioactive substances are nonessential, since the body can function properly without them.

bioavailability amount of nutrient available to the body based on its absorption.

bioinformation the language of communication of biological information in an organism, including the transfer of biological information from deoxyribonucleic acid (DNA) to ribonucleic acid (RNA) to protein.

biological value measure of protein quality, with a higher score for proteins of higher quality.

biomolecule any molecule that is produced by a living cell or organism and other organic compounds found in living organisms.

bisphosphonates medications primarily prescribed for osteoporosis, multiple myeloma, and used intravenously during cancer chemotherapy; they decrease bone turnover and inhibit the bone's reparative ability.

body mass index (BMI) mathematical calculation using a person's height and weight to determine weight status and to predict health risks that increase at higher levels of overweight and obesity (see p. 6).

bolus mass of food that is swallowed and passed into the stomach.

botanical plant or plant part valued for its medicinal or therapeutic properties, flavor, and/or scent.

bradycardia low or slow heart rate.

bradykinesia slowness of movement.

Bruxism clenching and grinding of teeth that erodes and diminishes the height of dental crowns.

calcitonin polypeptide hormone regulating the balance of calcium and phosphate in the blood by direct action on bone and kidney; secreted by the parathyroid, thyroid, and thymus tissue.

calorie amount of heat needed to increase the temperature of 1 kg of water to 1°C; measurement of the potential energy value of foods and energy within the body, equivalent to 1000 cal; more accurately called kilocalorie.

calorie-dense foods term used for food usually high in fats (or fat and sugar) and low in vitamins, minerals, and other nutrients. A characteristic of calorie-dense foods is that less volume of food is needed to furnish energy requirements.

calorimeter device used to measure kilocalories.

cancellous bone internal bone that appears spongy.

Candida invasive fungal microorganism.

carbohydrate a biomolecule containing carbon, hydrogen, and oxygen with twice as much hydrogen as oxygen; 1 g yields 4 cal; produced by plants through photosynthesis.

cardiovascular disease (CVD) condition involving the heart and blood vessels and producing various pathologic effects; also referred to as coronary heart disease (CHD) or coronary artery disease (CAD).

Caries Management by Risk Assessment (CaMBRA) used by dental professionals to identify risk of caries and to determine preventive and therapeutic goals for both children and adult patients.

cariogenic fermentable carbohydrate that causes a reduction of salivary pH to less than 5.5, resulting in demineralization of enamel and dental caries.

cariostatic (also see noncariogenic) carbohydrates that are caries-inhibiting; not metabolized by microorganisms in plaque biofilm; do not cause a reduction of salivary pH to less than 5.5.

casein principal protein in cow's milk and chief constituent of cheese.

catabolism breakdown of complex substances into simpler ones.

catecholamine an organic compound that consists of a single amine and a catechol; obtained from dietary tyrosine and/or phenylalanine.

cation ion carrying a positive charge as a result of a deficiency of electrons.

Chronic disease risk reduction intake (CDRR) nutrient intakes that are expected to reduce the risk of developing chronic disease.

celiac disease malabsorption syndrome in which individuals are hypersensitive to gluten, a protein inherent to wheat, rye, barley, and triticale.

cheilosis unilateral or bilateral presence of cracks and dry scaling around the vermilion border of lips and corners of the mouth; the skin is scaly with red fissures.

chelation therapy use of specific chemicals to bind and eliminate heavy metals from the body.

chemical bonds hold atoms together in a compound.

chemotherapy treatment of disease by chemical agents.

cholesterol waxy lipid found in all body cells; found only in animal products.

cholinergic parasympathetic (autonomic) nerves stimulated by acetylcholine.

chyme bolus entering the stomach, a semifluid material produced by gastric juices on ingested food.

circumvallate lingual papillae 8 to 10 large and distinctive structures forming a V shape on the posterior end of the anterior two-thirds of the dorsum of the tongue.

cis **isomer** the geometric arrangement of hydrogen atoms on the same side of the plane of a C=C double bond.

cleft lip/palate split where parts of the upper lip or palate fail to grow together.

clinical attachment loss (CAL) loss of periodontal attachment.

coenzyme molecule needed to activate an enzyme.

cofactor element similar to an enzyme necessary to activate reactions, but the molecule required is a mineral or electrolyte.

Coliforms a bacterial indicator of sanitation, universally present in the feces of animals.

Collagen basic protein substance of connective tissue helping support body structures such as skin, bones, teeth, and tendons.

colonics a method to cleanse the lower intestine based on the assumption that years of bad diet causes the colon to become caked with layers of accumulated toxins.

complementary feeding period first introduction of solid foods to an infant occurring at 4 months of age when neither breastmilk nor formula adequately meets all the nutrient requirements to promote growth and development.

complementary medicine use of untraditional medical and health care systems and products along with conventional medical treatments.

complex carbohydrates see *polysaccharides*.

compound lipids triglycerides with at least one of the fatty acids replaced with carbohydrate, phosphate, or nitrogenous compounds.

compressional forces actions in which the pressure attempts to diminish a structure's volume, which usually increases density.

condensation reaction biochemical reaction in which two molecules combine, eliminating water or some other simple molecule.

conditionally essential amino acids amino acids that are essential in the diet during certain stages of development or in certain nutritional or disease states.

conditionally indispensable amino acids amino acids normally not required by the body, but in certain physiological conditions become indispensable.

conjugated linoleic acid (CLA) family of at least 13 isomers (or forms) of linoleic acid, found especially in meats and dairy products.

constipation having a bowel movement fewer than three times per week with hard, dry, small, and difficult-to-pass stools.

covalent bond bond formed when electrons are equally shared between two nonmetals.

crepitus crackling or grating sound made by a joint, such as the temporomandibular joint.

cretinism stunting of growth often characterized by mental deficits and deaf mutism; a result of inadequate iodine intake during pregnancy.

dietary pattern is a focus on the diet as a whole rather than individual nutrients or foods.

Daily Value (DV) term used on food labels indicating the percentage of the DV provided by a serving to show the amount of nutrients provided as a percentage of established standards; based on a 2000-cal diet.

demineralization removal or loss of calcium, phosphate, and other minerals from tooth enamel, causing tooth enamel to dissolve.

dental erosion chemical removal of minerals from the tooth structure that occurs when an acidic environment causes the enamel to dissolve gradually; occurs with frequent exposure to foods with a pH below 4.2.

dental stomatitis traumatization and chronic inflammation of mucus membranes supporting a removable denture.

dentin hypersensitivity extremely painful feeling of exposed dentin resulting from a stimulus, such as temperature or tactile.

detoxification ("detox") the biochemical process that transforms non-water-soluble toxins and metabolites into water-soluble compounds that can be excreted in urine, sweat, bile, or stool.

dextrins intermediate products of the digestive enzymes on starch molecules; they are long glucose chains split into shorter ones.

dialysate material that passes through the membrane during dialysis.

diaphoresis excessive sweating.

diet history detailed dietary record; may include 24-hour recall; food frequency questionnaire; and other information such as weight history, previous diet changes, use of supplements, and food intolerances.

dietary acculturation dietary changes that occur as a result of adapting to food resources of a new location.

dietary fiber several different types of nondigestible carbohydrates and lignin intrinsic and intact in plants.

Dietary Reference Intakes (DRIs) set of nutrient-based reference values that identify amounts of required nutrients for various stages of life.

dipeptide two amino acids together.

diplopia perception of two images of a single object; also known as double vision.

disaccharides double sugars (two simple sugars joined together) containing 12 carbon atoms.

disease a condition of a living animal or plant body or of one of its parts that impairs normal functioning and is typically manifested by distinguishing signs and symptoms.

dispensable amino acids are nonessential amino acids that are essential for the body, but they can be produced by the body from indispensable (essential) amino acids so are not required in normal conditions.

docosahexaenoic acid (DHA) omega-3 fatty acid with 22 carbons and 6 double bonds synthesized by the body from linolenic acid; present in fish oils.

dysesthesia condition in which a burning sensation is produced by ordinary stimuli.

dysgeusia persistent, abnormal distortion of taste, including sweet, sour, bitter, salty, or metallic.

dysphagia difficulty in swallowing.

early childhood caries (ECC) early rampant tooth decay associated with inappropriate feeding practices.

edentulous without teeth or lacking some or all teeth.

eicosapentaenoic acid (EPA) omega-3 fatty acid with 20 carbon atoms and 5 double bonds synthesized by the body from linolenic acid; present in fish oils.

emulsification the breakdown of fats into smaller particles by lowering the surface tension.

enamel hypoplasia developmental disturbance of the teeth characterized by defective formation of the enamel matrix.

energy ability or power to do work.

enrichment process of restoring nutrients removed from food during processing.

enteral feedings feeding that delivers liquid food through a tube; may be used for infants and children with a functioning gastrointestinal tract unable to ingest nutrients orally to meet their metabolic needs.

enteric general term for the intestines.

enzymes complex proteins enabling metabolic reactions to proceed at a faster rate without being exhausted themselves.

epigenetics the scientific study of how nutrition and environmental factors regulate gene activity without changing the underlying DNA sequence.

epilepsy transient disturbance of brain function that results in episodic impairment or loss of consciousness.

epinephrine the "fight or flight" hormone secreted in time of immediate energy need; activates glycogen degradation for energy.

epiphyses growing points at the ends of long bones.

epithelialization natural healing process in which the area is covered with or converted to epithelium.

ergogenic enhanced physical performance, stamina, or recovery.

erosion permanent depletion of tooth surfaces due to the action of an external or internal chemical substance.

erythema marginated redness of mucous membranes caused by inflammation.

erythropoiesis formation of red blood cells.

esophagitis inflammation of the lower esophagus.

essential amino acids (EAAs) amino acids that must be supplied by the diet. Also known as indispensable amino acids.

essential fatty acids (EFAs) fatty acids (linoleic acid and linolenic acid) that must be supplied by the diet.

essential hypertension elevated blood pressure of unknown cause.

Estimated Average Requirement (EAR) amount of a nutrient estimated to meet the needs of half of the healthy individuals in a specific age and gender group.

Estimated Energy Requirement (EER) dietary energy intake predicted to maintain energy balance in healthy normal-weight individuals of a defined age, gender, weight, height, and physical activity level consistent with good health.

Evidence Analysis Library (EAL) a process in which an expert work group identifies practice-related questions, performs a systematic literature review, and develops and rates a conclusive statement for each question; such a library was developed by the Academy of Nutrition and Dietetics (AND).

evidence-based medical practices that have been thoroughly evaluated using scientific methods.

extracellular fluid (ECF) fluid outside the cells.

fatty acids structural component of fats.

fermentable carbohydrate carbohydrates that can be metabolized by bacteria in plaque biofilm to decrease the pH to a level causing demineralization; this includes all sugars and cooked or processed starches.

fibroblasts collagen-forming cells.

fibrotic formation of fibrous tissue of the gingiva and other mucous membranes because of chronic inflammation; tissue may clinically appear to be healthy, concealing the disease.

filiform papillae smooth, threadlike structures that are covered by a nonkeratinized epithelium, on the anterior two-thirds of the dorsum of the tongue.

flavin adenine nucleotide (FAD/FADH2) a redox coenzyme derived from riboflavin.

flexitarian person who primarily follows a plant-based diet, but occasionally eats small amounts of meat, poultry or fish; also known as a *semivegetarian.*

fluid volume deficit (FVD) relatively equal losses of sodium and water in relation to their gains.

fluid volume excess (FVE) relatively equal gains of water and sodium in relation to their losses.

fluorapatite fluoride-containing crystalline substance produced during bone and tooth development; resistant to acid.

fluorosis hypomineralization of enamel, caused by excessive fluoride intake during the formation of enamel.

foliate papillae vertical ridges or grooves scattered along the lateral borders of the tongue.

follicular hyperkeratosis condition characterized by the appearance of cone-shaped, horny, hyperkeratinized, scaly eruptions resulting from blocked pores as a result of vitamin A deficiency.

food deserts located in lower-income, inner-city, and rural areas, with few supermarkets but numerous small stores that stock limited nutritious food items, particularly produce, at affordable prices.

food fad catch-all term covering all aspects of nutritional nonsense, characterized by exaggerated beliefs about the value of nutrition in health and disease.

food frequency questionnaire checklist of many foods used to determine how often specific foods are consumed.

food insecurity lack of access to enough food to fully meet basic needs at all times.

food jags refusing to eat anything except one food for several days.

food quackery promotion of nutrition-related products or services having questionable safety or effectiveness, or both, for the claims made.

fortification process of adding nutrients not present in the natural product or to increase the amount above that in the original product.

full liquid diet nutrients provided in a liquid form when solid food is not tolerated; a transition between a clear liquid and soft diet.

functional fiber isolated, nondigestible carbohydrates with beneficial physiological effects in humans.

functional foods foods that contain potentially healthful products, including any modified food or food ingredients providing a health benefit beyond its traditional nutrients.

functional group a group of atoms that gives a family of molecules its characteristic chemical and physical properties.

fungating producing fungus-like growth.

fungiform papillae red, knoblike structures on the tongue scattered throughout the filiform papillae.

gastroesophageal reflux disease (GERD) return of gastric contents into the esophagus, causing a severe burning sensation under the sternum.

gene region of DNA sequence that contains the instructions to produce a specific protein required for life.

genome all of the DNA contained in an organism or cell, which includes chromosomes in the nucleus and DNA in the mitochondria.

genomics scientific discipline of mapping, sequencing, and analyzing the genome.

gingivitis inflammation of the gingival tissue.

ginseng fleshy root of a plant; stimulant used in energy drinks that may improve concentration and thinking, physical stamina, and athletic endurance, but may cause abdominal pain and headaches.

glossitis chronic inflammation of the tongue, characterized by the loss of filiform papillae on the dorsum of the tongue.

glossodynia pain in the tongue.

glossopyrosis pain, burning, itching, and stinging of the tongue with no apparent lesions.

glucagon a signal of the "starved" state; secreted when blood glucose levels are low.

glucogenic amino acids can be converted into glucose as a fuel for the body.

gluconeogenesis synthesis of glucose from noncarbohydrate sources.

gluten protein found mainly in wheat and to a lesser degree in rye, oat, and barley.

gluten sensitivity a condition in which individuals are unable to tolerate gluten; not an allergic or autoimmune response.

glycemic index a measure of the effect of different carbohydrate foods on blood glucose levels.

glycogen carbohydrate storage form of energy in humans.

glycogenesis process by which sugars, including fructose, galactose, sorbitol, and xylitol, are stored as glycogen.

glycolysis anaerobic conversion of glucose to produce energy in the form of adenosine triphosphate (ATP).

glycosidic bond a bond that combines two monosaccharides into a disaccharide.

goiter chronic enlargement of the thyroid gland occurring most frequently in areas with low iodine in the soil.

goitrogens naturally occurring substances in foods that interfere with the synthesis of thyroid hormone production; may cause goiter if consumed in large amounts.

gravida pregnant female; gravida followed by a Roman numeral or preceded by a Latin prefix (e.g., "primi-," "secundi-") designates the number of pregnancies for the female (e.g., gravida I or primigravida is a female in her first pregnancy).

guarana a seed containing four times as much caffeine as coffee beans.

gustatory sense of taste.

health claim claim that describes a health relationship between a food, food component, or dietary supplement ingredient and reduced risk of a disease or a health-related condition.

Healthy U.S.-Style Eating Pattern (U.S.-Pattern) an eating pattern introduced in the *2015-2020 Dietary Guidelines for Americans* indicating the number of food equivalents from each food group and subgroups for 12 caloric levels to be consumed each week for an adequate healthful diet.

hematopoiesis formation of red blood cells.

heme iron iron provided from animal sources.

hemochromatosis an uncommon disorder in which iron is absorbed at a high rate despite elevated iron stores in the liver.

hemosiderin storage form of iron in the liver when the amount of iron in the body exceeds storage capacity.

herbs leafy green parts of a plant.

herpetic related to the herpes virus; ulceration on the tongue or esophagus or both.

hiatal hernia partial protrusion (herniation) of the stomach through the diaphragm.

high-energy phosphate compounds instant source of energy for cells; also called *ATP.*

high-quality proteins foods that contain adequate amounts of the nine essential amino acids to maintain nitrogen balance and permit growth.

hirsutism excessive hair growth.

homeopathy treatment of diseases and conditions with minute doses of drugs that cause symptoms of a disease in healthy people to cure similar symptoms in sick people.

homeostatic mechanisms body's ability to correct nutritional imbalances, for instance, decreased nutrient intake accompanied by an increase in absorption or efficiency, or use.

hormone compound produced and secreted by cells of the body, transported in the blood to another site where it has a specific regulatory function.

hormone replacement therapy (HRT) therapy using medication that contains one or more female hormones, usually estrogen and progestin.

hunger physiological drive to eat or an uneasy or painful sensation caused by lack of food.

hydrocarbon the hydrophobic chain "tail" of a fatty acid that contains only carbon and hydrogen atoms.

hydrolysis splitting of a large molecule into smaller water-soluble ones that can be used by cells; the reaction requires water.

hydrolysis reactions cleavage of a compound with the addition of water.

hydrolyzed protein proteins broken down into amino acids.

hydrophilic "water-loving" biomolecules.

hydrophobic "water-fearing" compounds that do not readily combine with water.

hydroxyapatite inorganic component of bones and teeth.

hypercalcemia excessive levels of calcium in the blood.

hypercalciuria high levels of calcium in the urine.

hypercarotenemia excessive levels of carotene in the blood, characterized by yellowing of the palms of the hands and soles of the feet.

hypergeusia heightened taste acuity.

hyperglycemia elevated blood sugar.

hyperkalemia elevated potassium concentrations in the blood.

hyperlipidemia elevated concentrations of any or all of the serum lipids, especially triglycerides or cholesterol or both.

hypernatremia elevated serum sodium level.

hypertension persistent high arterial blood pressure; considered a risk factor for heart and kidney disease, and stroke.

hypervitaminosis A condition resulting from the ingestion of excessive amounts of vitamin A.

hypocalcemia deficient levels of calcium in the blood.

Hypochlorhydria reduced stomach acid production, specifically low hydrochloric acid.

hypodipsia diminished thirst.

hypogeusia loss of taste.

hypoglycemia low blood sugar (less than 70 mg/dL).

hypokalemia low potassium concentrations in the blood.

hyponatremia low or zero sodium levels in the blood.

hypotonic solution having less osmotic pressure than another solution.

iatrogenic adverse condition resulting from treatment (e.g., medications, irradiation, or surgery) by a health care provider.

immune response body's ability to protect itself from destructive bacteria and infection present in the body.

immunocompromised immune response weakened by a disease or pharmacologic agent.

immunoglobulins antibodies, the body's main protection from disease.

incontinence inability to control urinary or fecal excretion.

indispensable amino acids essential amino acids required in the diet; there are nine indispensable amino acids.

indirect calorimetry method to estimate metabolic energy by measuring oxygen consumption, carbon dioxide production, respiratory quotient, and resting energy expenditure as a means to assess and manage a patient's nutrition.

innate inborn.

insulin hormone that lowers blood sugar levels.

interesterified fats a new type of customized fat suitable for commercial preparation produced to replace *trans* fats; they affect blood lipids, but not as much as *trans* fats.

interstitial spaces between cells within a tissue or organ.

interstitial fluid fluid located between cells and in body cavities, including joints, pleura, and gastrointestinal tract.

intracellular fluid (ICF) liquid within cells.

intrinsic factor glycoprotein synthesized by parietal cells in the stomach; required for vitamin B$_{12}$ absorption.

ionic bond bond formed between a positively charged metal ion and a negatively charged nonmetal ion.

irradiated foods process of treating food with controlled amounts of ionized radiation to kill the spoilage-causing and disease-causing bacteria and molds in food.

ischemia inadequate blood flow and lack of oxygen because of constriction or obstruction of arteries.

Kaposi sarcoma malignant tumor of blood vessel origin that occurs on skin and oral mucosa.

Kayser-Fleischer ring greenish-yellow pigmented ring encircling the cornea; consists of copper deposits in the Descemet membrane.

keratinized epithelium a protein, main component of epidermis and horny tissues on the skin.

Keshan disease cardiomyopathy (disease of the heart muscle) resulting from deficiency of selenium found in females and children, primarily in Keshan, China.

ketoacidosis accumulation of ketone bodies in the blood.

ketogenic formation of ketone bodies.

ketogenic amino acids certain amino acids degrade into acetyl CoA and are converted into ketone bodies.

ketone bodies soluble forms of lipids that can be used as fuel for the body.

ketones normal products of lipid metabolism in the liver; can be used by muscles for energy if adequate amounts of glucose are available.

ketonuria ketones excreted in the urine as a result of high levels in the blood.

ketosis accumulation of ketone bodies in the blood.

kilocalorie see calorie.

kwashiorkor nutritional deficiency disease due to inadequate protein but adequate calories.

lactovegetarian person who consumes only products from plants and dairy products.

large intestine cecum, colon, and rectum.

leukemia generalized malignant disease characterized by distorted proliferation and development of white blood cells.

leukoplakia white, yellow, or gray thickened patches on mucous membranes of the oral mucosa that cannot be wiped away; appearance may be wrinkled, fissured, nodular, or smooth.

lichen planus a chronic inflammatory disease presenting as an itchy rash, mostly in the oral cavity.

linoleic acid essential fatty acid with 18 carbon atoms and 2 double bonds; also called omega-6 fatty acid.

lipase an enzyme that begins the process of digesting dietary lipids.

lipids compounds that contain carbon, hydrogen, and oxygen, with less oxygen in proportion to hydrogen and carbon than carbohydrates; provide 9 cal/g; a biomolecule that is produced by a living cell or organism.

lipoatrophy loss of fat from specific areas of the body, especially the face, arms, legs, and buttocks.

lipodystrophy rearrangement of fat cells in the face.

lipogenesis process of converting glucose to fats.

lipohypertrophy accumulation of fat on the back or the neck between the shoulders.

lipolysis fat breakdown.

lipoprotein compound lipids composed of triglycerides, phospholipids, and cholesterol combined with protein; produced by the body.

Listeriosis serious infection caused by food contaminated with the bacterium *Listeria monocytogenes*, which principally affects infants and adults with weakened immune systems.

long-chain fatty acids fatty acid that contains 12 or more carbon atoms.

longitudinal fissure slits or wrinkles that extend lengthwise on the tongue.

low birth weight (LBW) weighing less than 5½ lb (2500 g) at birth.

lower esophageal sphincter (LES) group of very strong circular muscle fibers located just above the stomach.

low nutrient density foods having a high fat, alcohol, or sugar content with nominal amounts of vitamins and minerals.

low-quality proteins plant proteins that lack one or more essential amino acids or may lack a proper balance of amino acids; also called incomplete proteins.

lymphatic system comprised of lymph (plasma-like tissue fluid), the lymph nodes, and lymph vessels that are not connected to the blood system; carries fat-soluble nutrients through the thoracic duct and into venous blood at the left subclavian vein.

lysosomes intracellular bodies containing hydrolytic enzymes that promote breakdown of materials taken into the cells.

macrodontia larger than normal teeth.

macroglossia large, protruding tongue.

macronutrients nutrients needed in large amounts by the body to provide energy—carbohydrates, protein, and fats.

macules flat lesions of abnormal color.

manganese madness severe psychotic and neuromuscular symptoms that resemble symptoms of parkinsonism.

marasmus nutritional deficiency caused by inadequate protein and calorie intake.

mastication process in which teeth crush and grind food into smaller pieces to initiate digestion.

masticatory efficiency how well a person prepares the food for swallowing.

mechanically altered diet regular diet altered in consistency during periods when chewing is difficult; a transition between a full liquid diet and a regular diet.

medium-chain fatty acids fatty acid with 6 to 10 carbon atoms.

megaloblastic anemia condition in which red blood cells are extra large in size but fewer in number.

melting point temperature at which a product becomes a liquid.

menopausal gingivostomatitis changes in the oral mucosa resulting in a dry, shiny gingiva that bleeds easily; color ranging from an abnormally pale pink to a deep red may be alleviated with estrogen hormone replacement.

menopause cessation of the menses; occurs when production of the hormones estrogen and progesterone ceases.

meta-analysis systematic analysis that is applied to separate experiments on a related topic involving pooling the data to provide larger study samples that generate information about statistically significant results from the cumulative research on a topic.

metabolism continuous processes whereby living organisms and cells convert nutrients into energy, body structure, and waste.

microflora microorganisms living in the large intestine.

microbiome all microbial cells in the human body, including bacterial, fungal, protozoal, and other single-cell microorganisms.

micrognathia abnormally small jaw.

micronutrients nutrients needed by the body in small amounts (e.g., vitamins and minerals).

microvilli minute cylindrical processes located on the surface of intestinal cells, greatly increasing their absorptive surface area.

mineralization deposition of inorganic minerals on an organic matrix.

mitochondria power source of the cell.

modified barium swallow assessment to measure physiological and anatomical abnormalities associated with swallowing.

molecule the smallest particle of a substance that retains all the properties of the substance.

monomer the smallest repeating unit present in a polymer.

monosaccharides simple sugars containing two to six carbon atoms.

monounsaturated fatty acid (MUFA) fatty acid containing one double bond; found in olive, peanut, and canola oil.

motivational interviewing an educational tool for changing behaviors involving a respectful, collaborative conversation.

mucositis ulcerations and sores of the mucous membrane in the mouth or throat, usually caused by chemotherapy or radiation.

myelin lipid substance that insulates nerve fibers and affects transmission of nerve impulses.

myxedema severe hypothyroidism.

nanotechnology the ability to measure and detect molecular structures in nanometers or smaller, allowing determination and manipulation of minute amounts of substances in the food supply.

naturopathy support of the body's inherent ability to maintain and restore health, using noninvasive treatments with minimal use of surgery and drugs.

necrosis degeneration and death of cells.

necrotizing enterocolitis (NEC) condition in neonates with development of cellular dead patches in the intestines interfering with digestion and absorption.

necrotizing ulcerative gingivitis (NUG) oral condition caused by nutritional deficiencies, stress, infection, and depressed immune responses; characterized by erythema and necrosis of the interdental papillae.

neoplasia an abnormal mass of tissue, more frequently referred to as a tumor.

neural tube defects (NTD) birth defects of the skull, brain, and spinal cord.

neutropenia diminished number of neutrophils in the blood; also called leukopenia or agranulocytosis.

nicotinamide adenine dinucleotide (NAD+/ NADH) a redox coenzyme derived from niacin.

night blindness inability to adapt to bright lights when the eyes are adapted to darkness.

nitrogen balance balance of reactions in which protein substances are broken down and rebuilt.

nocturia excessive urination at night.

noma severe gangrenous process usually manifesting as a small ulcer on the gingiva that becomes necrotic and spreads to the lips, cheek, and tissues covering the jaw; caused by inadequate amounts of protein.

noncariogenic (also see cariostatic) foods and beverages that do not decrease salivary pH below 5.5 and are not a factor in demineralization.

non-celiac gluten sensitivity (NCGS) intestinal and other symptoms related to ingesting gluten-containing foods but without celiac disease or wheat allergy.

nondigestible enzymes in the gastrointestinal tract cannot digest and absorb the substance; plant cells that remain largely intact through the digestive process.

nonessential amino acids (NEAAs) amino acids essential to the body, but not required in the diet. Also known as dispensable amino acids.

nonheme iron iron provided primarily from plant sources and supplements; less efficiently absorbed than heme iron.

nonnutritive sucking sucking on objects that do not provide nutrition (i.e., pacifier, fingers).

normoglycemia normal blood glucose range.

nucleic acid a biomolecule that is produced by a living cell or organism forms the genetic material in the cell; synthesizes cellular protein.

nucleotide building blocks for nucleic acids.

nutrient content claim characterizes the level of a nutrient in a food; terms used are "free," "low," "high," and "reduced."

nutrient-dense containing a high percentage of nutrients in relation to the number of calories provided.

nutrient density amount of nutrients in a food relative to its calories.

nutrients biochemical substances that can be supplied in adequate amounts only from an outside source, normally from food.

nutrigenomics/nutritional genomics scientific study of how foods or their components interact with genes and how individual genetic differences affect prevention or treatment of disease with regard to nutrients (and other naturally occurring compounds).

nutrition study of foods and nutrients and their effect on health, growth, and development.

nutrition and dietetic technician, registered (NDTR) nutritional professional having completed a 2-year degree in a Dietetic Technician Program or a 4-year degree from an approved (Accreditation Council for Education in Nutrition and Dietetics) program.

Nutrition Facts panel label on food products providing nutrient content of food and the number of servings in the package.

nutritional deficiency inadequate amounts of a nutrient available to sustain biochemical functions.

nutritional insult deficiency or excessive amounts of specific nutrients.

nutritionist person who may have a 4-year degree in foods and nutrition and usually works in a public health setting; may be legally defined in some states denoting licensure or certification.

nystagmus involuntary rapid movement of the eyeball.

obesity excess weight for height, with a BMI above 30.0.

observational studies epidemiologic research studies with no type of intervention or experiment.

odontoblasts tissue cells that deposit dentin and form the outer surface of dental pulp adjacent to the dentin; dentin-forming cells.

odynophagia pain associated with swallowing.

oils fats liquid at room temperature.

olfactory nerves receptors for smell.

omega-3 fatty acid unsaturated fatty acid with its first double bond at the third carbon atom from the methyl end; includes eicosapentaenoic acid and docosahexaenoic acid.

omega-6 fatty acid unsaturated fatty acid with its first double bond at the sixth carbon atom from the methyl end; includes linoleic acid and linolenic acid.

organic foods that meet U.S. Department of Agriculture (USDA) standards and do not contain parts of other slaughtered animals, were not given growth hormones or antibiotics, and allowed outdoors; not genetically engineered or irradiated; grown on land that has not been fertilized with sewage sludge or chemical fertilizers or treated with pesticides.

osmoreceptors neurons in the hypothalamus stimulated by increased osmolality, enhancing the release of ADH.

osmosis movement of water from an area of lower solute concentration to a higher solute concentration. When solute concentrations in the body are different, water moves across the membrane.

osteoblasts assist in production of collagen; help in building and reformation of new bone.

osteocalcin vitamin K–dependent, bone-specific protein that is released into blood from resorbed bone matrix and originating osteoblasts.

osteoclasts resorbed bone in microscopic cavities.

osteodystrophy abnormal bone development, similar to osteomalacia.

osteoid young bone that has not undergone calcification.

osteomalacia softening of bones.

osteonecrosis a condition in which bone dies or undergoes necrosis.

osteoporosis age-related disorder characterized by decreased bone mass, causing bones to be more susceptible to fracture.

overjet horizontal projection of upper teeth beyond the lower teeth.

overweight excess accumulation of body fat or a BMI between 25.0 and 29.9.

ovolactovegetarian vegetarian diet supplemented with milk, eggs, and cheese.

ovovegetarian type of vegetarian whose diet consists of foods from plants with the addition of eggs (no meat, poultry, fish, or dairy products).

oxidation process of hydrolyzing triglycerides into two-carbon entities to enter the TCA (Krebs) cycle for energy production.

oxidation-reduction reaction a chemical reaction that can convert functional groups into other functional groups.

oxidative phosphorylation a metabolic process that synthesizes phosphoric bonds from the energy released by the oxidation of various substrates.

pancreatic enzymes enzymes that hydrolyze carbohydrates, protein, and fats.

papillae epithelium surrounding taste buds; papillae appear on the tongue as little red dots, or raised bumps, and are most prevalent on the dorsal epithelium.

parasympathetic nerves division of autonomic nervous system.

Parkinson disease progressive neurologic condition characterized by involuntary muscle tremors, muscular weakness, rigidity, stooped posture, and peculiar gait.

parotitis inflammation of the parotid gland.

passive diffusion passage of a permeable substance from a more concentrated solution to an area of lower concentration.

pathogenic harmful.

pedometer instrument used by a walker; measures approximate distance walked by recording steps.

pellagra deficiency resulting from inadequate intake of niacin, which results in the four Ds (diarrhea, dermatitis, dementia, and death).

peptide bond a strong covalent bond that forms polypeptides.

periapical area around the root apex.

perimenopause time leading up to menopause, in which the ovaries begin to shut down, making less amounts of certain hormones, such as estrogen and progesterone.

periodontal disease infections and lesions affecting tissues that form the attachment apparatus of a tooth or teeth.

periodontitis inflammatory process involving interproximal and marginal areas of two or more adjacent teeth.

periodontium hard and soft tissues that surround and support teeth: gingiva, alveolar mucosa, cementum, periodontal ligament, and alveolar bone.

peripheral edema in the extremities, such as the legs and feet.

peristalsis involuntary rhythmic waves of contraction traveling the length of the alimentary tract.

pernicious anemia megaloblastic anemia with a decrease in red blood cells; occurs when the body cannot properly absorb vitamin B_{12} in the gastrointestinal tract.

petechia (pl. petechiae) small, pinpoint, round red spot caused by submucous hemorrhage.

phantom taste dysgeusia without identifiable taste stimuli.

phenylketonuria genetic disorder characterized by inability to metabolize the amino acid phenylalanine.

phospholipid fat-related substances that contain phosphorus, fatty acids, and a nitrogen-containing base; constituent of every cell.

photosynthesis compounding or building up of chemical substances under the influence of light; green plants use chlorophyll and energy from sunlight to produce carbohydrates from water and carbon dioxide and to liberate oxygen.

physical activity any bodily movement produced by skeletal muscles resulting in energy expenditure.

physical fitness ability to perform physical activity.

phytochemical biologically active substances found in plants.

pica abnormal consumption of specific food and nonfood substances, such as dirt, clay, starch, or ice; occurs more frequently during pregnancy.

plant sterols essential components of plant membranes resembling the chemical structure of cholesterol that perform similar cellular functions in plants; naturally present in small quantities in fruits, vegetables, nuts, seeds, legumes, and oils.

plaque biofilm well-organized community of bacteria embedded in a slime layer that adheres tenaciously to tooth surfaces, restorations, and prosthetic appliances.

plethora red appearance resulting from an excess of blood.

pocketed foods foods retained in the mouth, especially in the vestibule.

polycythemia sustained increase in number of red blood cells; may result in iron-deficiency anemia.

polymer a large molecule containing numerous repeating units.

polyols sugar alcohols formed from or converted to sugar; sorbitol, xylitol, and mannitol are present in the body or added to foods.

polypeptide several amino acids joined together.

polypharmacy use of at least 5 or more prescription medications.

polysaccharides (complex carbohydrates) sugars containing more than 12 carbon atoms.

polyunsaturated fatty acid (PUFA) fatty acid containing two or more double bonds.

portal circulation passage of nutrients from the gastrointestinal tract and spleen through the portal vein to the liver.

postabsorptive state time when digestive and absorptive processes are minimal, not affecting the basal metabolic rate.

ppb parts per billion.

prebiotics nondigestible food ingredients having beneficial effects on the host by stimulating growth or activity of probiotics in the colon.

precursor substance from which another biologically active substance is formed.

preeclampsia development of hypertension as a result of pregnancy or the influence of recent pregnancy; usually occurs after the 20th week of pregnancy.

premature born before the state of maturity, occurring with a gestational age (length of pregnancy) of less than 37 weeks.

primigravida female in her first pregnancy.

probiotics products containing live bacteria that aid in restoring and maintaining an intestinal balance of healthful bacteria.

prognathism overgrowth of the mandible.

prostaglandins hormone-like compounds derived from unsaturated fatty acids.

protease an enzyme that begins the process of digesting dietary proteins.

protein a biomolecule that is produced by a living cell or organism; chains of amino acids joined by peptide linkage; essential for physiological structure and function; contains nitrogen.

protein-energy malnutrition (PEM) nutritional deficiency condition caused by consistently consuming inadequate amounts of energy and protein.

protein-sparing energy source that allows protein to be used for building and repairing (i.e., fats and carbohydrates).

proteolytic enzymes enzymes that hydrolyze proteins.

prothrombin first stage in forming an insoluble clot; a deficiency results in impaired blood coagulation.

purging use of laxatives, enemas, emetics, diuretics, or exercise to negate effects of overindulgence.

purpura condition characterized by hemorrhaging into tissues, under the skin, and through the mucous membranes; the three types are petechiae, ecchymoses, and hematomas.

purulent exudates consisting of or containing pus; generally the result of inflammation.

pyogenic producing pus.

qualified health claims statements on food labels that are supported by some evidence but do not meet the scientific standard; must be accompanied by a disclaimer specified by the U.S. Food and Drug Administration (FDA).

quality of life an individual's perception of one's position in life in the context of the culture and value systems and in relation to the person's goals, expectations, standards, and concerns.

quercetin bioflavonoid reported to energize muscles (unsubstantiated claim).

radical group of atoms forming a fundamental constituent of a molecule.

R-binder protein produced by salivary glands necessary for absorption of vitamin B_{12}.

Recommended Dietary Allowances (RDAs) specific amounts of essential nutrients that adequately meet the known nutrient needs of 97% to 98% of healthy Americans.

redox coenzymes coenzymes that capture and transfer electrons.

reduction a gain of electrons, a decrease in charge, a loss of oxygen atoms, or a gain of hydrogen atoms.

registered dietitian-nutritionist (RDN) person who has completed a bachelor's degree in foods and nutrition with training in normal and clinical nutrition, food science, and food service management, and advanced training in medical nutrition therapy.

remineralization restoration or return of calcium, phosphates, and other minerals into areas that have been damaged, as by incipient caries, abrasion, or erosion.

remodeling resorption and reformation of bone.

renal failure inability of the kidneys to maintain normal function of excreting toxic waste materials.

renin enzyme synthesized in the kidney; released in response to low blood pressure.

residue total amount of fecal solids, including undigested or unabsorbed food, and metabolic (bile pigments) and bacterial products.

respiration a process in which animals hydrolyze glucose into carbon dioxide and water, and plants use these products for photosynthesis.

retinoic acid form of vitamin A that can be produced by the body and can be made in the laboratory; used in combination with other drugs to treat leukemia and acne.

retrognathic mandible posterior to its normal relationship with other facial positions.

rhodopsin light-sensitive pigment that allows the eye to adjust to changes in light.

rickets condition resulting from vitamin D deficiency, especially in infancy and childhood; causes disturbance of normal bone formation.

sarcopenia progressive loss of muscle mass, strength, and function due to the aging process.

satiety feeling of fullness.

saturated fatty acid fatty acid that does not contain any double bonds.

scorbutic similar to scurvy.

sealants clear or shaded plastic material applied to the occlusal surfaces of permanent teeth.

secretory immunoglobulin antibody present in oral, nasal, intestinal, and other mucosal secretions; provides the first line of defense in the oral cavity.

sensory neuropathy impairment of the ability to feel.

severe early childhood caries (SECC) see early childhood caries (ECC).

severe sensory neuropathy impairment of the ability to sense touch, vibration, temperature, and pinprick.

short-chain fatty acid fatty acid that contains fewer than six carbon atoms.

side chain (R group) the part of the amino acid that varies to form 22 different amino acids that varies from one amino acid to another.

signs objective evidence of disease perceptible to the clinician.

silver diamine fluoride (SDF) colorless ammonia solution containing silver and fluoride ions. The silver ion acts as an antibacterial agent. SDF is showing to be effective in inhibiting demineralization.

small intestinal bacterial overgrowth (SIBO) impaired gastric and intestinal emptying due to overuse of probiotics, causing excessive bacteria in the gastrointestinal tract, resulting in nausea, vomiting, bloating, flatulence, and diarrhea.

small intestine duodenum, jejunum, and ileum.

soluble dietary fiber dietary fibers that become viscous (sticky, thick) in solution (oats, legumes, psyllium seeds).

solutes dissolved substances in fluid.

solvent fluid in which substances are dissolved.

sphincter muscles any of the ringlike muscles encircling an opening that is able to contract to close the opening, such as the sphincter pylori between the stomach and small intestine.

spices botanical seasonings from seeds, berries, fruit, bark, or roots.

squamous metaplasia change in oral cavity cell structures with keratin production in the duct cells of salivary glands, caused by vitamin A deficiency.

stable nutrients nutrients of which more than 85% is retained during processing and storage.

stannous containing tin.

stomatitis inflammation of the oral mucosa.

Streptococcus mutans bacteria found in dental plaque biofilm.

structural lipids fats that are a component of cell membranes, tooth enamel, and dentin (e.g., phospholipids).

structural polysaccharides see dietary fiber.

substrate the substance acted upon and changed by an enzyme.

suckling process the infant uses to extract breastmilk by moving the jaws back and forth and squeezing with the gingiva; this encourages mandibular development by strengthening the jaw muscle.

sugar alcohols formed from or converted to sugar; also called polyols.

suppuration discharge or formation of pus.

symbiotic intimate relationship of two dissimilar organisms in a mutually beneficial relationship; for example, prebiotics stimulate growth or activity of beneficial bacteria from probiotics in the gut.

sympathetic nerves exhibiting a mutual relationship between two organ systems or parts of the body.

symptoms subjective evidence of abnormality as perceived by the patient.

synergistic effect for example, combined sweeteners yield a sweeter taste than each sweetener alone.

syrup of ipecac cardiotoxic drug induces vomiting after accidental ingestion of a chemical or poison.

systematic reviews reliable information based on all relevant published and unpublished evidence, selecting studies for inclusion, assessing the quality of each study, then compiling the findings and interpreting them to present a balanced and impartial summary while defining limitations of the evidence.

systemic condition disease or disorder that affects the whole body.

tachycardia rapid heartbeat.

taste buds receptors for sense of taste.

taurine an amino acid with antioxidant properties.

temporomandibular disorder (TMD) group of symptoms that cause pain and dysfunction in the head, face, and temporomandibular region.

tensional forces actions in which pressure stretches or strains the structure.

tetany neuromuscular disorder of uncontrollable muscular cramps and tremors.

thermic effect increase in metabolism that occurs during digestion, absorption, and metabolism of energy-yielding nutrients.

thiaminase active enzyme found naturally in foods (e.g., raw fish) inactivating thiamin.

thromboembolism plug or clot in a blood vessel formed by coagulation of blood.

thrombus blood clot.

tinnitus noise in the ears, which sometimes may be heard by others.

tocopherols name given to vitamin E and compounds chemically related to it.

tocotrienols component of vitamin E.

Tolerable Upper Intake level (UL) maximum daily level of nutrient intake that probably would not cause adverse health effects or toxic effects for most individuals.

total fiber sum of dietary fiber and added fiber.

total parenteral nutrition (TPN) nutrition provided to a patient with impaired digestive tract; special liquid food mixture administered into the blood through a vein.

toxoplasmosis infection caused by a parasite; gravida may be symptom-free because the immune system prevents the parasite from causing illness, but the infection is passed on to the fetus.

trabecular bone internal bone.

trans **fatty acid** unsaturated fatty acid that is usually monounsaturated; may be formed during hydrogenation, in which the hydrogen ions rotate so that the hydrogens stick out on opposite sides of the bond.

trans **isomer** the geometric arrangement of hydrogen atoms on opposite sides of the plane of a C=C double bond

transferrin serum protein transports iron in the blood.

tricarboxylic acid cycle (TCA cycle) the central metabolic pathway that produces energy, also known as the citric acid cycle or Krebs cycle.

triglycerides major form of lipid in the body and food composed of three fatty acids bonded to glycerol, an alcohol.

24-hour recall a method of assessing everything a person has consumed (foods, supplements, and beverages) in a 24-hour period; may or may not reflect a typical day.

umami flavorful, pleasant taste detected in foods containing L-glutamine present in amino acids and proteins.

unqualified health claims statements allowed on food labels by FDA; must be supported by qualified experts agreeing that scientific evidence is available determining a relationship between a nutrient and a specific disease.

unsaturated fatty acid (UFA) of or related to an organic compound, especially fatty acids, containing one or more double or triple bonds between carbons.

Upper Level (UL) see tolerable upper intake level.

uremic condition in which too much urea and other nitrous waste products are present in the blood.

valves/sphincter muscles circular muscles regulating the flow of bolus between different segments of the gastrointestinal tract.

variants different forms of genes.

varicose veins unnaturally and permanently distended veins.

vegan person who eats only plant foods.

vegetarian person who purposefully does not eat meat (beef, pork, poultry, seafood, and the flesh of any animal, and sometimes animal by-products).

very low food security at times, food intake of household members is reduced and normal eating patterns are disrupted because of insufficient funds or other resources to obtain food.

vitamins organic compounds which are essential for normal growth and nutrition and are required in small quantities in the diet because they cannot be synthesized by the body.

wheat allergy adverse immunologic reaction to wheat proteins.

whole grains grains and grain products made from the entire grain seed, usually called the kernel (consisting of bran, germ, and endosperm); a cracked, crushed, or flaked kernel must retain nearly the same relative proportions of bran, germ, and endosperm as the original grain, to be called whole grain.

xeroderma dry, rough, scaly skin.

xerophthalmia abnormally dry and thickened surface of the conjunctiva and cornea of the eye.

xerostomia dryness of the mouth resulting from inadequate salivary secretion.

xylitol sugar alcohol used as a sugar substitute; considered a nutritive sweetener; provides four calories per gram.

Answers to Nutritional Quotient Questions

Chapter 1: Overview of Healthy Eating Habits

1. False. No single food contains all the essential nutrients in amounts needed for optimal health.
2. False. Only consumption of added sugars should be reduced. Naturally occurring sugars, especially from milk and fruits, are desirable.
3. True.
4. False. DRIs are a set of nutrient-based reference values that include the Estimated Average Requirements, Recommended Dietary Allowances, Adequate Intakes, and Tolerable Upper Intake Levels intended to be used for planning and assessing diets of healthy Americans and Canadians.
5. True.
6. False. Three to five servings of vegetables and two to four servings of fruits are recommended.
7. True.
8. False. Sugar is implicated as a cause of dental caries but not in other major diseases, such as hypertension, cardiovascular disease, or diabetes mellitus.
9. True.
10. False. The nutrients that provide energy are fats, carbohydrates, and proteins.

Chapter 2: Concepts in Biochemistry

1. False. A hydrolysis reaction requires H_2O as a reactant to degrade molecules. A condensation reaction produces H_2O as a product.
2. False. Amino acids are the building blocks of proteins. Nucleotides are the building blocks of nucleic acids.
3. True.
4. False. Sucrose is a disaccharide containing glucose and fructose.
5. True.
6. True.
7. True.
8. False. Catabolism involves the oxidation of carbohydrates into CO_2 and H_2O. Oxidation is the loss of electrons. The electrons released in catabolism are captured by NADH and $FADH_2$ and used to synthesize ATP in oxidative phosphorylation.
9. False. Insulin is a signal of the "fed" state and is secreted when blood glucose levels are high. It activates metabolic pathways that will lower blood glucose levels, like glycolysis and glycogen biosynthesis, not glycogen degradation.
10. True.

Chapter 3: The Alimentary Canal: Digestion and Absorption

1. True.
2. False. Gurgling sounds, caused by air and fluid in the normal abdomen, indicate occurrence of peristalsis.
3. False. Absorption occurs primarily in the small intestine.
4. False. Long-chain triglycerides enter the lymphatic system; short-chain and medium-chain triglycerides enter the portal circulation.
5. True.
6. False. Door-like mechanisms between the digestive segments are called valves or sphincter muscles.
7. True.
8. False. Villi are located in the small intestine.
9. True.
10. True.

Chapter 4: Carbohydrate: The Efficient Fuel

1. False. The FDA has labeled raw sugar as unfit for direct use as a food or a food ingredient because of the impurities it contains.
2. True.
3. False. Oral bacteria are unable to metabolize xylitol, which is a calorie-containing sugar alcohol.
4. False. The desire for sweetness is not considered an acquired taste because newborn infants exhibit a preference for it.
5. True.
6. True.
7. False. Excessive calorie intake leads to obesity, whether from carbohydrates, proteins, fats, or alcohol.
8. False. Sucrose is table sugar.
9. False. Many other factors, including consumption of other fermentable carbohydrates, contribute to the development of caries.
10. True.

Chapter 5: Protein: The Cellular Foundation

1. True.
2. False. Malnourished children are highly susceptible to dental caries possibly related to alterations in the structure of tooth crowns and diminished salivary flow, or changes in saliva composition.
3. False. Gelatin does not contain all the indispensable amino acids.
4. False. The protein requirement for an older adult is at least equal to that of a young adult and may be increased.

5. False. Adequate amounts of protein are needed for the development of healthy teeth, but increasing protein beyond the RDA would not have any effect on tooth enamel.
6. False. Excessive amounts of protein without decreasing intake of other energy-containing nutrients may lead to an increase in fat stores and possibly lead to obesity.
7. True.
8. False. Marasmus is caused because of protein and calorie deficiency.
9. True.
10. True.

Chapter 6: Lipids: The Condensed Energy

1. False. The overall average of fat intake is important with respect to total energy intake; but foods such as margarine and oils, which are 100% fat, can be used safely in the diet.
2. False. As an antioxidant, vitamin E protects the oil to which it is added to some degree; however, in doing so, vitamin E may be inactivated, so it cannot be used by the body.
3. True.
4. False. The AMDR for fat is estimated to be 20% to 35% of energy intake for adults.
5. False. Bananas contain a trace of fat; avocados are 88% fat. However, they are both plant products, so they do not contain any cholesterol.
6. False. All fats produce 9 kcal/g.
7. True.
8. False. Even though they are nutritious foods, for most Americans, their use may need to be limited because of their high concentration of calories.
9. True.
10. True.

Chapter 7: Use of the Energy Nutrients: Metabolism and Balance

1. True.
2. True.
3. False. BMR stands for basal metabolic rate, which is the amount of energy needed to maintain involuntary physiologic functions.
4. True.
5. True.
6. False. Hunger is the physiologic drive to eat, whereas appetite implies a desire for specific types of food.
7. False. Fats are stored by the body for energy, but they must first be converted into a form that the body can use. Glycogen stores, which depend on carbohydrate intake, are readily available for energy.
8. True.
9. True.
10. False. Only fats, carbohydrates, proteins, and alcohol provide energy (cals).

Chapter 8: Vitamins Required for Calcified Structures

1. True.
2. True.

3. True.
4. True.
5. False. Retinol is obtained from animal foods; beta carotene is found in fruits and vegetables.
6. True.
7. True.
8. False. The deficiency of vitamin D causes rickets.
9. False. Vitamin K is essential for blood clotting; vitamin D functions to regulate blood calcium and phosphorus levels.
10. True.

Chapter 9: Minerals Essential for Calcified Structures

1. True.
2. False. Many nutrients work together for building strong healthy bones, including protein, calcium, phosphorus, magnesium, fluoride, and vitamins C and D.
3. True.
4. True.
5. False. Based on the DRIs, teenagers need 1300 mg of calcium. If milk is the only calcium source, a teen would need to consume 4 1/2 cups.
6. False. Fluoridation of community water supplies is the most effective method of preventing dental caries.
7. False. Although many females take calcium supplements to prevent osteoporosis, they are not essential for all females. Excessive calcium intake may increase the risk of CHD and symptoms including dizziness, kidney stone formation, and irregular heartbeat.
8. True.
9. False. Caffeine decreases calcium absorption.
10. False. Bottled waters vary in fluoride content.

Chapter 10: Nutrients Present in Calcified Structures

1. False. The National Academy of Medicine has established ULs for copper, manganese, and molybdenum, but not for chromium.
2. True.
3. True.
4. False. Although the evidence is not conclusive, some research studies suggest a possible association between aluminum toxicity and Alzheimer disease.
5. True.
6. False. Unrefined foods generally provide more trace minerals.
7. False. Aluminum is cariostatic, especially in combination with fluoride.
8. True.
9. False. Sugar is not a good source of any nutrients except calories. Good sources of chromium include meats, whole-grain cereals, mushrooms, green beans, and broccoli.
10. False. Selenium supplements are not recommended because selenium can be toxic.

Chapter 11: Vitamins Required for Oral Soft Tissues and Salivary Glands

1. True.
2. False. Vitamin D is called the sunshine vitamin because sun facilitates the body's production of vitamin D; vitamin B$_6$ is also called pyridoxine, pyridoxal, and pyridoxamine.
3. False. Beriberi is caused by a thiamin deficiency; niacin deficiency causes pellagra.
4. True.
5. False. Flushing and intestinal disturbances are symptoms of niacin toxicity. No toxicity symptoms have been observed for thiamin.
6. True.
7. True.
8. False. Liver, leafy vegetables, legumes, grapefruit, and oranges are rich sources of folate.
9. True.
10. True.

Chapter 12: Water and Minerals Required for Oral Soft Tissues and Salivary Glands

1. True.
2. True.
3. True.
4. True.
5. False. The National Academy of Medicine has established an AI for total fluid (beverages, water, and food) requirements to be 15 to 16 cups per day for males and 11 to 12 cups per day for females.
6. False. The minimum requirement for sodium is 500 mg per day for adults, but no RDA has been established for sodium. The *Dietary Guidelines* recommend less than 2300 mg sodium daily.
7. True.
8. False. Potassium is principally within the cells (intracellular).
9. True.
10. False. Oral pallor is a sign of iron-deficiency anemia.

Chapter 13: Nutritional Requirements Affecting Oral Health in Females

1. False. These cravings do not reflect natural instincts for required nutrients.
2. True.
3. False. If the diet is deficient in calcium, the fetal calcium requirements would be met first, but some of the calcium may come from her bones, not from her teeth.
4. False. Although she is "eating for two," normal energy requirements are not doubled. Depending on the prepregnancy weight, approximately 300 cal more than her usual calorie requirement are needed during the second and third trimesters.
5. True.
6. False. Iron and folate are usually the nutrients needing supplementation.
7. True.
8. False. Breast milk is normally thin and is nutritionally adequate.

9. False. The more often an infant nurses, the more milk is produced. Milk production is most active during infant sucking.
10. True.

Chapter 14: Nutritional Requirements During Growth and Development and Eating Habits Affecting Oral Health

1. True.
2. False. Fluoride supplements are not recommended for infants before age 6 months even though breast milk and artificial breast milk are low in fluoride.
3. False. Solid foods are introduced between 4 and 6 months of age, not at 6 weeks.
4. False. The previous recommendation to withhold foods that most commonly cause allergies until after 12 months of age has been replaced with new recommendations to introduce high allergenic foods (including peanuts) between 4 and 6 months of age along with introduction of other solid foods. However, they are a choking hazard; thus small nuts should be withheld or closely monitored until the molars erupt.
5. True.
6. True.
7. False. Breastfed infants need a supplement of 200 IU vitamin D beginning during the first 2 months to prevent rickets.
8. False. Suckling, as occurs when extracting milk from the breast, encourages maximum development of the genetically defined jaw and chin; breastfed infants are less likely to develop malocclusion.
9. False. Milk and dairy products are essential components of children's and adolescent's diets because of the high calcium requirement to increase bone mineral density and other important components of these products.
10. False. Toddlers and children need snacks because of their high energy needs; however, wholesome snacks (e.g., cheese cubes, fresh fruit, raw vegetable sticks, milk, or yogurt) that do not promote tooth decay are recommended.

Chapter 15: Nutritional Requirements for Older Adults and Eating Habits Affecting Oral Health

1. False. Because of changes in nutrient requirements secondary to physiologic changes, the National Academy of Medicine has developed DRIs for individuals 51 to 70 years old and older than 70 years.
2. True.
3. True.
4. False. The texture for edentulous patients is determined by their own preferences.
5. False. Dehydration is a frequent occurrence in elderly individuals for many reasons—impaired homeostatic mechanisms, decreased thirst sensation, inability of the kidney to concentrate urine, changes in functional status, side effects of medications, and mobility disorders.
6. True.
7. False. Iron intake requirement is lower after menopause.
8. True.
9. False. Although it is highly likely that an elderly individual may benefit from taking a dietary supplement, toxicity or

nutrient imbalances may occur. An older individual should consult a health care provider before deciding to take a vitamin supplement.

10. False. Physical activity can help ameliorate some chronic health problems, improve physiological well-being, and relieve symptoms of depression and anxiety.

Chapter 16: Food Factors Affecting Health

1. True.
2. False. Patterns and attitudes internalized during childhood promote a sense of stability and security for older patients.
3. False. No culture has ever been known to make food choices solely on the basis of nutritional values of food. The factors that seem to predominate in food choices are cultural and economic.
4. False. Only about 10% of the American food dollar is spent on food.
5. False. Fad diets may be physically harmless, but they are usually not based on sound nutritional principles.
6. False. Scientific research to date has not shown any nutritional benefits from the use of organically grown foods.
7. False. Although some food processing is detrimental to the nutritive value of foods, the goal of food processing is to maintain optimum qualities of color, flavor, texture, and nutritive value.
8. True.
9. True.
10. True.

Chapter 17: Effects of Systemic Disease on Nutritional Status and Oral Health

1. True.
2. True.
3. False. Supplements for anemia should not be prescribed without the results of blood testing to determine the type of anemia. High intakes of iron could possibly complicate the situation.
4. False. Because of the various considerations involved in constructing a meal plan and lifestyle changes for a patient with diabetes, the patient must be referred to a certified diabetes educator.
5. True.
6. True.
7. False. Kaposi sarcoma is a tumor that occurs frequently in immunocompromised patients.
8. True.
9. False. Although a patient with an eating disorder should be referred to a physician or an eating disorder program, it is the dental hygienist's responsibility to approach the patient with the objective findings.
10. False. Patients with bulimia are generally of normal weight or sometimes above recommended body weight.

Chapter 18: Nutritional Aspects of Dental Caries: Causes, Prevention, and Treatment

1. False. A combination of diet, host, environment, and saliva are necessary for initiation of dental decay.

2. True.
3. True.
4. True.
5. False. Sugar alcohols are fermented slowly by oral bacteria, and they are noncariogenic. Xylitol is cariostatic because of its ability to inhibit production of *Streptococcus mutans*.
6. False. An acid environment is required to demineralize a tooth; a cariogenic food causes the plaque pH to decrease to less than 5.5.
7. False. It is the least important factor to consider. Identifying frequency of intake, physical form, and the timing and sequence in a meal would provide a more accurate assessment.
8. True.
9. False. Although the RDAs provide a lot of factual information, they are too overwhelming for most patients. *MyPlate* website and *Dietary Guidelines for Americans* provide practical and general nutrition information relevant to preventing dental decay and improving overall health.
10. False. Information alone does not guarantee a behavioral change.

Chapter 19: Nutritional Aspects of Gingivitis and Periodontal Disease

1. True.
2. False. Indirectly, firm, fibrous foods reduce the amount of bacterial plaque biofilm by stimulating salivary flow, which promotes oral clearance of food and lessens food retention.
3. False. A nutrient deficiency can be a contributing factor to gingivitis, but local irritants (plaque biofilm and calculus) must be present. The inflammation can be exaggerated by a nutrient deficiency and by reduced resistance and recovery time.
4. True.
5. False. A patient may interpret this advice as condoning ice cream, gelatin, and chicken noodle soup, which would not provide enough nutrients or calories for quick recovery. The dental hygienist should provide a specific list of nutrient-dense foods for the patient to purchase before the periodontal surgery.
6. True.
7. True.
8. True.
9. True.
10. False. If surgery is indicated for a periodontal patient, optimally, the nutritional assessment and counseling should be completed before the procedure to increase nutrient reserves that would expedite the recovery period.

Chapter 20: Nutritional Aspects of Alterations in the Oral Cavity

1. False. Although root surface caries can be a complication of xerostomia, other causes are possible, such as frequent intake of hard candy. Also, a complete and thorough assessment of the patient is essential. No single factor is adequate to diagnose the presence, extent, or cause of root caries. An inaccurate evaluation can lead to inappropriate recommendations.
2. False. Although xerostomia is a common complaint in an older adult, the changes in saliva in a healthy older individual

are minimal. Xerostomia has been strongly associated with multiple factors, such as use of medications, one or more systemic diseases, and radiation, all of which are common to this population.

3. True.

4. False. Root caries appear on the root surface, in areas of gingival recession. This condition is seen more often in older adults who have experienced periodontal disease or toothbrush trauma.

5. False. Spongy cancellous bone is the major component of alveolar bone.

6. True.

7. True.

8. True.

9. False. It is important to have nutrient-dense foods available, but in different consistencies. A full liquid diet progressing to a mechanically altered diet and on to a regular diet would allow the patient to adjust to swallowing, chewing and biting with the new appliance.

10. True.

Chapter 21: Nutritional Assessment and Education for Dental Patients

1. False. Although the health and dental histories provide valuable information, they are not enough to determine the patient's nutritional status. Other evaluation tools include clinical assessment and dietary intake.

2. False. Clinical oral examinations detect physical signs and symptoms of many nutrient deficiencies. However, deficiencies generally do not appear until an advanced state exists. An oral examination, and dental histories could be used as an adjunct in identifying potential nutritional deficiencies.

3. True.

4. True.

5. False. Dietary counseling must be documented and other staff members must be informed about the nutritional counseling for consistency and reinforcement of the information at future appointments.

6. False. Changing a dietary habit is difficult and requires a meal plan and lifestyle behavioral changes tailored to meet the patient's needs. A thorough assessment identifies many factors that should be considered. Active involvement of the patient in establishing a meal pattern enhances compliance.

7. False. The dental hygienist is responsible for providing information and guiding the patient to make healthier decisions. Active participation, problem-solving, and decision-making allow for greater compliance. The patient should highlight the fermentable carbohydrates.

8. False. Changing food habits is very difficult. The first attempt established by the dental hygienist and patient may not have been successful, and other alternatives may need to be established. Follow-up is an essential component of the nutritional counseling process.

9. True.

10. True.

11. False. The patient's behavior is "explored" by building rapport and not being confronted; the patent is then "guided" by the dental professional and the patient "chooses" the course of treatment.

12. True.

Index

Page numbers followed by "*f*" indicate figures, "*t*" indicate tables, and "*b*" indicate boxes.